Residential, Home and Community Aged Care Workbook 3e

Designed as a companion to *Long-Term Caring: Residential, Home and Community Aged Care 5e,* the workbook contains questions, activities and assessments to assist you in meeting the requirements of Certificate III Individual Support.

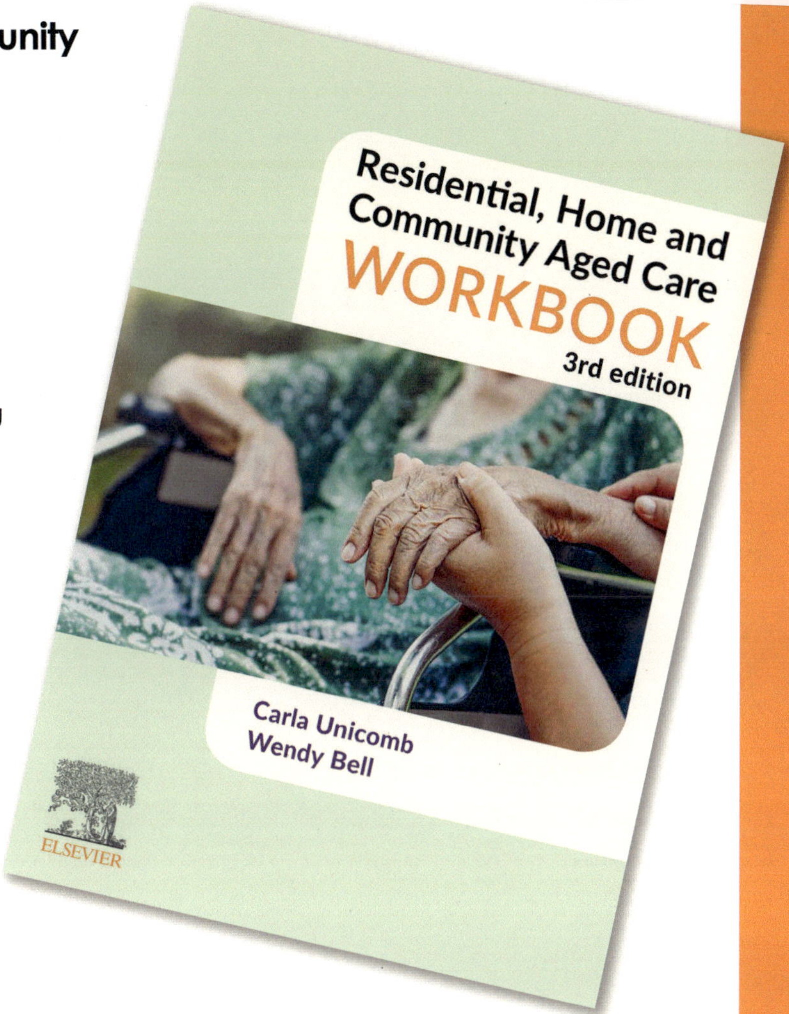

The workbook:

- Directs you to foundational knowledge in specific chapters and pages in *Long-Term Caring: Residential, Home and Community Aged Care 5e*
- Contains a variety of questions, activities and assessments to assist you in achieving skill and knowledge development.

For Instructors the *Residential Home and community Aged Care Instructors' Resource Pack* is available via Evolve with the workbook. Available online and fully customisable, the resource pack contains PowerPoint slides, final assessments and model answers.

To find out more, visit **www.elsevierhealthonline.com.au/agedcare3e/**

AUSTRALIA AND NEW ZEALAND EDITION

LONG-TERM CARING

Residential, Home and Community Aged Care

5th edition

Karen Scott
Margaret Webb
Clare Kostelnick

ELSEVIER

ELSEVIER

Elsevier Australia. ACN 001 002 357
(a division of Reed International Books Australia Pty Ltd)
Tower 1, 475 Victoria Avenue, Chatswood, NSW 2067

4th edition 2018; 3rd edition 2015; 2nd edition 2011.

ISBN: 978-0-7295-4398-9

National Library of Australia Cataloguing-in-Publication Data

NATIONAL LIBRARY OF AUSTRALIA

A catalogue record for this book is available from the National Library of Australia

Content Strategist: Melinda McEvoy
Content Project Manager: Shravan Kumar
Edited by Margaret Trudgeon
Proofread by Tim Learner
Copyrights Coordinator: Regina Lavanya Remigius
Cover Designer: Lisa Petroff
Index by Innodata
Typeset by GW Tech
Printed in China

Last digit is the print number: 9 8 7 6 5 4 3 2 1

Brief Contents

Contents

Study tips

This book was designed for you. It was designed to help you learn and understand the area of practice that you have chosen. The book is a useful resource as you gain experience and expand your knowledge.

This preface gives some study guidelines and helps you use the book. When given a reading assignment, do you read from the first page to the last page without stopping? How much do you remember? You will learn more if you use a study system. A useful study system has these steps:

1. Survey or preview
2. Question
3. Read and record
4. Recite and review.

PREVIEW

Before you start a reading assignment, preview or survey it. This gives you an idea of what the assignment covers. It also helps you recall what you already know about the subject. Carefully look over the assignment. Preview the chapter title, headings, subheadings and terms or ideas in bold print or italics. Also survey the objectives, key terms, first paragraph, boxes and review questions at the end of the chapter. Previewing only takes a few minutes. Remember, previewing helps you become familiar with the material.

QUESTION

After previewing, you need to form questions to answer while you read. Questions should relate to what might be asked on a test or how the information applies to giving care. Use the title, headings and subheadings to form questions. Avoid questions that have one-word answers. Questions that begin with *what*, *how* or *why* are helpful. While reading, you may find that a question does not help you study. If so, just change the question. Remember, questioning sets a purpose for reading. So changing a question only makes this step more useful.

READ AND RECORD

Reading is the next step. Reading is more productive after determining what you already know and what you need to learn. Read to find answers to your questions. The purpose of reading is to:

- gain new information
- connect the new information to what you already know.

Break down the assignment into smaller parts. Then answer your questions as you read each part. Also, mark important information. The information can be marked by underlining, highlighting or making notes. Underlining and highlighting remind you what you need to learn. You need to go back and review the marked parts later. Making notes results in more immediate learning. When making notes, write down important information in the margins or in a notebook. Use words and summary statements that will jog your memory about the material.

After reading the assignment, you need to remember the information. To remember the material, you must work with the information. This step involves organising information into a study guide. Study guides have many forms. Diagrams or charts help show relationships or steps in a process. Much of the information in this text is organised in this manner to help you learn. Note-taking in outline format is also very useful. The following is a sample outline:

1 Main heading
  A. Second level
  B. Second level
    i. Third level
    ii. Third level
2 Main heading

RECITE AND REVIEW

Finally, recite and review. Use your notes and the study guides. Answer the questions you formed earlier. Also answer any other questions that might have come up during the reading and the review questions at the end of the chapter. Answer all questions out loud (recite).

Reviewing is more about *when* to study rather than *what* to study. You will have already determined what to study during the preview, question and reading steps. The best times to review the material are straight after the first study session, one week later and regularly before a quiz or test, or a mid-term or final examination.

We hope you enjoy learning and your work. You and your work are important. You and the care you give may be bright spots in a person's day.

This book was also designed to help you study. It includes the special design features explained in the section "Text features".

Text features

CHAPTER 4

Workplace documentation and communication

By Ellie Kirov

AFTER READING THIS CHAPTER, YOU SHOULD BE ABLE TO:

- define the key terms listed in this chapter
- identify why care team members need to communicate
- state the rules for good communication
- state the purpose, parts and information found in the medical record
- identify the legal and ethical aspects of medical records
- discuss your role in the nursing process
- describe how information about a person is collected using the five senses
- describe the information you need to report to the registered nurse or the supervisor
- state the rules for recording and documenting
- demonstrate how to use a 24-hour clock
- describe the breakdown of medical terms and how they are constructed, and abbreviations
- discuss the use of computers and electronic networks in aged and disability care
- discuss how to protect the person's right to privacy when using computers and electronic networks
- state the rules for answering the telephone
- describe how to solve problems and deal with conflict.

Learning Objectives list what you should be able to do after reading the chapter.

Key terms are the important words and phrases in the chapter. Definitions are given for each term. The key terms introduce you to the chapter content. They are also a useful study guide.

Chapter 4: Workplace documentation and communication

a nurse to explain its meaning. You may also want to buy a medical dictionary so you can learn new words. Ensure it is an English, not US, version as US spelling frequently omits letters used in words in Australia and New Zealand; for example, use colour rather than color and haemoglobin, not hemoglobin.

Prefixes, roots and suffixes

Medical terms are formed by combining **word elements** – that is, prefixes, roots and suffixes (Table 4.?). Most come from Greek or Latin.

A **prefix** is placed at the beginning of a word. The prefix changes the word's meaning. As an example, the prefix *olig* (meaning 'scant', a small amount) is placed before the word *uria* (urine) to make *oliguria*, which means 'a scant amount of urine'. Prefixes are always combined with other word elements. They are never used alone.

The **root** contains the basic meaning of the word. Roots can be combined with other roots, with prefixes and with suffixes. A vowel (an 'o' or an 'i') is added when two roots are combined or when a suffix is added to a root. The vowel makes pronunciation easier.

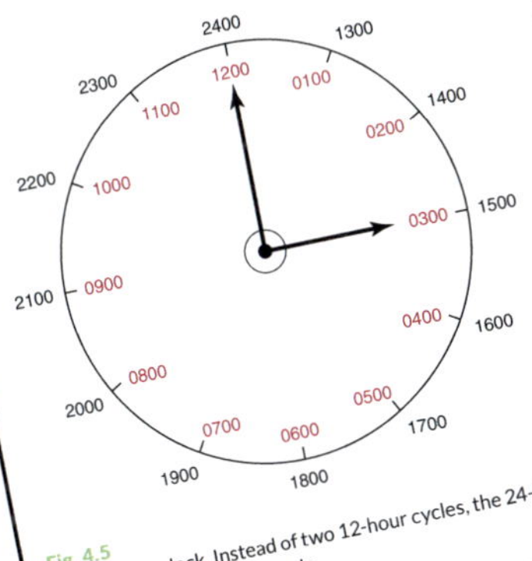

Fig. 4.5
The 24-hour clock. Instead of two 12-hour cycles, the 24-hour clock is one 24-hour time cycle.

Key terms

abbreviation: A shortened form of a word or phrase
admission sheet: A sheet which is completed when a person is first admitted to a facility and contains important information about the person
assessment: Collecting information about the consumer
care plan/comprehensive care plan: A written guide about the care a consumer should receive
communication: The exchange of information; a message ... received and interpreted by the intended person
...ct: A clash between opposing interests and ideas
...se: A collection of data or information that is stored ...ically in a structured format
...ntation: The process of creating written records ...ses, care and observation; also known as written
...communication: When a message sent is received ...reted by the intended person
...: A review of whether the goals in the planning ...ursing process have been met
...d aim by a person who requires nursing care
...tion: Performing or carrying out nursing ... in the care plan
...nosis: The identification of a disease or ... doctor
...d: A written account of a consumer's illness ... the treatment and care given by the health
...is: A statement describing a health problem ...d by nursing measures

nursing intervention: An action or measure taken by the nursing team to help the consumer reach a goal
nursing process: The method used by registered nurses to plan and deliver nursing care; its five steps are assessment, nursing diagnosis, planning, implementation and evaluation
objective data: Information that can be seen, heard, felt or smelt by another person; signs; also known as factual data
observation: Using the senses of sight, hearing, touch and smell to collect information about a consumer
prefix: A word element placed at the beginning of a word that alters its meaning
progress notes: A written description of the care given and the consumer's response and progress
recording: Writing an account of care and observations
reporting: Giving an oral account of care and observations
root: A word element containing the basic meaning of the word
signs: An indication or characteristic based on physical observation, examination or treatment of a consumer; objective data
subjective data: What is reported by a consumer and cannot be observed by using the senses; symptoms; also considered as a person's opinion
suffix: A word element placed at the end of a root to change the meaning of the word
symptoms: A consumer's description of what they are experiencing
triggers: Clues for the consumer assessment
word element: A part of a word

98

Bolded type is used to highlight key terms in the text. You see the key term in context and can turn to the Key terms to read its definition. This helps reinforce learning.

LONG-TERM CARING: Residential, Home and Community Aged Care

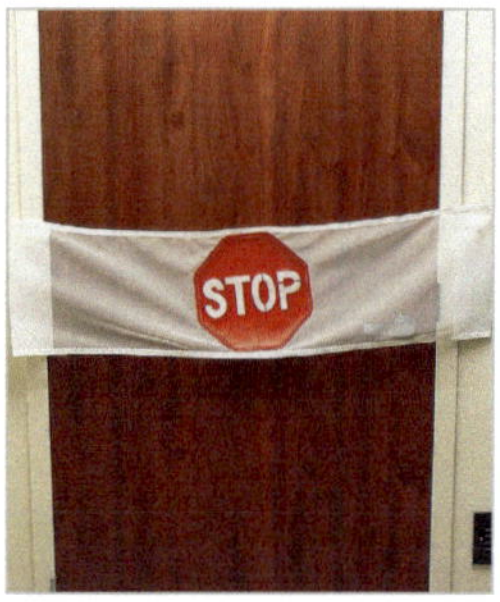

Fig. 2.2
Barriers prevent wandering.

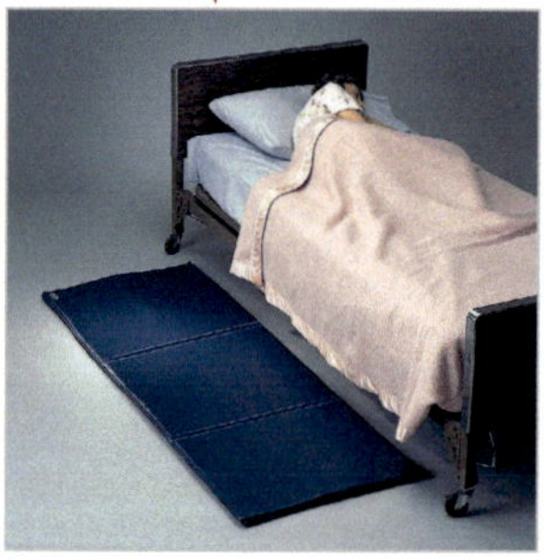

Fig. 2.3
A sensor mat beside the bed.

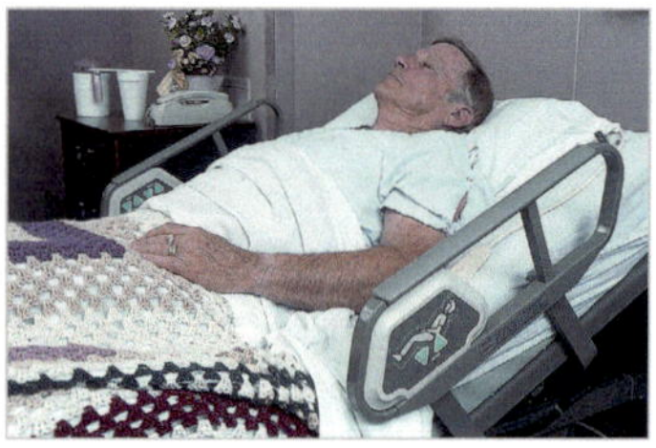

Fig. 2.4
Bed rails.

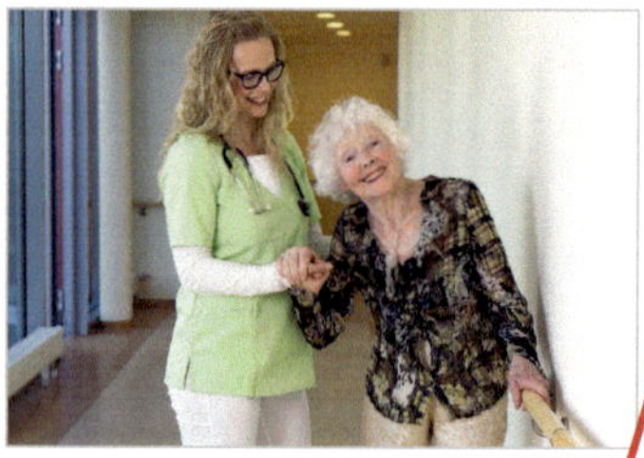

Fig. 2.5
Handrails provide support when walking.

three-quarters or the full length of the bed. When half-length rails are used, each side may have two rails. One is for the upper part of the bed, the other for the lower part. The care plan will tell you when to raise bed rails. They are usually needed for a client who is unconscious or sedated with medications. Some confused or disoriented clients may also need them. If a client needs bed rails keep them up at all times except when giving bedside care.

For an adult's safety, it is recommended that gaps be 10 cm or less between:

- the bed rail bars
- an upper and lower bed rail
- the bed rail and the mattress
- the upper bed rail and the headboard
- the lower bed rail and the footboard (Fig. 2.6).

Bed rails are a hazard for a clie
without help. Entrapment is a ris
ent can be caught, trapped or ent
or bed rail gaps. Gaps occur b
between the rail and the headbo
tween the bed rail and the matt
occur if the client's head, neck, c
trapped. Please note that in most
to be a form of restraint and
must be obtained prior to using t

Clients at greatest risk are thos

- are confused or disoriented
- are small in size
- have poor muscle control
- are restrained.

Check for the 10 cm rule wher
report any concerns to your sup

30

Colour illustrations and photographs visually present key ideas, concepts or procedure steps. They help you apply and remember the written material.

Safety Alerts focus your attention on the need to be safe and cautious when giving care.

LONG-TERM CARING: Residential, Home and Community Aged Care

SAFETY ALERT

Back massage

Back massages can be dangerous for people with certain heart diseases, back injuries, back surgery, skin diseases and some lung disorders. Check with the agency supervisor, nurse and care plan before giving back massages to any person.

Also, do not massage bony areas that are reddened. Reddened areas signal skin breakdown and pressure ulcers. Massage can lead to further tissue damage.

If the person's skin is not intact, you need to wear gloves. Follow Standard Precautions.

DELEGATION GUIDELINES

Back massage

Before giving a back massage, you need the following information from the care plan:

- Can the person have a back massage?
- How should you position the person?
- Does the person have position limits?
- When should the person receive a back massage?
- Does the person need frequent back massages for comfort, relaxation and/or skin management?
- What observations to report:
  - bruising
  - reddened areas
  - signs of skin breakdown.

GIVING A BACK MASSAGE

Quality of life

Remember to respect the person's privacy while doing any procedure. Address the person by name and ensure they know your name.

Pre-procedure

1 Call the person by name and introduce yourself.
2 Explain the procedure to the person before starting and ensure that you verbalise each step as it is carried out during the procedure.
3 Wash your hands.
4 Collect the following:
 - bath blanket
 - bath towel
 - lotion.
5 Provide for privacy and maintain warmth.
6 Raise the bed to a height that facilitates good body mechanics.

Procedure

7 Position the person in the prone or side-lying position. The back is towards you.
8 Expose the back, shoulders, upper arms and buttocks. Cover the rest of the body with the bath blanket.
9 Lay the towel on the bed along the back.
10 Apply the pre-warmed lotion to your hands or rub some between your hands.
11 Explain that the lotion may feel cool and wet.
12 Apply lotion to the lower back area.
13 Stroke up from the buttocks to the shoulders (Fig. 12.22). Then stroke down over the upper arms. Stroke up the upper arms, across the shoulders and down the back to the buttocks. Use firm strokes. Keep your hands in contact with the person's skin.
14 Repeat step 13 for at least 3 minutes.
15 Knead by grasping skin between your thumb and fingers (Fig. 12.23). Knead half of the back, starting at the buttocks, and move up to the shoulder. Then knead down from the shoulder to the buttocks. Repeat on the other half of the back.
16 Apply lotion to bony areas. Use circular motions with the tips of your index and middle fingers. (Do not massage bony areas that are reddened.)
17 Use fast movements to stimulate and slow movements to relax the person.
18 Stroke with long, firm movements to end the massage. Tell the person you are finishing.
19 Cover the person. Remove the towel and bath blanket.

Post-procedure

20 Provide for comfort.
21 Lower the bed to its lowest position.
22 Place the call bell within reach.
23 Return lotion to its proper place.
24 Remove the screens from around the person.
25 Follow agency policy for dirty linen.
26 Wash your hands.
27 Report any observations of concern to the nurse on duty.

270

Delegation Guidelines describe what information you need from the nurse and care plan before performing a procedure. They also tell you what information to report and record.

Procedures are written in a step-by-step format. They are divided into pre-procedure, procedure and post-procedure sections for easy studying.

Quality of Life in the procedure boxes, reminds you to respect the person's privacy, to call the person by name and to introduce yourself by name. These simple courtesies show respect for the resident as a person.

Focus on Community Care boxes are a reminder that caring practice occurs in a multitude of contexts.

Quality of Life box at the end of each chapter bridges the focus of the chapter with how to promote the resident's rights and enhance quality of life when giving care.

Case Studies are useful in assisting you to link what you have learnt from this text to a practical caregiving situation.

LONG-TERM CARING: Residential, Home and Community Aged Care

to your supervisor your observations about how the person slept. This helps them evaluate whether the goal of a regular sleep pattern was met.

Many people have rituals and routines before bedtime. These are often important to the person. These include some of those rituals and routines as described for rest. Always remember, it is the person's choice when to nap or go to bed, and the measures that promote comfort, rest and sleep. Always follow the person's wishes.

Check linen for crumbs after meals and remove them. Change linen whenever it becomes wet, soiled or damp.

When you are handling linen and making beds, always use safe handling practices and hold linen away from your body and clothing. Never shake linen in the air, as shaking it spreads microbes. Clean linen is always placed on a clean surface, such as a chair or table, and never placed on the floor. Never put dirty linen on the floor.

Clients with dementia

Sleep problems are common in people with Alzheimer's disease and other dementias. Night wandering is common. Restlessness and confusion often increase at night. This increases the risk of falls. It often helps to quietly and calmly direct the person to his or her room. Allowing night-time wandering in a safe and supervised setting is the best approach for some people. Follow the care plan.

FOCUS ON COMMUNITY CARE

When caring for a client within their home, you may be responsible for assisting them to prepare for bed at night. Always ask your client what their bedtime routine is and follow this. Ensure that items such as uridomes are applied securely, because if they leak or come off during the night your client may have to stay in a wet bed until help arrives the next day. Not only can this result in skin breakdown and damage, but also considerable discomfort, both physical and emotional, for your client.

Once your client is in bed, there will be times when they are unable to move or get out of it until a carer arrives the following morning to assist them to get up. It is your responsibility to ensure that not only are they safely positioned and have all their needs attended to, but that you have also secured their home well before you leave. Always check lights, electrical appliances, windows and doors. Ensure that they have appropriate emergency call devices accessible.

QUALITY OF LIFE

Comfort, rest and sleep are needed for quality of life and wellbeing. Aged Care Accreditation Standards require care strategies that promote comfort, rest and sleep. These relate to the bed, mattress, room temperature, noise level, lighting, linen, odours and the number of people in each room. The right to personal choice and taking part in planning care also promote comfort, rest and sleep.

Clients have the right to have their pain assessed and managed. Untreated pain decreases quality of life. You must report signs and symptoms of pain. This helps the nurse meet the person's needs.

CASE STUDY

Mina Chowdry lives by herself within the community in her own home. Her family is becoming increasingly concerned about her tiredness, lethargy and lack of willingness to do anything requiring any effort. She used to enjoy going to her grandchildren's sports days and concerts, but nowadays she says that 'she just doesn't have the energy to do so'. Her daughter contacted her GP about their worries. He sent his practice nurse to see her, who conducted an assessment. Mina admitted to not eating well at all and was just making jam sandwiches for most of her meals. Her fluid intake was also limited to just a few cups of tea during the day. She also advised the nurse that it hurt her to eat as her dentures moved around when she chewed. Meals on Wheels was immediately organised for Mina, providing her with a substantial and nutritious meal once a day. Her family bought her some water bottles, which Mina was able to fill and carry round the house with her. She also went to see her dental prosthetist, who remoulded her dentures so that they no longer moved around.

Within a few weeks Mina had improved considerably and her family were pleased to see her taking an interest in her home and grandchildren once again.

The regular meals, increased fluid intake and better-fitting dentures all contributed to her being able to achieve a better nutritional status. This subsequently improved both her physical and her psychological wellbeing.

Chapter 12: Caring for the person

- recognise the signs, symptoms and precautions relating to aspiration
- be aware of the fluid requirements for adults
- know what to do when a person has special fluid orders
- understand the purpose of intake and output records
- know what to count as fluid intake
- know how to assist with food and fluid needs
- be aware of the purpose, methods and comfort measures for enteral nutrition.

Food and water are physical needs that are necessary for life. The amount and quality of foods and fluids in the diet affect our physical and mental wellbeing. Older and disabled people may have special dietary needs. Poor diet and poor eating habits:

- increase the risk of infection
- increase the risk of chronic diseases
- cause chronic illnesses to become worse
- cause healing problems
- cause changes in physical and mental function, increasing the risk of accidents and injuries.

Eating and drinking provide pleasure (Fig. 12.96). They are often a part of social times with family and friends. A friendly, social setting for meals is important. It is important to remember that eating should be enjoyed and that it may be one of the few pleasures for older people. People may eat poorly when eating alone or in an unpleasant setting.

Many factors affect people's dietary practices. They include culture, finances and personal choice. Dietary practices also include selecting, preparing and serving food. The health team considers these factors when planning to meet the person's nutrition needs.

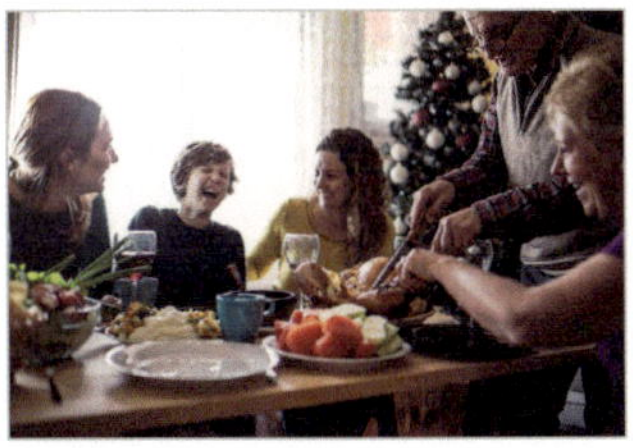

Fig. 12.96
Meals are enjoyed when shared with family and friends.

BASIC NUTRITION

Although nutrition is discussed elsewhere within this text in greater detail, a basic summary is presented here. **Nutrition** is the many processes involved in the ingestion, digestion, absorption and use of foods and fluids by the body. Good nutrition is needed for growth, healing and body functions. A well-balanced diet and correct kilojoule intake are needed. A high-fat and high-kilojoule diet causes weight gain and obesity. Weight loss occurs with a low-kilojoule diet.

Foods and fluids contain nutrients. A **nutrient** is a substance that is ingested, digested, absorbed and used by the body. Nutrients are grouped into fats, proteins, carbohydrates, vitamins and minerals.

Fats, proteins and carbohydrates give the body fuel for energy. The amount of energy provided by a nutrient is measured in kilojoules. A **kilojoule** is the amount of energy produced when the body burns food. More information about nutrition can be found in Chapter 13.

CARING ABOUT CULTURE

Food practices vary between religious groups and are often an important part of religious observance.

- *Christianity* – religious preference varies from faith to faith. Variations of fasting are observed by Roman Catholics on holy days such as Good Friday and during Lent. A majority of Seventh Day Adventists don't eat meat or dairy products. Mormons avoid coffee and alcohol.
- *Judaism* – can be liberal or Orthodox, depending on the degree of adherence to Jewish Law. Kosher food is permitted, and 'unclean' foods, such as pork and shellfish, are forbidden. Food preparation and consumption rules can be strict.
- *Islam* – prohibited foods are called *haram* and are believed to make the Creator deaf to a Muslim who eats them. This list can include pork, alcohol, bread products made with dried yeast and caffeinated drinks. Many Muslims choose to fast on certain days and during religious holidays.
- *Hinduism* – Hindus do not eat meat and often avoid foods that may have caused pain to animals. Many Hindus believe that food contains energy, such as sound waves, and can literally believe the saying 'You are what you eat'. Many Hindus fast, depending on their caste or social status.
- *Buddhism* – the dietary rules of Buddhism vary according to country and which branch of Buddhism is being practised. Some avoid meat and dairy products, others avoid only beef. Some Buddhists practise fasting, while others fast for religious festivals.

Source: Encyclopedia.com (2019). Religion and dietary practices. Online 30 Sept 2021. Available: www.encyclopedia.com/food/news-wires-white-papers-and-books/religion-and-dietary-practices

339

Caring about Culture boxes contain information to help you learn about the various practices of other cultures.

Hint boxes offer guidance on assisting people with mental health issues.

Boxes and tables contain important rules, principles, guidelines, signs and symptoms, nursing measures and other information in a list format. They identify important information and are useful study guides.

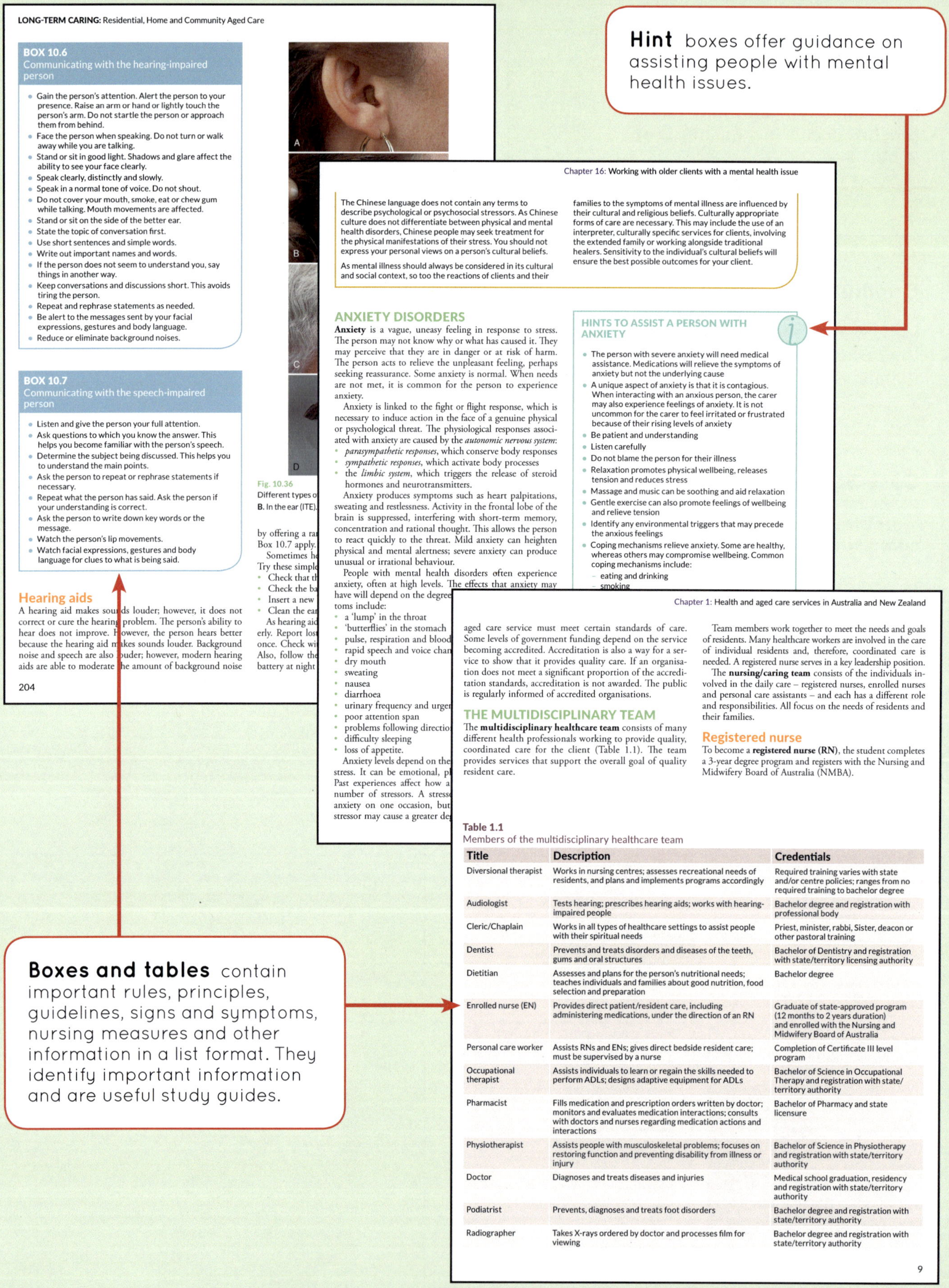
LONG-TERM CARING: Residential, Home and Community Aged Care

BOX 10.6
Communicating with the hearing-impaired person

- Gain the person's attention. Alert the person to your presence. Raise an arm or hand or lightly touch the person's arm. Do not startle the person or approach them from behind.
- Face the person when speaking. Do not turn or walk away while you are talking.
- Stand or sit in good light. Shadows and glare affect the ability to see your face clearly.
- Speak clearly, distinctly and slowly.
- Speak in a normal tone of voice. Do not shout.
- Do not cover your mouth, smoke, eat or chew gum while talking. Mouth movements are affected.
- Stand or sit on the side of the better ear.
- State the topic of conversation first.
- Use short sentences and simple words.
- Write out important names and words.
- If the person does not seem to understand you, say things in another way.
- Keep conversations and discussions short. This avoids tiring the person.
- Repeat and rephrase statements as needed.
- Be alert to the messages sent by your facial expressions, gestures and body language.
- Reduce or eliminate background noises.

BOX 10.7
Communicating with the speech-impaired person

- Listen and give the person your full attention.
- Ask questions to which you know the answer. This helps you become familiar with the person's speech.
- Determine the subject being discussed. This helps you to understand the main points.
- Ask the person to repeat or rephrase statements if necessary.
- Repeat what the person has said. Ask the person if your understanding is correct.
- Ask the person to write down key words or the message.
- Watch the person's lip movements.
- Watch facial expressions, gestures and body language for clues to what is being said.

Hearing aids
A hearing aid makes sounds louder; however, it does not correct or cure the hearing problem. The person's ability to hear does not improve. However, the person hears better because the hearing aid makes sounds louder. Background noise and speech are also louder; however, modern hearing aids are able to moderate the amount of background noise

204

Chapter 16: Working with older clients with a mental health issue

The Chinese language does not contain any terms to describe psychological or psychosocial stressors. As Chinese culture does not differentiate between physical and mental health disorders, Chinese people may seek treatment for the physical manifestations of their stress. You should not express your personal views on a person's cultural beliefs.

As mental illness should always be considered in its cultural and social context, so too the reactions of clients and their families to the symptoms of mental illness are influenced by their cultural and religious beliefs. Culturally appropriate forms of care are necessary. This may include the use of an interpreter, culturally specific services for clients, involving the extended family or working alongside traditional healers. Sensitivity to the individual's cultural beliefs will ensure the best possible outcomes for your client.

ANXIETY DISORDERS
Anxiety is a vague, uneasy feeling in response to stress. The person may not know why or what has caused it. They may perceive that they are in danger or at risk of harm. The person acts to relieve the unpleasant feeling, perhaps seeking reassurance. Some anxiety is normal. When needs are not met, it is common for the person to experience anxiety.

Anxiety is linked to the fight or flight response, which is necessary to induce action in the face of a genuine physical or psychological threat. The physiological responses associated with anxiety are caused by the *autonomic nervous system*:
- *parasympathetic responses*, which conserve body responses
- *sympathetic responses*, which activate body processes
- the *limbic system*, which triggers the release of steroid hormones and neurotransmitters.

Anxiety produces symptoms such as heart palpitations, sweating and restlessness. Activity in the frontal lobe of the brain is suppressed, interfering with short-term memory, concentration and rational thought. This allows the person to react quickly to the threat. Mild anxiety can heighten physical and mental alertness; severe anxiety can produce unusual or irrational behaviour.

People with mental health disorders often experience anxiety, often at high levels. The effects that anxiety may have will depend on the degree ... toms include:
- a 'lump' in the throat
- 'butterflies' in the stomach
- pulse, respiration and blood ...
- rapid speech and voice chan...
- dry mouth
- sweating
- nausea
- diarrhoea
- urinary frequency and urge...
- poor attention span
- problems following directio...
- difficulty sleeping
- loss of appetite.

Anxiety levels depend on the ... stress. It can be emotional, p... Past experiences affect how a... number of stressors. A stress... anxiety on one occasion, but ... stressor may cause a greater de...

HINTS TO ASSIST A PERSON WITH ANXIETY
- The person with severe anxiety will need medical assistance. Medications will relieve the symptoms of anxiety but not the underlying cause
- A unique aspect of anxiety is that it is contagious. When interacting with an anxious person, the carer may also experience feelings of anxiety. It is not uncommon for the carer to feel irritated or frustrated because of their rising levels of anxiety
- Be patient and understanding
- Listen carefully
- Do not blame the person for their illness
- Relaxation promotes physical wellbeing, releases tension and reduces stress
- Massage and music can be soothing and aid relaxation
- Gentle exercise can also promote feelings of wellbeing and relieve tension
- Identify any environmental triggers that may precede the anxious feelings
- Coping mechanisms relieve anxiety. Some are healthy, whereas others may compromise wellbeing. Common coping mechanisms include:
  - eating and drinking
  - smoking

Fig. 10.36
Different types o...
B. In the ear (ITE)...

by offering a ra... Box 10.7 apply. Sometimes h... Try these simpl...
- Check that th...
- Check the ba...
- Insert a new ...
- Clean the ea...

As hearing aid... erly. Report lost... once. Check wi... Also, follow the... battery at night...

Chapter 1: Health and aged care services in Australia and New Zealand

aged care service must meet certain standards of care. Some levels of government funding depend on the service becoming accredited. Accreditation is also a way for a service to show that it provides quality care. If an organisation does not meet a significant proportion of the accreditation standards, accreditation is not awarded. The public is regularly informed of accredited organisations.

THE MULTIDISCIPLINARY TEAM
The **multidisciplinary healthcare team** consists of many different health professionals working to provide quality, coordinated care for the client (Table 1.1). The team provides services that support the overall goal of quality resident care.

Team members work together to meet the needs and goals of residents. Many healthcare workers are involved in the care of individual residents and, therefore, coordinated care is needed. A registered nurse serves in a key leadership position.

The **nursing/caring team** consists of the individuals involved in the daily care – registered nurses, enrolled nurses and personal care assistants – and each has a different role and responsibilities. All focus on the needs of residents and their families.

Registered nurse
To become a **registered nurse (RN)**, the student completes a 3-year degree program and registers with the Nursing and Midwifery Board of Australia (NMBA).

Table 1.1
Members of the multidisciplinary healthcare team

Title	Description	Credentials
Diversional therapist	Works in nursing centres; assesses recreational needs of residents, and plans and implements programs accordingly	Required training varies with state and/or centre policies; ranges from no required training to bachelor degree
Audiologist	Tests hearing; prescribes hearing aids; works with hearing-impaired people	Bachelor degree and registration with professional body
Cleric/Chaplain	Works in all types of healthcare settings to assist people with their spiritual needs	Priest, minister, rabbi, Sister, deacon or other pastoral training
Dentist	Prevents and treats disorders and diseases of the teeth, gums and oral structures	Bachelor of Dentistry and registration with state/territory licensing authority
Dietitian	Assesses and plans for the person's nutritional needs; teaches individuals and families about good nutrition, food selection and preparation	Bachelor degree
Enrolled nurse (EN)	Provides direct patient/resident care, including administering medications, under the direction of an RN	Graduate of state-approved program (12 months to 2 years duration) and enrolled with the Nursing and Midwifery Board of Australia
Personal care worker	Assists RNs and ENs; gives direct bedside resident care; must be supervised by a nurse	Completion of Certificate III level program
Occupational therapist	Assists individuals to learn or regain the skills needed to perform ADLs; designs adaptive equipment for ADLs	Bachelor of Science in Occupational Therapy and registration with state/territory authority
Pharmacist	Fills medication and prescription orders written by doctor; monitors and evaluates medication interactions; consults with doctors and nurses regarding medication actions and interactions	Bachelor of Pharmacy and state licensure
Physiotherapist	Assists people with musculoskeletal problems; focuses on restoring function and preventing disability from illness or injury	Bachelor of Science in Physiotherapy and registration with state/territory authority
Doctor	Diagnoses and treats diseases and injuries	Medical school graduation, residency and registration with state/territory authority
Podiatrist	Prevents, diagnoses and treats foot disorders	Bachelor degree and registration with state/territory authority
Radiographer	Takes X-rays ordered by doctor and processes film for viewing	Bachelor degree and registration with state/territory authority

9

Chapter 3: Working within a legal and ethical environment

ACCREDITATION

You are working in residential or home care and accreditors are at your service. Can you answer the following questions?

- You are working in a client's home and they confide in you that they are worried that one of their children is taking money from their bank account. What do you do?
- You are working in a residential aged care service, and one of your consumers has bed rails applied for their safety. Does a restraint authorisation form have to be completed with EPOA or consumer consent?

REVIEW QUESTIONS

Circle T if the statement is true or F if the statement is false:

1 T / F Legislation is a guide only. It still leaves the worker the ability to choose what they prefer.
2 T / F It is okay to leave a computer screen showing the details of a care plan for a consumers open in an area that other people, including visitors and other residents, can view it if it is in a workplace.
3 T / F Harassment is illegal in the workplace, even if the staff want to use it on a client to make them have a shower that is scheduled on the care plan.
4 T / F Negligence can still be proved if a person did not intend to cause injury.
5 T / F Residents in an aged care service still have a definite set of rights, just as people within their homes.
6 T / F Restraint is a term which relates only to those which are physically applied.
7 T / F Placing a person in a chair close to a table in order to prevent them from moving out of the chair is NOT considered restraint.

Circle the BEST answer:

8 Ethics is:
a a set of laws
b the policies of your service
c knowledge of what is right and wrong conduct
d knowledge of how to give good care
9 Which of the following is not harassm
a Using touch to comfort a person
b Joking about a person's religion
c Asking for a sexual favour
d Imitating a person's disability
10 A document that gives instructions a future health is referred to as:
a an advance health directive
b a will
c a statement of intent
d a testament

Answers to these questions are on p.

Further reading

Advance Care Planning Australia (2021). Have the conversation across healthcare services. Online 28 February 2021. Available: www.advancecareplanning.org.au/for-health-and-care-workers/roles-and-responsibilities-in-healthcare
Australian Commission on Quality and Safety in Health Care (2021). Report on person-centred care organisations. Online February 28 2021. Available: Report on person-centred healthcare organisations | Australian Commission on Safety and Quality in Health Care
Australian Government (2021). Powers of Attorney: State Agencies. Online 28 February 2021. Available: www.australia.gov.au/information-and-services/family-and-community/wills-and-powers-of-attorney/powers-of-attorney
Australian Government, Department of Health (2012). Ageing and Aged Care. Decision-making tool: Supporting a restraint free environment in residential aged care. Online 28 February 2021. Available: Decision-Making Tool – Supporting a restraint-free environment.pdf (agedcarequality.gov.au)
Australian Government, Department of Health (2021). Charter of Care Recipients' Rights and Responsibilities – Residential Care. Online February 28 2021. Available: charter_of_care_recipients_rights_responsibilities_-_residential_care.pdf (dss.gov.au)
Australian Government, Department of He ing consumers and their families and care and partnerships. Online 28 February 202 au/internet/publications/publishing.nsf/C mono-toc,mental-pubs-p-mono-inc,mental
Australian Government, Fair Work Ombudsm harassment. Online 28 February 2021. A gov.au/employee-entitlements/bullying-and
Australian Government, Federal Register of L Act 1988. Online 28 February 2021. Availa au/Details/C2016C00979
Australian Government, Federal Register of L Amendment (Enhancing Privacy Protection February 2021. Available: www.legislation.gov.
Australian Government, My Aged Care (2021 ministration. Online 28 February 2021. A care.gov.au/legal-information/guardianship
Australian Government, My Aged Care (202 sibilities: Home Care. Online 28 February myagedcare.gov.au/quality-and-complain consumer-rights/rights-and-responsibilities-
Australian Institute of Patient and Family-Cen 28 February 2021. Available: www.aipfcc.or

Accreditation boxes help you start to consider the importance of understanding the accreditation process.

ACCREDITATION

You are working in residential or home care and accreditors are at your service. Can you answer the following questions?

- As a carer, how would you treat a consumer with dignity and respect if they are from a different culture than you?
- What would you consider discrimination in care delivery within a service?
- How can you support a person's identity when providing care?

REVIEW QUESTIONS

Circle T if the statement is true or F if the statement if false:

1 T / F Australia has a White Australia migration policy.
2 T / F According to the ABS, in 2020 29.8 per cent of all Australians were born overseas.
3 T / F Asylum seekers are illegal immigrants.
4 T / F Culture, race and ethnicity are the same thing.
5 T / F All cultures consider their elders to be wise.
6 T / F In some cultures it is inappropriate to hug a person of the opposite sex.

Circle the BEST answer:

7 The current Australia population comes from approximately how many countries?
a 50
b 100
c 200
d 240
8 There are approximately how many different languages spoken in Australia (excluding Indigenous languages)?
a 50
b 100
c 200
d 240
9 The major religions in Australia are:
a Christianity, Hinduism and Buddhism
b Christianity, Islam and Buddhism
c Christianity, Buddhism and Islam
d Christianity, Shintoism and Islam
10 The basic fundamentals of Islam are called:
a The Five Pillars of Islam
b The Four Cornerstones of Islam
c The Five Rules of Islam
d The Five Cornerstones of Islam

Answers to these questions are on p. 454.

Further reading

Aged Care Quality and Safety Commission (2019). Guidance and resources for providers to support the Aged Care Quality Standards. Online 10 September 2021. Available: https://agedcare.royalcommission.gov.au/system/files/2020-06/CTH.0001.4000.4927.pdf
Doutrich D, Arcus K, Dekker L et al (2012). Cultural safety in New Zealand and the United States: looking at a way forward together, Journal of Transcultural Nursing, 23(2):143.
Nursing Council of New Zealand (2011). Guidelines for Cultural Safety, the Treaty of Waitangi and Māori Health in Nursing and Midwifery Practice.
Raukawa-Tait M (2012). Cultural safety an issue for all NZ's elderly. The Daily Post (Rotorua). 1 May, A8.
Australian Government, Department of Home Affairs (2021). Migration program planning levels. Online 10 September 2021. Available: https://immi.homeaffairs.gov.au/what-we-do/migration-program-planning-levels
Islamic Council of Victoria (2021). Taking care of Muslim patients. Online 10 September 2021. Available: www.icv.org.au/media/icv-policy-research/taking-care-of-muslim-patients/
Parliament of Australia (2020). Temporary migration figures: the quarter before COVID-19 hit June 2020. Available: www.aph.gov.au
Refugee Council of Australia (2021). How do refugees come to Australia under its Refugee and Humanitarian program? Online 10 September 2021. Available: www.refugeecouncil.org.au/coming-to-australia/
Stats NZ Tatauranga Aotearoa (2020). New Zealand's population passes 5 million. Online 18 May 2020. Available: www.stats.govt.nz/news/new-zealands-population-passes-5-million

References

Australian Bureau of Statistics (ABS) (2021). Migration Australia. Online 10 September 2021. Available: www.abs.gov.au/statistics/people/population/migration-australia/latest-release

164

Review Questions are a useful study guide. They help you to review what you have learnt. They can also be used when studying for a test or the competency evaluation. Answers can be found at the back of the book.

CRITICAL THINKING ACTIVITY

You are a carer working for a community agency on the outskirts of a city. You have been assigned the care of Mrs Angha Patel. Mrs Patel is a southern Indian migrant and a practising Hindu. She has only recently started receiving care after she had a fall at home and required surgery for a fractured hip. You are required to prepare a meal for her, wash and vacuum the tiled floors, vacuum all carpets, clean the bathroom and toilet and hang out her washing. You are also required to assist her with her shower and dressing. All carers who have cared for Mrs Patel have reported that she shouts at them in Hindi, speaks minimal English only, gets angry with them very quickly and often cries. When she does speak of her family, it is very derogatory and she blames them for why she is not getting better quickly. She often does not eat the meals that you prepare.

Questions

1 Considering her cultural background, what do you believe could be some of the reasons why Mrs Patel is behaving this way?
2 What steps could you take to try and assist Mrs Patel without her becoming angry?
3 What could you do to ensure that she eats the prepared meals?
4 Who would you ask for advice to better understand Mrs Patel?
5 What government and non-government organisations and services are available in your local area to assist you?
6 Once you have completed questions 2–5, develop a care plan for Mrs Patel that all carers could use when assisting her.

163

Critical Thinking Activities and related questions help you apply your learning to situations you may encounter.

Online resources

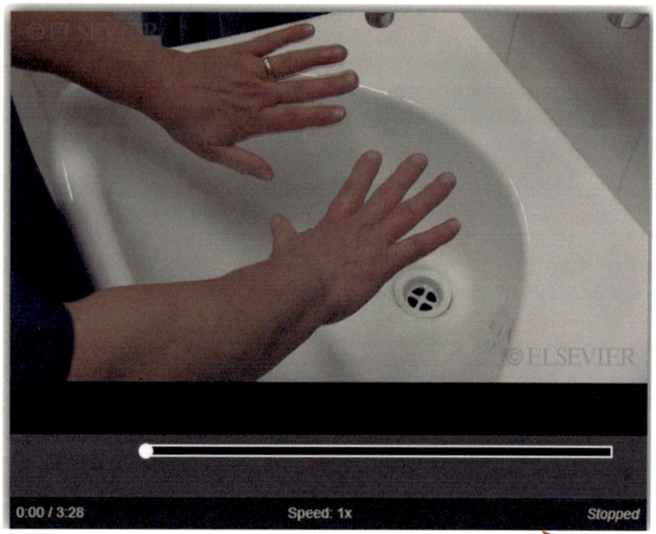

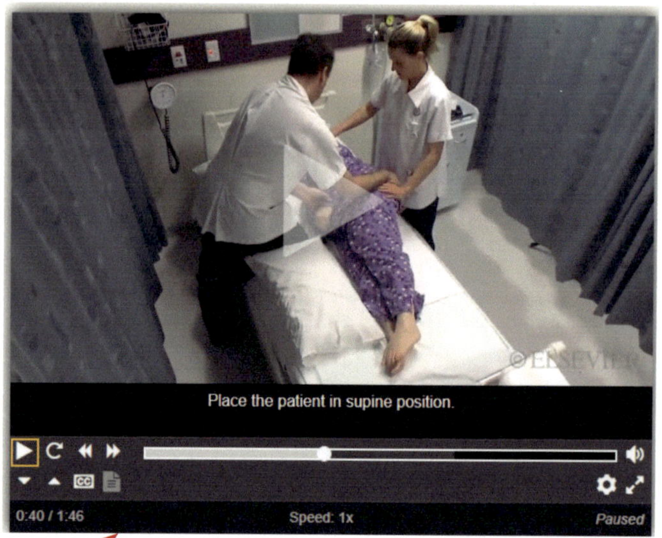

Videos demonstrating important skills and procedures can be viewed at Evolve; see inside front cover for access information. The list of videos can be found in the Brief contents list.

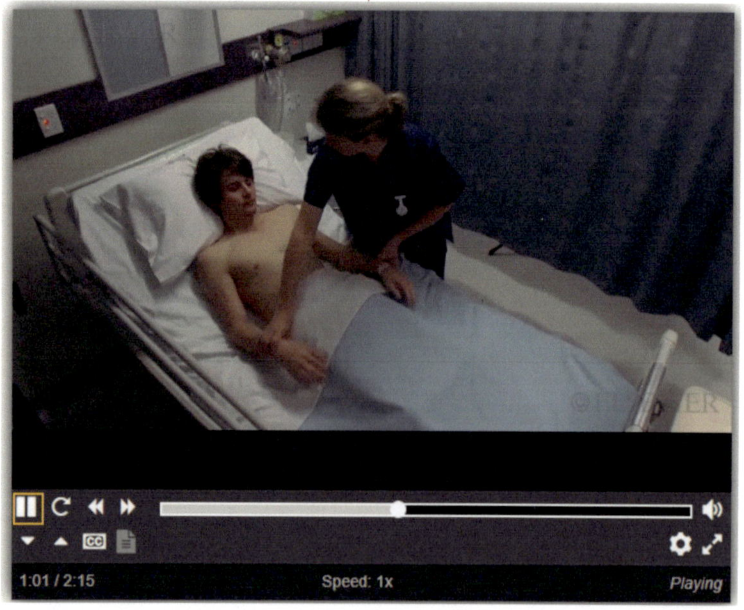

Preface

This fifth edition of *Australian and New Zealand Long-Term Caring: Residential, Home and Community Aged Care* has been a joint effort by the many people involved. The contributing writers have used their vast experience and professional networks to bring to the text a comprehensive and professional view of the aged care industry within Australia and New Zealand. Acknowledging all those who assisted the writers would be a momentous task, and naming each one individually would risk omitting some who have made significant contributions. We therefore dedicate this acknowledgment to all those who assisted by sharing with us their information, insights and resources.

It is also essential to acknowledge the role that many past and current clients and consumers of care have played. Without their wisdom and presence within our professional lives, no accurate and informative text could have been brought to publication.

We are also especially grateful to the people at Elsevier Australia, Melinda McEvoy, Shravan Kumar and Margaret Trudgeon for their support in this fifth edition.

Karen Scott, RN, BNurs, BA, BDementiaCare, GradDipTrainDev, MEd
Clinical Nurse Consultant, Residential Aged and Home Care, Churches of Christ Qld, Australia

Margaret Webb, RN, RM, BNurs, GradCertTESOL, GradDipFET, AdvDipBusMgt, MEd(AWE)
Manager/Consultant MW Projects, Brisbane, Qld, Australia

ABOUT THE EDITORS

Karen Scott and **Margaret Webb** are registered nurses with experience in the vocational education and training sector, along with the aged care sector. They have a passion for the development and delivery of long-term care, and the principles of normalisation and individualised care are foremost in their beliefs. Recognised as leaders in the field of curriculum development for carers and enrolled nurses within Australia, they are well suited to edit this Australasian text. They have both been asked on numerous occasions to provide consultancy advice throughout Australia on aspects of vocational education and training and the roles of both carers and enrolled nurses.

Using their professional and personal networks, they have assisted in drawing together and developing a team of writers for this text, to realise their understanding of excellence within aged care practices. Wanting this text to reflect many voices, they have striven to maintain an eclectic view of aged care practices across Australasia.

Contributors

Odette Best RN, BHSc, MPh, PhD
Professor and Associate Head, Indigenous Research and Community Engagement
School of Nursing and Midwifery, University of Southern Queensland, Qld, Australia

Dianne Cheeseman BNurs, CertGenNus, CertChildHealth, GradDipEdNurs, DipBTTM
Education Consultant, Brisbane, Qld, Australia

Ali Drummond RN, BSc(Nurs)

Will Edwards DipTOL, BA, BHort, MPh, PhD
Director, Taumata Associates, Hawera, New Zealand

Tara Kent BSocSc, BLaw(LLB), DipDisability, DipLifestyleLeisure, GradCertLegalP, MEd(LitNum), MHumServ(Disability), MEd(ABA)
Developmental Educator, Director of Instinct CBT, Brisbane, Qld, Australia

Janet Kerswell RN, GradDipMentHlth(Dist)
Inpatient Unit, New Farm Clinic, Brisbane, Qld, Australia

Ellie Kirov BSc(Hons)(BiolSc), PhD(BiomedSc)
Unit Coordinator & Lecturer (Health Sciences), School of Science, Edith Cowan University, Perth, WA, Australia

Penny Kraemer BPharm, MPS
Pharmacist, Port Macquarie, NSW, Australia

Suzanne Meehan CRN, BSocSc, BSocWk, CertVocEd, DipPrimHlthCare, MGerontol
Team Leader, Aged Care – SBIT (retired), Brisbane, Qld, Australia

Mihi Ratima BSc, DPH, DipMaoDev, PhD
Maori Health and Development, Taumata Associates, Hawera, New Zealand

Rangimahora Reddy BBS, DipAcc, MBS(Acc)
CEO, Rauawaawa Kaumātua Charitable Trust, Hamilton, Waikato, New Zealand

Melanie Robinson BSc(Nurs), GradDip (PaedOncol), MNursRes
Child and Adolescent Health Service WA Health, Perth, WA, Australia
Adjunct Senior Lecturer, Ngangk Yira Research Centre for Aboriginal Health and Social Equity
Murdoch University, Perth, WA, Australia

Karen Scott RN, BNurs, BA, BDementiaCare, GradDipTrainDev, MEd
Clinical Nurse Consultant, Residential and Home Care, Churches of Christ, Qld, Australia

Carla Unicomb RN, BHSc(Nurs), CertIVTAE, GradCertOHS, GradCertVocEdTrain
Director Training Beyond 2000, Manly, NSW, Australia

Margaret Webb RN, RM, BNurs, GradCertTESOL, GradDipFET, AdvDipBusMgt, MEd(AWE)
Manager/Consultant, MW Projects, Brisbane, Qld, Australia

Figure credits

Fig. 1.1: Modified from Cambridge Research Institute: Trends affecting the US health care system 262. Health Planning Information Series, Human Resources Administration, Public Health Service, Department of Health, Education and Welfare, Washington, DC; 1976, revised and updated 1992, US Government Printing Office;

Figs 1.2, 2.4, 2.6, 2.7, 2.9, 2.10, 2.11, 2.13, 2.14, 2.21, 2.22, 2.23, 2.24, 2.25, 2.26, 2.27, 2.28, 2.29, 2.30, 2.31, 2.32, 2.33, 2.34, 2.35, 2.36, 2.42, 2.47, 2.51, 2.52, 2.54, 3.1, 3.2, 4.4, 9.1c, 9.4, 9.7, 10.26, 10.52, 10.56, 11.4, 11.6, 11.7, 11.12, 11.13, 12.2, 12.4, 12.16, 12.18, 12.21, 12.22, 12.29, 12.30, 12.37, 12.40, 12.45, 12.47, 12.52, 12.55, 12.56, 12.58, 12.59, 12.60, 12.62, 12.64, 12.70, 12.76, 12.80, 12.81, 12.82, 12.83, 12.95, 12.97, 12.103, 12.104, 12.105, 12.116, 12.142, 13.4, 14.1, 14.2, 14.7, 14.8, 14.9, 17.1, 17.2: Reproduced with permission from Sorrentino A & Gorek B (2003) Mosby's textbook for long-term care assistants (4th edn), Mosby, St Louis;

Figs 2.1, 2.2, 2.3, 2.44, 2.45, 12.114, 12.115: © Posey Products (a TIDI Products Company);

Fig. 2.5: iStockphoto/Horsche;

Figs 2.8, 2.16, 2.20, 2.37, 2.38, 2.39, 2.40, 2.41, 2.43, 2.48, 2.49, 5.1, 5.2, 8.4, 9.1a, 9.5, 10.1, 10.3, 10.4, 10.8, 10.9, 10.10, 10.11, 10.27, 10.28, 10.29, 10.33, 10.34, 10.35, 10.37, 10.41, 10.43, 10.44, 10.45, 10.46, 10.47, 10.48, 10.55, 10.59, 10.60, 10.61, 10.62, 10.63, 10.64, 10.65, 11.1, 11.5, 11.8, 11.9, 11.10, 11.11, 12.1, 12.3, 12.5, 12.6, 12.7, 12.8, 12.9, 12.10, 12.11, 12.13, 12.14, 12.15, 12.19, 12.20, 12.23, 12.24, 12.25, 12.26, 12.27, 12.28, 12.31, 12.32, 12.33, 12.35, 12.36, 12.38, 12.39, 12.41, 12.42, 12.43, 12.44, 12.48, 12.49, 12.50, 12.51, 12.54, 12.57, 12.61, 12.63, 12.65, 12.67, 12.68, 12.69, 12.71, 12.72, 12.73, 12.74, 12.75, 12.84, 12.85, 12.86, 12.88, 12.92, 12.93, 12.94, 12.99, 12.101, 12.106, 12.108, 12.109, 12.110, 12.111, 12.112, 12.113, 12.117, 12.118, 12.119, 12.120, 12.121, 12.122, 12.123, 12.124, 12.125, 12.126, 12.127, 12.128, 12.130, 12.131, 12.134, 12.135, 12.136, 12.137, 12.138, 12.139, 12.140, 12.144, 13.5, 14.6: Reproduced with permission from Sorrentino A & Gorek B (2011) Mosby's textbook for long-term care nursing assistants (6th edn), Mosby, St Louis;

Fig. 2.12 Reproduced with permission from Cook AM, Polgar JM, Encarnação P (2020) Assistive technologies: principles and practice (5th edn), Elsevier;

Fig. 2.15: Crisp J & Taylor C (2005) Potter & Perry's fundamentals of nursing (2nd edn), Elsevier, Sydney;

Fig. 2.17: Shutterstock.com/Dmitry Kalinovsky;

Figs 2.18, 2.19: Used with permission from Briggs Healthcare;

Fig. 2.46, 12.91: Potter PA, Perry AG (2009) Fundamentals of nursing: concepts, process and practice (5th edn), Mosby, St Louis;

Fig. 2.50: Courtesy of 3M Health Care, St Paul, MN;

Fig. 2.53: de-Vitry Smith S & Bayes S (2019) Skills for midwifery practice, ANZ edition, Elsevier Australia;

Fig. 4.1: iStockphoto.com/Pamela Moore;

Fig. 4.5: Perry AG, Potter PA, Ostendorf WR (2018). Clinical nursing skills and techniques (9th edn), Elsevier, St Louis;

Fig. 4.6: iStockphoto/MonkeyBusinessImages;

Fig. 6.1: Australian Bureau of Statistics, Cat no. 2071.0 Census of Population and Housing: Reflecting Australia – Stories from the Census, 2016 © Commonwealth of Australia;

Fig. 6.2: © Newspix/Kelly Barnes;

Fig. 8.1: iStockphoto/Obencem;

Fig. 8.2: ©Paula Solloway/Alamy;

Fig. 8.3: iStockphoto/HearttoHeart0225;

Fig. 8.5: iStockphoto/DrAbbate;

Fig. 8.6: Adam.J.W.C./Wikipedia/CC BY 3.0;

Fig. 9.1b: © 2017 Tobii Dynavox. All rights reserved;

Fig. 9.2a: Shutterstock/Vladimir Mucibabic;

Fig. 9.2b: iStockphoto/humonia;

Fig. 9.3: Reproduced with permission from Tobii Dynavox, LLC ©2021 Tobii Dynavox. All rights reserved;

Fig. 9.6: Maslow's hierarchy of needs Created by J. Finkelstein;

Fig. 9.8: Shutterstock.com/fizkes;

Fig. 10.2: Yanoff M, Duker JS (2009) Ophthalmology (3rd edn), St Louis, Mosby;

Figs 10.5, 10.6, 10.7: Courtesy of Department of Dermatology, School of Medicine, University of Utah;

Fig. 10.12: Goldman L (2008) Cecil medicine (23rd edn), Saunders, Philadelphia;

Fig. 10.13: Kamal A, Brockelhurst JC (1991) Colour atlas of geriatric medicine (2nd edn), Mosby, St Louis;

Figs 10.14, 10.66: Damjanov I (2006) Pathology for health professionals (3rd edn), Elsevier, St Louis;

Fig. 10.15: © Zimmer Biomet;

Fig. 10.16: Klatt EC (2010) Robbins and Cotran atlas of pathology (2nd edn), Saunders, Philadelphia;

Fig. 10.17: Thompson JM et al (eds) (2002) Mosby's clinical nursing (7th edn), St Louis, Mosby;

Fig. 10.18, 10.32: Thibodeau GA, Patton KT (2002) The human body in health and disease (3rd edn), Mosby, St Louis;

Fig. 10.19: Beare PC, Myers JL (1998) Principles and practice of adult health nursing (3rd edn), Mosby, St Louis;

Fig. 10.20, 10.42: Lewis SM, Heitkemper MM, Dirksen SR (2007) Medical–surgical nursing: assessment and management of clinical problems (7th edn), Mosby, St Louis;

Fig. 10.21: Malarvizhi S, Renuka G (2019) Black's medical–surgical nursing: clinical management for positive outcomes. First South Asia edition, Elsevier;

Fig. 10.22: Phipps WJ, Sands JK, Marek JF (1999) Medical–surgical nursing: concepts and clinical practice (6th edn), Mosby, St Louis;

Fig. 10.23: Modified from Christensen BL, Kockrow EO (2011) Adult health nursing (6th edn), Mosby, St Louis;

Fig. 10.24: Courtesy Cameron Bangs, MD. From Auerback PS (1995) Wilderness medicine: management of wilderness and environmental emergencies (3rd edn) Mosby, St Louis;

Fig. 10.25: iStockphoto/Horsche;

Figs 10.30, 10.53: Thibodeau GA, Patton KT (2010) The human body in health and disease (5th edn), Mosby, St Louis;

Fig. 10.31: Modified from Thibodeau GA, Patton KT (2010) The human body in health and disease (5th edn), Mosby, St Louis;

Fig. 10.32: Thibodeau GA, Patton KT (2002) The human body in health and disease (4th edn), Mosby, St Louis;

Fig. 10.36: Potter PA, Perry AG et al (2017) Fundamentals of nursing (9th edn), Elsevier.

Fig. 10.38: iStockphoto.com/nkbimages;

Fig 10.39: Reproduced courtesy of Sam Simons;

Figs 10.40, 10.49, 10.50: Phipps WJ, Cassmeyer VL, Sands JK, Lehman MK (1995) Medical–surgical nursing: concepts and clinical practice (5th edn), Mosby, St Louis;

Fig. 10.51: Lewis SM, Heitkemper MM, Dirksen SR (2000) Medical–surgical nursing: assessment and management of clinical problems (5th edn), Mosby, St Louis;

Fig. 10.52: Sorrentino SA, Remmert MS, Wilk MJ (2018) Mosby's Canadian textbook for the support worker (4th edn), Elsevier Canada;

Fig. 10.56: Damjanov I (2009) Pathology (3rd edn), Saunders, Philadelphia;

Fig. 10.57: Gould BE (2006) Pathophysiology for the health professions (3rd edn), Saunders, Philadelphia;

Fig. 11.2: Adapted from deWit SC (2009) Fundamental concepts and skills for nursing (3rd edn), St Louis, Saunders;

Fig. 11.3: Remmert, L & Sorrentino SA (2021) Mosby's textbook for nursing assistants (10th edn), Elseiver;

Fig. 12.17: © ArjoHuntleigh. Reproduced with permission;

Fig. 12.34: Reproduced with permission from Sorrentino A & Gorek B (2020) Mosby's textbook for long-term care nursing assistants (8th edn), Mosby, St Louis;

Fig. 12.46: Cabot Health, Bristol Stool Chart – https://en.wikipedia.org/wiki/Bristol_stool_scale#/media/File:BristolStoolChart.png. CC BY SA 3.0;

Fig. 12.66: Dover is a trademark of a Covidien company. © Covidien;

Fig. 12.77: Photos reprinted with permission Gordian Medical, Inc. DBA American Medical Technologies. NPUAP copyright & used with permission. Illustrations copyright and used with permission of National Pressure Ulcer Advisory Panel, December 2017;

Fig. 12.78: Bryant RA et al (eds) (1992) Acute and chronic wounds: nursing management, Mosby, St Louis;

Fig. 12.79: Wilk M (2021) Sorrentino's Canadian textbook for the support worker (5th edn), Elsevier, Canada;

Fig. 12.87: Belch et al (1996) Colour atlas of peripheral vascular diseases (2nd edn), Wolfe Medical, London;

Figs 12.89, 12.90, 12.107: Potter PA, Perry AG (2009) Fundamentals of nursing (7th edn), Mosby, St Louis;

Fig. 12.96: iStockphoto/MilosStankovic;

Fig. 12.98: © Performance Health, www.performhealth.com.au;

Fig. 12.129: Perry, A, Potter P, Ostendorf et al (2021) Clinical nursing skills and techniques (10th edn), Elsevier;

Figs 12.132, 12.133 Sehgal M, Jacobs J, Briggs WS (2021) Mobility assistive device use in older adults, American Family Physician, 15 June; 103(12), 737–744;

Fig. 12.102: iStockphoto/shapecharge;

Fig. 12.141: iStockphoto/xavierarnau;

Fig. 12.143: iStockphoto/FamVeld;

Fig. 13.1: National Health and Medical Research Council © Commonwealth of Australia;

Fig. 13.2: iStockphoto/a_namenko;

Fig. 13.3: iStockphoto/FredFroese;

Fig. 14.3: Alzheimer's Orange County (2020) Rain demonstration. Online. Available: www.alzoc.org/wp-content/uploads/2015/11/Rain-demo.png;

Fig. 14.4: US National Library of Medicine. Dementia with Lewy Bodies. Photo by Kondi Wong, Armed Forces Institute of Pathology;

Fig. 14.5: © BrightFocus Foundation;

Figs 15.1, 15.3: Science Photo Library;

Fig. 15.2: Shutterstock.com/In the Light Photography

Fig. 18.1: Courtesy of Manrex Pty Ltd Webstercare, www.webstercare.com.au.

CHAPTER 1
Health and aged care services in Australia and New Zealand

By Suzanne Meehan

AFTER READING THIS CHAPTER, YOU SHOULD BE ABLE TO:

- define the key terms listed in this chapter
- briefly describe the Australian and New Zealand healthcare systems
- describe the health and aged care services available in Australia and New Zealand
- describe the types, purpose and organisation of aged care in Australia and New Zealand
- describe the make-up of the healthcare team
- discuss the aged care structure within which you work
- identify the diversity of roles and responsibilities of a personal care assistant (paid carer)
- describe the strategies that assist in the delegation of tasks and responsibilities of a carer
- define 'quality care' and explain how it is provided
- promote quality of life.

Key terms

accountable: Being responsible for one's actions and the actions of others who perform delegated tasks; answering questions about and explaining one's actions and the actions of others

accreditation: A series of standards and processes that aged care services must meet and go through in order to ensure continued admission of clients to that service. It ensures standards of care for older people

Aged Care Assessment teams (ACATs): Teams of medical, nursing and allied health professionals who assess the physical, psychological, medical, restorative, cultural and social needs of frail older people and help them and their carers to access appropriate levels of support

acute illness: A sudden illness from which the person is expected to recover

aged care service: A service that provides healthcare services to residents who require regular or continuous care; licensed nursing care is required

Alzheimer's disease: A disease that is the most common form of dementia and causes progressive damage to brain cells that results in impaired memory, thinking and behaviour.

Australian National Aged Care Classification (AN-ACC) Funding: This funding is designed to provide equitable funding to approved residential aged care services, by linking subsidy to the characteristics of services and residents that drive costs

Carer Counselling Program: Works to improve the health, wellbeing, resilience and financial security of carers and to ensure that caring is a shared responsibility of family

chronic illness: An illness, slow or gradual in onset, for which there is no known cure; the illness can be controlled and complications prevented

Commonwealth Home Support Programme (CHSP): Entry-level support at home for older people who need some help with daily tasks so they can live independently

Consumer Directed Care (CDC) model: A way of delivering care that gives individuals choice and flexibility.

deconditioning: The process of becoming weak from illness or lack of exercise

delegating: Authorising another person to perform a task

duty of care: A legal term based on the principle of reasonableness; founded in the law of negligence

Enable New Zealand: An organisation that supports disabled people to access health and disability services, equipment and information, enabling them to live the lives they want to lead

enrolled nurse (EN): An individual who has studied nursing and is registered with a national authority to practise as an EN; also called a registered nurse (Division 2) in some states of Australia; also called a nursing assistant in New Zealand

healthcare assistant: Staff member who provides basic task-oriented care under a nurse's supervision

home care packages (HCP): Coordinated care that enables older people to continue living at home, who might otherwise require residential aged care services

hospice: A healthcare agency or program for people who are dying

job description: A list of the responsibilities and functions the centre expects you to perform

Medicare: The Australian federal health insurance program for Australian citizens, New Zealand citizens and permanent visa holders

Multi-Purpose Services (MPS) Program: Provides integrated health and aged care services to regional and remote communities in areas that can't support both a separate aged care home and a hospital

multidisciplinary healthcare team: The many healthcare workers whose skills and knowledge focus on the person's total care

My Aged Care: An Australian Commonwealth government website and contact centre facilitating access to all government subsidised aged care services

National Aboriginal and Torres Strait Islander Aged Care Strategy: The National Aboriginal and Torres Strait Islander Health Plan 2013–2023 is an evidence-based policy framework designed to guide policies and programs to improve Aboriginal and Torres Strait Islander health over the decade from 2013 to 2023.

National Disability Insurance Scheme (NDIS): Australian Commonwealth Government scheme providing a range of supports for people under 65 with a permanent disability to help them live an ordinary life; may include personal care and support, access to the community, therapy services and essential equipment. This may be at home or in residential aged care

National Relay Service: The person placing the call accesses TRS from any TTY or standard phone by calling 711. The caller is connected to a communications assistant, who relays communication between the caller and the recipient.

National Respite for Carers Program: aims to give the carer a break; achieved by taking the carer or care recipient out of the carer environment.

nursing/caring team: The individuals involved in providing nursing or persona care, e.g. registered nurses, enrolled nurses and personal carers

personal care worker: A person who provides basic personal care under a nurse's supervision; also called personal care assistant, personal carer or personal care attendant

private hospital: A service owned by a for-profit, not-for-profit or charitable organisation

private insurance: Insurance bought by individuals and families

public hospital: A service owned, operated or funded by the state/territory/country

Regional Assessment Service (RAS): A service for older people who have lower care needs, but still require a little help around the home

registered nurse (RN): An individual who has studied nursing for a minimum of 3 years and is registered with a national licensing authority to practise as an RN

residential aged care service: A service that provides 24-hour aged care services

retirement village: A complex made up of self-care accommodation; this may or may not include hostel-type accommodation and an aged care service

Royal Flying Doctor Service: A non-profit organisation that provides emergency and primary health care services for those living in rural, remote and regional areas of Australia

serviced apartment: An apartment in a safe setting, where supervision is provided with support but not 24-hour nursing care for residents assessed as requiring a low level of care

short-term restorative care: Supports people to be independent again after a setback, such as an illness or a fall, allowing them to stay in their own home

standard of care: The skills, care and judgement required to be demonstrated by health team members under similar conditions

Support Needs Assessment Unit: Successful health needs assessments require a practical understanding of what is involved, the time and resources necessary to undertake assessments and sufficient integration of the results into planning and commissioning of local services

Support Services for Remote and Indigenous Aged Care: Services that provide specialised care services that respect culture as well as meeting care needs. These include employing Aboriginal or Torres Strait Island people to provide care; including the local community in aged care planning and providing care; having buildings for cultural ceremonies and family visits

task: A function, procedure, activity or work that does not require the knowledge or judgement of a registered nurse

transition care: Time-limited, goal-oriented and therapy-focused services available to eligible older people after a hospital stay

INTRODUCTION

It is important for those working in any aspect of healthcare to understand the basics of the Australian and New Zealand healthcare systems, to recognise how employers, employees, their work processes and clients are affected by these arrangements. Health-care systems operate within the broader social and economic environments of each country. The differences between how Australia and New Zealand have approached healthcare delivery is the result of the way in which the government systems of each country are organised. In Australia, there is a federal and state split in healthcare service provision, while in New Zealand one national government organises healthcare services for the entire country.

AUSTRALIA

Settlement of Australia occurred tens of thousands of years ago by groups of people now referred to as Aboriginal and Torres Strait Islander people, or Indigenous Australians. White settlement commenced in 1788 with convicts from Great Britain, and people of other nationalities followed. As a result, Australia's current population (around 25.5 million people) has a wide ethnic diversity.

In 1901, Australia became an independent, federated nation comprising six states and two territories. With Federation, the Constitution established the Commonwealth (federal) Government. Each state or territory retains its own parliament, and has local governments, such as municipal or shire councils.

GOVERNMENTS, THE PRIVATE SECTOR AND HEALTH

The major role of the Commonwealth in healthcare is to provide leadership in policy-making, particularly on national issues, such as public health, research and national information management. The Commonwealth funds most medical services out of hospitals, and most health research.

The states and territories are primarily responsible for the delivery and management of **public hospitals** and services, and the regulation of health professionals. The states and territories deliver public acute and psychiatric hospital services, and a wide range of community and public health services, including school health, dental health, maternal and child health and environmental health programs.

The Commonwealth, states and territories jointly fund public hospitals and community care for aged and disabled persons. The Commonwealth Government manages **aged care services** and the states manage disability services, and some aged care services.

Residential aged care is financed and regulated by the Commonwealth Government and provided mainly by the non-government sector (religious, charitable and for-profit providers). The Commonwealth, some state, territory or local governments provide some community services.

There is a large private sector in health services. Private health insurance can cover private and public hospital charges (public hospitals only charge patients who elect to be private patients in order to be treated by the doctors of their choice), and a portion of medical fees for inpatient services. **Private health insurance** can also cover allied health and paramedical services (such as the services of physiotherapists and podiatrists), and some aids and appliances (such as spectacles).

Non-government religious and charitable organisations play a significant role in health services, public health and health insurance.

HEALTH STATUS

The Australian population generally has a good health status, with life expectancy at birth of 80.9 years for boys born in 2017–19 and 85 years for girls born in that period. However, the health status of Aboriginal and Torres Strait Islander people leads to a life expectancy which is approximately 8 years shorter. Otherwise, the pattern of disease is similar to that of other developed countries (AIHW 2021).

HEALTH SERVICES DELIVERY

Australia has a mix of public and private sector providers of health services. Most doctors are self-employed, although some are salaried employees of Commonwealth, state or local governments. Salaried specialist doctors in public hospitals often have rights to treat some patients in these hospitals as private patients. In some allied health and paramedical professions, a significant proportion are self-employed; others are employed by state and local government health organisations.

Public hospitals include those established by governments and some initially established by religious or charitable bodies, but now directly funded by government. There are a small number of hospitals built and managed by private firms providing public hospital services under arrangements with state governments. Most acute-care beds and emergency outpatient clinics are in public hospitals. Large urban public hospitals provide most of the more complex hospital care, such as intensive care, major surgery, organ transplants, renal dialysis and specialist outpatient clinics.

Private hospitals are owned by for-profit or not-for-profit organisations, such as large corporate operators, religious organisations and private health insurance funds. In the past, private hospitals tended to provide less complex non-emergency care, such as simple elective surgery. However, in the past decade the services offered by some private hospitals have become increasingly complex, as they have moved to providing a range of high-technology services.

Specialised mental healthcare in the public sector is provided in separate psychiatric hospitals, general hospitals and community-based settings. Historically, mental health services have operated separately from mainstream health services, but the Commonwealth, state and territory governments are currently working under the National Mental Health Strategy to incorporate mental health services into mainstream health. Other key reforms are focusing on replacing separate psychiatric hospitals with community-based and general hospital services, and integrating mental healthcare provided in different settings.

Australia's aged care system focuses on two main forms of care delivery: residential and community care (ranging from Meals on Wheels, home help and transport to care for people who would otherwise need residential care). Residential services are mainly in the non-government sector, with many operated by religious and charitable organisations.

My Aged Care was introduced on 1 July 2013 and is made up of the My Aged Care website (myagedcare.gov.au) and My Aged Care contact centre (1800 200 422). The **My Aged Care Regional Assessment Service (RAS)** is a national assessment workforce, operating at a regional level in all states and territories, and responsible for conducting face-to-face assessments of older people who are seeking entry-level support at home provided under the **Commonwealth Home Support Programme (CHSP)**. This was originally established as the Community Home Support Programme in 2015. The CHSP consolidated the **Commonwealth Home and Community Care (HACC) program**, Planned Respite from the National Respite for Carers Program, The Day Therapy Centres Program and The Assistance with Care and Housing for the Aged Program. My Aged Care makes it easier for older people, their families and carers to have their aged care needs assessed and be supported to locate and access services.

Carers' needs are supported through in-home and day respite, which can be accessed through CHSP or **home care packages (HCPs)**, as well as emergency respite and subsidised residential care respite.

HCPs cater for the more complex needs of older people who want to stay at home and provide them with access to a range of ongoing personal services, support services and clinical care that help them with their day-to-day activities. The program is part of the Australian Government's continuum of care for older people in Australia, providing services between the CHSP and residential aged care. Clients contribute fees to both CHSP and HCP services. Both daily and means-tested fees are part of the fees connected with HCP. All packages are delivered using a Consumer Directed Care model. The aim of this approach to planning and managing care and services is to give consumers choice and flexibility in the supports they access, based on need and how they are delivered. At every level, providers will need to work with consumers to balance their duty of care with an individual's right to make choices that are reasonable risks.

Flexible care acknowledges that the needs of aged care recipients may require a different care approach to that provided through mainstream residential and home care. For example, **transition care** provides time-limited, goal-oriented and therapy-focused packages of services to eligible older people after a hospital stay. **Short-term restorative care** can support people to be independent again after a setback, such as an illness or a fall, allowing them to stay in their own home. The **Carer Counselling Program** provides short-term counselling and support services around specific areas of concern; and people who are deaf or have a hearing or speech impairment can contact My Aged Care Centre using the **National Relay Service**. The **National Respite for Carers program** provides respite information and other support to allow a break from the caring role.

Australia provides several specific services based on its unique geographical and population needs. These include: the Royal Flying Doctor Service, which delivers care to remote areas by aircraft; the **Multi-Purpose Services Program**, which provides integrated health and aged care services, allowing services to exist in regions that could not viably support stand-alone hospitals or aged care homes; and the **National Aboriginal and Torres Strait Islander Aged Care Strategy**, which aims to improve access to and quality of culturally appropriate care for older people age 50 years and over from Aboriginal and Torres Strait Islander communities.

Organisations are funded to provide culturally appropriate aged care for older Aboriginal and Torres Strait Islander people close to home and community; **Support Services for Remote and Indigenous Aged Care** allows aged care providers to deliver services to Aboriginal and Torres Strait Islander people located in remote and very remote areas.

THE NATIONAL HEALTHCARE FUNDING SYSTEM

The aim of the national healthcare funding system is to give all citizens access to healthcare while allowing choice for individuals. The major part of the national healthcare system is called **Medicare**. Medicare was established to provide healthcare to all Australians. It is financed largely from general taxation, which includes a Medicare levy based on a person's taxable income. Commonwealth funding for Medicare is mainly provided as:

- subsidies for prescribed medicines. Medicines or pharmaceuticals prescribed by doctors and dispensed by pharmacies are directly subsidised by the Commonwealth Pharmaceutical Benefits Scheme (PBS) with a safety net providing partially free medicines for the chronically ill and free or subsidised treatment by practitioners, such as doctors, participating optometrists or dentists
- grants to state and territory governments to help cover the costs of providing access to public hospitals at no cost to patients
- specific-purpose grants to state/territory governments and other bodies.

The Commonwealth also funds some special categories, such as members of the armed forces and veterans, who have additional arrangements while remaining eligible for mainstream Medicare coverage. Some injuries and illnesses are covered by compulsory workers' compensation insurance, and injuries from motor vehicle accidents may be covered by compulsory third party motor vehicle insurance. However, Medicare has wide gaps when it comes to ancillary services and Medicare-provided hospital cover does not give individuals the choice of hospital, doctor or admission time, unlike private health insurance, which generally does.

Another new initiative of the Commonwealth Government is the progressive implementation of the **National Disability Insurance Scheme (NDIS)**. This is a new way of providing support to people with intellectual, physical, sensory, cognitive and psychosocial disability, their families and carers in Australia. The NDIS provides all Australians under the age of 65 who have a permanent disability with the reasonable and necessary supports they need to live an ordinary life. This may include personal care and support, access to the community, therapy services and essential equipment. It aims to support people to live in the community setting or other settings that are suitable for their age and may pay for modifications to make their homes accessible. It may also assist them to live independently with supports, such as personal care to help with showering or dressing, or help preparing meals and cleaning. Fees for support services will apply. Those with NDIS can carry that into residential aged care, and continue this support, even when over 65.

Before 1997, aged care services in Australia were funded by the Commonwealth government. Funding was divided into nursing care, support services and infrastructure. Care services were required to spend this money during a 12-month period and to validate how this was spent.

After the reform of the aged care sector in Australia in 1997 and the introduction of the *Aged Care Act 1997*, the way in which aged care services received money was changed. Services were required to account for the funding they received and the **standard of care** they provided to older people.

On 27 February 2017, **Aged Care Assessment Teams (ACATs)** were given the responsibility of assessing individuals for specific home care packages, as below:

Level 1 – supports people with basic care needs

Level 2 – supports people with low-level care needs

Level 3 – supports people with intermediate care needs

Level 4 – supports people with high-level care needs.

Through the assessment process, the client will have the option of indicating the minimum home care package level they would accept as an interim measure in the event a package is not available at their approved higher level. Additionally, the client will need to indicate if they are seeking or not seeking home care services. ACATs will also assign priority for home care services based on a client's individual needs and circumstances. A client's date of approval and priority for care will determine their place in the national queue for home care packages. Once the client reaches the top of the national queue, they receive a letter confirming they have been assigned a home care package and at what level. It may be an offer below the approved level, allowing commencement of care while they await the approved level to become available. Home care package funding will follow the consumer, allowing them to choose and direct package funding to the provider that best meets their needs, and giving home care providers the opportunity to expand their businesses to meet local demand and consumer expectations. If a consumer chooses to change providers, any unspent funds within their package will follow them to the new provider, although exit fees may apply. To receive funding:

- Services had to document the care being given (care plans, assessment and progress notes had to reflect the care being given).
- Care staff were required to be trained; those not already trained were required to undertake training at Certificate III level.

In October 2022, the new system of funding **Australian National Aged Care Classification Funding (AN-ACC)** was initiated. This residential care subsidy is a payment by the government to certain approved providers for providing residential care to certain care recipients, through residential aged care services. Residential care subsidy under AN-ACC can only be paid if:

- the provider is approved
- the resident has been assessed and approved for residential respite or permanent residential care by an ACAT or Aged Care Assessment Service (ACAS) in Victoria
- the care is provided by accredited residential aged care service
- the service has an allocation of places
- there is not a restriction on subsidy.

Most residents or consumers pay daily care fees and accommodation payments related to their level of care, with some provision for those residents who cannot pay these charges. A means-tested care fee or fees for extra or additional services may apply. With the increased ageing of the population there is an increasing demand for trained staff and for both residential and community services, especially for those clients living with dementia. The increasing number of people with dementia has indicated a need for changes to our communities to make them dementia-friendly and to support people with dementia to continue to live well and remain involved in the things they enjoyed before their diagnosis.

HEALTHCARE SETTINGS

The healthcare industry includes a multitude of services provided by many different health professionals and

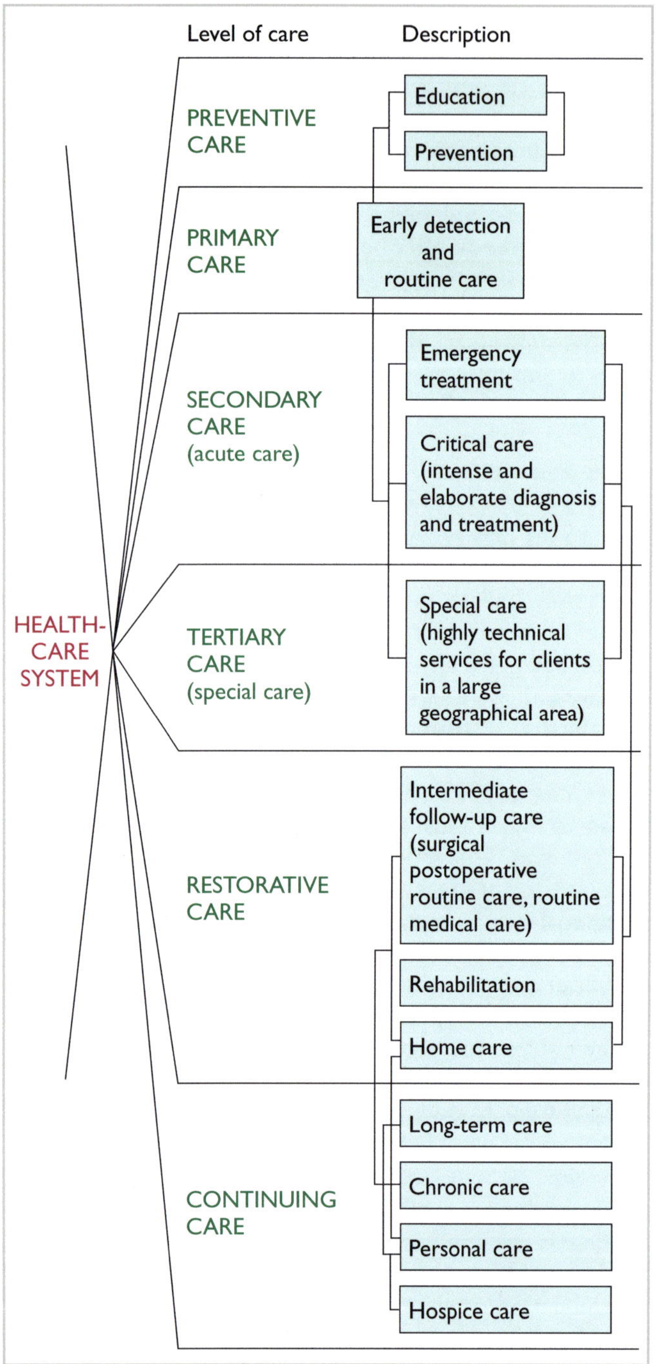

Fig. 1.1
Trends affecting the healthcare system.

agencies (Fig. 1.1). Services can be broadly classified as those that provide:

- *preventive care* – health promotion and illness prevention in settings such as community clinics, schools, industries and medical practices
- *primary care* – diagnosis and treatment of disease and illness, usually in a medical practice, hospital, clinic or outpatient service
- *tertiary care* – rehabilitation or long-term care provided by rehabilitation centres, hospitals and residential aged care services.

FACTORS AFFECTING HEALTHCARE DELIVERY

In recent decades there has been a shift in healthcare away from the diagnosis and treatment of disease towards an approach of health promotion and disease prevention. People within the community are now more knowledgeable about health and preventing illness, and are prepared to accept some responsibility for their own health. As a result, healthcare providers have developed and initiated several health promotion programs.

PROVISION OF AGED CARE

Several sectors provide aged care services, including private providers and charitable organisations. All are bound by the *Aged Care Act 1997* and their respective state laws. The Act also details what services must be provided to any client who receives a community care package, identified as high care, low care or respite care. The Act identifies three areas of care:

- residential aged care
- community or home care
- flexible care.

Overall, at a legislative level the work of personal care assistants is primarily unregulated; however, the policies and procedures of the service or organisation regulate practice.

The Aged Care Act also identifies the need for carers to receive training in aged care, to develop the knowledge and skills needed to provide basic care.

Areas of study include:

- communication
- providing individual support
- working with diverse people
- working legally and ethically
- supporting independence and wellbeing
- resident/client rights
- infection control
- safety and emergency procedures
- personal care skills
- feeding methods
- elimination procedures
- skin care
- transferring, positioning and turning methods
- dressing
- ambulating the person
- range-of-motion exercises
- signs and symptoms of common diseases
- how to care for cognitively impaired persons (those who have problems with thinking and memory).

These requirements help ensure that personal care assistants (carers) have appropriate, current knowledge and skills to give safe, effective care.

AGED CARE SERVICES

The number of aged care services in Australia has grown in the past few decades. This has been partly due to the ageing population, improving technologies, better treatment strategies and an increasing emphasis on healthy lifestyles.

Many aged people are able to remain in their own homes for longer periods than those in previous generations, or until they die. A relatively small percentage of the aged population requires care in an aged care service. Some retirement villages include serviced apartments and a **residential aged care service** within their grounds.

Purpose and goals

Residential aged care services are there to provide a supportive, caring home where the individual needs of the residents are catered for and where families and the community are welcome to interact. The purpose of aged care services is to promote physical and mental health.

When an older person 'moves in' to a residential aged care service, this becomes not only the place where they are cared for, but also their home. By respecting the different needs, interests, preferences, personalities and lifestyles of each client, nurses and carers work with frail older people in ways that promote a sense of individuality. They need to take into account the client's right to make choices and decisions, such as choosing their own bedtimes and meals, and involvement in healthcare decisions. Older people believe that respecting a person incorporates the following major elements: empathy, care, autonomy, provision of information, recognition of individuality, dignity and attention to needs.

Most residents have one or more chronic illnesses, and all are helped and encouraged to:

- accept the limits of their diseases
- function within those limits
- focus on abilities, not disabilities
- do as much for themselves as possible
- change habits that can make their illnesses worse
- eat properly and exercise.

The goals of aged care services include:

- *promoting understanding of changes*: It is important for the resident and their family to accept and understand the physical and mental changes that occur, and families are taught how to assist their loved ones to maintain the highest possible level of functioning. They are also taught how to accept the limits of chronic illness.
- *preventing communicable diseases*: A communicable disease is one that can spread from one person to another. Colds and influenza (flu), for example, can cause major health problems for older and disabled people. The care assistant may be the first person to detect signs and symptoms of a communicable disease.
- *treating chronic illness*: A **chronic illness** is slow or gradual in onset and has no cure. Chronic illness can be controlled, and complications can be prevented with proper treatment. An **acute illness**, on the other hand, begins suddenly and the person should recover, but may require hospital care.
- *providing rehabilitation or restorative care*: People are helped to return to their highest possible level of physical and mental functioning to become or remain as independent as possible. Rehabilitation begins when a person is admitted to the service. Often residents are deconditioned after an acute illness. **Deconditioning** is the process of becoming weak from illness or lack of exercise. Disabilities can result from strokes, fractures or surgery. All staff follow the rehabilitation program.

People living in aged care services are called 'residents' or 'consumers'; they are not called 'patients'. The service is their permanent or temporary home. Aged care services are designed to meet the special needs of people who are older or disabled. They provide services to those who cannot care for themselves at home but do not need hospital care. Services range from supportive care to very complex care. Medical, nursing, personal care, dietary, recreational, rehabilitative and social services are provided. Housekeeping and laundry are included.

With the growth and ageing of Australia's population, and an increase of chronic and generally incurable illnesses, the types of patient groups requiring palliative care has broadened. The goal of palliative care is to improve the quality of life of patients with an active, progressive disease that has little or no prospect of a cure. Palliative care is delivered in almost all settings where healthcare is provided: acute hospitals, general practices, community settings (such as people's own homes) and residential aged care services. Most aged care services follow the Eden Alternative or a similar model, to direct the residents' experiences. This philosophy of care aims to ensure that the residents have a vibrant and interactive home environment. This includes supporting valued routines and skills, respecting culture, accessing companion animals, indoor plants and gardens and encouraging children to visit.

Serviced apartments provide a safe setting, and supervision is provided with support but not 24-hour nursing care for residents, who are assessed as requiring low levels of care. Residents can usually dress themselves, and usually tend to their grooming and bathroom needs with little help. Services include three meals a day, housekeeping, laundry and transportation. There is a 24-hour caregiver and an emergency call system. Residents or consumers receive help with personal care and medication reminders. The caregiver may be a personal care worker. Historically, the residents or consumers of hostels were largely independent; however, with the increase in availability of community care services, older people now recognise that they may need supervision with many of their care needs.

A **retirement village** is a complex made up of self-care accommodation and may or may not have attached serviced apartments and/or a residential aged care service.

Other services

Some aged care services provide learning experiences for students who are studying to become nurses, carers, doctors or other health team members. All students focus on the centre's purposes and goals, and assist in promoting health, treating illness and preventing communicable disease, and in rehabilitation. Many services have special care units, including hospice and dementia care units.

Hospices

In **hospice** care, the main guardians are the family care giver and a hospice nurse who makes periodic stops. Hospice care can be administered in a residential aged care service, a hospice building or sometimes a hospital; however, it is most commonly practised in the home. To be considered for hospice care, one has to be terminally ill or is expected to die before long. The person's physical, emotional, social and spiritual needs are met in a setting that allows a response to the will of the ill person. The family's needs are met too. Children and pets can visit, and family and friends can assist with care.

Units for people living with dementia

A unit for people living with dementia is for people with **Alzheimer's disease** and other diseases that cause dementia signs and symptoms. These diseases cause progressive damage to brain tissue. Currently there is no cure for dementia. Depending on what area of the brain is damaged, memory, language, problem-solving, personality, behaviour and functional skills are among changes that occur. Behavioural and psychological symptoms of dementia that may distress the resident, family or carers can include repetitive questions, wandering, apathy, anxiety, calling out, disinhibited behaviour, agitation, aggression and psychosis. Due to the increased and special needs of residents or consumers who have dementia, staffing levels are generally higher. Staff are trained to recognise and identify the possible cause of any behaviour that is distressing for the resident.

In the late stages of dementia, people may be totally dependent on carers to survive. The course of decline varies considerably across patients and different types of dementia. The time from diagnosis to death typically ranges from 2 to 10 years. In liaison with substitute decision-makers, it may be decided to support the resident in another unit in the service for palliative care.

Respite care

Respite care (also known as 'short-term care') is a form of support for both client and carer. It gives the carer the opportunity to attend to everyday activities or go on holidays while ensuring the client's needs are supported. Respite care may be given informally by family friends or neighbours, or by formal respite services.

Respite care may be for a few hours or days or for longer periods, depending on the client's needs, the needs of the carer, eligibility and what services are available in the area. It can happen in your home or at services, such as an overnight respite cottage, a day centre or residential aged care service. Some aged care services and hospitals provide respite care. This care may be provided in special units. Often the length of stay is short – a few weeks or months. If problems occur, the person may need long-term permanent residential care.

With the ageing of the 'baby boomer' generation, the demand for aged care services is growing. Some of the factors affecting this sector are: a shortage of acute-care beds; an increasing percentage of older people in the population; a reduction in community services available to assist people; changes in the family structure, with more women taking up paid employment and, therefore, not being available at home to take on a carer role. Respite care is a responsibility of the CHSP.

Quality improvement and accreditation

Healthcare services have a responsibility to provide quality care to clients and their families. Providers are responsible and held accountable for the care and services they provide. Quality-control systems are used to ensure that specified levels of care are met. In Australia, the Aged Care Quality and Safety Commission (ACQSC) (2020) assesses the performance of residential aged care homes to ensure the rights of residents are protected, i.e.:

1. Consumer dignity and choice
2. Ongoing assessment and planning with consumers
3. Personal care and clinical care
4. Service and supports for daily living
5. Organisational service environment
6. Feedback and complaints
7. Human resources
8. Organisational governance.

If these and legislated accreditation standards are met, the service can then receive Australian Government subsidies. The process of accreditation is outlined as follows:

- Self-assessment by the provider of the service against the Quality Standards.
- Submission of an application for accreditation of a commencing service.
- Submission of an application for re-accreditation of an accredited service or recommencing service.
- Assessment by a team of registered quality assessors at a site audit and development of a site audit report.
- Development of a performance assessment report outlining compliance with the Quality Standards.
- A decision about the service's accreditation by a decision-maker (delegate of the Aged Care Quality and Safety Commissioner).
- Issue of an accreditation certificate; the certificate of accreditation may be displayed at the accredited service.
- Publication of the performance report and accreditation decision on the ACQSC website.
- Monitoring the quality of care and service at the service and managing any non-compliance with the Quality Standards (ACQSC 2020).

Health services are assessed for accreditation by approved accreditation agencies against the National Safety and Quality Health Service (NSQHS) Standards. The NSQHS has standards and practices for hospitals, aged care services and home care agencies, and serves to improve the quality of care to the public. To become accredited, a residential aged care service must meet certain standards of care. Some levels of government funding depend on the service becoming accredited. Accreditation is also a way for a service to show that it provides quality care. If an organisation does not meet a significant proportion of the accreditation standards, accreditation is not awarded. The public is regularly informed of accredited organisations.

THE MULTIDISCIPLINARY TEAM

The **multidisciplinary healthcare team** consists of many different health professionals working to provide quality, coordinated care for the client (Table 1.1). The team provides services that support the overall goal of quality resident care.

Team members work together to meet the needs and goals of residents. Many healthcare workers are involved in the care of individual residents and, therefore, coordinated care is needed. A registered nurse serves in a key leadership position.

The **nursing/caring team** consists of the individuals involved in the daily care – registered nurses, enrolled nurses and personal care assistants – and each has a different role and responsibilities. All focus on the needs of residents and their families.

Registered nurse

To become a **registered nurse (RN)**, the student completes a 3-year degree program and registers with the Nursing and Midwifery Board of Australia (NMBA).

Table 1.1
Members of the multidisciplinary healthcare team

Title	Description	Credentials
Diversional therapist	Works in nursing centres; assesses recreational needs of residents, and plans and implements programs accordingly	Required training varies with state and/or centre policies; ranges from no required training to bachelor degree
Audiologist	Tests hearing; prescribes hearing aids; works with hearing-impaired people	Bachelor degree and registration with professional body
Cleric/Chaplain	Works in all types of healthcare settings to assist people with their spiritual needs	Priest, minister, rabbi, Sister, deacon or other pastoral training
Dentist	Prevents and treats disorders and diseases of the teeth, gums and oral structures	Bachelor of Dentistry and registration with state/territory licensing authority
Dietitian	Assesses and plans for the person's nutritional needs; teaches individuals and families about good nutrition, food selection and preparation	Bachelor degree
Enrolled nurse (EN)	Provides direct patient/resident care, including administering medications, under the direction of an RN	Graduate of state-approved program (12 months to 2 years duration) and enrolled with the Nursing and Midwifery Board of Australia
Personal care worker	Assists RNs and ENs; gives direct bedside resident care; must be supervised by a nurse	Completion of Certificate III level program
Occupational therapist	Assists individuals to learn or regain the skills needed to perform ADLs; designs adaptive equipment for ADLs	Bachelor of Science in Occupational Therapy and registration with state/territory authority
Pharmacist	Fills medication and prescription orders written by doctor; monitors and evaluates medication interactions; consults with doctors and nurses regarding medication actions and interactions	Bachelor of Pharmacy and state licensure
Physiotherapist	Assists people with musculoskeletal problems; focuses on restoring function and preventing disability from illness or injury	Bachelor of Science in Physiotherapy and registration with state/territory authority
Doctor	Diagnoses and treats diseases and injuries	Medical school graduation, residency and registration with state/territory authority
Podiatrist	Prevents, diagnoses and treats foot disorders	Bachelor degree and registration with state/territory authority
Radiographer	Takes X-rays ordered by doctor and processes film for viewing	Bachelor degree and registration with state/territory authority

Table 1.1
Members of the multidisciplinary healthcare team *continued*

Title	Description	Credentials
Registered nurse (RN)	Assesses, makes nursing diagnoses, plans, implements and evaluates nursing care; supervises and delegates care tasks to ENs and personal care attendants	Bachelor degree and registration with Nursing and Midwifery Board of Australia
Social worker	Helps residents and families deal with social, emotional and environmental issues affecting illness and recovery; coordinates community agencies to assist patient/resident and family	Bachelor of Social Work and registration with state/territory authority
Speech pathologist	Evaluates speech and language, and treats voice, hearing and communication disorders; evaluates and treats swallowing disorders	Bachelor degree and registration with state/territory authority
Natural therapist	Specialises in a range of complementary medical techniques and remedies (including homeopathy, herbalism and aromatherapy) to assist in the diagnosis, treatment and prevention of physical illness or dysfunction.	Graduate of a state-approved program or bachelor degree within a specific area of practice

ADLs: activities of daily living

RNs assess, make nursing diagnoses, plan, implement and evaluate all care. An RN develops a care plan with the person and makes sure that the team follows the plan. The RN also delegates care and tasks to team members. The RN then evaluates with the resident or substitute decision-maker how the care plan and care are affecting the person. The person is supported to maintain or improve their health and independence, and family teaching is provided.

The RN carries out the doctor's orders. He or she may delegate the order to a member of the team. RNs do not diagnose diseases or illnesses, and do not prescribe treatments or medications.

Enrolled nurse

The scope of practice for an **enrolled nurse (EN)** comes under the NMBA. Duties are performed under the direction and supervision of a registered nurse. To be entered on to the roll, the student completes a program of 12 months to 2 years' duration, with medication administration as part of their diploma program.

Personal care worker

A **personal care worker (PCW)** provides basic personal care under a nurse's supervision; other titles for this are personal care attendant, care worker and **healthcare assistant**. The term assistant in nursing (AIN) is being phased out and replaced by personal care worker. PCWs provide much of the care in aged care services. To work in an aged care service, they must have formal training (Certificate III level) (Fig. 1.2) and pass a competency evaluation.

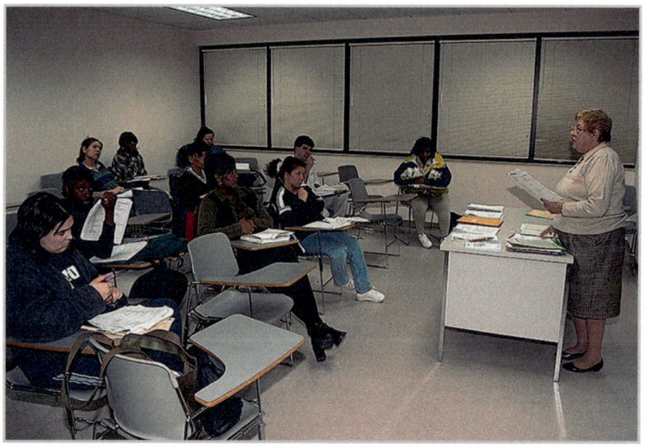

Fig. 1.2
Students attending a Certificate III in Individual Support training program.

EMPLOYEE ORIENTATION

Once you have been employed by an organisation as a carer, you will need to take part in an orientation program. Most services have these for new employees. At orientation sessions, the service's policies and procedures are explained. Your skills may also be checked; that is, the service may ask you to demonstrate some procedures in your job description, such as manual handling. This is to make sure you do them safely and correctly. You will also be shown how to use the centre's supplies and equipment.

Some services have preceptor or mentor programs. A preceptor or mentor is a staff member who guides and supports a new employee. The purpose of this program is to

help you succeed in your new role and to help ensure quality client care. A preceptor/mentor will:
- help you to learn the centre's layout, so you can find what you need
- introduce you to clients and other staff
- help you to organise your work
- help you to feel comfortable as part of the team
- be available to support you where necessary.

A preceptor or mentor is not your supervisor.

Roles and responsibilities

Policy and procedure direct the roles and responsibilities of the carer, both in residential aged care services and in the community. Carers are primarily unregulated workers. To protect the clients in your care from harm you must understand what you can do, what you cannot do and the legal limits of your role. In some states, this is called 'scope of practice'.

Your supervisor may be an RN or a non-nurse manager with an RN overseeing the client's care. As a carer, you will often work independently and without supervision. You will be required to report changes to your supervisor and document all care you have given during your shift or while visiting someone in their home. The rules listed in Box 1.1 will help you understand your role.

While working in a carer role, you will undertake duties related to a person's hygiene, safety, comfort, nutrition, exercise, elimination and, in some areas, medications. You will also undertake **tasks** that require manual handling, observation and the collection of specimens. Observations you may have to perform are temperature, pulse, respiration and blood pressure. (These procedures are detailed later in this text.) You will also have to safeguard the psychological comfort of the person in your care.

BOX 1.1
Rules for carers

- You work independently.
- Your supervisor will assign your work.
- Report any changes in a person's physical or mental status to your supervisor. Report the changes as soon as possible.
- Document changes in the client's progress notes.
- Review the client's care plan prior to commencing care.
- Perform no function or task that you are not trained to do.
- Perform no function or task that you are not comfortable doing without supervision.
- Perform only those functions and tasks that you are legally allowed to do and that are included in your job description.

Your training prepares you to carry out certain duties, but the organisation for which you work will define what you can or cannot do in your role. Although you may have training in a particular task, you should not carry out that task unless it is within organisational guidelines. However, you may, on occasion, be asked to carry out tasks for which you have had no training. You should not carry out these tasks until you have received training and are confident and competent in undertaking them.

It is important that before you start in your new role as a carer you are familiar with your job description, as it reflects the laws and regulations that affect your practice.

Job description

The **job description** is a list of the responsibilities and functions the organisation expects you to perform (see Table 1.2 for an example). It also states educational requirements. In some organisations, the job description is written in a way that forms part of your performance appraisal (see Fig. 1.3 for an example).

When applying for a position it is important to obtain a copy of the job description. If there is any duty you are unsure of, you should discuss this with your potential employer. You should also discuss opportunities for further training, especially in the tasks that you are not trained to do.

Before accepting a job, ask yourself the following questions:
- Does the employer want me to work beyond the legal limits of a carer role?
- Will I be working beyond my training limits?
- Am I expected to perform acts that are against my moral or religious principles?

Remember that it is up to you, not your employer, to decide whether you maintain your personal work ethics. No employer can force you to do something beyond your legal role. It is important that you are not threatened or harassed by your supervisor or employer if you decide not to carry out a task or procedure. If you work under an individual workplace agreement, make sure you know what wage and conditions you want written into your agreement before you sign. Understanding the ethical and legal aspects of your role is equally important. Guidelines for working within these aspects are discussed in Chapter 3.

CARER GUIDELINES

Residents or consumers, clients, families and visitors expect the health team to look and act in a certain way, and you are a member of the health team. Therefore, you should pay careful attention to your personal health and appearance. How you address the client and how you speak are also very important (see Box 1.2).

Personal health

The work of a carer can be physically demanding, and you will need to maintain your own personal health – ensure

Table 1.2
Job description

Title	Personal Care Assistant
Location	Cedar Nursing Home
Responsibilities	The delivery of proficient personal care. The Personal Care Assistant (carer) acts as an assistant with the client in ensuring their care needs are met. The classification is service-based and the Personal Care Assistant (carer) is identified as performing them competently and consistently.
Qualifications	*Essential:* Certificate III in Individual Care *Desirable:* A personal care assistant with relevant qualifications and 2–3 years' experience working in aged care Demonstrated experience in caring for the older person Demonstrated knowledge of care of the older person Demonstrated effective communication, problem solving and advocacy skills Documented participation in education and staff development Demonstrated knowledge and involvement in quality management Demonstrated knowledge of infection control Demonstrated knowledge of and commitment to carry out safe working practices.
Award	Aged Care General Service (State) Award
Conditions of employment	As per award
Salary	As per award
Annual leave	As per letter of appointment
Hours of attendance	As per letter of appointment
Notice of resignation	One week

you get sufficient sleep and rest and follow good dietary rules. Do not come to work in an aged care service if you are suffering from a communicable disease, such as a cough, the flu or diarrhoea. The older person is highly susceptible to these diseases, and they can spread very rapidly through any residential service.

Hygiene

Personal cleanliness needs careful attention. Bathe daily. Use a deodorant or antiperspirant to prevent body odours. Brush your teeth after meals and use a mouthwash to prevent breath odours. If you have been eating garlic or other odorous foods, ensure you use a mouthwash regularly throughout the day. If you are a smoker, ensure that you rinse your mouth or brush your teeth after each cigarette break. Some strong smells can make the older person feel nauseated and unwell.

Appearance

Your appearance is extremely important when working with people. An unkempt and generally untidy appearance can make it difficult for clients to have confidence in your ability to assist them to look and feel good. Most aged care services do not expect staff to wear a 'traditional' healthcare uniform. Often carers are expected to wear street clothes or a corporate uniform. Corporate uniforms are often colourful, casual and give a professional appearance. If you are to wear your own clothes, the following guidelines may help you decide what to wear. However, always be guided by your service's guidelines, as it may have explicit expectations in relation to appearance.

- *Shoes* – as you will be on your feet for most of the day it is essential to have good, supportive shoes. These should be comfortable and enclosed, with a good gripping sole and a small heel, and should preferably be made of leather.
- *Stockings/socks* – these are optional.
- *Skirt* – this should come to your knees or lower. As you will be doing a great deal of bending and stretching, anything shorter may not be discreet.
- *Blouse/shirt/top* – it is best to wear a top that has an action back, as you will be using your arms and stretching. Avoid low-cut tops that show cleavage.
- *Trousers* – avoid wearing tight-fitting trousers.
- *Jewellery* – avoid dangling jewellery as it may be pulled and broken, or may harm the client. Plain band-style rings can be worn, but any ring with a stone, claw or raised decoration should be avoided. Some older people have very fragile skin and these rings will cause the skin to rip and tear. Some older people may be disturbed by the appearance of facial jewellery; out of respect for their views, you should refrain from wearing it.
- *Hair* – all hair longer than shoulder length should be tied back. It is not very pleasant for the older person if your hair is hanging over their food as you assist them with meals, or if it brushes against their face as you attend to their needs.

Staff member: ____________________ Supervisor: ________________________

Date: _________________

Competency	Demonstrated
Delivers care within the guidelines of the organisation's philosophy and mission statement. Knows the significance of the organisation's mission statement. Can give a practical application of the mission statement to an everyday care situation.	
Complies with policies and procedures. Knows where policies and procedures can be accessed. Can tell you the policy for managing work safety risk. Can tell you the policy for managing an emergency with a client. Observes client confidentiality, privacy and dignity in accordance with privacy policy and procedures. Is familiar with compliments, concerns and complaints policy and procedures.	
Complies with the organisation's specified standards. Knows the Commonwealth Department of Health and Ageing standards for client care facility's therapeutic relationship. Can explain how a standard affects day-to-day care. Can explain their responsibilities for administering medications to a client.	
Participates in meetings and education as directed. Is able to incorporate education into daily practices and contribute at meetings. Has attended mandatory education requirements for the organisation (medication management, fire safety, manual handling, safe food handling and hand-washing technique).	
Is involved in the organisation's continuous quality improvement activities. Understands the organisation's quality improvement activities. Has actively been involved in carrying out audits when requested.	
Is accountable for safe working practices and environment within WorkCover guidelines and legislation. Knows the WorkCover Occupation Health and Safety (OH&S) guidelines and legislation. Can recognise, and reports to supervisor, significant hazards in the workplace, both indoors and outdoors. Observes proper use of equipment. Follows manual handling procedures. Adopts safe working practices at all times. Implements practices to prevent or minimise risk. Reports all incidents/accidents to the coordinator and completes relevant documentation.	
Provides care to the organisation's clients as prescribed in the care plan and in cooperation with the Director of Care. Delivers competent and high-quality care to clients as per care plan and to the standard required by the organisation. Obtains advice and direction when appropriate, in response to changes in clients' needs. Reports any difficulties in carrying out client care and seeks advice. Changes and updates documentation as required, following correct organisational policy and procedure. Identifies situations of risk, potential risk or urgent need, and promptly reports these to the appropriate person.	
Immediately reports all client incidents/accidents to the Director of Care and completes relevant documentation.	
Works cooperatively in a team environment. Works in cooperation with other team members.	

Fig. 1.3
Performance appraisal.

Works independently without direct supervision. Is able to demonstrate the ability to work independently without direct supervision.	
Is able to plan daily work schedule within reasonable time frames. Demonstrates good time management skills.	
Communicates appropriately with clients and colleagues. Communication is clear and relevant to situation/activities undertaken. Seeks advice about communication difficulties with clients or colleagues from the Director of Care or an appropriate person. All forms of communication with clients and colleagues reflect an understanding and respect for individual differences and needs. Seeks clarification in understanding work instructions when required, and reports any difficulties to the appropriate person. Completes reports to the standard expected. Reports are clear and accurate.	
Encourages social and physical independence of clients. Provides necessary information and support for client to maintain social and physical independence, by referring to coordinator for advice if required (e.g. physiotherapy assessment/diversional therapy). Identifies potential risk of social isolation. Encourages clients to make independent decisions regarding their care and activities of daily living where possible.	
Knows where to access policies and procedures relating to infection control. Observes infection control procedures in all aspects of care delivery.	

Comments:

Appraisal Action Plan

Issue	**Goal**	**Actions**	**Evaluation & evaluation date**

Staff member: ____________________ Supervisor: ________________________

Signature: ________________________ Signature: ________________________

Date: ________________

Fig. 1.3

Performance appraisal *continued.*

BOX 1.2
Rules of conduct for personal care assistants

- Respect each person as an individual.
- Perform no act that is beyond the legal limits of your role.
- Perform only those acts that you have been prepared to do.
- Assist with medications only when delegated and under the supervision of the RN.
- Carry out the directions and instructions of the supervisor to the best of your ability.
- Follow the service's policies and procedures.
- Complete each task safely.
- Follow the client's care plan, to ensure that you carry out the care in accordance with the client's needs.
- Act as a responsible person at all times.
- Recognise the limits of your role and knowledge.
- Keep the person's information confidential.
- Protect the person's privacy.
- Perform no action that will cause the person harm.
- If unsure or unclear about care, ask your supervisor.

Speech and language

Your speech and language must be professional. The speech and language you use at home and in social settings may be unacceptable at work. Words that you may commonly use with family and friends, especially slang expressions and swear words, may offend clients, visitors and co-workers. Be kind and courteous at all times to the clients in your care.

DELEGATION

In residential services the RN is responsible for **delegating** tasks to personal care workers, assistants in nursing (AINs) or carers. In the community an RN or the supervisor delegates care tasks to the carer. The supervisor should ensure that the carer is carrying out tasks for which they have been trained and ensure that only RNs or ENs carry out complex nursing tasks.

The person must be competent to perform the task in a given situation. For example, a carer would not be expected to be able to undertake a complex wound dressing.

Who can delegate?

Supervisors or RNs can delegate tasks to carers, and these delegated tasks must be within the carer's scope of practice. Delegation decisions must protect the health and safety of the client. The delegating person is then accountable for the tasks. To be **accountable** means to be responsible for one's actions and the actions of others who perform delegated tasks. It also involves answering questions about and explaining one's actions and the actions of others.

The delegating supervisor must make sure that the task is completed safely and correctly. Hence, the supervisor is accountable for the tasks that they have delegated to the carer. As a carer, you cannot delegate tasks to another carer. You can ask someone to help you. However, you cannot ask or tell someone to do your work. Carers are also accountable for their own practice. 'Accountability' is about taking responsibility for your actions, always ensuring you are competent to do the activity you've been asked to perform and always putting patients'/clients' interests first. You should be doing it as part of an agreed plan of care for the patient/client.

The delegation process

Tasks are not always delegated to a carer. If the health status of a client changes and with that change your client needs to be attended to by a carer and an RN, you need to inform your supervisor of this change, to ensure continuity of care. For example, say Mrs Ali has had a fall and now has a dressing to her shin. You are not trained in dressings and so the RN or EN and your supervisor need to be informed of the dressing. Therefore, in accepting care for Mrs Ali you have accepted all care except responsibility for the dressing, because you have informed the RN/EN and your supervisor that you cannot do that task.

Delegated tasks must be within your scope of practice.

As a carer you must know:

- what tasks your state allows personal care assistants to perform
- the tasks in your job description
- what you were taught within your training
- what skills you have learned
- how your skills were assessed
- what relevant work experience you have.

Your supervisor/manager should be kept up to date with your abilities and your concerns. The service's policies and your job description state the tasks that can be delegated to you. These documents must follow state laws, rules and legal opinions relating to carers. To make delegation decisions, nurses need to review the questions in Box 1.3.

The roles and responsibilities of AINs and carers are now very similar. Both are also able to assist clients taking medication if they have the appropriate competency. In the aged care sector, supervision of medication is the concern of professional nurses. However, if medication assistance is in your job description and you have not received education in this area, you are strongly advised to be assessed for competence.

Another factor that may influence whether or not you can give medication is state legislation, such as the *Poisons*

BOX 1.3
Factors affecting delegation decisions

- What is the person's condition? Is it stable or likely to change?
- What are the person's basic needs at this time?
- What is the person's mental function at this time?
- What are the person's emotional and spiritual needs at this time?
- Can the person assist with their own care? Does the person depend on others for care?
- Is the task something the supervisor can delegate?
- For this person, does the task require the knowledge, judgement and skill of a registered nurse?
- How often will the care staff have to assess the person?
- Can the task harm the person? If yes, how?
- What effect will the task have on the person?
- Is it safe for the person if the task is delegated to you?
- Do you have the training and experience to perform the task, given the person's current condition?
- Is your training documented? How were your training and skills assessed?
- How often have you performed the task?
- What other tasks have been delegated to you?
- Do you have the time to perform the task safely?
- Is a registered nurse or manager available to supervise you?
- How much supervision will you need?
- Will you need more directions as you perform the task?
- Is a registered nurse or manager (supervisor) available to help or take over if the person's condition changes or problems arise?

and Therapeutic Goods Act 1966. You should be aware of the legislation requirements in your own state or territory, as well as the policies of the service, as these also identify the boundaries within which you work. (Assisting with medications is discussed in detail in Chapter 18.)

Do not get offended or angry if you cannot perform a task that is usually delegated to you; you should not do something that requires a nurse's judgement. The supervisor should discuss with you what is best for the person at the time, and that decision is also best for you at that time. For example, say you always care for Mrs Melovi: you take her vital signs, you assist her with bathing, dressing and grooming, and you also help her walk. However, Mrs Melovi becomes ill – she is weak and not eating well, and the supervisor wants to observe and evaluate the changes in her condition.

The person's circumstances are central factors in making delegation decisions, which should always result in the best care for the person. Poor delegation decisions by a supervisor can put a person's health and safety at risk. The supervisor may also face serious legal problems. If you perform a task that places a person at risk, you can also face serious legal problems.

The 'Five Rights of Delegation' sum up the delegation process effectively. They are important for supervisors, but you can also use this list to assist you in knowing whether you have been delegated appropriate tasks/duties.

1. The *right task* – Can the task be delegated? Is the nurse allowed to delegate the task? Is the task in your job description?
2. The *right circumstances* – What are the person's physical, mental, emotional and spiritual needs at this time?
3. The *right person* – Do you have the training and experience to perform the task for this person?
4. The *right directions and communication* – Ensure that you have been given clear directions. The supervisor should tell you what observations to make and when to report back, and allow questions and help you set priorities.
5. The *right supervision* – The supervisor/manager should guide, direct and evaluate the care you give. They should demonstrate tasks as necessary and be available to answer questions. The less experience you have with a task, the more supervision you need. Complex tasks require more supervision than basic tasks. The person's circumstances also affect how much supervision you need. The supervisor will assess how the task has affected the person and how well you performed the task and will tell you what you did well and how you can improve your work. This will help you to give the best care possible.

BOX 1.4
The five rights of delegation

The right task
- Does your state allow you to perform the task?
- Were you trained to do the task?
- Do you have experience performing the task?
- Is the task in your job description?

The right circumstances
- Do you have experience performing the task, given the person's condition and needs?
- Do you understand the purpose of the task for the person?
- Can you perform the task safely under the current circumstances?
- Do you have the equipment and supplies to complete the task?
- Do you know how to use the equipment and supplies?

The right person
- Are you comfortable performing the task?
- Do you have concerns about performing the task?

The right directions and communication
- Did the nurse give clear directions and instructions?
- Did you review the task with the supervisor?
- Do you understand what the supervisor expects?

The right supervision
- Is a supervisor available to answer questions?
- Is a nurse available if the person's condition changes or if problems occur?

YOUR ROLE IN DELEGATION

To protect the person from harm, you must perform the task safely. When a task is delegated to you, you have two choices: you can agree, or you can refuse to do the task. To decide, use the Five Rights of Delegation (Box 1.4).

Accepting a task

When you agree to perform a task, you are responsible for your own actions. What you do or fail to do could harm the person, so you must complete the task safely. If you are unsure or have questions about a task, ask for help. Report to the supervisor what you did and your observations, and document this in the progress notes and on the care plan.

Duty of care

Duty of care is based on the principle of reasonableness and is founded in the law of negligence. Negligence can occur if anything care staff do, or anything they fail to do, falls below the required standard of reasonableness, and results in foreseeable harm to an older person.

Refusing a task

You have the right to say no. Sometimes refusing to follow directions is your right and duty.

You should refuse to accept a task when:

- the task is beyond the legal limits of your role
- the task is not in your job description

- you are not prepared to perform the task
- the task could harm the person
- the person's condition has changed
- you do not know how to use the supplies or equipment
- the directions are unethical, illegal or against service policy
- the directions are unclear or incomplete
- a nurse is not available for supervision.

Use common sense. This protects you and the person. Ask yourself if what you are doing is safe for the person.

Never ignore an order or request to do something. Tell the nurse about your concerns. If the task is within the legal limits of your role and in your job description, a supervisor can help increase your comfort with the task. The supervisor can:

- answer your questions
- demonstrate the task
- show you how to use supplies and equipment
- help you as needed
- observe you performing the task
- check on you often
- arrange for training as needed.

You cannot refuse a task just because you do not like or do not want to do it. You need sound reasons for refusing, otherwise you place the person at risk of harm. You could also lose your job. However, you must always be aware that if you attend to a client with whom you do not wish to work, or undertake a task that you do not want to do, you may unwittingly display this feeling to the client you are caring for. This will make your client feel uncomfortable and possibly upset. Always discuss your reasons for refusal with your supervisor or the registered nurse.

FOCUS ON COMMUNITY CARE

Much of the care provided for the person with a disability is delivered within the community or within their own home. Always remember that when you are caring for anybody within their home, you do so as an invited guest and need to adapt to the person's individual standards. You are the guest of the person you care for, and your appearance, demeanour, attitudes and actions must reflect this.

CASE STUDY

Alice McTalley has just completed a Certificate III in Individual Care and is now applying for jobs within the aged care sector. During her course Alice worked in a large aged care service. This service has independent living units, a secure dementia unit and a residential aged care service. The manager of the service suggests that Alice apply for a part-time position at the service, as he has received excellent reports from Alice's supervisors.

Alice enjoyed her time at this service and has obtained an application package (including a job description). She obtains some help from her teachers in completing her résumé and application. Following an interview, Alice is offered a position at the service. She will work in a number of the areas in the complex, to gain experience.

Before Alice starts working, an induction plan is completed, with goals detailed for the first 3 months of her employment. This plan is to be reviewed regularly. Alice finds the work challenging but feels confident in the career she has chosen.

Within 12 months of commencing employment, Alice is helping new staff settle into the service and has decided to continue with further study in aged care.

NEW ZEALAND

New Zealand has a system of public and private health services. Public healthcare is subsidised by the New Zealand Government, while private healthcare is paid for by the individual consumer. There are both public and private hospitals. Public hospitals are available to any New Zealand citizen or resident; private hospitals are available to anyone who holds appropriate health insurance.

HEALTH STATUS

The New Zealand population generally enjoys good health. However, the health status of the Māori and Pacific Islander people is poorer than that of other New Zealanders. The life expectancy for European New Zealanders is on average 10 years longer than Māori and six to seven years longer than Pacific Islander people. Factors that affect the health of New Zealanders include smoking, exercise and alcohol consumption.

HEALTH OF OLDER PEOPLE STRATEGY

New Zealand's Healthy Ageing Strategy was released in December 2016. It set the strategic direction for the next 10 years for the delivery of services to people into and throughout their later years. The vision for the strategy is that older people live well, age well and have a respectful end of life in age-friendly communities.

The Healthy Ageing Strategy and detailed action plan were developed through extensive collaboration with the health and social sectors in New Zealand and are aligned to the World Health Organisation's Global Strategy and Action Plan on Ageing and Health 2016.

The Healthy Ageing Strategy's key strategic themes are:

1. Prevention, healthy ageing and resilience throughout people's older years
2. Living well with long-term health conditions
3. Improving rehabilitation and recovery from acute episodes
4. Better support for older people with high and complex needs
5. Respectful end-of-life care.

Key achievements over the first two years

- Implementation of a nationwide program of falls and fracture prevention and treatment initiatives, led by the Accident Compensation Corporation (ACC) and District Health Boards (DHBs)
- Improved remuneration, training and employment conditions for care and support workers in aged care
- Initial work on a National Framework to improve consistency and quality for home and community support sector services
- Significant progress by the Office for Seniors in supporting the establishment of age-friendly cities and communities, and Hamilton and New Plymouth being accepted into the WHO Global Network for Age-Friendly Cities and Communities.

The focus for 2019–22

There are 26 priority actions for 2019–22, which sit under nine key focus areas, and complement the ongoing work related to the priorities of the first 2 years:

1. Maintain and enhance older people's capacity through supportive environments, health promotion and disease minimisation and prevention.
2. Improve the wellbeing of people by coordinating assistance to socially isolated older people.
3. Prevent unnecessary acute hospitalisations and emergency department attendances.
4. Support rehabilitation closer to home.
5. Implement models of care that are needs based, person-centred and equitable.
6. Support the capacity and capability of the workforce to provide care and support for older people with a more complex and diverse range of health and support needs.
7. Improve support for informal carers.
8. Monitor the performance of the system in implementing the Strategy. A priority action to enable this is the development of an outcomes and measurement framework for this purpose.
9. Strengthen implementation of the New Zealand Dementia Care Framework and cognitive impairment pathways (Ministry of Health 2020).

ASSESSMENT, TREATMENT AND REHABILITATION SERVICES

The aim of assessment, treatment and rehabilitation (AT&R) services is to identify and treat potentially reversible conditions, manage symptoms and restore clients to their maximum level of function. Any person over the age of 65 years who requires assistance with activities of daily living (ADLs) is referred to a gerontology specialist team in order to undergo a comprehensive assessment of their needs. These specialist units are attached to DHBs and are interdisciplinary. Referrals to the unit may be made by general practitioners (GPs) who might have concerns about the safety of a client, or by the medical team in a public hospital where an older person has been receiving care. The assessment process may be carried out in a hospital setting or in the individual's home. The latter is often desirable because it allows the specialist team to assess how well the individual is managing at home. Furthermore, older people often become disoriented when taken out of their home environment, making it difficult to assess their cognitive abilities. Following the assessment, the gerontology specialist team recommends the type and level of care required (Box 1.5). This may include:

- a rehabilitation program
- ageing in place with support
- sheltered housing
- continuing care in a rest home, hospital or dementia unit.

Rehabilitation programs

Rehabilitation programs take place in specialist units in public hospitals and are interdisciplinary. The focus is on assisting clients to regain sufficient functional ability to return to their own homes.

Ageing in place

Most people prefer to remain in their own homes as they age. Following a rehabilitation program, some people may be able to live independently in their own homes, while others may require some assistance to do so. Support (information and financial) is available for home modification and funding for equipment that will allow people with disabilities to return to or remain in their own homes.

BOX 1.5
Gerontology specialist teams

Gerontology specialist teams include:

- geriatricians
- gerontology nurse specialists
- physiotherapists
- occupational therapists
- continence nurse specialists
- speech therapists

BOX 1.6
Providing care at home

Healthcare assistants provide hands-on care for those individuals who are able to remain at home with support. Typically, support includes assistance with bathing or showering, dressing, undressing, housekeeping and shopping. Healthcare assistants are expected to be aware of and report significant changes in an individual's status.

Funding for this assistance is managed on a contractual basis from the Ministry of Health by **Enable New Zealand**. Some people may require ongoing daily assistance in order to remain at home. The success of this option depends on the availability of and access to support services. Subsidies are available on a scale of need determined by the **Support Needs Assessment Unit**. Services available in New Zealand include assistance with ADLs, Meals on Wheels, cleaning and laundry. Most older people in New Zealand do remain in their own homes, with or without support (Box 1.6). Carers are crucial to New Zealand society. At least one in 10 people in New Zealand is a carer. Carers are people who care for friends, family, whānau and *aiga* (Samoan: clan) members with a disability, health condition or illness who need help with everyday living. The care role is often hidden within families and communities, in part because many consider it to be just 'what families do'. Carers:

- enable people to live and participate in their communities.
- also help reduce dependence on health and aged care systems.

Mahi Aroha – Carers' Strategy Action Plan 2019–2023

Mahi Aroha includes a range of actions that we will help carry out with other government agencies and sector organisations over the next 5 years. These actions are focused on:

- Recognising carers and their contributions
- Improving the way carers can navigate the support and services available to them
- Supporting the wellbeing of carers
- Helping carers who want to balance their caring role with paid work or study (Ministry of Social Development 2019).

REST HOME MANAGEMENT

Some rest homes are on the same site as or are attached to a continuing care hospital. This ensures the availability of an RN at all times. Stand-alone rest homes are not legally obliged to have an RN on site at all times. The ratio of RNs is determined by the number of residents in the rest home. DHBs are responsible for ensuring that the needs of older adults are met and that they are appropriately cared for. Gerontology nurse specialists, employed by DHBs, consistently monitor the care provided by continuing care services.

QUALITY IMPROVEMENT

All health and disability providers in New Zealand, including continuing care rest homes and hospitals, must be certified by the Ministry of Health under the *Health and Disability Services (Safety) Act 2001*. In order to be certified, services must comply with the Health and Disability Sector Standards (2001). These Standards are designed to establish consistent, safe and acceptable levels of care for all consumers of health and disability services in New Zealand and provide the framework for each service to develop a continuous quality improvement program. The government has recently conducted a study into the respite services offered to disabled people. Quality audits are conducted within a specified period (maximum of 3 years), with surveillance audits taking place halfway through certification. Whereas meeting sector standards may be open to individual interpretation, the DHB contracts are more specific about the standards that providers are expected to meet. The most definitive difference between rest homes and hospitals is staffing levels and staff qualifications. Table 1.3 summarises the requirements for each, as specified in health fund contracts. It should be noted that these are minimum standards and will be exceeded by many services.

HEALTH AND DISABILITY SECTOR STANDARDS

Health and Disability Sector Standards (Standards New Zealand 2021) comprise six outcomes to be achieved. Each outcome is expanded into several standards and includes criteria required to achieve the outcome. DHBs base their service specifications on these standards. Now called Ngā Paerewa Health and Disability Services, the six outcomes to be achieved are:

1. Our rights
2. Workforce and structure
3. Pathways to wellbeing
4. Person-centred care and safe environment
5. Infection prevention and antimicrobial stewardship
6. Restraint and seclusion (NZ Standard Health and Disability Services 2021).

Each of these outcomes and the standards it encompasses is summarised below.

Our rights

This outcome recognises the right of clients to receive safe services that demonstrate respect for their cultural and individual values and beliefs. The standards for achieving this outcome include: providing services in accordance with consumer rights legislation; recognition of Māori values and beliefs; recognition of individual values and beliefs; maintaining consumer confidentiality; advocacy and consumer support; assistance to maintain contact

Table 1.3
Management and healthcare staffing

	Rest home	Hospital
Manager qualifications	Must hold a current qualification or have experience relevant to management and care of older people. Evidence of at least 8 hours annually of relevant professional development.	Must be either a GP or a registered general or comprehensive nurse. Must hold a qualification or have experience relevant to both management and the care of older people. Evidence of at least 8 hours annually of relevant professional development.
Staff qualifications	Registered nurse for a specified number of hours each week, depending on numbers and dependency of residents.	There must be at least one registered general or comprehensive nurse on duty at all times. The prescribed formula for nurse hours per week is for one full-time equivalent for every five patients. A 30-bed hospital would then have 240 RN hours per week.
Care staff numbers	For 10 or fewer residents: one care staff on duty at all times. Up to 29 residents: one care staff on duty at all times and one on call at all times. More than 30 residents: at least two care staff at all times. More than 60 residents: at least three care staff at all times.	A minimum of two care staff at all times. The RN determines the number and distribution of care staff required according to the needs of residents.
Medical officers	24-hour, 7 days a week on-call cover. It is usual for a doctor to be contracted to provide a service to a rest home. All residents must be visited and medications reviewed at least 3-monthly.	24-hour, 7 days a week on-call cover. Service is usually contracted to a doctor or group of doctors. Doctors visit the service weekly and see each patient fortnightly or as required. Medications must be reviewed 3-monthly.
Physiotherapist	Registered physiotherapist contracted to provide required services.	
Dietitian	Food service planned and audited by a registered dietitian.	

with family/whānau and community; respect for and maintenance of privacy and dignity at all times; and informed consent.

Workforce and structure

People receive quality services through effective governance and a supported workforce. This outcome recognises the client's right to efficient, effective and well-managed services that comply with legislation. The standards for achieving this include:

- efficient management that ensures appropriate and well-planned services
- a documented and maintained quality and risk management system that reflects continuous quality improvement principles, recording of adverse events and operating problems
- notification to statutory agencies where applicable; a complaints management system that is accessible and complies with legislation; efficient and effective management of the service, ensuring the provision of safe and appropriate services to clients
- human resource management processes that are conducive to good employment practice and meet current legislative requirements, and the provision of timely, appropriate and safe services from sufficient suitably qualified, skilled and experienced healthcare staff.

Pathways to wellbeing

People participate in the development of their pathway to wellbeing and receive timely assessment followed by services that are planned, coordinated and delivered in a manner that is tailored to their needs. The standards for achieving this outcome encompass each stage of service provision (assessment, planning, service provision, evaluation and review), including: care that is timely, competent and appropriate to the client's assessed needs, goals and desired outcomes; assessment of needs that is comprehensive and timely; care planning that is client-focused, integrates services and promotes continuity of care; regular evaluation of care plans; and the maintenance of planned activities and interests appropriate to the client's needs and age. Management of the standard provides a service that is planned and coordinated and complies with current legislation and meets the needs of clients. The standards for achieving this outcome include: compilation of information for each client that is identifiable, accurate, current, confidential and accessible when required; maintenance of client records that are accurate, reliable, authorised and comply with current legislative and regulatory requirements; safe and timely administration of medication in accordance with legislative and regulatory requirements; provision of food and nutrition according to individual needs (including special diets); infection control management that protects clients, visitors, staff and the community from exposure to infection; and management systems that protect clients, visitors and staff from exposure to hazardous substances.

Person-centred and safe environment

Health and disability services are provided in a safe environment that ensures physical privacy, safety, adequate space and amenities to facilitate independence, is in an appropriate setting and meets the needs of people with disabilities. The standards for achieving this outcome include: respect for the client's physical privacy when delivering care; adequate space to promote safe mobility and freedom of movement; provision of habitable, appropriately furnished areas; provision of adequate personal hygiene services that take account of physical privacy; adequate personal living space; accessible areas for relaxation, activity and efficient emergency and security systems; safe and appropriate external areas; adequate light and ventilation; and an environment that is maintained at a safe and comfortable temperature.

Infection prevention and anti-microbial stewardship

Health and Disability service provider infection prevention (IP) and anti-microbial stewardship (AMS) strategies define a clear vision and purpose with quality of care, welfare and safety at the centre. The IP and AMS programs are up-to-date and informed by evidence and are a strategy that seeks to maximise quality of care and minimise infection risk and adverse effects from antibiotic use such as anti-microbial resistance. There are adequate human, physical and information resources to implement the infection control program and meet organisational needs. Documented policy and procedures reflect correct accepted good practice. Policy and procedures are practical, safe and appropriate and suitable for the type of service provided. Education on infection control is provided for all service providers, support staff and consumers. Surveillance for infection control is carried out in accordance with agreed objectives, priorities and methods specified in the infection control program.

Restraint and seclusion

The outcome of this standard demonstrates that services maintain a policy of minimisation and a process for determining approval of all types of restraint used, restraint processes (including policy and procedures), duration of restraint and ongoing education on restraint use. The process is made known to service providers and others. Rigorous assessment of consumers is undertaken where indicated in relation to use of restraint. Regular evaluation of all forms of restraint and monitoring and quality reviews are important.

Seclusion is to be for safety reasons only. It must take place only in an approved and designated secure room.

THE CARE TEAMS IN CONTINUING CARE SERVICES

The direct care staff in a continuing care service consist of RNs, ENs and healthcare assistants (also known as caregivers or support workers). In New Zealand, healthcare assistants are the predominant direct care staff in both rest homes and hospitals. However, in rest homes they may be the only direct care staff on duty. In both rest homes and hospitals, the RN is responsible for the planning of care and for ensuring that quality assurance activities are maintained. The roles of RNs, ENs and healthcare assistants are as follows:

- Registered nurses assess, make nursing diagnoses, plan, implement and evaluate nursing care. The registered nurse develops the care plan and ensures that it is implemented. They are also responsible for delegation and evaluation of care, for liaising with patients and their families, for ensuring patients and their families are fully informed and for promoting autonomy. They are responsible for ensuring that treatments, including medication, are administered correctly and on time. In some instances, the registered nurse is wholly responsible for the smooth operation of the service and for ensuring that the legislative requirements of the service are met.
- Enrolled nurses assist RNs in delivering nursing care to individuals in community, residential and hospital settings. They perform delegated interventions to provide care and comfort for individuals and groups. ENs do not practise independently.
- Healthcare or assistants or carers provide basic task-oriented care under a nurse's supervision. Most assistants are trained onsite by the service, and formal training is not compulsory. However, there are courses available for those who wish to advance to more senior positions within the service.

EDUCATION

The Bachelor of Health Science (Nursing) is a full-time 3-year degree. Additionally, some tertiary institutions have developed flexible postgraduate gerontology programs that allow participants to start at certificate level and pursue a pathway to diploma, masters or doctorate level if they wish. Increasing numbers of RNs are choosing postgraduate studies in gerontology.

Nursing assistants undergo a one-year training program, comprising 350 hours of theory and 650 hours of practice. Some, but not all, tertiary institutions provide nursing assistant courses.

The Community Support Services Industry Training Organisation (CSSITO), in collaboration with the Ministry of Health, has developed a national certificate that offers foundation-level training for disability support workers (home support and residential care). The foundation course can be built on to in order to attain higher skill levels. Courses are provided by some tertiary teaching organisations and are also available online.

FOCUS ON COMMUNITY CARE

Services are provided within the home and community sectors to assist the older person or those people with a disability to stay within their own homes or in the community for as long as practicable. Approximately 70,000 care workers provide care for people within a community or home-based environment. To receive this care, the client can call My Aged Care Contact Centre directly or their doctor or a health professional can make a referral online, or family and friends can approach a healthcare professional who contacts My Aged Care on the client's behalf. All referrals to RAS and ACATs must come via this method. Family may refer to My Aged Care if they are authorised to do so and EPOA has been enacted, or the client has given consent to My Aged Care.

QUALITY OF LIFE

Care of the elderly is high on the agenda for both Australia and New Zealand. The care provided in aged care services is always focused on the residents, who have the right to a comfortable and safe setting. To protect them from harm you must understand your roles and responsibilities. What you do and how you do it affects their quality of life. You need to ensure that the way you look or act does not cause concern or distress to clients in your care.

Aged care services must care for residents in a manner that promotes dignity and self-esteem, and must also promote residents' physical, psychological and emotional wellbeing. Residents are shown respect, are spoken to in a polite and courteous manner and are provided with good, honest and thoughtful care. Box 1.7 lists actions that show concern for the person's dignity and privacy. The multidisciplinary healthcare team helps all residents to become or remain as independent as possible.

Accreditation requires training and competency evaluation programs that provide the knowledge and skills needed to give basic care for all workers involved in direct care. You must always practise within the legal limits of your role. Although the RN or supervisor delegates your tasks to you, they must be done under the guidance of the relevant federal and state laws, and the service's guidelines and procedures.

Activities

To promote quality of life, aged care services must provide activity programs that allow personal choice. They must promote physical, intellectual, social, spiritual and emotional wellbeing. Many residential aged care services provide religious services for spiritual health. Residents may need to be assisted to and from activity programs and may require assistance with the activities.

Environment

To promote quality of life, the residential aged care service environment must be clean, safe and as home-like as possible, and this includes allowing residents to have personal items.

BOX 1.7
Actions to promote dignity and privacy

For courteous and dignified interactions:

- use the right tone of voice
- use good eye contact
- stand or sit close enough as needed
- use the person's proper name and title
- gain the person's attention before interacting with them
- use touch if the person approves
- respect the person's social status
- listen with interest to what the person is saying
- do not yell, scold or embarrass the person.

For courteous and dignified care:

- groom the person's hair, beard and nails as they wish
- assist with dressing the person in appropriate clothing for the time of day and in accordance with their personal choice
- promote independence and dignity in dining
- respect the person's private space and property
- assist with walking and transfer without interfering with the person's independence
- assist with bathing and hygiene preferences without interfering with the person's independence

BOX 1.7
Actions to promote dignity and privacy *continued*

- provide a neat and clean appearance:
  - clean-shaven or groomed beard
  - nails trimmed and clean
  - dentures, hearing aid, glasses and other prostheses used correctly
  - clean clothing
  - clothing properly fitted and fastened
  - shoes, hose and socks properly applied and fastened.
  - provide extra clothing for warmth as needed, such as a sweater or a lap blanket.

For privacy and self-determination:

- drape the person properly during care and procedures to avoid exposure and embarrassment
- drape the person properly when in a chair. Use curtains or screens during care and procedures
- close the room door during care and procedures or as the person desires
- knock on the door before entering. Wait to be asked in
- close the bathroom door when the person uses the bathroom.

To maintain personal choice and independence:

- the person smokes in designated areas if that is available
- the person takes part in activities according to their interests
- the person is involved in scheduling their activities and care.

REVIEW QUESTIONS

Circle T if the statement is true or F if the statement is false:

1 T / F A person in a long-term care service can refuse a treatment or procedure.

2 T / F In New Zealand, the enrolled nurse develops the care plan and ensures that it is implemented.

3 T / F Personal care workers provide basic care under supervision.

4 T / F A small percentage of older people live in aged care services.

5 T / F In New Zealand, services shall aim for a restraint- and seclusion-free environment

6 T / F Personal choice is important for quality of life.

7 T / F In New Zealand, all health and disability providers, including continuing care rest homes and hospitals, must be certified.

8 T / F In Australia, aged care services must be accredited by the Australian Aged Care and Quality Agency.

9 T / F It is important for those working in any aspect of healthcare to understand the basics of the Australian and New Zealand healthcare system.

10 T / F An aged care service provides healthcare services to residents who require continuous care.

Answers to these questions are on p. 454.

Further reading

Aged Care Quality and Safety Commission (ACQSC) (2021). Aged Care Quality Standards. Australian Government. Online 23 August 2021. Available: www.agedcarequality.gov.au/consumers/standards/resources

Australian Government (2021). My Aged Care. Online 21 February 2021. Available: www.myagedcare.gov.au/

Australian Government Department of Health (2021). Initiatives and programs: My Aged Care. Online 21 February 2021. Available: my.gov.au and www.health.gov.au

Australian Government Department of Health and Aged Care (2022). The Australian National Aged Care Classification (AN-ACC) Funding Guide Online 3rd February 2023. Available: https://www.health.gov.au/resources/publications/the-australian-national-aged-care-classification-an-acc-funding-guide

HealthCare New Zealand (2021). New Zealand's most trusted healthcare, disability and wellbeing support. Online 21 February 2021. Available: www.healthcarenz.co.nz/

Health Insurance Consultants Australia (HICA) (2021). Online 21 February 2021. Available: www.hica.com.au/content/health-care-funding-in-australia

MND New South Wales (2021). Multidisciplinary care team. Online February 2021. Available: www.mndnsw.asn.au/index.php?option=com_content&view=article&id=228:multi-disciplinary-care-team&catid=106:living-better-for-longer&Itemid=214

New Zealand Aged Care Association (2021). Online February 2021. Available: nzaca.org.nz/

References

Aged Care Quality and Safety Commission (ACQSC) (2020). About accreditation. Australian Government. Online 23 August 2021. Available: www.agedcarequality.gov.au/consumers/about-accreditation

Australian Institute of Health and Welfare (AIHW) (2021). Life expectancy and deaths. Online 23 August 2021. www.aihw.gov.au/reports-data/health-conditions-disability-deaths/life-expectancy-deaths/overview

Ministry of Health NZ (2020). Healthy Ageing Strategy: update. Online 23 August 2021. Available: www.health.govt.nz/our-work/life-stages/health-older-people/healthy-ageing-strategy-update

Ministry of Social Development (2019). Mahi Aroha – Carers' Strategy Action Plan 2019–2023. Online 23 August 2021. Available: www.msd.govt.nz/documents/about-msd-and-our-work/work-programmes/policy-development/carers-strategy/carers-strategy-action-plan-2019-2023.pdf

New Zealand Standard Health and Disability Services (2021). Ngā Paerewa Health and Disability Services Standard. Online 23 August 2021. Available: www.standards.govt.nz/shop/nzs-81342021/

Standards New Zealand (2021). Health care services standards. Online 19 October 2021. Available: www.standards.govt.nz/get-standards/sponsored-standards/health-care-services-standards/

CHAPTER 2
Protecting the person and the carer

By Ellie Kirov

AFTER READING THIS CHAPTER, YOU SHOULD BE ABLE TO:

- define the key terms listed in this chapter
- understand the requirements for adhering to legislation
- understand accident risk factors and identify common hazards
- understand the safety measures to prevent falls, burns, poisoning and suffocation
- understand why clients are identified before receiving care and know how to identify clients
- understand how to prevent equipment accidents and handle hazardous substances
- understand the safety measures for fire prevention, fire management and using oxygen
- know how to report accidents and errors
- know how to protect yourself from workplace violence
- understand your role in risk management
- understand the purpose and rules of using good body mechanics
- identify the causes, signs and symptoms of back injuries
- understand the comfort and safety measures for turning, moving and positioning a client
- know how to safely perform transfers involving beds, chairs, wheelchairs and toilets
- know why good body alignment and position changes are important
- recognise the importance of infection control and understand the chain of infection
- know how to minimise nosocomial infections
- recognise the importance of cleanliness and know how to wash your hands appropriately
- understand the safety procedures described in this chapter
- know how to promote quality of life.

Key terms

additional precautions: Infection control precautions that are applied in the care of a client who is known to have a communicable disease or to be in an infectious state

base of support: The area on which an object rests

body alignment: The way in which the head, trunk, arms and legs are aligned with each other

body mechanics: Using the body in an efficient and careful way

burn: Injury to the skin or mucous membranes caused by heat, cold, electricity, chemicals, gases, friction or radiation

carrier: A human or animal reservoir for microorganisms not showing signs or symptoms of infection

chair position: A position that ensures good body alignment for a client sitting in a chair

code of practice: Practical guidance for people with work-related health and safety duties on how to achieve the standards required under the *Work Health and Safety Act 2011*, and effective ways to identify and manage risks

coma: The state of being unaware of one's surroundings and unable to react or respond to people, places or things

communicable disease: A disease that can be spread from person to person; caused by pathogens

contamination: The process of becoming unclean and contaminated with microorganisms

dementia: A set of chronic signs and symptoms in which memory and the ability to think and reason are lost

disaster: A sudden catastrophic event in which many people are injured and killed, and property is destroyed

disinfectant: A liquid chemical that destroys microorganisms and viruses, as opposed to an antiseptic, which prevents the growth and spread of microorganisms

dorsal recumbent position: The back-lying or supine position

earth: Lead that carries leaking electricity to the earth and away from an electrical item

electric shock: When electric current passes through the body

Fowler's position: A semi-sitting position; the head of the bed can be raised between 45 and 90 degrees

friction: The rubbing of one surface against another

hazardous substance: Any chemical that presents a physical hazard or a health hazard in the workplace

hygiene: A set of practices performed for the promotion and preservation of health

immunity: Protection against a certain disease, either through the human body's own mechanism or through vaccination

infection: A disease state resulting from the invasion and growth of microorganisms in the human body

lateral or side-lying position: Lying on one side or the other

log rolling: A method of turning a person as a unit, in alignment, with one motion

manual handling: Any activity in which force is exerted to lower, carry, push, pull or otherwise manipulate a person or an object

mechanical lifter or hoist: A piece of equipment that is used to raise the client from their bed, chair, bath or the floor

microorganism: A small (micro) living plant or animal (organism) seen only with a microscope; a microbe

modified left lateral recumbent position: A left side-lying position in which the upper leg is sharply flexed so that it is not on the lower leg and the lower arm is behind the person

monkey bar: Triangular-shaped attachment that hangs over the client's bed, used by the client to shift their weight in the bed or to steady themselves as they get into or out of bed

neutral detergent: A cleaning fluid that is used to maintain high standards of cleanliness for reusable items

non-pathogen: A microbe that does not usually cause an infection. Non-pathogens can and do become pathogens

normal flora: Microorganisms that live and grow in a certain area and cause no harm if undisturbed

nosocomial infection: An infection acquired after admission to an aged care service, hospital or healthcare service

pathogen: A microbe that is harmful and can cause an infection or a disease

personal protective equipment (PPE): Gloves, protective eye wear and a plastic apron to protect from body fluids or hazardous chemicals

poisoning: Occurs when a substance that is harmful to the body is swallowed, inhaled, injected or absorbed

posture: Body alignment

prone position: Lying on the abdomen with the head turned to one side

reservoir: The environment in which microorganisms live and grow (e.g. a host)

safe patient handling: Formerly known as the no lift policy, where manual lifting in all but exceptional cases is replaced by the use of lifting machines, people-moving aids and self-mobilisation

safety: To achieve an acceptable level of risk by identifying and controlling recognised hazards

shearing: When skin sticks to a surface and the muscles slide in the direction the body is moving in

side-lying position: Lying on one side or the other; also known as the lateral position

signs: What you observe when caring for a client

slide sheet: A sheet used to slide and reposition the client without unnecessary pulling or dragging of the client in their bed, chair or other surface

Standard Precautions: Precautions that prevent the spread of infection within a healthcare setting

standing lifter: A lifter used for clients who can bear their weight and stand up

suffocation: When breathing stops from lack of oxygen

supine position: The back-lying or dorsal recumbent position

symptoms: A physical or mental feature that may indicate a person has a disease or a condition

transfer belt: A belt used to transfer a person who is unsteady or disabled; also known as a walking belt

trapeze: Triangular-shaped attachment that hangs over the client's bed, used by the client to shift their weight in the bed or to steady themselves as they get into or out of bed; also known as a monkey bar

vaccine: A preparation that contains dead or weakened microorganisms given to produce immunity against an infectious disease

walking belt: A belt used to transfer a person who is unsteady or disabled

workplace-related violence: Any act or threat of physical violence, harassment, intimidation or other threatening behaviour that occurs at work and can affect and involve employees, clients and visitors

INTRODUCTION

Safety is a basic need for both the client and the carer. The entire care team must provide for client safety. Ordinary and sometimes extraordinary measures are needed to prevent accidents and keep clients safe. The goal is to decrease the client's risk of accidents and injuries without limiting their mobility and independence, and to keep clients, visitors and staff safe without interfering with the client's rights. As a carer, however, you must also ensure that your own safety is maintained. You will often move and reposition clients, moving and turning them in bed, for example, or transferring them to and from chairs and wheelchairs. During these and other tasks, you must use your body correctly to protect yourself and the client from injury.

It is in everyone's interests to include safe manual handling as an integral part of modern work practice. Manual handling is any activity in which force is exerted to lower, carry, push, pull or otherwise manipulate a person or an object. It involves activities such as moving and repositioning clients, pushing wheelchairs, pulling to position shower chairs, lowering clients into the bed or chair and regularly carrying heavy loads, such as bundles of linen.

As a carer, it is also important to maintain the highest standards of hygiene and infection control, because this is the best preventive measure to keep the environment free from disease. Infection is a major health and safety hazard for your clients and their visitors, and for you and your colleagues. Minor infections cause short illnesses; other infections are serious and can cause death. Older and disabled clients are at an increased risk, as they may have a lowered immunity due to poor nutrition, their disease state and the medications they take. It is essential to understand and appreciate the importance of infection control regardless of the setting.

LEGISLATION

Maintaining a safe workplace and adhering to safe work practices is not simply a matter of choice or solely determined by policies and procedures of the workplace. Workplace health and safety is legislated, and in both Australia and New Zealand there are laws that demand that all workplaces must adhere to the relevant legislation to ensure the **safety** of workers, clients and visitors. In Australia, the main objective of the *Work Health and Safety Act 2011* is to 'provide for a balanced and nationally consistent framework to secure the health and safety of workers and workplaces'. Take time to visit the Australian Government Federal Register of Legislation website and peruse the legislation (see Further reading at the end of the chapter).

Advice on how to apply this legislation in the workplace is offered in the various state and territory codes of practice. A **code of practice** provides practical guidance for people who have work health and safety duties about how to achieve the standards required under the Act, and effective ways to identify and manage risks.

THE SAFE ENVIRONMENT

In a safe environment a person has a very low risk of illness or injury. The client feels safe and secure, both physically and mentally. The risk of infection, falls, burns, poisoning or other injuries is low. Temperature and noise levels are comfortable, smells are pleasant and there is enough light and room to move about safely. The client is not afraid and has few worries or concerns for their safety. The client must receive the right care and treatment and be protected from falls, burns, poisoning, suffocation and infection. To protect the client from harm, you need to follow the client's care plan and practise the safety measures outlined in this chapter.

Consider all the hazards in the home (Box 2.1).

ACCIDENT RISK FACTORS

Some clients cannot protect themselves; they rely on others for safety. You need to know the factors that increase a client's risk of accidents and injury. You also need to follow the client's care plan.

Some of the major risk factors for injury for aged care clients are listed below.

- *Age* – Older people have decreased strength and move slowly. Some are unsteady. If balance is affected, they may fall easily. These changes prevent quick reflexes to avoid dangers. Older clients are also less sensitive to heat and cold. They have poor vision and hearing, and a dulled sense of smell.
- *Awareness of surroundings* – People need to know their surroundings to be able to protect themselves from injury. An illness or injury can lead to **coma**. Coma is a state of being completely unaware of one's surroundings and unable to react or respond. A person in a coma cannot react or respond to people, places or things, and relies on others for protection.
- *Agitated and aggressive behaviour* – Pain can cause these behaviours, and lead to confusion, decreased awareness of one's surroundings and fear of what may happen. These clients present dangers to themselves and others.
- *Impaired vision* – People with poor vision have problems seeing things. They can fall or trip over equipment, furniture or cords. Some have problems reading labels. They may mistakenly eat or drink such things as perfume, aftershave lotion, hand lotion or cleaning agents.
- *Impaired hearing* – People with impaired hearing have problems hearing explanations and instructions. They may not hear warning signals or fire alarms. Some cannot hear approaching meal carts, medication carts,

BOX 2.1
Home hazard assessment

Home exterior

- Are footpaths even and unbroken?
- Are steps easy to see and in good repair?
- Do steps have securely fastened, easy-to-grip handrails?
- Is there adequate lighting at night?
- Is outdoor furniture sturdy?
- Are garden tools and hoses stored safely?
- Are pools and ponds fenced appropriately?

Home interior

- Do all rooms, stairways and halls have adequate non-glare lighting?
- Are night-lights available?
- Are rugs secured with slip-resistant backing?
- Do rugs lie flat without curled edges?
- Are wooden and tiled floors slip-resistant?
- Are furniture, fans, heaters and electrical cords placed appropriately to permit mobility?
- Is furniture of the correct height and sturdiness to provide support for getting up and down?
- Are there any steps or thresholds that may pose a hazard?
- Are step edges clearly marked with coloured tape?
- Are handrails available and secure?
- In homes with young children, are window guards installed?
- In homes with young children, are barriers installed to prevent toddler access to stairs?
- Are temperature and humidity within normal range?

Kitchen

- Are handwashing services available?
- Is the pilot light on for the gas stove?
- Are the stovetop and oven clean?
- Can the dials on the stove be read clearly?
- Are storage areas within easy reach?
- Are workbenches at a comfortable height?
- Are fluids, such as cleaners and bleach, in original containers and stored properly?
- Is the lighting over bench tops and work areas adequate?
- Is the water temperature within normal range?
- Are there clean areas for food storage and preparation?
- Are the refrigerator and freezer temperatures correct?
- Is the refrigeration adequate?

Bathroom

- Are handwashing services available?
- Are there slip-resistant mats or surfaces in the bath or shower?
- Are bath mats secured?
- Are handrails needed near the bath, shower and toilet?
- Is an elevated toilet seat needed?
- Are medications in their original containers?
- Are medication containers child-resistant if children live in their home or visit?
- Have out-dated medications been discarded?
- Is water temperature regulated?

Bedroom

- Are beds of adequate height to allow getting on and off easily? Is the bed stable?
- Is day and night lighting adequate?
- Is there a light within reach of the bed?
- Is there a telephone beside the bed?
- Is the floor free of telephone and electrical cords?
- Are emergency numbers visible near the telephone?
- In children's bedrooms, do bunk beds have a safety rail?

Electrical and fire hazards

- Are smoke detectors installed?
- Are the batteries for all detectors tested every month and changed annually on a specific date, such as a birthday?
- Have chimneys and stoves been checked for proper ventilation?
- Are extension cords in good condition and used appropriately?
- Are appliances in good working order?
- Are electrical appliances located away from water sources?
- Is there a fire extinguisher near the cooking area?
- Are combustible items, such as oil-based paints, petrol and oily rags, stored in a garage and/or basement?
- Are torches available?
- Is there a first-aid kit available to adult members of the household?
- Does everyone in the family have easy access to emergency telephone numbers?

Source: J Crisp, C Douglas, G Rebeiro et al. (2020). Potter and Perry's Fundamentals of nursing 6th edn. Elsevier, Sydney; Government of Western Australia. Department of Health (2020). Stay on your feet. Move, improve, remove. Home safety checklist. Online. Available: www.stayonyourfeet.com.au/over60/remove-hazards/homesafetychecklist/; TA Touhy & KF Jett (2019). Ebersole & Hess' Toward healthy aging: Human needs and nursing response, 10th edn. Mosby, St Louis.

stretchers or clients in wheelchairs. They do not know that they need to move to safety.

- *Impaired smell and touch* – Illness and ageing affect the senses of smell and touch. When smell is reduced, a person may not detect smoke or gas fumes. When touch is reduced, burns are a risk, as the person has problems sensing heat and cold. Some people have a decreased sense of pain and can be injured without realising it. For example, if Mrs Parks has new shoes, and this causes a blister, she may not feel this blister as she may have poor circulation in her legs and feet. The blister can then become a serious wound.

- *Impaired mobility* – Some disabling diseases or injuries make it impossible to move away from danger. The person may be aware of danger but unable to move to safety. Some people cannot walk or propel wheelchairs. Some are paralysed.
- *Medications* – Medications have many side-effects, especially in older people. These include loss of balance, drowsiness and lack of coordination. Reduced awareness, confusion and disorientation can also occur. These changes may cause the person to be fearful and uncooperative. Report changes in a person's behaviour to your supervisor or the nurse.

PREVENTING FALLS

Falls are the most common type of accident in aged care services and in clients' own homes. Most occur in those over the age of 65. The risk increases with age. A history of falls increases the risk of falling again. In consumer settings, most falls occur between 9.00 a.m. (0900) and 11:00 a.m. (1100), as this is when clients tend to mobilise and attend to personal care; and between 6.00 p.m. (1800) and 9.00 p.m. (2100), as this is when there is increased activity by clients attending to their personal toileting needs. Falls are also more likely to occur during shift changes, because at this time staff are busy coming on and going off duty. Confusion can occur about who is giving care and answering call bells. Shift change times vary among aged care services, but usually occur between the hours of:

- 6.00 a.m. and 8.00 a.m. (0600 and 0800)
- 2.00 p.m. and 4.00 p.m. (1400 and 1600)
- 10.00 p.m. and midnight (2200 and 2400).

In addition to accident risk factors, clients can have other problems that increase their risk of falling (Box 2.2). Aged care services have fall prevention programs, but common sense and simple measures can also prevent many falls. The measures listed in Box 2.3 are part of an aged care service's fall prevention program and the client's care plan. The care plan also lists measures for the person's specific risk factors. Some agencies have bed alarms (Fig. 2.1). Within consumer settings, the home can be assessed for risks to ensure that, as in consumer services, clients are as safe as possible in all settings. The home environment is variable and must be assessed in every case.

Some falls will occur. The aged care team works with the person and family to reduce the risk of falls without decreasing quality of life. In the event that a fall should occur, it is essential to undertake recognised management strategies and follow with immediate post-fall care. Post-fall management strategies are listed in Box 2.4 (p. 31).

Handrails and grab bars

Handrails can be in hallways, stairways and bathrooms. They provide support for clients who are weak or unsteady when walking (Fig. 2.5). They also provide support for sitting down on or getting up from a toilet. Grab bars are installed along bathtubs to help getting into and out of the bath. These can be installed in a home environment to help with safety in the home.

BOX 2.2
Factors that increase the risk of falling

- A history of falls
- Weakness and unsteadiness
- Slow reaction time
- Confusion, disorientation, fainting
- Decreased mobility
- Foot problems and/or shoes that fit poorly
- Elimination needs and urinary incontinence
- Dizziness and light-headedness
- Joint pain and stiffness
- Muscle weakness
- Low blood pressure
- Balance problems and vision problems
- Drowsiness
- Poor muscle coordination
- Alcohol and medication side-effects
- Depression
- Unfamiliar environment, poor judgement and memory problems
- Improper use of wheelchairs, walkers, canes or crutches

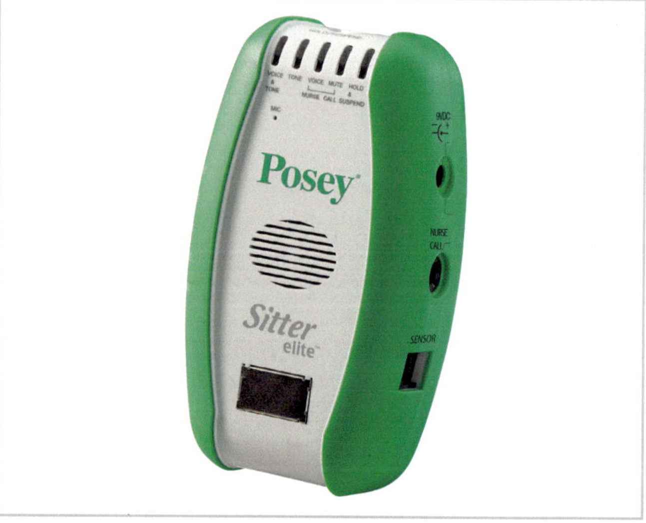

Fig. 2.1
Bed alarm.

Bed rails

Some hospital-type beds have bed rails (side rails) that can be raised and lowered (Fig. 2.4). They lock in place with levers, latches or buttons. Bed rails can be half,

BOX 2.3
Safety measures to prevent falls

- The client is checked regularly. Careful and frequent observations are very important.
- Rooms, hallways and bathrooms have good lighting.
- Light switches (including those in bathrooms) are within reach and easy to find.
- Night-lights are installed in bedrooms, hallways and bathrooms.
- Handrails are on both sides of stairs and hallways, as well as in bathrooms.
- Safety rails and grab bars are in showers and bathtubs, and by the toilet.
- Scatter, area and throw rugs are not used.
- Floor coverings are one colour. Bold designs can cause dizziness in older clients.
- Floors have non-glare, non-slip surfaces.
- Non-skid wax is used on hardwood, tiled or linoleum floors.
- Floors and stairs are free of clutter and items that can cause tripping.
- Floors are free of spills. Wipe up spills immediately.
- Floors are free of excess furniture and equipment.
- Electrical and extension cords are out of the way.
- Furniture is placed for easy movement.
- Furniture is not rearranged.
- Chairs have armrests. The armrests give support when sitting and standing.
- A telephone and bedside light are by the bed.
- Baths and showers have non-slip surfaces or non-slip bath mats.
- Non-skid footwear is worn. Long shoelaces are avoided.
- Clothing fits properly, is not loose and does not drag on the floor. Belts are tied or secured in place.
- Fluid needs are met.
- Glasses and hearing aids are worn as needed. Reading glasses are not worn when the client is up and about.
- The client is taught how to use the call bell.
- The call bell is always within the client's reach.
- The client is asked to call for assistance when help is needed in getting out of bed or a chair, or when walking.
- Call bells are answered promptly. The client may need assistance right away. They may not wait for help.
- Frequent checks are made on clients with poor judgement or memory.
- Clients at risk of falling are in rooms close to the supervisors' station.
- Companionship is provided. Sitters, companions or volunteers are with the client.
- Bed and chair alarms are used. These devices sense when a client tries to get up from a bed or chair. Respond to these alarms promptly.
- Carers explain procedures before and while performing them.
- Clients are properly positioned in beds, chairs and wheelchairs. Pillows, wedge pads or seats are used as directed by the supervisor and the care plan.
- Non-slip strips are on the floor next to the bed and in the bathroom. They are intact.
- The client is assisted with elimination needs at regular times and whenever a request is made. The client is assisted to the bathroom, or the bedpan, urinal or commode is provided.
- The bedpan, urinal or commode is kept within easy reach of those who can use the device without assistance.
- A warm drink, soft lights or a back massage is used to calm the client who is agitated.
- Barriers are used to prevent wandering (Fig. 2.2).
- The bed is in the lowest horizontal position, except when giving bedside care. This reduces the distance from the bed to the floor if the client falls or gets out of bed.
- A mattress or special sensor mat is placed on the floor beside a client's bed. This reduces the chance of injury if the client falls or gets out of bed (Fig. 2.3).
- Bed rails are used according to the care plan. Please note that in most areas, bed rails are deemed to be a form of restraint and the appropriate authorisation must be obtained prior to using them (Fig. 2.4).
- Wheelchairs, walkers and canes fit properly. Do not let anyone use another client's equipment.
- Wheelchairs, walkers and canes work properly. Wheelchair brakes are in working order.
- Crutches, canes and walkers have non-skid tips.
- The correct procedures and equipment are used to transfer clients from bed to chair. Follow the client's care plan.
- Bed, wheelchair and stretcher wheels are locked for transfers.
- The client's feet are positioned on wheelchair footrests.
- The client is kept involved in meaningful activities. Follow the client's care plan.
- Caution is used when turning corners, entering corridor intersections and going through doors. You could injure a client coming from the other direction.
- A safety check is made of the room after visitors leave. They may have lowered a bed rail, removed the call bell or moved a walker out of reach. Or they may have brought an item that could harm the client.

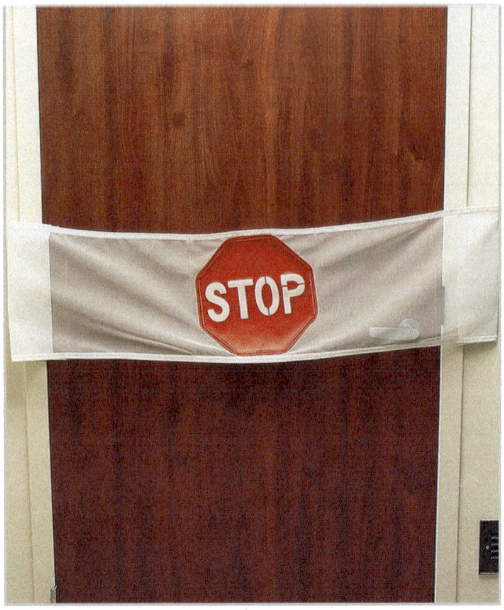

Fig. 2.2
Barriers prevent wandering.

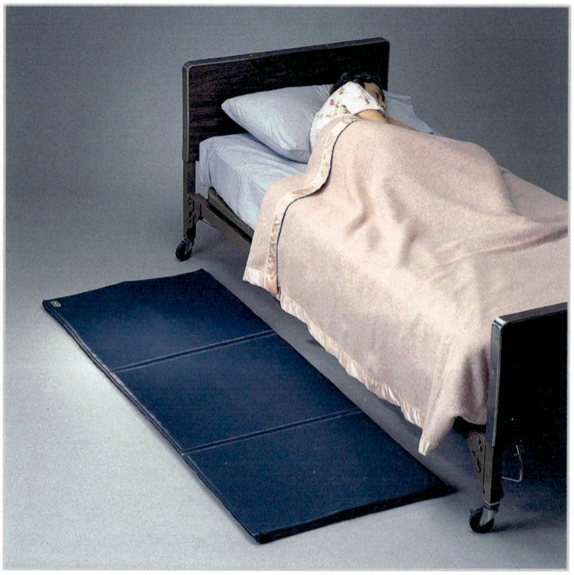

Fig. 2.3
A sensor mat beside the bed.

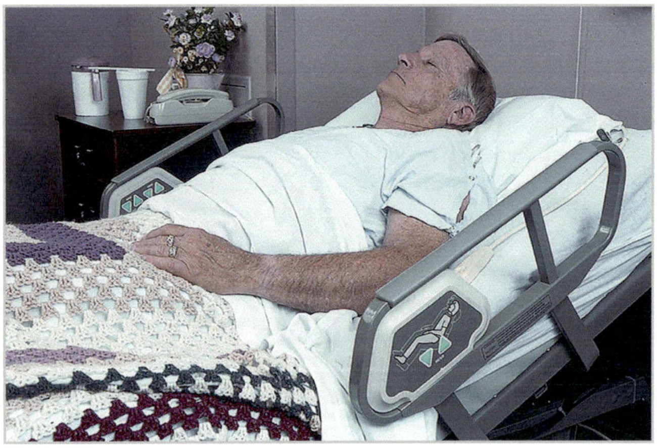

Fig. 2.4
Bed rails.

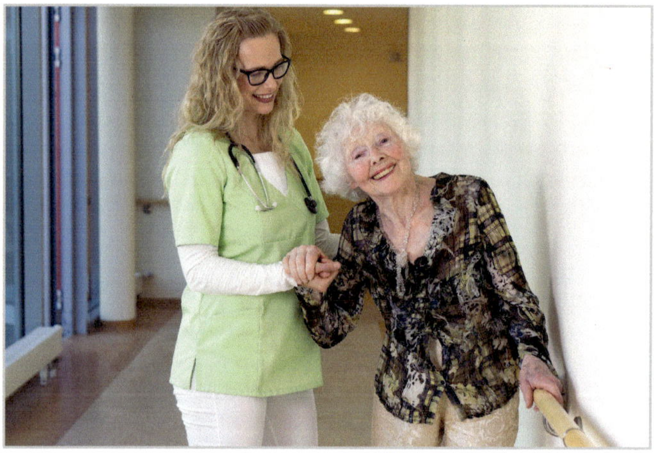

Fig. 2.5
Handrails provide support when walking.

three-quarters or the full length of the bed. When half-length rails are used, each side may have two rails. One is for the upper part of the bed, the other for the lower part. The care plan will tell you when to raise bed rails. They are usually needed for a client who is unconscious or sedated with medications. Some confused or disoriented clients may also need them. If a client needs bed rails keep them up at all times except when giving bedside care.

For an adult's safety, it is recommended that gaps be 10 cm or less between:

- the bed rail bars
- an upper and lower bed rail
- the bed rail and the mattress
- the upper bed rail and the headboard
- the lower bed rail and the footboard (Fig. 2.6).

Bed rails are a hazard for a client trying to get out of bed without help. Entrapment is a risk (Fig. 2.7). That is, a client can be caught, trapped or entangled in the bed rail bars or bed rail gaps. Gaps occur between half-length rails, between the rail and the headboard or footboard, and between the bed rail and the mattress. Injury or death can occur if the client's head, neck, chest, arm or leg becomes trapped. Please note that in most areas bed rails are deemed to be a form of restraint and appropriate authorisation must be obtained prior to using them.

Clients at greatest risk are those who:

- are confused or disoriented
- are small in size
- have poor muscle control
- are restrained.

Check for the 10 cm rule when giving care. Immediately report any concerns to your supervisor. Bed rails prevent

BOX 2.4
Management of falls (Post-fall management)

Immediate response

- Follow local Clinical Emergency Response Systems and protocols.
- Undertake rapid assessment and basic life support (if required).
- Signs of injury may include:
  - bruising
  - lacerations
  - swelling
  - redness
  - abrasions
  - shortening of limbs
  - restricted limb movement
  - external rotation of lower limbs
  - inability to bear weight
  - pain on applying pressure
  - deformity
- Complete observations.
- Notify the relevant senior nurse or medical officer of fall.

Observations and monitoring

- The client may develop symptoms later that can indicate serious changes in their condition.
- Undertake further observations and monitoring at least hourly for a minimum of 4 hours then 4-hourly for the next 24 hours or as clinically indicated.
- Review ongoing observations as required.
- Check for sepsis – risk factors or signs and symptoms of infection.
- Check for delirium – fluctuating changes in cognition, changes in behaviour and increasing confusion.
- Check for head injury – CT scan may be required in clients indicating risk factors (e.g. anticoagulant therapy, increasing confusion, nausea and vomiting, aged over 65 years).
- Continue monitoring.

Communicate

- Reassure the client and explain all treatment and investigations.
- Notify the person responsible (family, carer, friend) for permission and inform them of the fall.
- If the person is not able to communicate effectively, engage with a substitute decision-maker.
- Discuss appropriate treatment options and clarify if there is an advance care directive in place (symptom management is important).
- Implement plan of care and inform staff of care plan.
- Communicate at clinical handover (observations, falls risk and interventions in place).

Document

- Treatment, palliation/escalation process and outcome documented in the clinical record.
- Change fall status to: high-risk (record in clinical record and complete revised care plan).
- Complete Incident Information Management System (IIMS) report and note incident and IIMS number in the clinical record.
- Complete a review of fall event with ward clinical leadership team.

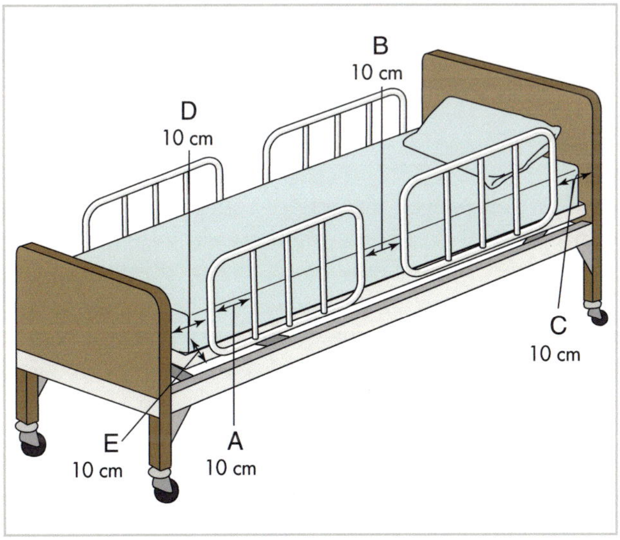

Fig. 2.6
The 10 cm rule.
Only 10 cm are recommended between: **A.** the bed rail bars; **B.** the upper and lower bed rails; **C.** the upper bed rail and the headboard; **D.** the lower bed rail and the footboard; and **E.** the bed rail and the mattress.

clients from getting out of bed. They are, therefore, considered restraints. Legislation forbids the use of any restraints unless they are needed to safeguard a client's safety. Some clients feel safer with bed rails up. Others use them to change positions in bed. All restraints must be ordered by the doctor, and regular checks must be made while they are up. The need for bed rails must be carefully noted in the client's care plan.

Wheel locks

Many bed legs have wheels, which allow the bed to be moved easily. Each wheel has a lock to prevent the bed from moving (Fig. 2.8). Wheels are locked at all times except when moving the bed. Make sure bed wheels are locked when giving bedside care and when you transfer a client to or from the bed. Wheelchair and stretcher wheels are also locked during transfers. You or the client could be injured if the bed, wheelchair or stretcher moves.

PREVENTING POISONING

Accidental **poisoning** is a health hazard in aged care services and in the home. Poor vision and confusion are major risk factors. Make sure the client cannot reach hazardous

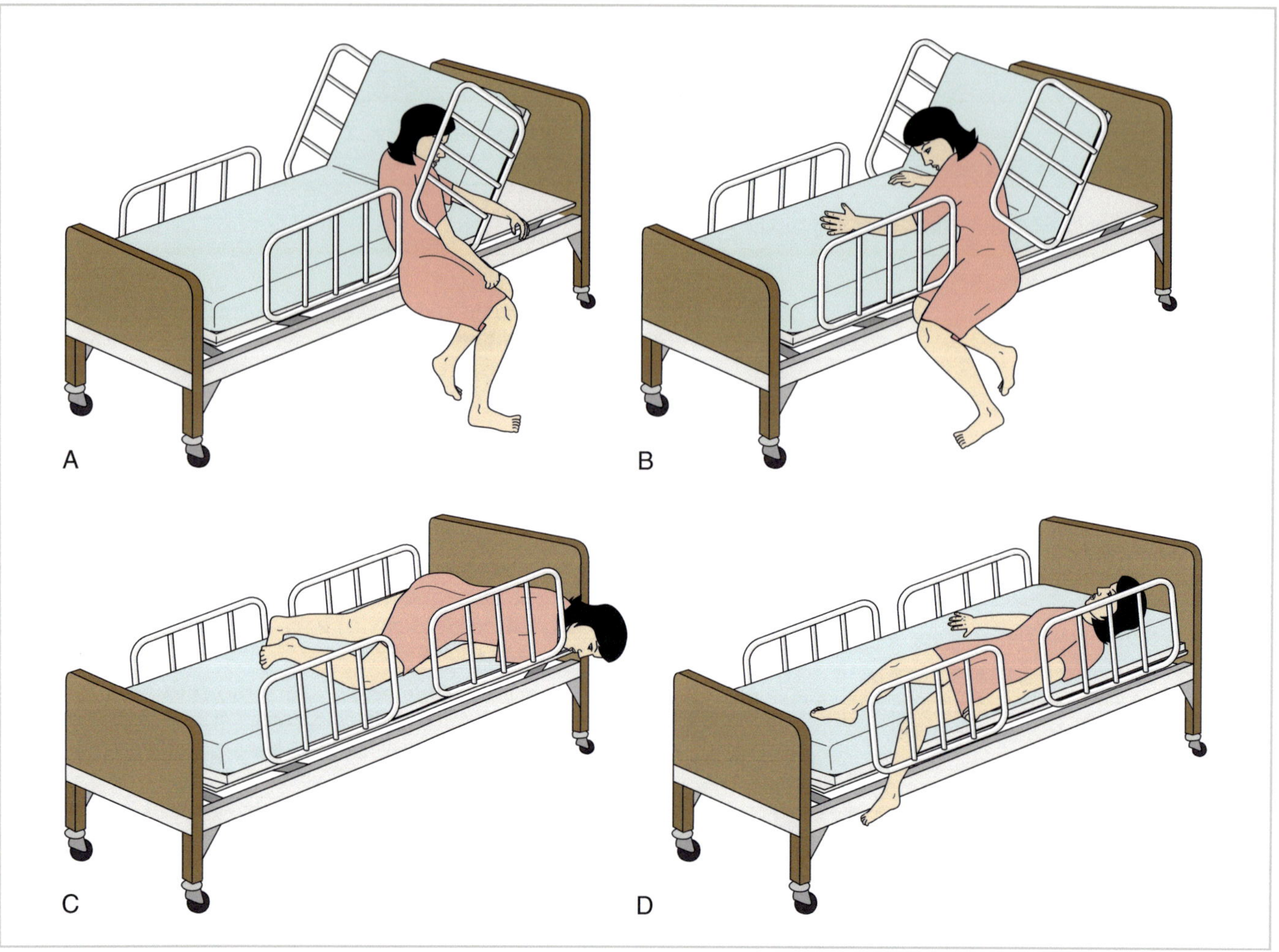

Fig. 2.7
Entrapment is a safety risk with bed rails.
A. The client is trapped between the bed rail bars. **B.** The client is trapped in between the bed rail gap. **C.** The client is trapped between the bed rail and the headboard. **D.** The client is caught between the mattress and the bed rail.

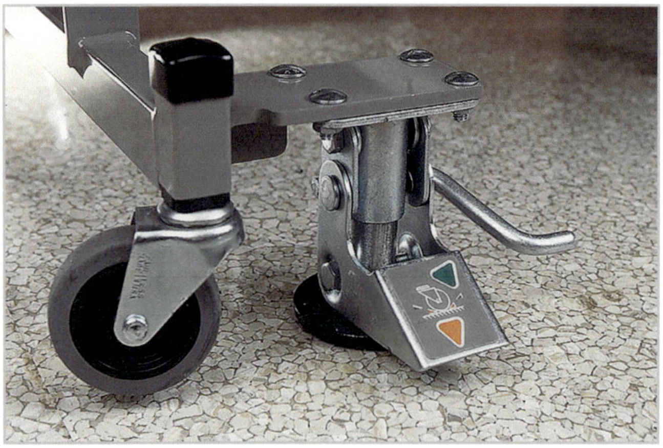

Fig. 2.8
Lock on a bed wheel.

materials. Follow aged care service policy and procedures for storing personal care items (mouthwash, lotion, deodorant and others). These items cause harm when swallowed. Within a home environment, ensure items are out of reach of children and stored securely. The home can be a very unsafe environment, so it is essential to monitor surroundings.

PREVENTING BURNS

Burns are a leading cause of death, especially among children and older people. Smoking, spilled hot liquids, electrical items and very hot bath water are common causes of burns in aged care services. The following safety measures can help prevent burns:

- Be sure clients smoke only in designated smoking areas.
- Supervise smoking by clients who cannot protect themselves.

- Do not allow smoking in bed.
- Do not allow smoking where oxygen is used or stored.
- Check equipment for frayed cords and proper working order.
- Do not use client-owned electrical items until they have been safety checked. The maintenance department of your aged care service or any registered electrician can do this.
- Do not allow the use of space heaters.
- Do not allow the client to sleep with a heating pad.
- Do not use electric blankets.
- Turn cold water on first, then hot water. Turn hot water off first, then cold water.
- Check bath water temperature before the client gets into the bath.
- Assist the client with eating and drinking as needed. Spilled hot food or fluids can cause burns.
- Follow safety guidelines when applying heat and cold.

PREVENTING SUFFOCATION

Suffocation occurs when breathing stops from lack of oxygen. Death occurs if the client does not start breathing again. Common causes of suffocation include choking, drowning, inhaling gas or smoke, strangulation and electrical shock. Carbon monoxide poisoning is another cause. It results from a lack of oxygen in the air. The client breathes in air filled with carbon monoxide, not oxygen. Faulty exhaust systems on cars and damaged furnaces and chimneys are common causes.

The following safety measures can help prevent suffocation:

- Cut food into small, bite-sized pieces for those who cannot do so themselves.
- Be sure the client's dentures are in place.
- Sit the client upright at 90 degrees
- Make sure the client can chew properly and swallow the food served.
- Report loose teeth or dentures to your supervisor.
- Check the client's care plan for swallowing problems before serving snacks or beverages.
- The client may ask for something that they cannot swallow.
- Tell your supervisor immediately if a client has difficulty swallowing.
- Do not give oral foods and fluids to a client with feeding tubes.
- Never leave a client unattended in the bathtub or shower.
- Move all clients and visitors from the area if you smell gas or smoke.
- Position the client in the bed properly.
- Use bed rails correctly.
- Use restraints properly.
- Make sure that all electrical cords and appliances are in good repair.

PREVENTING EQUIPMENT-RELATED ACCIDENTS

All equipment is unsafe if broken, not used correctly or not working properly. Inspect all equipment before use. Check glass and plastic items for cracks, chips and sharp or rough edges. These can cause cuts, stabs or scratches. Do not use damaged equipment or give it to clients.

Electrical items must work properly and be in good repair. Frayed cords (Fig. 2.9) and overloaded outlets (Fig. 2.10) can cause fires and electrical shocks. An **electric shock** is when an electric current passes through the body. It can burn the skin, muscles, nerves and other tissues. It can affect the heart muscle and cause death. Report frayed cords and broken equipment. Tag the item and send it for repair immediately.

Three-pronged plugs (Fig. 2.11) are used on all electrical items. Two prongs carry electric current. The third prong is

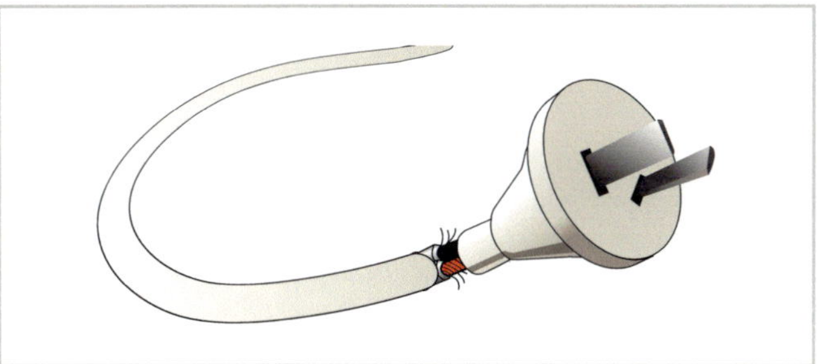

Fig. 2.9
A frayed electrical cord.

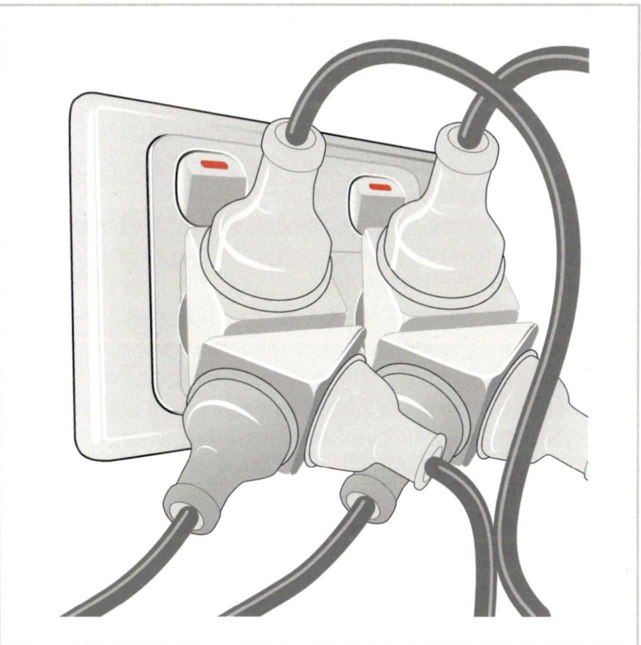

Fig. 2.10
An overloaded electrical outlet.

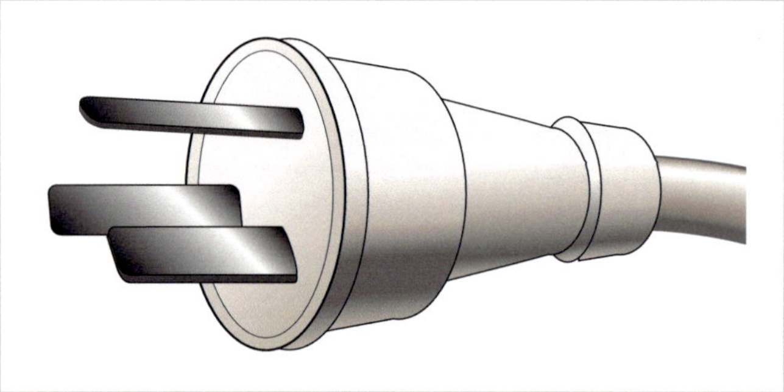

Fig. 2.11
A three-pronged plug.

called the **earth**. The earth carries leaking electricity to the earth and away from the item. If an earth is not used, leaking electricity can be conducted to a person. It can cause an electric shock and possible death. Immediately report a shock received while using an item. Tag the item and send it for repair immediately. Warning signs of a faulty electrical item include:

- shocks
- loss of power or a power outage
- dimming or flickering lights
- sparks
- sizzling or buzzing sounds
- a burning odour
- loose plugs.

An incident report is completed if a client, visitor or staff member has an equipment-related accident.

Consider the prevention of accidents related to equipment (Box 2.5).

WHEELCHAIR SAFETY

Some clients cannot walk or have severe problems walking. A wheelchair may be useful (Fig. 2.12). If able, the client propels the wheelchair using the hand-rims. Some clients use their feet to move the chair. Other wheelchairs have motors for self-propelling. They have hand, chin, mouth or other controls that let the client move the chair. If the client cannot propel the wheelchair, another person pushes it using the handgrips/push handles. Some services also use footrest covers to protect older consumers from skin tears.

Safety measures are needed when using wheelchairs (Box 2.6). A client can fall out of the chair or even fall during transfers to and from the chair. It is important to be aware of the risks and hazards associated with wheelchair use.

HANDLING HAZARDOUS SUBSTANCES

A **hazardous substance** is any chemical that presents a physical hazard or a health hazard in the workplace. Workplace health and safety regulations require that all aged care employees understand the issues associated with these substances. You should understand the risks of hazardous substances and know how to handle hazardous substances safely.

Physical hazards can cause fires or explosions. Health hazards are posed by chemicals that can cause acute or chronic health problems. Acute problems occur rapidly and

BOX 2.5
Preventing equipment accidents

- Follow aged care service policies and procedures.
- Follow the manufacturer's instructions. Read all caution and warning labels.
- Do not use unfamiliar equipment. Ask for training where needed. Also, ask your supervisor to supervise you when you first use the item.
- Use equipment only for its intended purpose.
- Make sure the item works before you begin.
- Make sure you have all required equipment. For example, if you need to plug in an item there must be an outlet.
- Place a 'Do not use' sticker on broken items. Complete a repair request form and explain the problem.
- Tell your supervisor about broken items.
- Do not try to repair broken items.
- Keep electrical items away from water.
- Keep work areas clean and dry. Wipe up spills immediately.
- Do not use electrical items if you are wet, your hands are wet or you are standing in water.
- Do not put your finger or any item into an electrical outlet.
- Turn off equipment before unplugging it. Sparks occur when electrical items are unplugged while turned on.
- Hold on to the plug (not the cord) when removing it from a wall outlet or extension power board. This prevents sparks.
- Do not give showers or baths during an electrical storm. Lightning can travel through pipes.
- Do not use electrical appliances or telephones during storms.
- Do not use water to put out an electrical fire. If possible, turn off or unplug the item.
- Do not touch a person who is experiencing an electric shock. If possible, turn off or unplug the item. Call for help immediately.
- Keep electrical cords away from heating vents and other heat sources.
- Turn off equipment when you have finished using it.

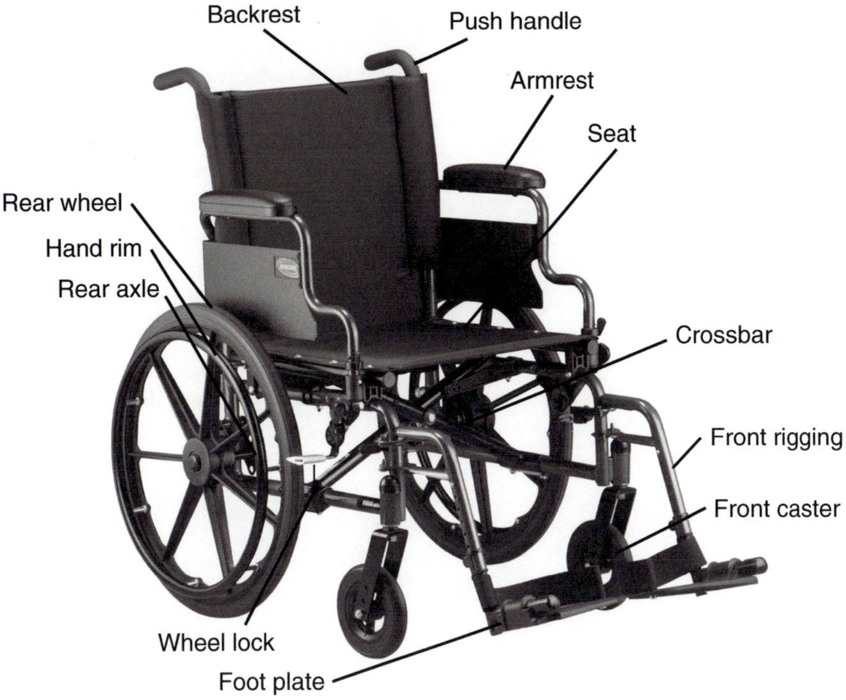

Fig. 2.12
Parts of a wheelchair.

BOX 2.6
Wheelchair safety

- Check brakes. Make sure you can lock and unlock them.
- Check for flat or loose tyres. A brake will not lock on to a tyre that is flat or loose.
- Make sure that wheel spokes are intact. Damaged, broken or loose spokes can interfere with moving the wheelchair or locking the brakes.
- Make sure the casters point forward. This keeps the wheelchair balanced and stable.
- Position the client's feet on the footrests before pushing or repositioning the chair. The client's feet must not touch or drag on the floor when the chair is moving.
- Push the chair forwards when transporting the client. Do not pull the chair backwards.
- Lock both brakes before you transfer a client to or from the wheelchair.
- Remind the client to keep the brakes locked when not moving the wheelchair. The brakes prevent the chair from moving if the client wants to move to or from the chair.
- Do not let the client stand on the footrests.
- Do not let the footrests fall back on to the client's legs.
- Make sure the client has wheelchair accessories where needed – safety belt, pouches, trays, lapboards, cushions.
- Remove the armrests (if removable) when the client transfers to the bed, commode, bath or car.
- Remove the armrests (if removable) when lifting the client from the chair.
- Swing footrests out of the way for transfers to and from the wheelchair. Some footrests detach for transfers.
- Clean the wheelchair according to aged care service policy.
- Ask a nurse or physiotherapist to show you how to propel wheelchairs up steps and ramps and over kerbs.

last a short time. They usually occur from a short-term exposure. Chronic problems usually result from long-term exposure and can occur over a long period of time.

Health hazards can:

- cause cancer
- affect the formation and function of blood cells
- damage the kidneys, nervous system, lungs, skin, eyes or mucous membranes
- cause birth defects, miscarriages and fertility problems from damage to the reproductive system.

Exposure to hazardous substances can occur under normal working conditions. It can also happen during certain emergencies, such as equipment failures, container ruptures or the uncontrolled release of a hazard into the workplace. Hazardous substances include:

- medications used in cancer therapy (chemotherapy, anticancer medications)
- anaesthetic gases
- gases used to sterilise equipment
- oxygen

- disinfectants and cleaning solutions
- radiation used for X-rays and cancer treatments
- mercury (found in older-type thermometers and blood pressure devices)
- common household chemicals, such as bleaches and cleaners.

Your employer provides hazardous substance training. You are told about hazards, exposure risks and protection measures. It is essential that you learn to read and use warning labels and material safety data sheets (MSDS). Each hazardous substance requires certain protection measures. Box 2.7 lists general rules for the safe handling of hazardous substances.

Labelling

Hazardous substance containers include bags, barrels, bottles, boxes, cans, cylinders, drums and storage tanks. All should have warning labels (Fig. 2.13) applied by the manufacturer. Warning labels include:

- physical hazards and health hazards (health hazards include the organs affected and potential health problems)
- precaution measures (e.g. 'Do not use near open flame' or 'Avoid skin contact')
- what personal protective equipment to wear
- directions for using the substance safely
- storage and disposal information.

BOX 2.7
Safety measures for handling hazardous substances

- Read all warning labels.
- Follow the safety measures on the warning label and the MSDS.
- Make sure each container has a warning label that is not damaged.
- Use a leak-proof container to carry or transport a hazardous substance.
- Wear PPE to clean spills and leaks. The warning label or MSDS tells you what to wear (mask, gown, gloves, eye protection and safety boots).
- Clean up spills immediately. Work from clean to dirty. Use circular motions.
- Dispose of hazardous waste in sealed bags or containers.
- Wash your hands after handling hazardous substances.
- Work in well-ventilated areas to avoid inhaling gases. Store hazardous substances according to the MSDS.

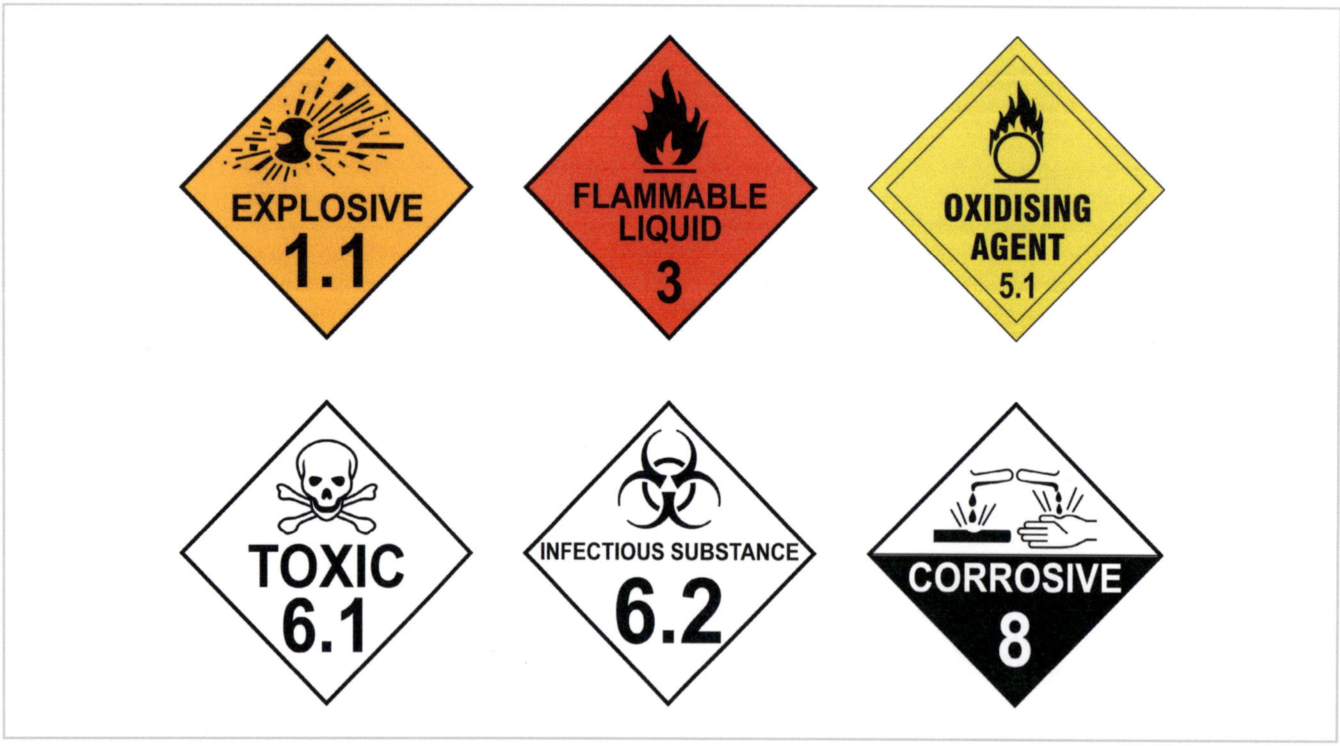

Fig. 2.13
Warning labels on hazardous substances.

Words, pictures and symbols communicate the warnings. A container must have a label. It must not be removed or damaged in any way. If a warning label is removed or damaged, do not use the chemical. Take the container to your supervisor and explain the problem. Do not leave the container unattended.

Material safety data sheets

Every hazardous substance has an MSDS, which provides the following information about each hazardous substance:

- the chemical name and any common names
- the ingredients contained in the substance
- physical and chemical characteristics (appearance, colour, odour, boiling point and others)
- potential physical effects (fire, explosion)
- conditions that could cause a chemical reaction
- how the chemical enters the human body (inhalation, ingestion, skin contact or absorption)
- health hazards, including signs and symptoms
- protective measures (how to use, handle and store the substance)
- emergency and first aid procedures
- explosion information and fire-fighting measures (including what type of fire extinguisher to use)
- how to clean up a spill or leak
- personal protective equipment needed during clean-up
- how to dispose of the substance
- manufacturer information (name, address and a telephone number for information). Employees must have ready access to all MSDS.

MSDS are kept alongside the chemical they relate to. Check the MSDS before using a hazardous substance, cleaning up a leak or spill or disposing of the substance. Tell your supervisor immediately about a spill or leak. Do not leave a spill or leak unattended.

FIRE SAFETY

Fire is a constant danger. Faulty electrical equipment and wiring, overloaded electrical circuits and smoking are major causes of fire. The entire aged care team must work to prevent fires. They must act quickly and responsibly if a fire occurs. Three conditions are needed for a fire – a spark or flame, a material that will burn and oxygen.

Preventing fires

Fire prevention measures require vigilant surveillance of client and staff surroundings. Most aged care services have a no-smoking policy and smoke-free areas. No smoking is allowed inside the buildings. Signs are posted on all entry doors. Conditions and items in a client's surroundings, such as if a client is receiving oxygen therapy, also pose a fire hazard. These and other fire safety measures are listed in Box 2.8.

What to do if there is a fire

It is important to know your aged care service's policies and procedures for fire emergencies. Know where to find fire alarms, fire extinguishers and emergency exits. Fire drills are held to practise emergency fire procedures. Remember the acronym RACE:

R – Rescue. Rescue people who are in immediate danger if it is safe to do so. Move them to a safe area.

A – Alarm. Sound the nearest fire alarm. Notify the switchboard operator.

BOX 2.8
Fire prevention measures

- Follow the fire safety measures for using oxygen. Special safety measures are needed where oxygen is used and stored (see the charting sample in Fig. 2.14).
- 'No Smoking' signs are placed on the door and near the bed. Smoking is dangerous in any healthcare service due to fire risks but smoking around oxygen is extremely dangerous.
- Smoke only outside, if and where it is allowed.
- Smoking materials – cigarettes, cigars and pipes, matches and lighters – are removed from the room.
- Empty ashtrays into a metal container partially filled with sand or water. Do not empty ashtrays into plastic containers or waste bins lined with paper or plastic bags.
- In the client's home, be sure all ashes, cigars and cigarettes are out before emptying ashtrays. Provide ashtrays to clients who are allowed to smoke.
- Supervise clients who smoke. This is very important for those who are confused, disoriented or sedated.
- Keep matches and lighters away from confused and disoriented clients.
- Clients should wear a cotton gown or pyjamas.
- Woollen blankets and synthetic fabrics that cause static electricity are removed from the room.
- Electrical items are turned off before being unplugged.
- Electrical items are in good working order. This includes shavers, fans, heating pads, televisions and radios.
- Do not leave cooking unattended on stoves, in ovens or in microwave ovens.
- Lit candles are not allowed.
- Store flammable liquids in their original containers. Keep the containers out of clients' reach.
- Materials that ignite easily are removed from the room. These include oil, grease, alcohol, nail polish remover and other things that ignite easily.
- Do not smoke or light matches or lighters around flammable liquids or materials.

Date	Time	
28/9/22	1400	Continuous O_2 started at 2 litres per nasal cannula. Smoking materials, electrical equipment,
		and other hazards were removed from the room. Resident and family were educated about the
		safety precautions used where O_2 is used. "No Smoking" signs posted on the room door and the
		wall at the head of the bed. Mary Martin, EN

Fig. 2.14
Charting sample.

C – Contain. Close doors and windows to contain the fire. Turn off oxygen or electrical items used in the general area of the fire.

E – Extinguish. Use a fire extinguisher on a small fire that has not spread to a larger area. If there is any doubt that the fire may be too difficult to extinguish, evacuate immediately to the nearest assembly area and act as directed by the service's fire warden.

USING A FIRE EXTINGUISHER

Procedure

1. Activate the fire alarm.
2. Get the nearest fire extinguisher.
3. Carry the extinguisher upright.
4. Take the extinguisher to the fire.
5. Remove the safety pin.
6. Direct the hose at the base of the fire.
7. Push the top handle down.

Also, clear equipment from all normal and emergency exits. Do not use lifts if there is a fire. Aged care services usually require that all employees demonstrate use of a fire extinguisher. Fire departments demonstrate their use once or twice a year. Different extinguishers are used for different kinds of fires. Fires can be oil, grease, electrical, paper or wood fires. A general procedure for using a fire extinguisher (Fig. 2.15) is given opposite.

Evacuation

All aged care services have evacuation policies and procedures. If evacuation is necessary, clients closest to the danger are taken out first. Those who can walk are given blankets to wrap around themselves. A staff member escorts them to a safe place. Fig. 2.16 shows how to rescue clients who cannot walk. Once the fire brigade arrives, the fire officers direct rescue efforts.

DISASTERS

A **disaster** is a sudden catastrophic event in which many people are injured and killed, and property is destroyed. Natural disasters include tornadoes, cyclones, blizzards, earthquakes, volcanic eruptions, floods and some fires. Human-made disasters include car, bus, train and aeroplane accidents, fires, bombings, power plant accidents, riots, gas or chemical leaks, explosions and wars.

All services have procedures for natural disasters that could occur in your area. Follow them to keep clients and yourself safe. The plan generally provides for:

- discharging clients who can go home
- assigning staff to an emergency area
- assigning staff to take equipment to the emergency area
- assigning staff to transport clients from the treatment area
- calling off-duty staff in to work.

A disaster may damage the aged care service. The disaster plan includes policies and procedures for evacuating the aged care service.

BOMB THREATS

All areas where there are several people together can be targeted for a bomb threat. Although unlikely, this can include aged care services. All services have policies and procedures for handling bomb threats. You will learn about them during your new employee orientation. You must follow them if a caller makes a bomb threat or if you find an item that sounds or looks strange. Bomb threats are usually received by telephone. However, they can be sent by mail, email, text message or other means. A person can also leave a bomb in the service. If you see a stranger in an aged care service, tell your supervisor immediately. You cannot be too safe.

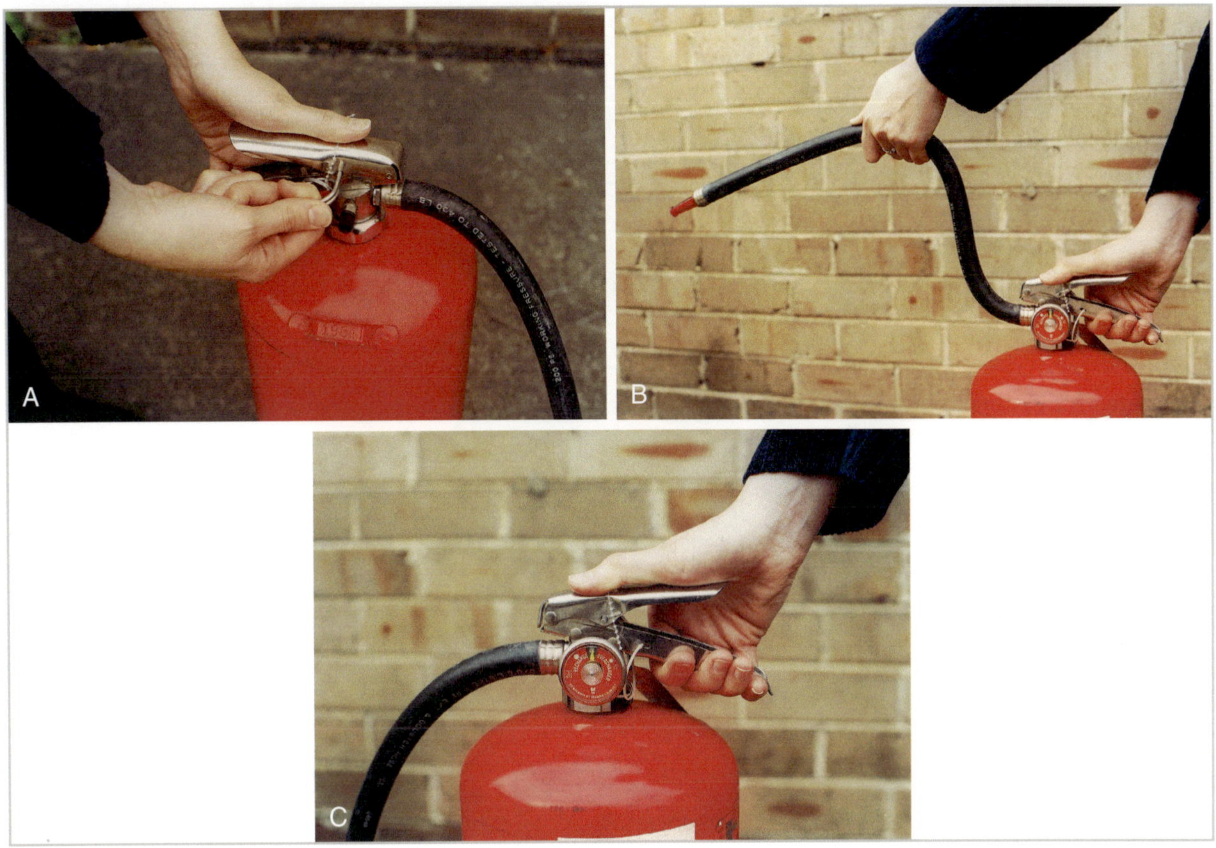

Fig. 2.15
Using a fire extinguisher.
A. Remove the safety pin. **B.** Direct the hose at the base of the fire. **C.** Push the top handle down.

WORKPLACE VIOLENCE

Violence in the workplace can happen, and the aged care service is no exception. Although most health **workplace-related violence** happens in acute healthcare settings, it can still occur in the aged care service. Factors associated with work-related assaults in aged care services include:

- consumers, families or friends who have weapons
- acutely disturbed clients
- mentally ill clients who do not take needed medications or do not receive appropriate follow-up care
- the perception that aged care services may carry medications that could be sold 'on the streets'
- some behavioural episodes of clients with dementia
- clients, visitors or workers at the aged care service who are substance abusers
- upset, agitated and disturbed family and visitors
- low staff levels during meals, emergencies and at night
- poor lighting in parking areas
- lack of training for staff in recognising and managing potentially violent situations.

Workplace health and safety goals are aimed at preventing or reducing employee exposure to situations that can cause death or injury. Worksite hazards are identified, and prevention measures are developed and followed. All employees should receive safety and health training. You need to:

- understand and follow the aged care service's workplace violence prevention program
- understand and follow safety and security measures
- voice any safety and security concerns
- report violent incidents promptly and accurately
- serve on health and safety committees that review workplace violence
- attend training programs that help you recognise and manage agitation, assault behaviour and criminal intent.

Box 2.9 lists some measures that can prevent or control workplace violence. Box 2.10 lists personal safety practices. Follow them in your everyday activities.

Also practise the following safety measures when dealing with an agitated or aggressive client:

- Stand away from the client. Judge the length of the client's arms and legs. Stand far enough away so the client cannot hit or kick you.
- Stand close to the door. Do not become trapped in the room.
- Know where to find panic buttons, call bells, alarms, closed-circuit monitors and other security devices (see Fig. 2.17).
- Keep your hands free.

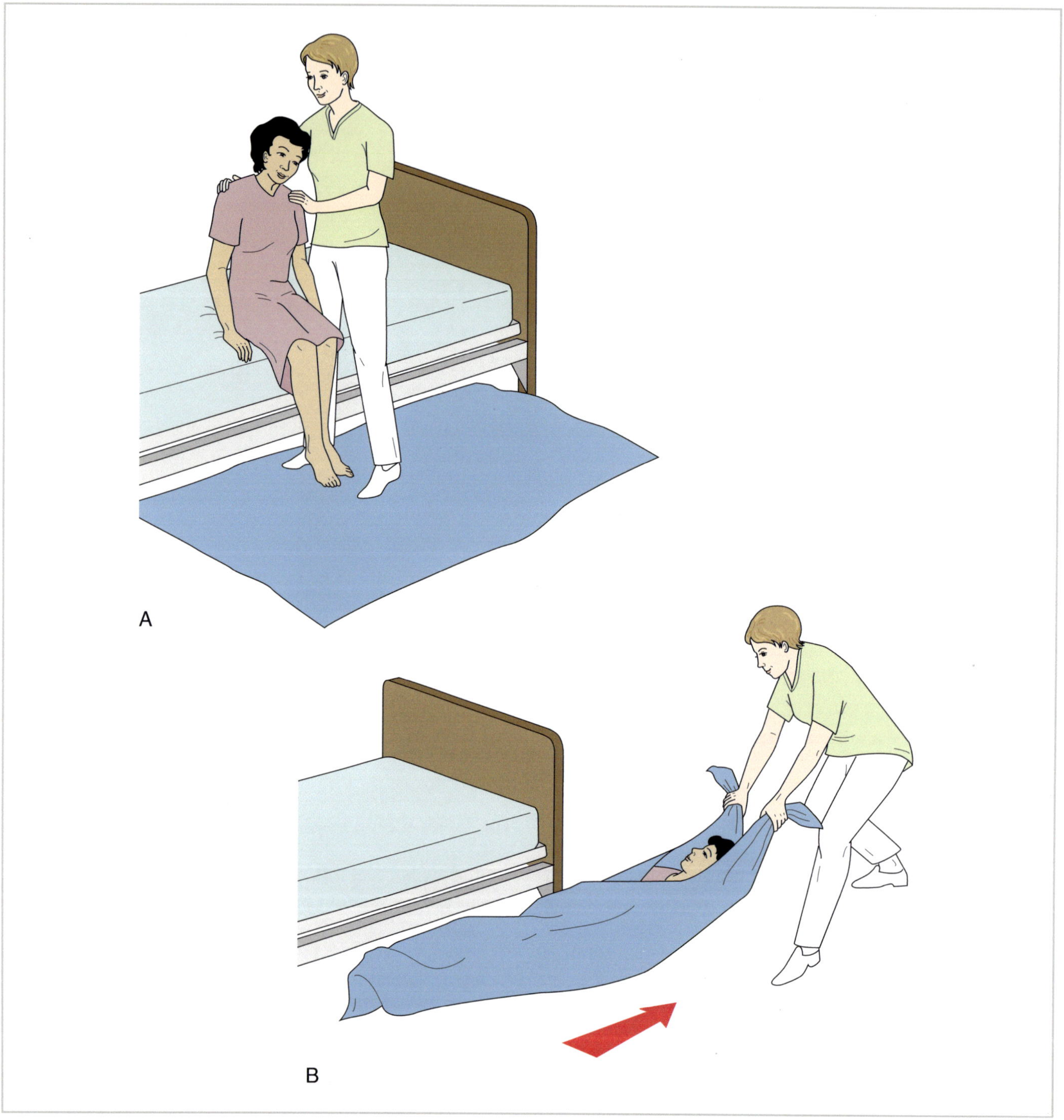

Fig. 2.16

One-rescuer carry.

A. Spread a blanket on the floor. Make sure that the blanket will extend beyond the client's head. Assist the client to sit on the side of the bed. Grasp the client under the arms and cross your hands over their chest. Lower the client to the floor by sliding them down one of your legs. **B.** Wrap the blanket around the client. Grasp the blanket over the head area and pull the client to a safe area.

- Stay calm. Talk to the client in a calm manner. Do not raise your voice or argue, scold or interrupt them.
- Do not touch the client.
- Tell the client that you will get a supervisor to speak to them.
- Leave the room as soon as you can. Make sure the client is safe.
- Tell your supervisor or security officer about the situation.
- Complete an incident report according to aged care service policy.

BOX 2.9
Measures to prevent or control workplace violence

- Alarm systems, closed circuit television (CCTV) monitoring (Fig. 2.18) and panic buttons, hand-held alarms, mobile or cordless phones, two-way radios and telephone systems are installed. These systems have a direct line to security staff or the police.
- Metal detectors are at entrances to identify guns, knives or other weapons.
- Curved mirrors are at hallway intersections and hard-to-see areas.
- Bullet-resistant, shatterproof glass is used at your supervisors' stations, reception areas and admitting areas.
- Waiting rooms are comfortable and reduce stress.
- Family and visitors are informed in a timely manner.
- Furniture is placed to prevent entrapment.
- Pictures, vases and other items that can serve as weapons are few in number.
- Staff restrooms lock and prevent access to visitors.
- Unused doors are locked.
- Bright lights are used inside and outside buildings.
- Burnt out lightbulbs are replaced or repaired.
- Broken lights, windows and door locks are replaced or repaired.
- Security escort services are used for walking to cars, bus stops or train stations.
- Vehicles are locked and in good repair.
- Security officers deal with agitated, aggressive or disruptive consumers or visitors.
- Consumers and visitors are restrained as per service policy, if they are a threat to themselves or others.
- Access to medication storage areas is controlled.
- A nurse assesses the behavioural history of new and transferred clients.
- Aggressive and agitated consumers are treated in open areas. Privacy and confidentiality are maintained.
- Staff are not alone when caring for clients with agitated or aggressive behaviours.
- Jewellery that can serve as a weapon is not worn (grabbing earrings and bracelets, strangling with necklaces).
- Long hair is worn up and off the collar. A client can pull long hair and cause head injuries.
- Keys, scissors, pens or other items that can serve as weapons are not visible.
- Tools or items left by maintenance personnel or visitors are removed if they can serve as weapons.
- Staff wear ID badges that verify employment.
- A 'buddy system' is used when using lifts, restrooms and low traffic areas.
- Uniforms fit well. Tight uniforms limit your ability to run. An attacker can grab a loose uniform.
- Shoes have good soles. Shoes that allow slipping limit your ability to run.

BOX 2.10
Personal safety practices

- Know the area you will visit. Ask questions about the area.
- Make a 'dry run' of the area. Know the route in advance. The shortest route is not always the safest.
- Have plenty of fuel in your car.
- Keep your car in good working order.
- Keep these in your car: torch with working batteries, a fire extinguisher and a first aid kit.
- If your car breaks down, raise the bonnet and use your emergency indicators. Stay in the car. Call the police if you have a mobile phone. If someone stops to help, ask that person to call the police.
- Check for places to park. Choose a well-lit area. If using a parking garage, park near the entrance, exit or on the lower level. Try to get close to the attendant if there is one. Remember that the closest space to your destination is not always the safest for parking.
- Park your car so that you can leave quickly and easily. Park at street corners so no one can park in front of you. In parking lots, back in. You can see more from your front windscreen than from the back window.
- Lock your car. However, sometimes you may want to leave it unlocked. If you need to get in the car fast, you do not want to fumble with keys. Use your judgement. Do not leave anything in the car if you leave it unlocked.
- Have your car key ready so you can get into the car quickly. Do not fumble for keys on the way to or at the car.
- Check the back seat before getting into the car. Make sure no one is in the car. If someone is in the car, leave immediately.
- Check under the car. A person hiding under the car can grab your ankle or leg. If someone is under the car, leave immediately.
- Lock your car doors when you get in the car. Keep the windows rolled up.
- Keep handbags and other valuables under the seat or at your side. Do not leave them on the seat. They are easy targets for smash-and-grab robberies.
- If you have to walk, use well-lit, busy streets. Avoid parks, vacant blocks, alleyways and construction sites. Again, the shortest way is not always the safest.

BOX 2.10
Personal safety practices *continued*

- Carry a mobile phone and note the location of phone booths. Know your location and keep telephone calls simple.
- Carry money or a phone card for public phone calls, and for bus, train or taxi fares (carry a transport card for public transport if necessary). Keep money in your pocket to avoid fumbling around in your handbag or wallet.
- If you think someone is following you, go to a police station, fire station or shop.
- Stand with others and near the ticket booth if using public transport. Sit near the driver or conductor.
- Do not hitchhike or pick up hitchhikers.
- Let someone know where you are at all times. Let someone know when you leave and when you arrive at your destination. If you do not call when expected, the other person will know that something is wrong.
- Make it known that you do not carry medications, needles or syringes.
- Do not carry valuables. Leave them at home or in the car boot. If someone wants what you have, give it to them. The only thing of value is you.
- Carry wallets and handbags safely. Men should carry their wallet in an inside coat or pants pocket. Never carry a wallet in the rear pocket. Keep a firm grip on a handbag. Keep the handbag close to your body.
- Do not wear headphones or use a mobile phone when walking. They stop you from hearing cars, trains, buses and people around you.
- Carry a whistle or shriek alarm.
- If you are attacked, scream as loudly and as long as you can. Keep screaming. Both men and women should scream.
- Use your car keys as a weapon. Carry them in your strong hand. Have one key extended. Hold the key firmly. If you are attacked, go for the person's face. Slash the person's face with the key. Do not use poking motions. Also, do not try for a certain target because you might miss. Do not be shy – your attacker will not be.
- Remember that you have two arms, two hands, two feet and two knees. This means that you can attack from four directions at once. Do not be shy – your attacker will not be. Push, pull, wrench and so on. You can attack the genital area of either a man or a woman.
- Use your thumbs as weapons. Go for the eyes and push hard.
- Carry a travel-sized aerosol hairspray. Spray it at the face.

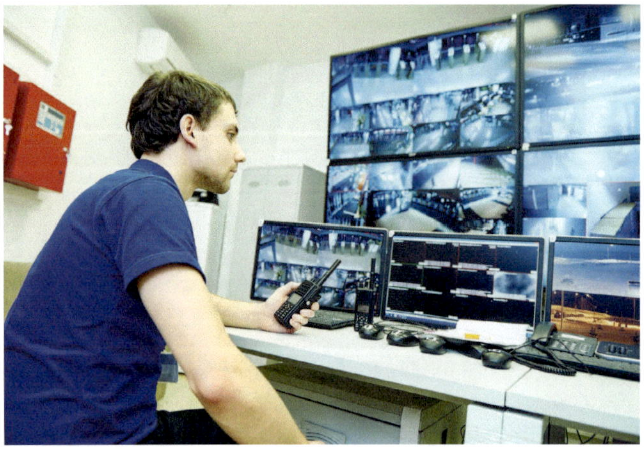

Fig. 2.17
People entering and leaving the aged care service are monitored on closed-circuit television (CCTV).

RISK MANAGEMENT

Risk management involves identifying and controlling risk and safety hazards that affect the aged care service. The intention is to:

- protect everyone in the aged care service (clients, visitors and staff)
- protect aged care service property from harm or danger
- protect client valuables
- prevent accidents and injuries.

Risk management deals with these and other issues:

- safety
- accident and fire prevention
- negligence and malpractice
- consumer abuse
- workplace violence
- federal and state requirements.

Risk managers work with all aged care service departments. They look for patterns and trends in incident reports, client and staff complaints and accident and injury investigations. Risk managers look for and correct unsafe situations. They also make procedural changes and training recommendations as needed.

Personal belongings

The client's belongings must be kept safe. A personal belongings list is completed when a client is admitted to an aged care service (Fig. 2.18). Each item is listed and described. The staff member and client sign the completed list.

A valuables envelope is used for jewellery and money the client does not want to keep with them (Fig. 2.19). Each jewellery item is listed and described on the envelope.

Form 883/2 BRIGGS, Des Moines, IA 50306 (800) 247-2343 PRINTED IN U.S.A.

INVENTORY LIST

ON DISCHARGE

QTY.	ARTICLES	QTY.	APPLIANCES	QTY.	PROSTHETIC DEVICES	ACQUIRED AFTER ADMISSION	
	Belts		T.V. - Ser. #:		Dentures: ☐ Upper		
	Blouses		Radio - Ser. #:		☐ Lower ☐ Partial	Date	Item
	Coats		Hair Dryer		Eye Wear		
	Dresses		Electric Razor		Cane		
	Gloves				Walker - Ser. #:		
	Hats				W/chair - Ser. #:		
	Housecoats - Robes		Jewellery		Brace		
	Jackets		Ring (Describe)				
	Nightgowns - Pyjamas						
	Purses		Watch (Describe)		OTHER		
	Shaving Kit						
	Shoes		Mobile phone				
	Shorts						
	Slacks						
	Slippers						
	Slips		FURNITURE				
	Socks/Hose						
	Suitcases						
	Suits				VALUABLES RELEASED FROM SAFE		
	Sweaters						
	Ties						
	Undershirts						
	Underwear						

I received on discharge in satisfactory condition the above articles and a copy of this list.
Disposition of belongings: ____________________

▶ ____________________ ____________ ▶ ____________________ ____________
Signature of Patient/Resp. Party | Date | Signature of Facility Representative | Date

NOTE Patient/Responsible Party is responsible for assuring that all personal belongings are properly marked. All items brought in after admission are added to this inventory at the request of Patient/Responsible Party.

ON ADMISSION

QTY.	ARTICLES	QTY.	APPLIANCES	QTY.	PROSTHETIC DEVICES	ACQUIRED AFTER ADMISSION	
	Belts		T.V. - Ser. #:		Dentures: ☐ Upper		
	Blouses		Radio - Ser. #:		☐ Lower ☐ Partial	Date	Item
	Coats		Hair Dryer		Eye Wear		
	Dresses		Electric Razor		Cane		
	Gloves				Walker - Ser. #:		
	Hats				W/chair - Ser. #:		
	Housecoats - Robes		Jewellery		Brace		
	Jackets		Ring (Describe)				
	Nightgowns - Pyjamas						
	Purses		Watch (Describe)		OTHER		
	Shaving Kit						
	Shoes		Mobile phone				
	Shorts						
	Slacks						
	Slippers						
	Slips		FURNITURE				
	Socks/Hose						
	Suitcases						
	Suits				VALUABLES LOCKED IN SAFE		
	Sweaters						
	Ties						
	Undershirts						
	Underwear						

I certify that this is a correct list of my clothes and belongings which I wish to retain in my possession and for which I take ENTIRE RESPONSIBILITY. I have received a copy of this list.

▶ ____________________ ____________ ▶ ____________________ ____________
Signature of Patient/Resp. Party | Date | Signature of Facility Representative | Date

If the patient is unable to sign, state reason: ____________________

▶ Signature of Witness: ____________________

PATIENT NAME—LAST	FIRST	MIDDLE	HOSP. NO.	ROOM NO.

Form 883/2 BRIGGS, Des Moines, Iowa 50306 PRINTED IN U.S.A. **INVENTORY LIST**

Fig. 2.18
Personal belongings list.

BRIGGS, Des Moines, Iowa 50306 PRINTED IN U.S.A.

PATIENT VALUABLES ENVELOPE

THIS FACILITY CANNOT ASSUME RESPONSIBILITY FOR ITEMS RETAINED IN YOUR POSSESSION. PATIENT UNDERSTANDS THAT BY SIGNING BELOW HE/SHE IS AWARE OF THIS POLICY AND VERIFIES THAT THE ITEMS LISTED BELOW AS INVENTORY ARE CORRECT AND THAT THE ENVELOPE HAS BEEN SEALED IN HIS/HER PRESENCE.

SIGNATURE OF PATIENT: ____________ DATE: ____

ACCEPTED BY: ____________ DATE: ____

NAME ____________

ROOM NO. ____________

HOSP NO. ____________

DOCTOR ____________

DATE ____________

CASH

CURRENCY:

NO.	VALUABLES (DESCRIPTION)	CHECK LIST (✓)
1.		
2.		
3.		
4.		
5.		
6.		
7.		
8.		
9.		
10.		
11.		
12.		
13.		
14.		
15.		

REPOSSESSION OF VALUABLES — PATIENT ACKNOWLEDGEMENT OF RECEIPT IN ENTIRETY

PATIENT/RELATIVE/OTHER	DATE	HOSPITAL REPRESENTATIVE	DATE

FORM 789 BRIGGS, Des Moines, Iowa 50306 800-247-2343

PRINTED IN U.S.A.

Fig. 2.19
Patient valuables envelope.

Describe what you see. For example, describe a ring as having a white stone with six prongs in a yellow setting. Do not assume that the stone is a diamond in a gold setting. For valuables:

- place each jewellery piece in the envelope with the client watching
- count money with the client
- put jewellery and money in the envelope
- seal the envelope. Sign it in the same way that you sign the personal belongings list
- give the envelope to your supervisor. Your supervisor will take it to the safe or send it home with the family.

Dentures, glasses, hearing aids, watches, some jewellery and radios are kept at the bedside. Items kept at the bedside are listed in the client's record. Clothing, shoes and other items brought from home are labelled with the client's name.

REPORTING ACCIDENTS AND ERRORS

Report accidents and errors to your supervisor immediately. This includes:

- accidents involving clients, visitors or staff
- errors in care – this includes giving the wrong care, giving care to the wrong client or forgetting to give care
- broken or lost items owned by the client (e.g. dentures, hearing aids or glasses)
- lost money or clothing
- hazardous substance accidents
- workplace violence incidents.

MANUAL HANDLING AND BODY MECHANICS

Mechanics is an anatomical term that is used when describing the way in which an object moves. The body has its own natural way of moving, but the way in which we move our bodies is not always efficient. **Body mechanics** refers to good **posture**, correct balance and using the strongest and largest muscles for work. Failing to use good body mechanics can result in injury, muscle strain and chronic fatigue. Using the body in an effective way is the key to preventing manual handling injuries. You must focus on the body mechanics of both your client and yourself. **Body alignment** means the correct position for the head, neck, arms, torso, legs and feet. It is concerned with the way in which the parts of your body are placed when you lie down flat on your back. If a client's body is placed in the wrong alignment, this will be easy to identify because it looks uncomfortable and it will definitely cause strain and stiffness. Body alignment is important for your clients, especially those who are disabled and, therefore, cannot reposition themselves.

CORRECT BODY ALIGNMENT

While standing, keep your chest high and your shoulders relaxed and pulled back slightly. Your spine, hips, knees and ankles should have symmetrical horizontal balance - with your hips level and your knees straight ahead. Your spine should have three curves, which create shock absorption while you walk, sit or stand. The cervical curve at your neck flexes towards the front of your body. The thoracic curve bends slightly backwards at the shoulder blade area, and the lumbar region of your spine should curve inwards towards the front of your body at your waist area.

Base of support

The **base of support** is the area on which an object rests. Your feet are your base of support when you are standing (Fig. 2.20). Your balance and, more importantly, your base of support will be good if your feet are placed hip-width apart. Understanding your base of support is important for moving people, even when there is a 'no lift' policy. It is better for your back if you stand with your feet apart when you know you are going to be standing for a long period; for example, queuing behind people. This uses your base of support effectively.

The strongest and largest muscles are in the shoulders, upper arms, hips and thighs. Use these muscles to lift and move heavy objects. Otherwise, you place strain and exertion on smaller and weaker muscles, which can cause fatigue and injury. Back injuries are a major risk. Good body mechanics are based on the following methods (Fig. 2.21):

- Bend your knees and squat to lift a heavy object.
- Do not bend from your waist. Bending from the waist places strain on the small back muscles.
- Hold items close to your body and base of support. This involves upper arm and shoulder muscles. Holding objects away from your body places strain on small muscles in your lower arms.

Good body mechanics are required for all activities, including cleaning, laundry, getting in and out of a car, holding a baby and gardening. Consider the lumbar spine when doing any activities (see Box 2.11). Follow the rules in Box 2.12 to safely and efficiently move clients and heavy objects. Carers are at great risk of back injuries, due to the fact that they regularly undertake manual handling activities.

It is essential that all carers working within consumers care services, hospitals, and when working within the home and community care settings, understand that there is generally a **safe patient handling** policy (formerly known as no lift policy) in place for all staff. This policy was developed as a means of addressing the high rates of injury suffered by nurses and care workers arising from the manual handling of people. Under this policy, manual lifting in all but exceptional cases is replaced by the use of lifting machines, people-moving aids and the encouragement of self-mobilisation of consumers or clients. Staff are not asked to physically support the weight of those they are assisting to transfer or move; mechanical and/or other aids are used instead.

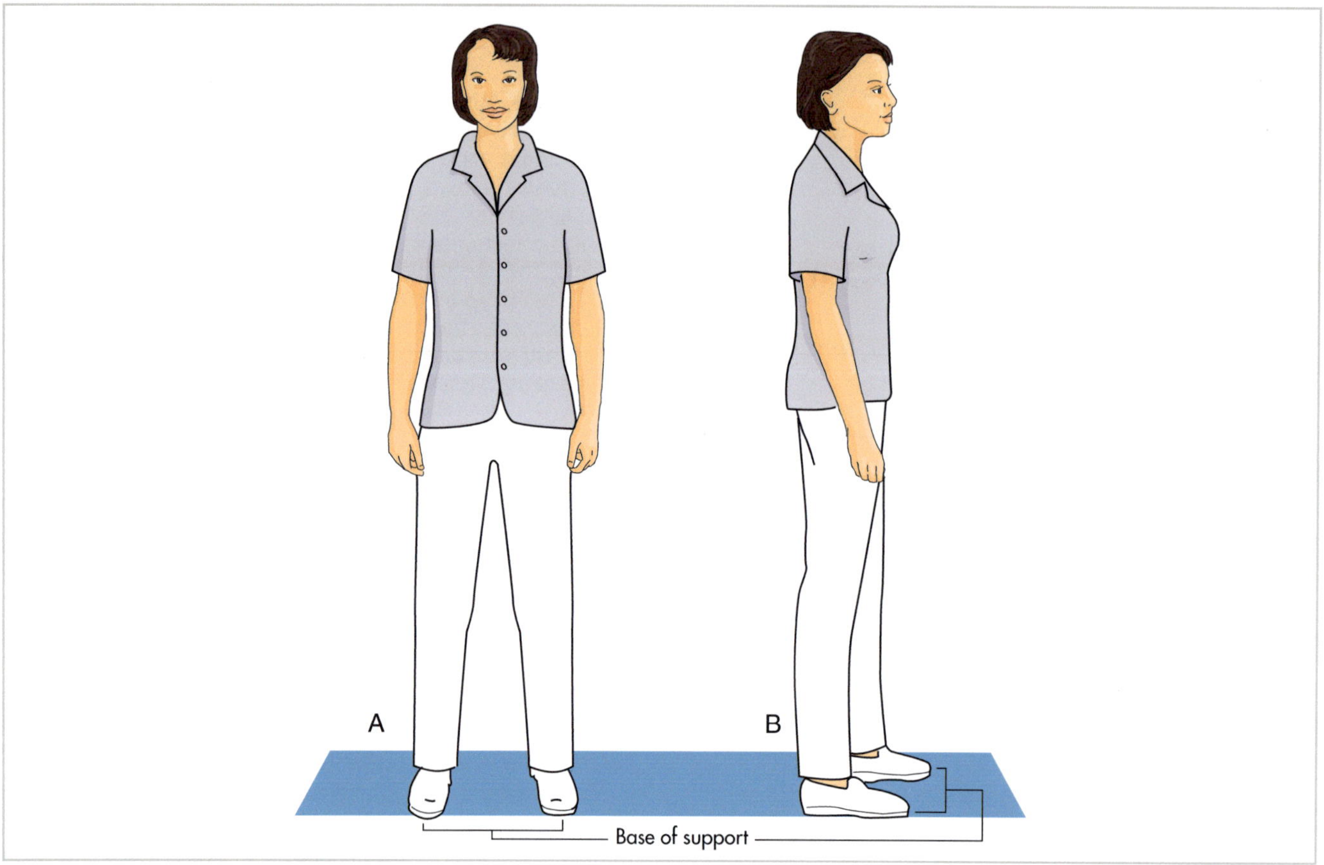

Fig. 2.20

A. Anterior (front) view of an adult in good body alignment with feet apart for a wide base of support. **B.** Lateral (side) view of an adult with good posture and alignment.

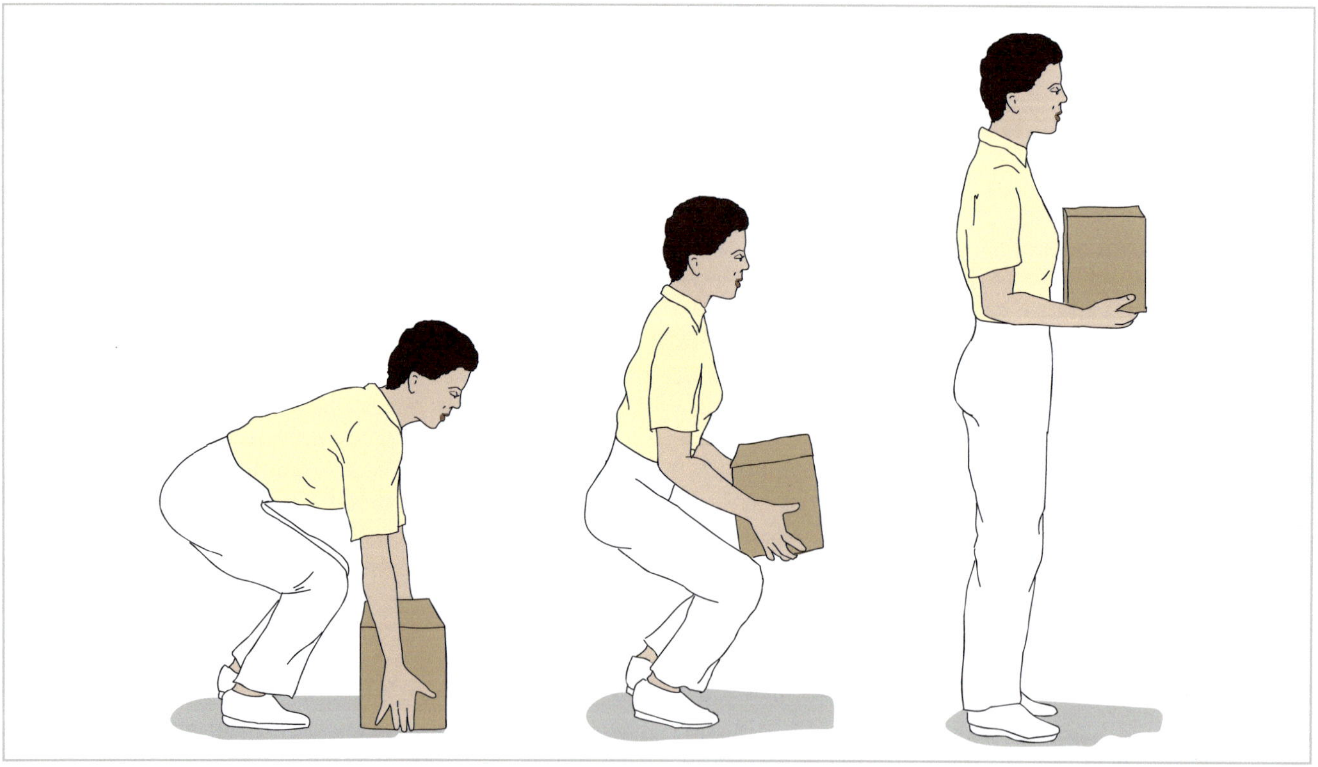

Fig. 2.21

Picking up a box using good body mechanics.

BOX 2.11
Rules for good body mechanics and manual handling techniques

- Keep your body in good alignment, with a wide base of support.
- Use the stronger and larger muscles in your shoulders, upper arms, thighs and hips. Keep objects close to your body when moving or carrying them.
- Ensure that you have adequate room to move. Remove any clutter that could impede manual handling.
- Avoid unnecessary bending and reaching. Raise the bed so it is close to your waist. Adjust the over-bed table so it is at your waist level.
- Face your work area. This prevents unnecessary twisting.
- Push, slide or pull heavy objects whenever you can, rather than lifting them. Pushing is better than pulling.
- Widen your base of support when pushing or pulling. Move your front leg forwards when pushing. Move your rear leg back when pulling.
- Use both hands and arms to move or carry heavy objects.
- Turn your whole body when changing the direction of your movement. Move and turn your feet in the direction of the turn, rather than twisting your body.
- Work with smooth and even movements. Avoid sudden or jerky motions.
- Get help from a co-worker if the client cannot assist you with turning or moving.
- Get help from a co-worker to move a heavy object or client. Do not lift or move them by yourself.
- Bend your hips and knees to move heavy objects from the floor. Straighten your back as the object reaches thigh level. Your leg and thigh muscles will work to raise the item off the floor and to waist level.
- Do not move objects higher than chest level. Do not move above your shoulders. Use a step stool to reach an object higher than chest level.

BOX 2.12
The functions of the lumbar spine

The lumbar spine bears the compressive weight of the body when we are upright and allows for flexibility when we move. The spinal column is the key support structure and it protects the spinal cord. It has a series of curves that allow for both shock absorption and flexibility. In addition, there are shock-absorbing discs above and below each spinal vertebra. Leaning to one side or bending forwards and twisting while lifting a heavy object can cause the soft interior of the disc to bulge out and protrude. This will pinch spinal nerves, causing pain and, sometimes, permanent damage.

Spinal ligaments are bands of tough fibrous tissue that act to prevent excessive movement of the joints. With prolonged strain and poor posture these ligaments will become overstretched and may even tear if placed under great strain. Ligament damage is permanent as there are no blood vessels to assist in repair, unlike muscle tissues.

The inward curve in the small of the back is known as the lumbar lordosis. This curve is lost when sitting or bending forwards. If this curve is lost for long periods, muscular problems will develop. Thus, poor postural habits make us prone to injury and back pain, and injury will develop if the soft tissues and joints of the spinal column are placed in a position that overstretches and distorts the natural alignment of the spine.

It is important to remember that the strongest and largest muscles of our body are in the shoulders, upper arms, abdomen and thighs. These are the muscles that we should use when manual handling, whether it is caring for our clients or picking up our groceries when shopping. Our spinal column, discs, ligaments and back muscles are not designed to take heavy loads and we must be vigilant in the care that we take to maintain a healthy lumbar spine.

SAFETY ALERT

Back injuries

The following activities are often associated with back injury in care services:

- moving a person who is totally dependent on others for care
- moving a person who is combative
- transferring a person who is on the floor to the bed or a chair
- repositioning a person in the bed or on a chair
- transferring a person from the bed to a chair, or from a chair to the bed
- transferring a person from one chair to another chair (includes transfers from wheelchair to toilet and toilet to wheelchair)
- bending to bathe a person or to change linen
- positioning a person on a bedpan
- changing an incontinence product
- trying to stop a person from falling.

Back care and injuries

The spine in the lower back (lumbar region) bears the compressive weight of the body when we are upright and allows for flexibility when we move. The spinal column is composed of bony spinal vertebrae alternated with shock-absorbing discs. This is the key support structure for the body and protects the spinal cord. The spinal column bears a series of curves that allow for both shock absorption and flexibility. The inward curve in the small of the back is known as the lumbar lordosis. If this curve is lost for long periods, such as during sitting or bending forwards, muscular problems will develop. Leaning to one side or bending forwards and twisting while lifting a heavy

BOX 2.13
Resting your back

One cause of back pain and manual handling injuries is failure to take a break from the task. At regular intervals during a working shift, when you are moving clients in bed or completing a series of manual handling tasks, you should stand up straight with hands on hips and gently bend backwards at least five or six times, then bend sideways gently to each side, five or six times. This allows the body to realign and helps to avoid fatigue and stress on the lumbar region. This recommendation also applies to people such as clerical workers and students who sit at the computer for prolonged periods.

object can cause the soft interior of the discs to bulge out and protrude. This will pinch spinal nerves, causing pain and sometimes permanent damage.

Being aware of your posture, especially during **manual handling**, and making an effort to rest and stretch your back regularly during your shift, will help you to maintain a healthy spine (see Box 2.13). Back injuries can occur from repeated activities over time, or from one event.

Signs and symptoms of back injury include:

- a clearly identified area of pain in the lumbar region
- pain when trying to resume a normal posture
- decreased mobility (i.e. a reluctance to move around, bend, walk)
- pain when standing or rising from a seated position
- pain that radiates to another area, such as the back of the thigh.

The most common underlying causes of back injuries include:

- lack of training, equipment or resources
- sudden or jerky movements
- repetitive movements that are prolonged, extreme and sustained, when the body is in poor alignment
- poor technique
- inadequate assistance (i.e. low staffing levels)
- reaching while lifting
- poor posture when sitting or standing
- staying in one position too long
- poor body mechanics when lifting, pushing, pulling or carrying objects
- poor physical condition – not having the strength or endurance to perform tasks without strain
- repeated lifting of awkward items, equipment or persons
- twisting while lifting
- bending while lifting
- maintaining a bent posture
- heavy lifting
- fatigue
- poor footing, such as on slippery floors
- lifting with forceful movement.

It is important to remember that our strongest and largest muscles are in the shoulders, upper arms, hips and thighs. These are the muscles that we should use when manual handling, whether it is caring for our clients or picking up our groceries when shopping. Poor postural habits make us prone to injury and back pain, and injury will develop if the soft tissues, joints and ligaments of the spinal column are placed in a position that overstretches and distorts the natural alignment of the spine. Spinal ligaments are bands of tough fibrous tissue that act to prevent excessive movement of the joints. With prolonged strain and poor posture, these ligaments will become overstretched and may even tear if placed under great strain. Ligament damage is permanent as there are no blood vessels to assist in repair, unlike muscle tissues. Our spinal column, discs, ligaments and back muscles are not designed to take heavy loads and we must be vigilant in the care that we take to maintain a healthy lumbar spine.

Back injury in care services is often associated with activities such as:

- moving a client who is totally dependent on others for care
- moving a client who is combative
- transferring a client who is on the floor to the bed or a chair
- repositioning a client in the bed or on a chair
- transferring a client from the bed to a chair, or from a chair to the bed
- transferring a client from one chair to another chair (includes transfers from wheelchair to toilet and toilet to wheelchair)
- bending to bathe a client or to change linen
- positioning a client on a bedpan
- changing an incontinence product
- trying to stop a client from falling.

It is important to practise good body mechanics and manual handling techniques to protect yourself and others from injury. Rather than working alone, it is always better to have a co-worker help you move or transfer a client. Pain will develop when a heavy load or object is moved incorrectly. Bending and twisting at the same time is a disastrous combination of movements.

Lifting devices should always be used when moving heavy or difficult objects. However, on those occasions when you do lift an object, even light and non-difficult ones, the rules are as follows:

- Plan the move. If the load is too heavy, get help.
- Position your feet apart if possible.
- Bend your knees and hold the load firmly with both hands.
- Raise your head and pull your chin in to keep your back straight.
- Move the load to your waist slowly by straightening your legs, keeping your elbows close to your body.
- To put the load down, bend your knees and keep your back straight.

Through continued exposure to stresses and strains, damage accumulates over time until eventually a single event or activity can trigger the onset of debilitating back pain or injury. Also, if manual handling is not done correctly, damage can occur to other parts of the body, such as the wrists, shoulder, neck and knees. The carer's whole body is at risk if manual handling is not done properly. To help prevent back injuries, follow the rules in Box 2.12 (see p. 47).

MOVING A PERSON IN BED

For all manual handling procedures, the carer is required to communicate with the client and explain clearly what is going to happen next. You must consider the needs of the client. At least two people are needed to move a heavy, weak or very elderly person up in bed. This protects the client and you from pain and injury (see Box 2.14).

BOX 2.14
Clients with dementia

Clients with **dementia** may not be able to understand what you are doing. They may resist your efforts to reposition them or to transfer them from the bed to the chair. The client may shout at you, grab you or try to hit you. In these situations, always get a co-worker to help you. Do not force the client, because this will not help but will escalate the situation. The client's care plan will also have measures to help you provide safe care. These measures may include:

- proceeding slowly – the client will need more time to comprehend what is happening; they should not be made to feel rushed or that they must think and move quickly, as this will create anxiety and a negative reaction
- using a calm, soothing and pleasant voice
- diverting the client's attention
- rescheduling the procedure to another time
- asking the registered nurse or enrolled nurse to assess the client
- getting assistance.

Adapted from Australian Nursing and Midwifery Federation (2018b). Safe Patient Handling. Online. Available: www.anmf.org.au/documents/policies/P_Safe_Patient_Handling.pdf.

Repositioning a person in their bed is important because it reduces the risk of pressure injury, which can develop on many areas of the body. Pressure injury will occur if your client is not repositioned regularly. You should check the care plan to see if this is required as often as every second hour.

Before you reposition the person, it is important to check the care plan. In general, if slide sheets are to be used you must have a co-worker to assist you. A carer working on their own can use a folded slide sheet, but only if the client is able-bodied enough to assist in the procedure. Also ensure that you do not lift when using a slide sheet – it is always a sliding movement, not a lifting one. Due to workplace health and safety policies, some services have strict protocols stating that pressure area care activities are to be conducted by staff members working in pairs. This ensures that two carers attend to clients who require regular repositioning. Some clients can move themselves up and down the bed and turn themselves onto their sides. Others need help from at least one person. Clients who are able to bend their knees and slowly roll to one side can help you to reposition them. Recognition and reward promotes a therapeutic relationship with your client. Most clients will demonstrate enthusiasm if they believe that they can assist you in your work.

Raising the person's head and shoulders

You may have to raise a person's head and shoulders to dress them, to turn them, to remove a pillow or to give care. You can raise the person's shoulders easily and safely by locking arms with them (Fig. 2.22A–D). It is best to have help with older clients to prevent pain or injury to fragile joints and bones. You also need help if the client is heavy or hard to move.

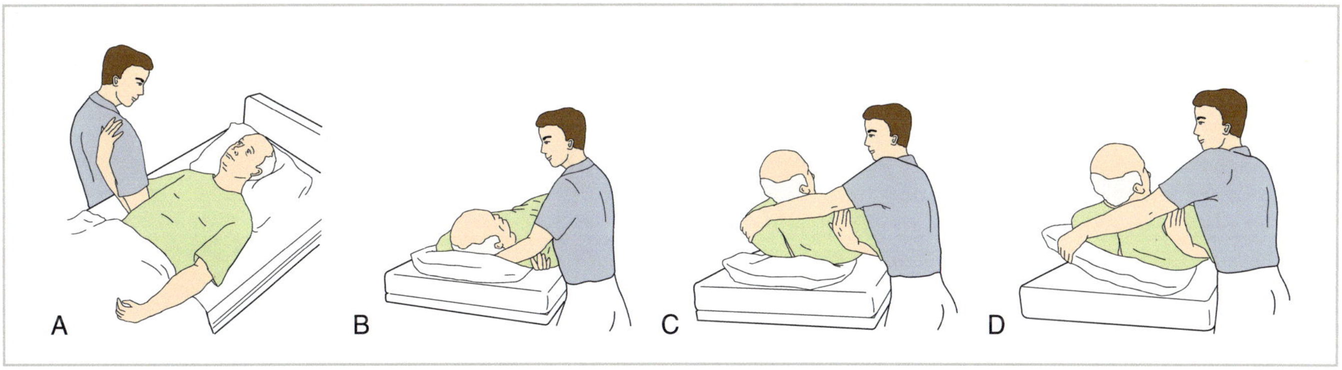

Fig. 2.22
Raising the client's head and shoulders by locking arms with the client.
A. The client's near arm is under the carer's near arm and behind the shoulder. **B.** The carer's far arm is under the client's neck and shoulders, with the near arm under the client's near arm. **C.** The client is raised to a semi-sitting position by locking arms. **D.** The carer lifts the pillow while the client is in a semi-sitting position.

RAISING THE PERSON'S HEAD AND SHOULDERS

Quality of life

Remember to respect the client's privacy while doing any procedure. Address the person by name and ensure they know your name. One staff member should take control of 'counting' during the log roll to ensure a coordinated approach.

Pre-procedure

1. Follow the delegation guidelines.
2. Ask a co-worker to help if you need assistance.
3. Wash your hands.
4. Call the client by name.
5. Explain what you are going to do.
6. Provide privacy.
7. Lock the bed wheels (if applicable).
8. Raise the bed for body mechanics (if applicable).

Procedure

9. Ask your co-worker to stand on the other side of the bed.
10. Ask the client to put their near arm under your near arm and behind your shoulder. Their hand rests on top of your shoulder. If you are standing on the right side, the client's right hand rests on your right shoulder (see Fig. 2.22). If you have help, the client does the same with your co-worker. The client's left-hand rests on your co-worker's left shoulder.
11. Put your arm nearest the client under their arm. Your hand is on the client's shoulder. Have your co-worker do the same.
12. Put your free arm under the client's neck and shoulders. If you have help, your co-worker does the same.
13. Help the client pull up to a sitting or semi-sitting position on the count of three.
14. Use the arm and hand that supported the client's neck and shoulders to give care. Your co-worker supports the client.

Post-procedure

15. Help the client lie down. Provide support with your locked arms. Support the client's neck and shoulders with your other arm.
16. Provide for comfort. Position the client in good body alignment.
17. Place the call bell within reach (if applicable).
18. Raise or lower bed rails (if applicable). Follow the care plan.
19. Lower the bed to its lowest position (if applicable).
20. Remove any privacy screens (if applicable).
21. Wash your hands.
22. Report and record your observations.

Sitting Up, Moving or Rolling the Person

Explain to the person that you will assist them to sit up on the count of three. If your client has a **trapeze** or **monkey bar**, check that they are permitted to use this. If so, encourage them to pull themselves up on the count of three, with some assistance from you. If there is no monkey bar for the client to use, they can assist you by using their elbows and their heels to move up the bed. Once again, explain to the person that you are going to count to three and that you will be asking them to carefully press their elbows and their heels into the mattress and to put their chin on their chest. If the intention is for the client to sit up in bed, arrange the pillows so that there is support for their head and shoulders. On the count of three, ask the client to push back. This way the person has helped you to reposition them and reduced their risk of muscle strain. Be sure to offer encouragement and to reward your client's efforts.

Older people have fragile skin that tears easily, so it is important to protect their skin during moving. Friction and shearing can injure the skin. Both cause infection and pressure ulcers. **Friction** is the rubbing of one surface against another. When moved in bed, the client's skin rubs against the sheet. **Shearing** is when the skin sticks to a surface and muscles slide in the direction the body is moving (Fig. 2.23). Shearing occurs when the client slides down in bed or is moved in bed. For example, when the head of the bed is raised to a sitting position, the skin on the buttocks stays in place. However, the hip bones move forwards as the client slides down in bed. The skin is pinched between the mattress and the hip bones. To reduce friction and shearing, roll or move the client. Use a slide sheet to move the client in bed and reduce friction. Remember to keep the client properly

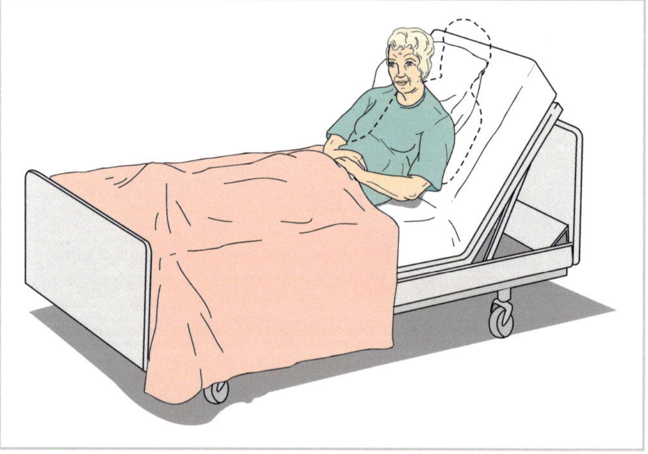

Fig. 2.23
A client in poor alignment after sliding down in bed.

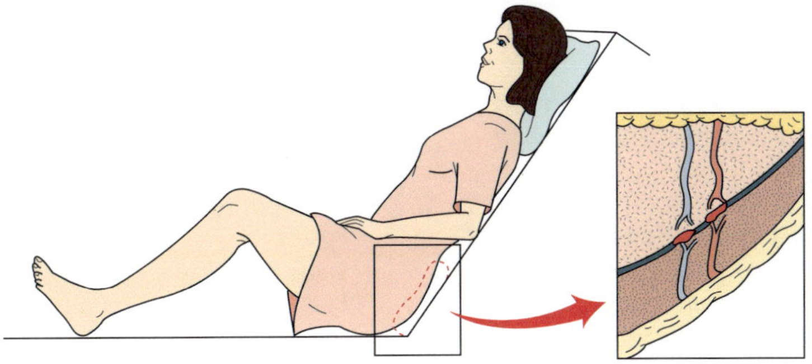

Fig. 2.24
Shearing.
When the head of the bed is raised to a sitting position, the skin on the buttocks stays in place. However, internal structures move forwards as the client slides down in bed. The skin is pinched between the mattress and the hip bones.

covered and screened. This protects their right to privacy. Also, many clients have severe arthritis or osteoporosis. Be very careful when moving them. Always ask a co-worker to help you. This protects the client and you from pain and injury.

When the head of the bed is raised, it is easy to slide down towards the middle and foot of the bed (Fig. 2.24). The client is moved up in bed to maintain good body alignment and comfort. Some clients can move themselves up in bed alone or with assistance. This helps them feel independent. You can sometimes move lightweight adults up in bed alone if they use a trapeze. However, it is best to have help and to use a lift or slide sheet to protect you and the client from pain and injury.

A **slide sheet** can be used if the client is unable to move effectively up the bed (Fig. 2.25). Slide sheets are used to slide and reposition the client without unnecessary pulling or dragging of the client in their bed, chair or other surface (Fig. 2.26). The sheet is made of viscose or 'parachute' material, which is very slippery. The key point with slide sheets is that there must be two layers underneath the client to achieve a successful 'slide' to a new position. The slide sheet must be folded in half as it is designed to 'slide' on itself in much the same way that a tractor tyre goes around in a circular fashion. You will need to place the slide sheet underneath the client's bottom.

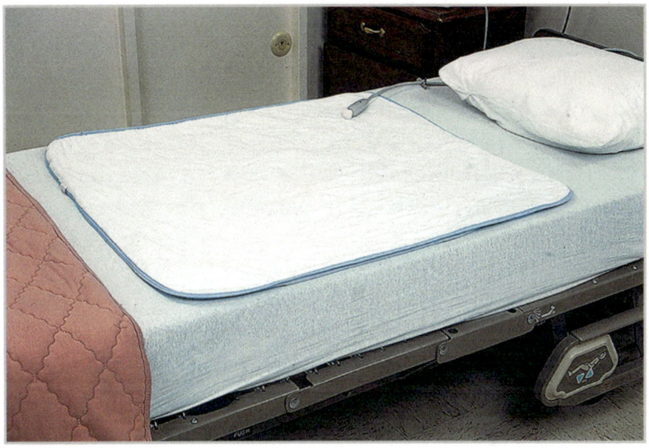

Fig. 2.25
Turning pad or slide sheet.

SAFETY ALERT

Moving a person to the side of the bed

When moving a person to the side of the bed, you must know which method to use. Agree on the care plan. Otherwise, you could seriously injure the person. This is very important for those who are frail, have arthritis or have spinal cord involvement.

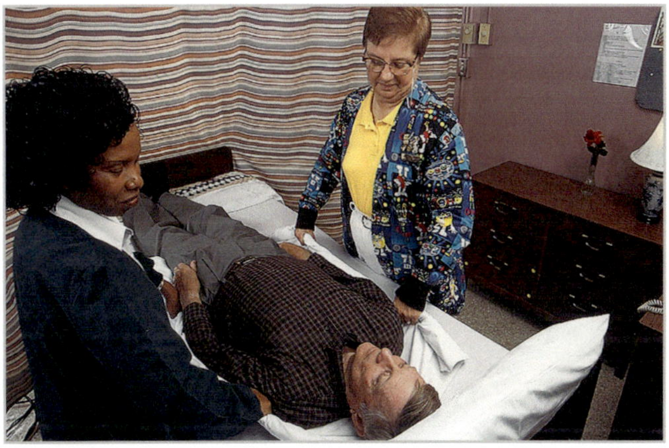

Fig. 2.26
A slide sheet is used to move the client up in bed.
The slide sheet extends from the client's head to above the knees. The slide sheet is rolled close to the client and held near the shoulders and buttocks.

DELEGATION GUIDELINES

Sitting, moving, rolling the person

Many delegated tasks involve moving the person in bed. Before moving or lifting a client, you need the following information from the care plan:

- Special position orders from the doctor (i.e. the client's comfort level and what body parts are painful).
- Limits in the person's ability to move or be repositioned (i.e. how much assistance the person needs).
- What procedure to use. For safety and efficiency, decide how you will move the client before starting the procedure.
- How many staff members are needed to safely move the client. If you need help from a co-worker, ask someone to help you before you begin. Also plan how you will protect drainage tubes or containers connected to the client.
- Whether special equipment is needed to move the client (e.g. trapeze, slide sheet).
- What supportive devices are needed for positioning.
- How to position the client.
- Whether the client uses bed rails when the bed is raised.
- Beds are raised horizontally to lift and move a client in bed. This reduces bending and reaching. You must:
  - use the bed correctly
  - protect the client from falling when the bed is raised
  - follow the rules of body mechanics and manual handling techniques
  - position the client in good body alignment after moving or turning.
  - keep the client in good body alignment
- What observations to report and record.

Slide sheets are indispensable when the client is partly or mostly unable to reposition or move themselves. When carrying out this procedure unassisted, it is important to place the bed rails 'up' on one side of the bed. This is the side that your client will roll towards so that you can place the folded slide sheet underneath their bottom. The bed rails will ensure that your client does not fall off the bed and has something to hold on to.

Note that unless the slide sheet is king size, it is difficult to use a single slide sheet. Using a single slide sheet involves folding it in half, which can mean that you and your colleague do not have enough material to hold on to so as to carry out the procedure safely and effectively. Therefore, it is recommended that two single-sized slide sheets are used to allow the procedure to be undertaken safely.

Sometimes you will have to reach over the client. If the client is close to you, you will not need to reach so far. One method of moving involves moving the client limb by limb. The slide or slide sheet method is used for very old people and those with arthritis. Using a slide or slide sheet helps prevent pain, skin damage and injury to the bones, joints and spinal cord. When using a slide sheet, you need a co-worker to help you.

Slide sheets can also be used to carefully position the client at the side of the bed, ready for transfer to the standing lifter or to a shower chair or wheelchair. With a walking belt in place, the client can be positioned with minimal effort at the side of the bed, allowing the legs to dangle and drop. This is a routine activity that allows the client time to adjust to sitting up, and then progress to standing once they feel that their blood pressure has adjusted. In some situations, the slide sheet is useful when a client has had a fall and is partly trapped beneath a piece of furniture or in a tight space in the bathroom.

USING A SLIDE SHEET

Quality of life

Remember to respect the person's privacy while doing any procedure. Address the person by name and ensure they know your name. One staff member should take control of 'counting' during the log roll to ensure a coordinated approach.

Pre-procedure

1. Follow the delegation guidelines.
2. Ask a co-worker to help you.
3. Wash your hands.
4. Call the client by name and explain the procedure to the person.
5. Provide for privacy.
6. Lock the bed wheels and raise the bed for body mechanics (if applicable).
7. Lower the head of the bed to a level appropriate for the client (if applicable). It should be as flat as possible. It will be impossible to move the client to a sitting position if the backrest is in the upright position. Ask the client if you can lower the back rest of the bed so that you can carefully lie the client down.
8. Stand on one side of the bed. Your co-worker will stand on the opposite side of the bed, ready to receive the client when she or he rolls over.
9. Lower the bed rails if up (if applicable).
10. The client must be rolled carefully onto their side so that you can place the slide sheets underneath their body.
11. The slide sheets are placed flat on the bed, one on top of the other. Note: If you have to use one slide sheet it must be folded in half, with the opening of the fold pointing towards the pillows.

12 When positioning the slide sheets on the bed, they must cover the area from the shoulders to mid-thigh, or the procedure will result in shearing and friction burns to your client. A single slide sheet is difficult to position correctly to cover this area and so is potentially harmful to your client.
13 Once the slide sheets are correctly aligned your co-worker will have to carefully roll the client back towards you so that the slide sheets can be fed under the client, collected and arranged on the other side of the bed.
14 Roll the client back on to the slide sheets, and once again check that the slide sheets reach underneath the shoulders down to mid-thigh.
15 Place the pillow against the headboard if the client can be without it. This prevents the head from hitting the headboard when they are moving up.
16 Ask your client to be ready to lift their head forwards, place their chin on their chest and their arms across their chest.

Procedure

17 Stand with a wide base of support. Point your foot near and towards the head of the bed. Face that direction. Your feet must be in the correct position before you slide the client up the bed. The foot closer to the pillows should be pointing in the same direction that the sliding transfer is headed. Your other foot remains in a neutral position.
18 Roll the sides of the slide sheet up close to the client. The top layer of slide sheet will be grasped in your hands as though you are holding bicycle handlebars. Do not turn your wrists upwards; they should be facing downwards.
19 Grasp the rolled-up slide sheet firmly near the client's shoulders and buttocks. You are going to keep your arms straight and stand so that you are touching the sides of the bed. Support the client's head.
20 Bend your hips and knees. To protect your back, you will be leaning towards the pillows in a sideways lunging position when you go ahead with the slide procedure. Your lower back and your bottom must not swing out and away from the side of the bed. Your co-worker must maintain the same position and be ready on the count of three. You must maintain correct lumbar lordosis during this procedure.
21 Explain that you will move on the count of three. You will move the client in time with your co-worker, and your client will slide up the bed with reasonable ease. Shift your weight from your rear leg to your front leg.
22 Slide the client up in bed on the count of three. The client pushes against the bed with their feet if able.
23 Slide sheets can create a fast movement, so take care not to rush this procedure. Moving too quickly may alarm your client and this will affect the level of trust that they have for future interactions.
24 If you need to turn the client on their side, turn them towards you or away from you. The direction depends on the client's condition and the situation.

Post-procedure

25 The sitting position can be achieved by asking the client to lean forwards and 'bend in the middle' while you arrange pillows and adjust the bed setting or back rest to the upright position.
26 Unroll the slide sheet.
27 Provide for comfort. Position the client in good body alignment.
28 Place the pillow under the client's head and shoulders. Straighten linen.
29 Place the call bell within reach (if applicable).
30 Raise or lower bed rails (if applicable). Follow the care plan.
31 Raise the head of the bed to a level appropriate for the client, and lower the bed to its lowest position (if applicable).
32 Remove any privacy screens (if applicable).
33 Wash your hands.
34 Report and record your observations.

SAFETY ALERT

Turning a person

When turning a person in bed, use good body mechanics and manual handling techniques to protect yourself from injury. The person must be in good alignment. Otherwise musculoskeletal injuries, skin breakdown or pressure ulcers could occur.

Log rolling with a slide sheet is often used to turn some clients. It helps prevent pain in those with arthritic spines and hips.

Log rolling

Certain procedures require the client to lie on their side. Turning a client onto their side also helps prevent complications from bed rest. When turning a client in bed, use good body mechanics and manual handling techniques to protect yourself from injury. The client must be in good alignment or musculoskeletal injuries, skin breakdown or pressure ulcers could occur.

With certain spinal conditions or diseases, a client's recovery depends on careful attention to how they are repositioned. The appropriate method is the log roll. Log rolling with a slide sheet is often used to turn some clients. It helps prevent pain in those with arthritic spines and hips. This method will be indicated on the care plan and must be observed. It means that the client cannot be simply rolled over by one carer, as this would allow the neck and back to flop in poor body alignment. **Log rolling** means turning the client as a unit, in alignment, with one motion (Fig. 2.27). The spine is kept straight. Log rolling is used in order to

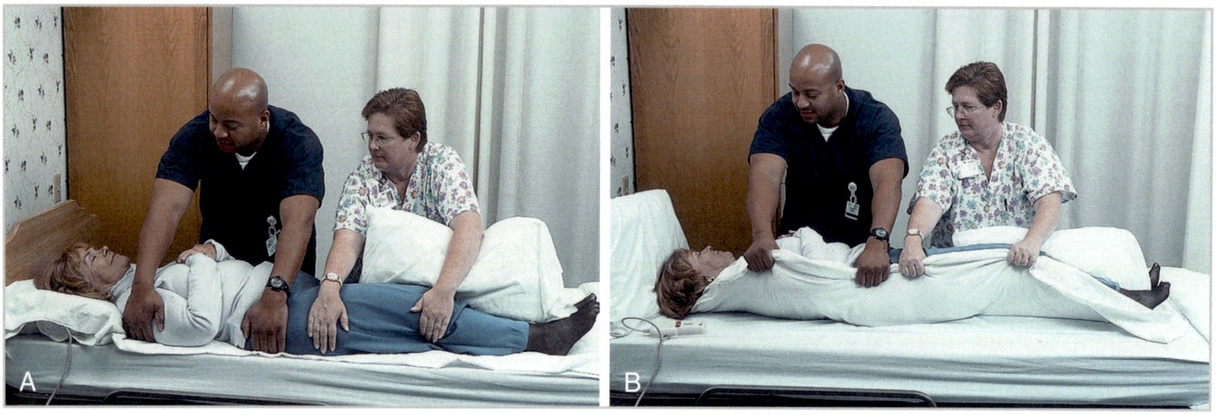

Fig. 2.27
Log rolling.
A. A pillow is placed between the client's legs, and the arms are crossed on the chest. The client is on the far side of the bed.
B. A turning sheet is used to log roll the client. Note: If you plan to move the client up in bed after log rolling them, place the pillow against the headboard.

maintain spinal alignment when changing the bed linen, removing a bed pan or washing a client's neck and back. It is also used for:

- older clients with arthritic spines or knees
- clients recovering from hip fractures
- clients with spinal cord injuries (the spine must be kept straight at all times after spinal cord injury).

Two or three staff members are needed to log roll a client. Three are needed if the client is tall or heavy. Sometimes a turning sheet is used. After the client is turned, position them in good body alignment. Pillows are used to support the client in the side-lying position. Some clients can turn and reposition themselves in bed. Others need some assistance. Some depend totally on the carer.

LOG ROLLING A PERSON

Quality of life

Remember to respect the person's privacy while doing any procedure. Address the person by name and ensure they know your name. One staff member should take control of 'counting' during the log roll to ensure a coordinated approach.

Pre-procedure

1 Follow the delegation guidelines.
2 Ask a co-worker to help you.
3 Wash your hands.
4 Call the person by name.
5 Explain the procedure to the person.
6 Provide for privacy.
7 Lock the bed wheels (if applicable).
8 Raise the bed for body mechanics (if applicable). Bed rails are up if used.

Procedure

9 Make sure the bed is flat.
10 Stand on the side opposite to which you will turn the person. Your co-worker stands on the other side.
11 Lower the bed rails, if used (if applicable).
12 Move the person as a unit to the side of the bed near you. Use the slide sheet.
13 Place the person's arms across their chest. Place a pillow between their knees.
14 Raise the bed rail if used (if applicable).
15 Go to the other side.
16 Stand near the person's shoulders and chest. Your co-worker stands near the buttocks and thighs.
17 Stand with a broad base of support, one foot in front of the other.
18 Ask the person to hold their body rigid.
19 Roll the person towards you, or use a slide sheet. Turn the person as a unit.

Post-procedure

20 Provide for comfort. Position the person in good alignment. Use pillows as directed by the nurse and the care plan. The following is a common method:
   a One pillow against the back for support.
   b One pillow under the head and neck if allowed.
   c One pillow or folded bath blanket between the legs.
   d A small pillow under the arm and hand.
21 Place the call bell within reach.
22 Raise or lower bed rails (if applicable). Follow the care plan.
23 Lower the bed to its lowest position (if applicable).
24 Remove any privacy screens (if applicable).
25 Wash your hands.
26 Report and record your observations.

MOVING THE PERSON TO THE SIDE OF THE BED (DANGLING)

Repositioning and care procedures will require you to move the client to the side of the bed. Clients sit on the side of the bed (dangle) for many reasons. Many older people become dizzy or faint if they get out of bed too fast. They need to sit on the side of the bed for one to five minutes before walking or transferring. Some clients increase their activity in stages – bed rest, then sitting on the side of the bed, then sitting in a chair and then walking. While dangling their legs, the client coughs and deep breathes. They also move their legs back and forth and in circles in order to stimulate circulation.

When moving a person to the side of the bed, you must know which method to use. Refer to the care plan or you could seriously injure the person. This is very important for those who are very old, have arthritis or have spinal cord involvement. Two workers may be needed. Clients with balance or coordination problems need support. If dizziness or fainting occurs, the client is laid down. Problems with sitting and balance often occur after illness, injury and bed rest. Some clients who are disabled also have problems with sitting and balance. Provide support when the client is sitting on the side of the bed. This protects them from falling and other injuries. Remember to respect the client's privacy while doing any procedure. Address the person by name and ensure they know your name.

SAFETY ALERT

Dangling

Problems with sitting and balance often occur after illness, injury and bed rest. Some people who are disabled also have problems with sitting and balance. Provide support when the person is sitting on the side of the bed. This protects them from falling and other injuries.

HELPING A PERSON TO SIT ON THE SIDE OF THE BED (DANGLE)

Quality of life

Remember to respect the person's privacy while doing any procedure. Address the person by name and ensure they know your name. One staff member should take control of 'counting' during the log roll to ensure a coordinated approach.

Pre-procedure

1. Follow the delegation guidelines.
2. Ask a co-worker to help if using a slide sheet.
3. Wash your hands.
4. Call the client by name.
5. Decide which side of the bed to use and move furniture to provide moving space.
6. Explain the procedure to the client.
7. Provide for privacy.
8. Position the client in a side-lying position facing you (Fig. 2.28). The client lies on their strong side.
9. Lock the bed wheels (if applicable).
10. Raise the bed for body mechanics (if applicable).
11. Raise the head of the bed to a sitting position (if applicable).

Procedure

12. Lower the head of the bed to a level appropriate for the client (if applicable). It should be as flat as possible.
13. Stand on the side of the bed by the client's hips. Face the foot of the bed.
14. Lower the bed rail near you if bed rails are used (if applicable).
15. Stand with your feet about 20 cm apart. The foot closer to the head of the bed is in front of the other foot. Bend your knees.
16. Cross the client's arms over their chest.
17. If using a slide sheet:
    - a. Roll the slide sheet up close to the client.
    - b. Grasp the rolled-up slide sheet near the client's shoulders and buttocks. Your co-worker does the same. Make sure you support the client's head.
    - c. Rock backwards on the count of three, moving the client towards you. Your co-worker rocks backwards slightly and then forwards towards you while keeping their arms straight.
    - d. Unroll the slide sheet. Remove any wrinkles.
18. If not using a slide sheet:
    - a. Slide one arm under the client's neck and shoulders. Place the other arm over the client's thighs, near the knees.
    - b. Pivot towards the foot of the bed while moving the client's lower legs and feet over the side of the bed. As the legs go over the edge of the mattress, the trunk is upright.
    - c. Ask the client to hold on to the edge of the mattress. This supports them in the sitting position.
19. Check the client's condition:
    - a. Ask how they feel. Also ask if they feel dizzy or light-headed.
    - b. Check for difficulty breathing.
    - c. Note if the skin is pale or bluish in colour (cyanotic).
20. Help the client lie down if necessary. Help them move to the centre of the bed.
21. Do not leave the client alone. Provide support if necessary.

Post-procedure

22. Provide for comfort. Position the client in good body alignment.

23 Follow the nurse's directions and the care plan. Reposition the pillow under the client's head and shoulders.
24 Place the call bell within the client's reach (if applicable).
25 Raise or lower bed rails (if applicable). Follow the care plan.
26 Lower the bed to its lowest position (if applicable).
27 Remove any privacy screens (if applicable).
28 Return furniture to its proper place.
29 Wash your hands.
30 Report and record your observations.

DELEGATION GUIDELINES

Dangling

The procedure for dangling is also part of other care activities – assisting the client to stand, transferring them from bed to chair, partial bath and others. When delegated the dangling procedure or tasks that involve dangling, you need the following information from the care plan:

- Areas of weakness – for example, if the client's arms are weak, the client cannot hold onto the side of the mattress for support. If the left side of the client's body is weak, you need to turn the client onto the stronger right side. The client can then use their right arm to help move from the lying to sitting position.
- The amount of assistance the client needs.
- Whether you need a co-worker to help you.
- How long the client needs to sit on the side of the bed.
- What exercises the client needs to perform while dangling.
- Leg and foot exercises.
- Coughing and deep breathing.
- Whether the client will walk or transfer to a chair after dangling.
- Pale or bluish skin colour (cyanosis).
- Complaints of dizziness, light-headedness or difficulty breathing.
- How well the activity was tolerated.
- The length of time the client dangled.
- The amount of help needed.
- Other observations or complaints.

TRANSFERRING THE CLIENT

To transfer a client means to move them from one place to another. Clients are often moved from their beds to chairs, wheelchairs, shower chairs, commodes or toilets. Some can transfer themselves or need only a little help. Some are transferred by one, two or three people. The rules of body mechanics and manual handling apply when transferring. Also, arrange the room so there is enough space for a safe transfer. Remove any clutter. Correct chair, wheelchair or stretcher placement is needed for a safe and efficient transfer.

The client wears non-skid footwear for transfers as this protects them from falls by preventing slipping and sliding. Remember to securely tie shoelaces or the client could trip and fall. The bed and stretcher wheels must be locked and the wheelchair and shower chair brakes must be on. Both

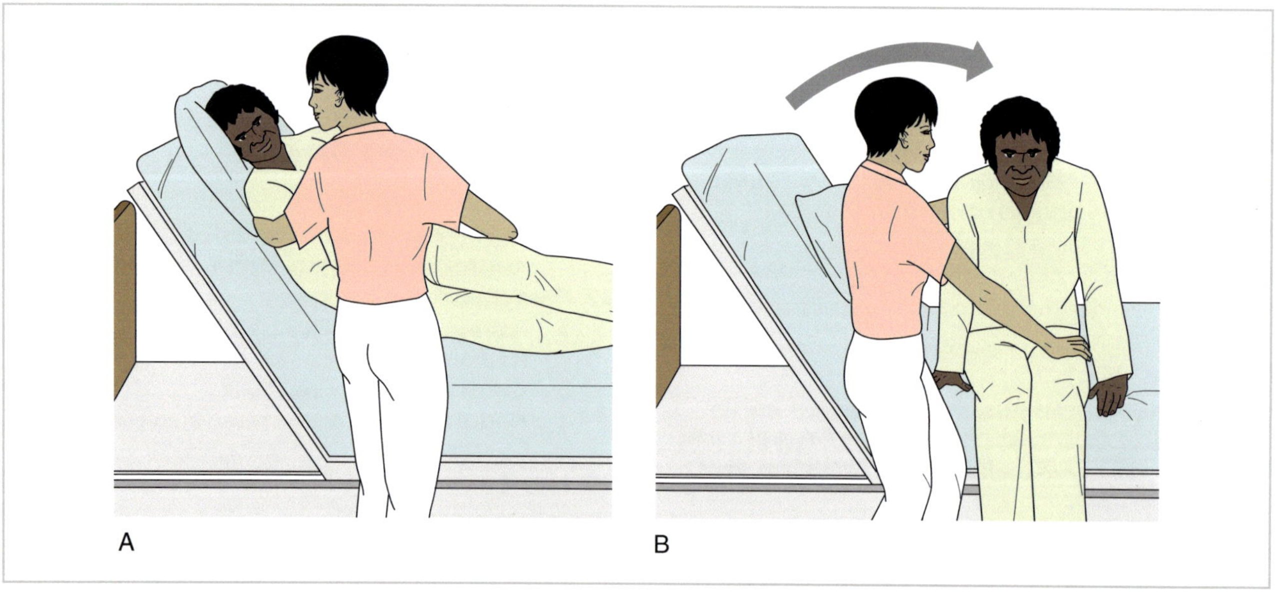

Fig. 2.28
Helping the client sit on the side of the bed.
A. The client's thighs are supported. **B.** The client sits upright as the legs and feet are pulled over the edge of the bed.

measures prevent the bed, stretcher, wheelchair or shower chair from moving during the transfer, which could cause the client to fall.

Most wheelchairs or bedside chairs have vinyl seats and backs. Vinyl holds body heat, so the client becomes warm and perspires more. You can cover the back and seat with a folded bath towel. This increases the client's comfort in the chair. Some clients have wheelchair cushions or positioning devices. These prevent pressure ulcers, maintain posture or prevent the client sliding forwards. Ask the nurse how to use and place the device.

DELEGATION GUIDELINES

Transferring a client

When you are delegated transferring procedures, you need the following information from the care plan:

- Which procedure to use for:
  - transferring the client to a chair or wheelchair
  - transferring the client to a wheelchair with assistance
  - transferring the client from the chair or wheelchair to bed
  - transferring the client using a mechanical lift
  - transferring the client to and from the toilet.
- Areas of weakness – for example, if the client's arms are weak, the client cannot hold onto the side of the mattress for support. If the client has a weak left side, they get out of bed on the stronger right side. The client can use their right arm to help move from the lying to the sitting position.
- What equipment is needed – such as walking belt, wheelchair, mechanical lift, positioning devices, wheelchair cushion.
- The amount of help the client needs.
- How many co-workers are needed to help you.
- Complaints of light-headedness, pain, discomfort, difficulty breathing, weakness or fatigue.
- The amount of help needed to transfer the client.
- How the client helped with the transfer.

Using a walking/transfer belt

A **walking belt**, or **transfer belt**, is a belt used to walk a client who is unsteady on their feet or who requires the assistance of one or two carers when attempting to ambulate (walk) (Fig. 2.29). It helps prevent falls and other injuries. The walking belt must never be used to lift or move a client from the floor. It is not designed to lift a client or to take their weight.

APPLYING A WALKING BELT

Quality of life

Remember to respect the client's privacy while doing any procedure. Address the person by name and ensure they know your name.

Procedure

1. Wash your hands.
2. Call the client by name.
3. Explain the procedure to the client.
4. Provide for privacy.
5. Assist the client to a sitting position.
6. Apply the belt around the client's waist over clothing. Do not apply it over bare skin.
7. Tighten the belt so it is snug. It should not cause discomfort or impair breathing. You should be able to slide four fingers between the belt and the client.
8. If the client is a woman, make sure that her breasts are not caught under the belt.
9. Place the buckle off-centre in the front or at the back, for the client's comfort. The buckle should not be over the spine.
10. Grasp the walking belt from underneath when using it to transfer the client.

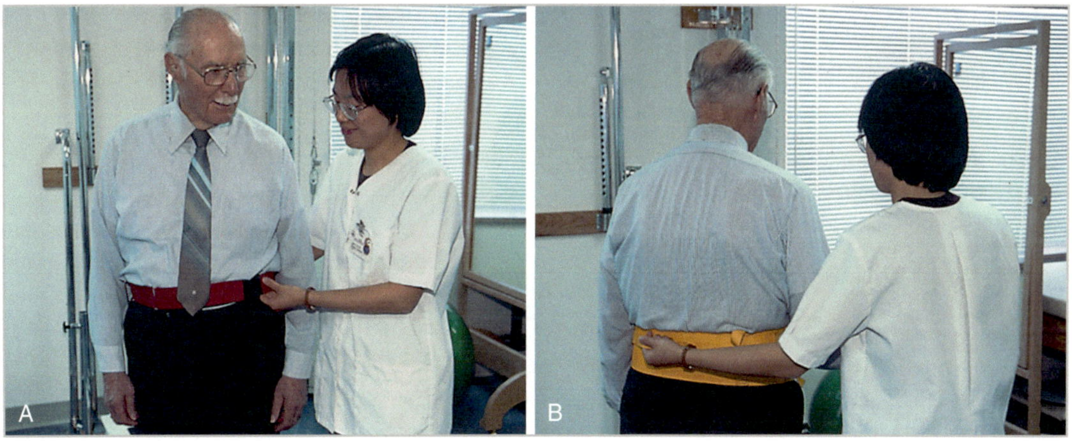

Fig. 2.29
Walking belt. Note the different types of walking belts.
A. The belt buckle is positioned off centre in the front. **B.** The belt buckle is positioned at the back. It is not over the spine.

The walking belt fits snugly around the waist of the client and is secured by large strips of Velcro and a safety buckle. There are several sizes: small, medium, large and extra-large. It is important that the belt fits the client properly and that it is not loose around their waist or too tight and restrictive. The belt must not ride up or restrict the client from breathing. Walking belts have handles at the front, sides and back. These handles are used by the carers when steadying the client on their feet or returning the client to their chair or bed. Carers should hold the first and third strap when walking clients.

The walking belt eliminates the need to hook your client underneath their arms (armpits) or to place pressure on their delicate skin. It is a simple but valuable piece of equipment and can be used for most clients. If the client needs help, a walking belt is required. To use a walking belt safely always follow the manufacturer's instructions. Whenever used, it is applied over clothing; it is never applied over bare skin. Also, it is applied under the breasts. Breasts must not be caught under the belt. Remember to respect the client's privacy while doing any procedure. Address the client by name and ensure they know your name.

The procedure used depends on the client's abilities, condition and size. If the client cannot assist, a mechanical lifter is used. Help the client out of bed on their strong side. If the left side is weak and the right side strong, get the client out of bed on the right side. In transferring, the strong side moves first. It pulls the weaker side along. Transfers from the weak side are awkward and unsafe.

Transferring the person from bed to chair or wheelchair

Safety is important when transferring a client from bed to a chair, wheelchair, commode or shower chair. It is possible to complete this task with no assistance from a colleague. However, the client must be fully independent, so that basic supervision only is required. A client who cannot support their own weight while being transferred from bed to chair must be managed using a hoist. In this situation, even a walking belt should not be used for this procedure, because the client could easily collapse on to the floor and suffer a serious injury. Staff would also be at significant risk of permanent and debilitating injury.

Transfers from a chair or wheelchair to bed have the same rules as transfers from a bed to a chair. If the client is weak on one side, transfer the client so that the strong side moves first. Therefore, the client is transferred to bed on the opposite side from which they transferred out of bed. For example, the client's right side is weak and the left side strong. To transfer the client from bed to the chair, the chair is placed on the left side of the bed. This allows the client's left side to move first. Now you will transfer the client back to bed. If you leave the chair on the left side of the bed, the client's right side – the weak side – is near the bed. The weak side will move first. This is unsafe for the client. Therefore, you need to move the chair to the other side of the bed. The client's stronger left side will be near the bed. The stronger left side moves first, for a safe transfer. Remember to respect the client's privacy while doing any procedure. Address the client by name and ensure they know your name.

TRANSFERRING THE PERSON TO A CHAIR OR WHEELCHAIR

Quality of life

Remember to respect the client's privacy while doing any procedure. Address the client by name and ensure they know your name.

Pre-procedure

1 Follow the delegation guidelines.
2 Explain the procedure to the client.
3 Collect:
- wheelchair or armchair
- seat cushion if needed
- robe and non-skid footwear
- paper or sheet
- walking belt if needed.

4 Wash your hands.
5 Call the client by their name.
6 Provide for privacy.
7 Decide which side of the bed to use. Move furniture to provide moving space.
8 Place the chair at the head of the bed.

Procedure

9 Place a folded bath towel or cushion on the seat if needed.
10 Lock wheelchair wheels. Raise the footrests. Remove the footrests or swing them out of the way.
11 Lower the bed to its lowest position. Lock the bed wheels.
12 Fan-fold top linen to the foot of the bed.
13 Place the paper or sheet under the client's feet. Put non-skid footwear on the client.
14 Help the client sit on the side of the bed. Make sure their feet touch the floor.
15 Help the client put on a robe if they are wearing sleepwear.
16 Apply the walking belt if needed.
17 **Method 1: Using a walking belt** (Some centres require the use of a walking belt when assisting a client to transfer (see Fig. 2.29).)
- a Stand in front of the client.
- b Have the client hold on to the mattress.
- c Make sure the client's feet are flat on the floor.
- d Have the client lean forwards.
- e Grasp the walking belt at each side.
- f Brace your knees against the client's knees. Block their feet with your feet (Fig. 2.30). Alternatively,

use the knee and foot of one leg to block the client's weak foot. Place your other foot slightly behind yourself for balance.

- g Ask the client to push down on the mattress and to stand on the count of three. Pull the client into a standing position as you straighten your knees (Figures 2.31, 2.32).

18 Method 2: No walking belt

- a Follow steps 17 a–c.
- b Standing in front of the client, place your right shoulder to the client's left shoulder. Your left arm is around the client and your right arm is on the client's right hip.
- c Have the client lean forwards.
- d Brace your knees against the client's knees. Block their feet with your feet. Alternatively, use the knee and foot of one leg to block the client's weak foot. Place your other foot slightly behind you for balance.
- e Ask the client to push down on the mattress and to stand on the count of three. Guide the client up into a standing position as you straighten your knees.

19 Support the client in the standing position. Hold the walking belt or keep your hands around the client's shoulder blades. Continue to block the client's feet and knees with your feet and knees.

20 Turn the client so they can grasp the far arm of the chair (Fig. 2.33). Their legs will touch the edge of the chair.

21 Continue to turn the client until the other arm rest is grasped.

22 Lower the client into the chair as you bend your hips and knees. The client assists by leaning forwards and bending their elbows and knees (Fig. 2.34).

23 Make sure the client's buttocks are to the back of the seat. Position the client in good alignment.

Post-procedure

24 Provide for comfort. Position the client's feet on the wheelchair footrests.

25 Cover the client's lap and legs with a blanket. Keep the blanket off the floor and the wheels.

26 Position the chair as the client prefers. Lock the wheelchair wheels.

27 Make sure the call bell and other necessary items are within reach.

28 Arrange room furniture to meet the client's needs.

29 Remove any privacy screens (if applicable).

30 Wash your hands.

31 Report and record your observations.

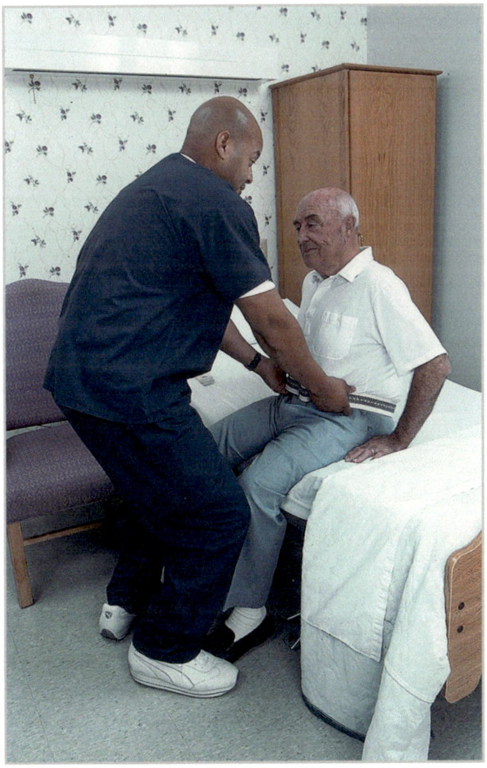

Fig. 2.30
Prevent the client from sliding or falling by blocking their knees and feet with your own knees and feet.

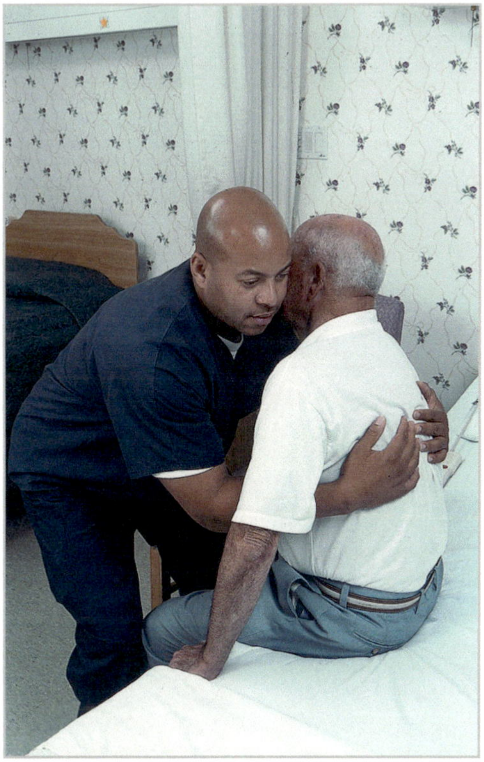

Fig. 2.31
A client being prepared to stand. The hands are placed under the client's arms and around the shoulder blades.

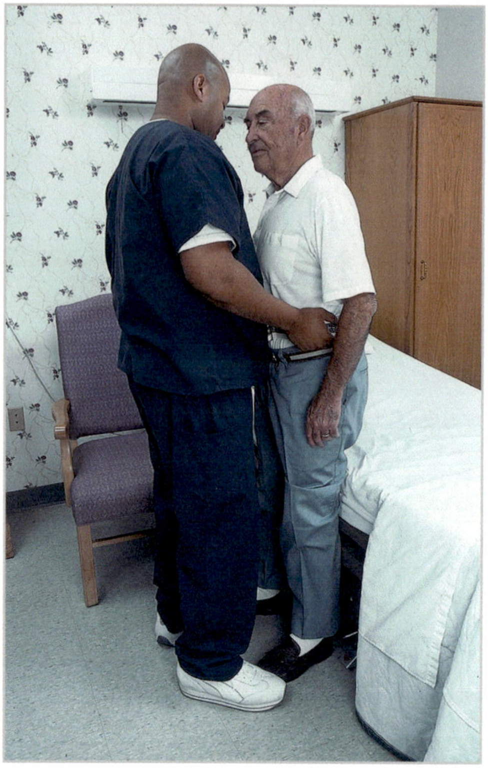

Fig. 2.32

The client is pulled up to a standing position and supported by holding the walking belt and blocking the client's knees and feet.

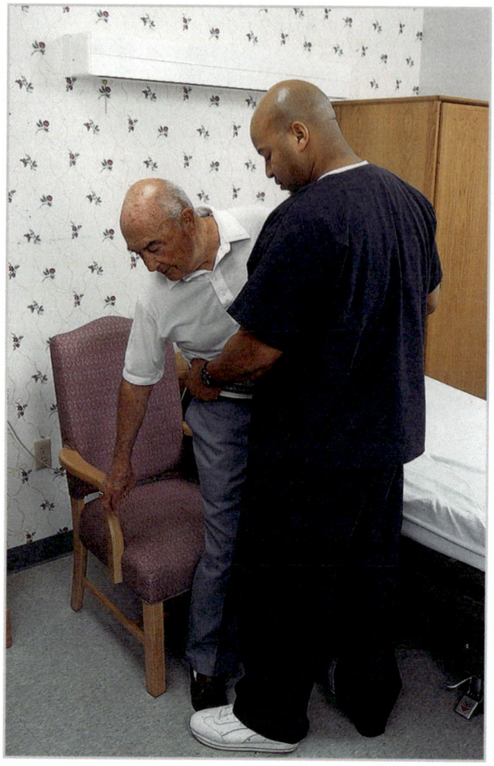

Fig. 2.33

The client is supported as he grasps the far arm of the chair. His legs are against the chair.

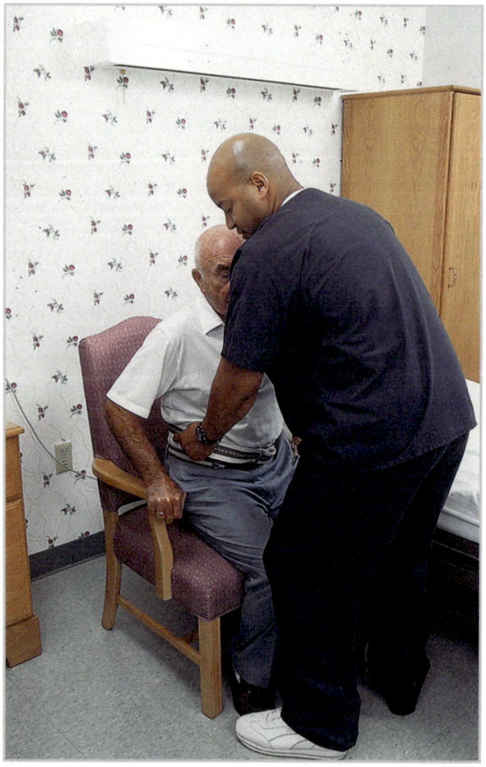

Fig. 2.34

The client holds the armrests, leans forwards and bends the elbows and knees while being lowered into the chair.

SAFETY ALERT

Chair or wheelchair transfers

The client wears non-skid footwear for chair transfers. These prevent slipping and sliding on the floor. Also, follow the measures for wheelchair safety.

Transferring the client to and from the toilet

Using the bathroom for elimination promotes the client's dignity, self-esteem and independence. It is also more private than using a bedpan, urinal or bedside commode. However, getting to the toilet is hard for clients who use wheelchairs (Fig. 2.35). Bathrooms are usually small, so there is little room for you and a wheelchair. Therefore, transfers involving wheelchairs and toilets are often difficult. The risk of falls is great.

Repositioning in a chair or wheelchair

The client in a chair or wheelchair can slide down into the chair. For good body alignment and safety, the client's back and buttocks must be against the back of the chair. If

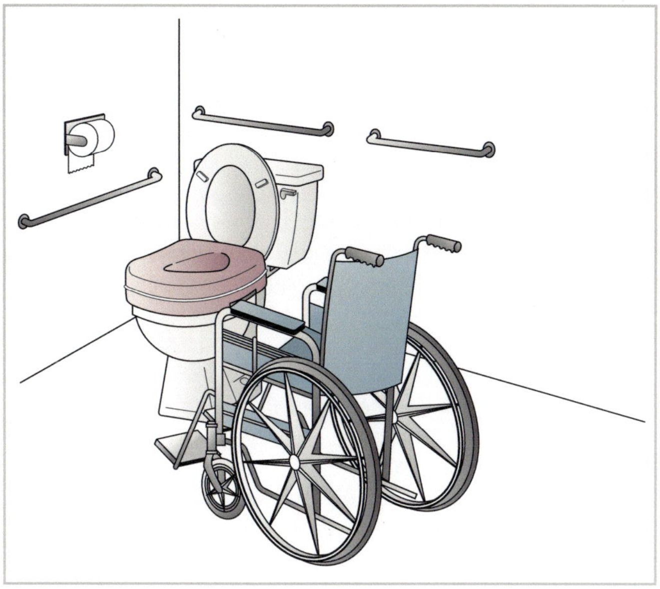

Fig. 2.35
The wheelchair is placed at a 90-degree angle to the toilet.

the client can assist, encourage them to move back in the chair by pushing down with their arms on the edge of the chair and easing their buttocks backwards. Place your hands on their knees and prevent their feet from sliding forwards. If the client is unable to assist you, you can use a slide sheet to assist with this procedure, or a mechanical lifter must be used.

WHEELCHAIR TRANSFERS WITH ASSISTANCE

Some wheelchair transfers involve assisting the client from the bed to the chair. To return the client to bed, assist them from the chair to the bed. Always use a mechanical lifter, as most services have a safe patient handling policy stating that manual lifting by staff is forbidden. Manual lifting by carers is dangerous for the carer and the client.

Lifters and hoists

The **mechanical lifter**, or **hoist** as it is sometimes referred to, is a piece of equipment that is battery operated and is used to raise the client from their bed, chair, bath or the floor. There are mechanical and electric lifts. The hoist is on wheels and has a sling that is positioned, with great care, underneath the client prior to them being lifted and moved. The most important rules associated with safe use of this piece of equipment is that staff must be trained in its use and must not operate the lifter on their own. Healthcare providers and aged care services have strict protocols regarding the safe use of hoists and lifters, and these should be understood before operating the equipment. Most services require new staff to be instructed and tested prior to being allowed to operate this equipment.

Standing lifters

The **standing lifter** is used for clients who can bear their weight and stand up. It is essential that the client is capable of doing this if the apparatus is to work correctly. The lifter is placed in front of the client, who is seated. A large belt is placed around the client's torso and under the arms. The belt is connected to the lifter. The client's feet must be resting on the platform of the lifting device. The client is encouraged to place their arms up on the frame of the lifter for security. The client is slowly and carefully raised from their chair or from the side of the bed. It is important to consider the client's dignity when operating the standing lifter, as exposure cannot be avoided.

Clients who cannot help themselves are transferred with mechanical lifts, as are clients who are too heavy for staff to transfer (Fig. 2.36). Lifts are used for transfers into chairs, stretchers, bath-tubs, shower chairs, toilets, pools or vehicles. Some centres use more than one type of lift.

Before using a lift:

- make sure you are trained in its use
- make sure the lift works
- make sure the sling, straps, hooks and chains are in good repair
- compare the client's weight and the lift's weight limit. Do not use the lift if a client's weight exceeds the lift's capacity
- ensure at least two staff members are available to provide assistance.

Mechanical lifters

Mechanical lifters vary among manufacturers. In addition, manufacturers have different models. Knowing how to use one lifter does not mean that you know how to use others. Always follow the manufacturer's instructions. If you have questions, ask the nurse. If you have not used a certain lifter before, ask the nurse to show you how to use it safely. Also ask the nurse to help you use it the first time and until you are comfortable using it.

TRANSFERRING A PERSON TO OR FROM THE TOILET USING A MECHANICAL LIFTER

Quality of life

Remember to respect the person's privacy while doing any procedure. Address the person by name and ensure they know your name.

Pre-procedure

1 Follow the delegation guidelines.
2 Make sure the person has an elevated toilet seat. That way, the toilet seat and wheelchair are at the same level.
3 Check the grab bars by the toilet. If they are loose, tell your supervisor. Do not transfer the client to the toilet if the grab bars are not secure.

Procedure

4 Have the client wear non-skid footwear.
5 Position the wheelchair next to the toilet if there is enough room. If not, position the wheelchair at a right angle to the toilet (see Fig. 2.35). It is best if the client's strong side is near the toilet.
6 Lock the wheelchair brakes.
7 Raise the footrests. Remove or swing them out of the way.
8 Apply the walking belt.
9 Help the client unfasten their clothing.
10 Use the walking belt to help the client stand and turn to the toilet. The client uses the grab bars to turn to the toilet.
11 Support the client with the walking belt while they lower their clothing. Alternatively, have the client hold on to the grab bars for support, while you lower their pants and undergarment.
12 Use the walking belt to lower the client on to the toilet seat.
13 Remove the walking belt.
14 Tell the client you will stay nearby. Remind them to use the call bell or call for you when help is needed.
15 Close the bathroom door to provide privacy.
16 Stay near the bathroom. Complete other tasks in the client's room.
17 Knock on the bathroom door when the client calls for you.
18 Help with wiping, perineal care, flushing and handwashing as needed.
19 Apply the walking belt.
20 Use the walking belt to help the client stand.
21 Help the client raise and secure their clothing.
22 Use the walking belt to transfer the client to the wheelchair.
23 Make sure the client's buttocks are to the back of the seat. Position the client in good alignment.
24 Position the client's feet on the footrests.
25 Cover the client's lap and legs with a blanket. Keep the blanket off the floor and wheels.
26 Position the chair as the client prefers. Lock the wheelchair wheels.

Post-procedure

27 Place the call bell (if applicable) and other necessary items within reach.
28 Remove any privacy screens (if applicable).
29 Wash your hands.
30 Report and record your observations.

SAFETY ALERT

Mechanical lifters

Mechanical lifters vary among manufacturers. In addition, manufacturers have different models. Knowing how to use one lifter does not mean that you know how to use others. Always follow the manufacturer's instructions.

If you have questions, ask the nurse. If you have not used a certain lifter before, ask the nurse to show you how to use it safely. Also ask the nurse to help you use it the first time and until you are comfortable using it.

POSITIONING

The client must be properly positioned at all times. Regular position changes and good body alignment promote comfort and wellbeing. Breathing is easier and circulation is promoted. Proper positioning also helps prevent many complications, such as pressure ulcers and contractures. When you are in bed or in a chair, you move and turn for your comfort. Many clients do too. Some need reminding to adjust their position and others need some help. Still others depend entirely on the nursing team for position changes.

Whether in bed or a chair, the client is repositioned at least every 2 hours. Some clients are repositioned more often. Pressure ulcers are a serious threat from lying or sitting too long in one place. Wet, soiled and wrinkled linen are other causes. Whenever you reposition a client, make sure the linen is clean, dry and wrinkle-free. Change or straighten linen as needed. Contractures can also develop from staying in one position too long. A contracture is the lack of joint mobility caused by abnormal shortening of a muscle. Repositioning, exercise and activity help prevent contractures. You must follow the care plan.

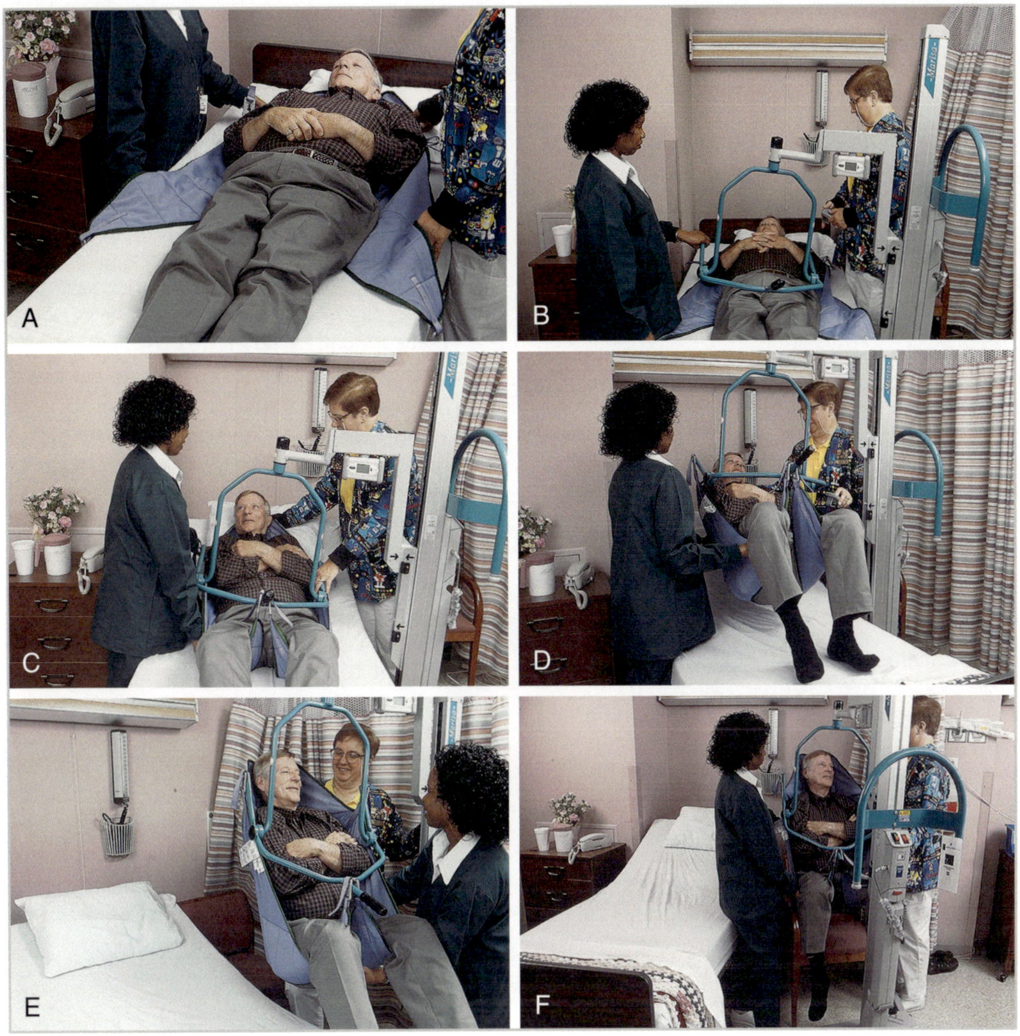

Fig. 2.36

Using a mechanical lifter.

A. The sling is positioned under the client. The lower edge is behind the client's knees. **B.** The lift is over the client. The lift's legs are spread to widen the base of support. **C.** The sling is attached to a swivel bar. **D.** The lift is raised until the sling and client are off the bed. **E.** The client's legs are supported as the client and lift are moved away from the bed. **F.** The client is guided into a chair.

SAFETY ALERT

Positioning

Pressure ulcers are a serious threat from lying or sitting too long in one place. Wet, soiled and wrinkled linen are other causes. Whenever you reposition a person, make sure the linen is clean, dry and wrinkle-free. Change or straighten linen as needed.

Contractures also can develop from staying in one position too long. A contracture is the lack of joint mobility caused by abnormal shortening of a muscle. Repositioning, exercise and activity help prevent contractures.

TRANSFERRING A PERSON USING A MECHANICAL LIFTER

Quality of life

Remember to respect the person's privacy while doing any procedure. Address the person by name and ensure they know your name.

Pre-procedure

1 Follow the delegation guidelines.
2 Ask a co-worker to help you.
3 Explain the procedure to the client.
4 Collect:
   - mechanical lifter
   - a chair or wheelchair
   - footwear
   - blanket or cushion.
5 Wash your hands.
6 Call the client by name.
7 Provide for privacy.

Procedure

8 Check the lifter carefully. Ensure that all moving parts can move freely. Check that the lifter will take the weight of the client being lifted. There is a maximum weight sign on the lifter and any client heavier than this maximum weight should never be lifted with the lifter. If the lifter has a battery, check this is charged and working. Ensure the lifter has been serviced within the past 12 months. If it has not, notify the nurse. Take note of where the emergency let-down button is in case the battery fails.
9 Inspect the sling. Ensure that it is the correct size for the client, and that it is in good condition. It should not be soiled or show any sign of fraying. Centre the sling under the client. To position the sling, turn the client from side to side as if making an occupied bed. Position the sling according to the manufacturer's instructions.
10 Lock the bed wheels (if applicable). Lower the bed.
11 Raise the lifter so you can position it over the client.
12 Attach the sling to the swivel bar. Some slings have straps and others have a plastic clip that clicks into place.
13 Ask the client to cross their arms over their chest.
14 Raise the lifter so that the harness is under tension. Check that all of the straps or clips are secured correctly. Ensure that the client's genital area is not being pinched by the sling. It may be necessary to place a small towel in the genital area.
15 Raise the lifter high enough until the client and sling are free of the bed.
16 Have your co-worker support the client's legs as you move the lifter and client away from the bed.
17 Position the lifter so that the client's back is towards the chair.
18 Position the chair so that you can lower the client into it.
19 Lower the client into the chair. (Follow the manufacturer's instructions.) Guide the client into the chair. It may be necessary to stand behind the client and pull the sling back to ensure the client is well back in the chair.
20 Lower the swivel bar to unhook the sling. Remove the sling from under the client unless otherwise indicated.
21 Put footwear on the client and position their feet on wheelchair footrests.
22 Cover the client's lap and legs with a blanket. Keep it off the floor and wheels.
23 Position the chair as the client prefers. Lock the wheelchair wheels.

Post-procedure

24 Place the call bell (if applicable) and other necessary items within reach.
25 Wash your hands.
26 Report and record your observations.
27 Reverse the procedure to return the client to bed.

DELEGATION GUIDELINES

Positioning

You are often delegated tasks that involve positioning and repositioning. You need the following information from the nurse and the care plan.

The doctor may also order certain positions or position limits. Follow these guidelines to position a client safely:

- Use good body mechanics.
- Ask a co-worker to help you if needed.
- Explain the procedure to the client.
- Be gentle when moving the client.
- Provide for privacy.
- Place the call bell within the client's reach after each positioning.
- Position or observe positioning limits ordered by the doctor.
- Know how often to turn and reposition the client.
- Decide how many co-workers need to help you.
- Know what skin care measures to perform.
- Know what range-of-motion exercises to perform.
- Know where to place pillows.
- Know what positioning devices are needed and how to use them.
- Know what observations to report and record.

Remember to respect the client's privacy while doing any procedure. Address the client by name and ensure they know your name.

Fowler's position

In **Fowler's position**, the head of the bed is raised to a semi-sitting position (Fig. 2.37). The head of the bed is raised between 45 and 90 degrees. In a semi-Fowler's position, the head of the bed is raised between 30 and 45 degrees. Good body alignment for Fowler's position involves:

- keeping the spine straight
- supporting the head with a small pillow
- supporting the arms with pillows.

Clients with heart and respiratory disorders can usually breathe more easily in Fowler's position.

Supine position

The **supine (dorsal recumbent) position** is the back-lying position (Fig. 2.38). The bed is flat, the head and shoulders are supported on a pillow and the client's arms and hands are at their side. You can support the arms with regular-sized pillows. Or you can support the hands on small pillows with the client's palms down. The nurse may ask you to place:

- a folded or rolled towel under the client's lower back
- a small pillow under the client's thighs
- a pillow under the lower legs. This lifts the heels off the bed to prevent them from rubbing on the sheets. Do not horizontally place a pillow under the client's calves. This significantly increases the risk of blood clots forming.

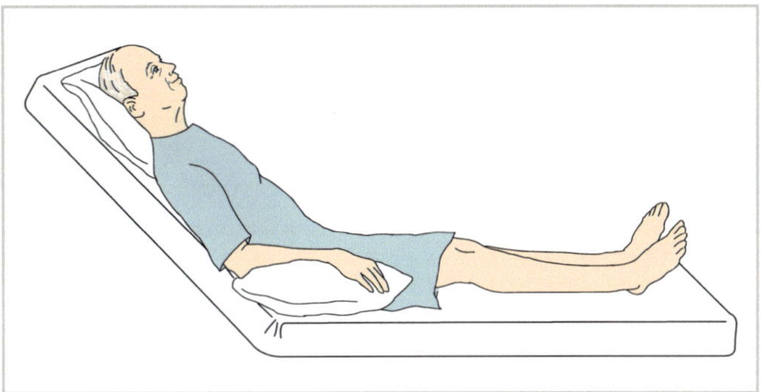

Fig. 2.37
Fowler's position.

Prone position

A client in the **prone position** lies on their abdomen with their head turned to one side (Fig. 2.39). Small pillows are placed under the head, abdomen and lower legs. The arms are flexed at the elbows, with the hands near the head. You also can position the client with their feet hanging over the end of the mattress (Fig. 2.40). If that is done, a pillow is not needed under the lower legs. Most older people do not tolerate the prone position. They have limited range of motion in their necks. Check with the nurse before placing any client in the prone position.

Lateral position

A client in the **lateral (side-lying) position** lies on one side or the other (Fig. 2.41).

- A pillow is placed under the client's head and neck.
- The upper leg is in front of the lower leg. (The nurse may ask you to position the upper leg behind the lower leg, not on top of it.)
- The upper leg and thigh are supported with pillows.
- A pillow is positioned against the client's back. The client rolls back against the pillow so that their back is at a 45-degree angle with the mattress.
- A small pillow is placed under the upper hand and arm.

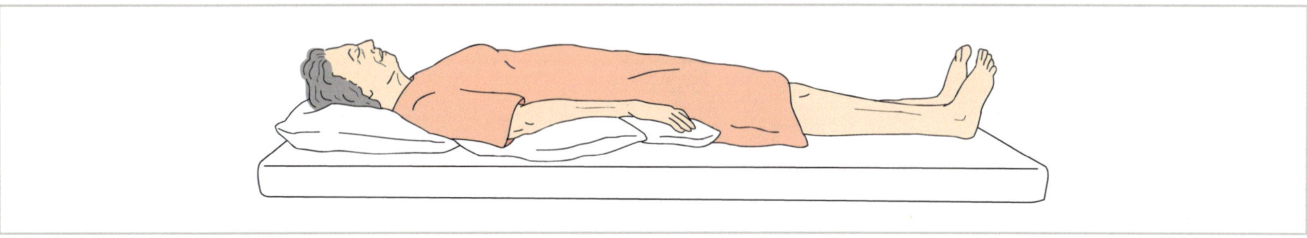

Fig. 2.38
Supine position.

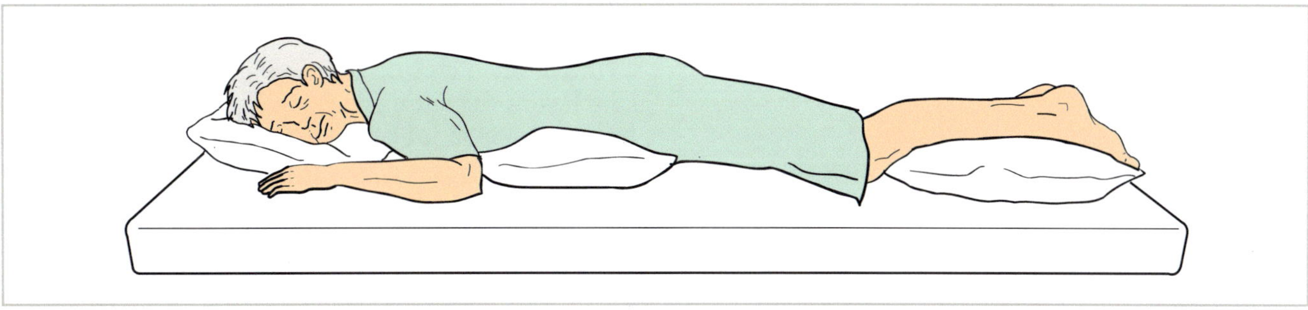

Fig. 2.39
Prone position.

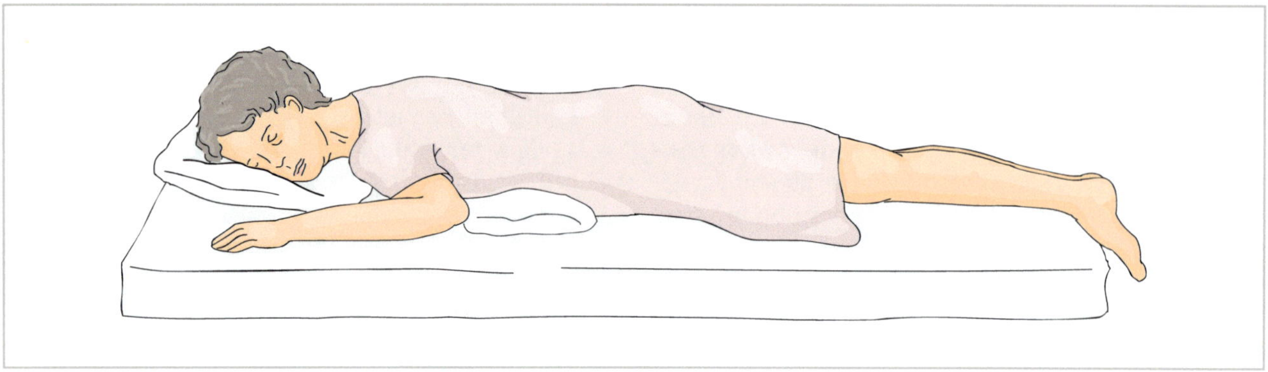

Fig. 2.40
Prone position with the feet hanging over the edge of the mattress.

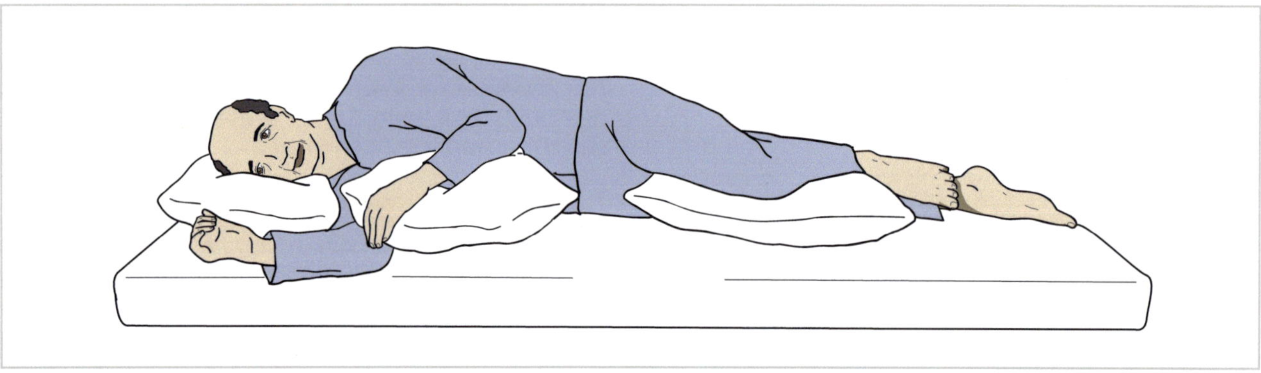

Fig. 2.41
Lateral position.

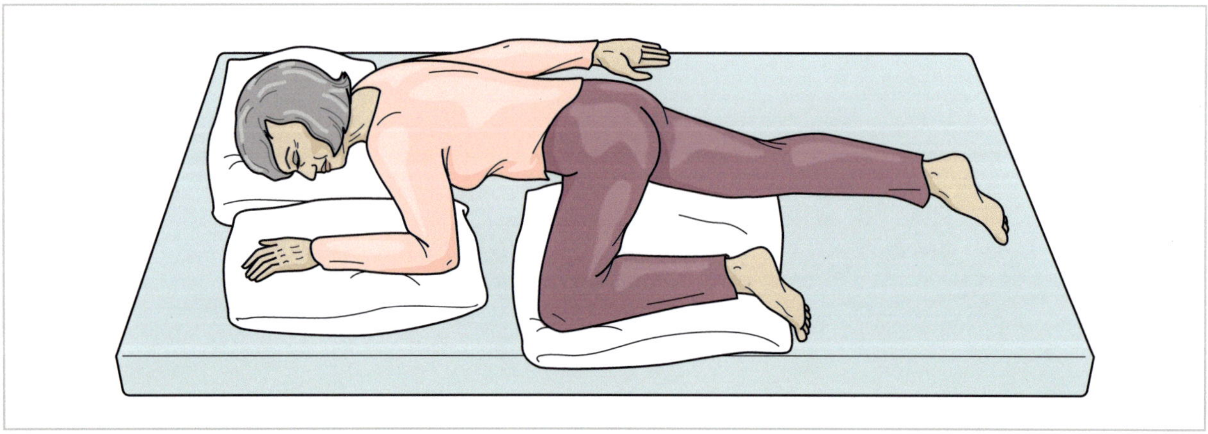

Fig. 2.42
Modified left lateral recumbent position.

Modified left lateral recumbent position

The **modified left lateral recumbent position** is a left side-lying position (Fig. 2.42). The upper leg is sharply flexed so that it is not on the lower leg. The lower arm is behind the client. For good body alignment:

- place a pillow under the client's head and shoulder
- support the upper leg with a pillow
- place a pillow under the upper arm and hand.

This position is usually not comfortable for older people. Check with the nurse before placing a client in the modified left lateral recumbent position.

Chair position

To enable good **chair position**, a sitting client must hold their head and upper body erect, otherwise poor alignment results (Fig. 2.43). To ensure good alignment the:

- client's back and buttocks are against the back of the chair

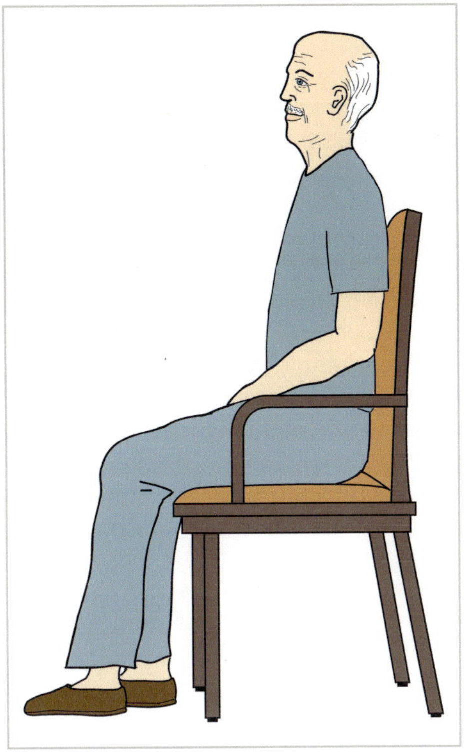

Fig. 2.43
Chair position.
The client is positioned in a chair. The feet are flat on the floor, the calves do not touch the chair and the back is straight and against the back of the chair.

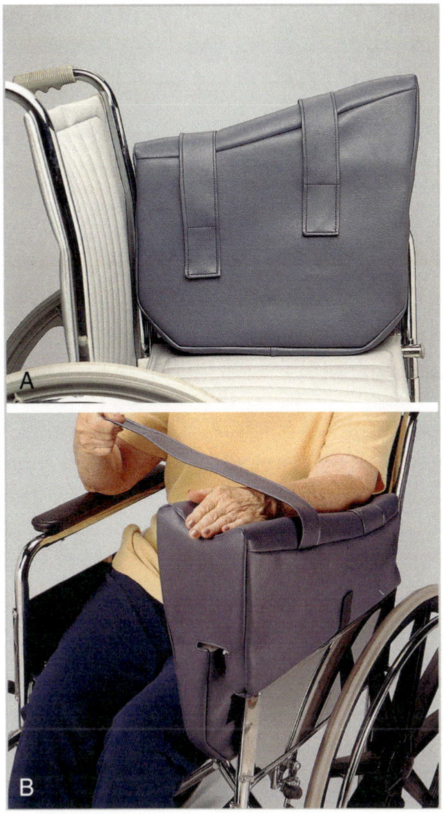

Fig. 2.44
Elevated armrest.

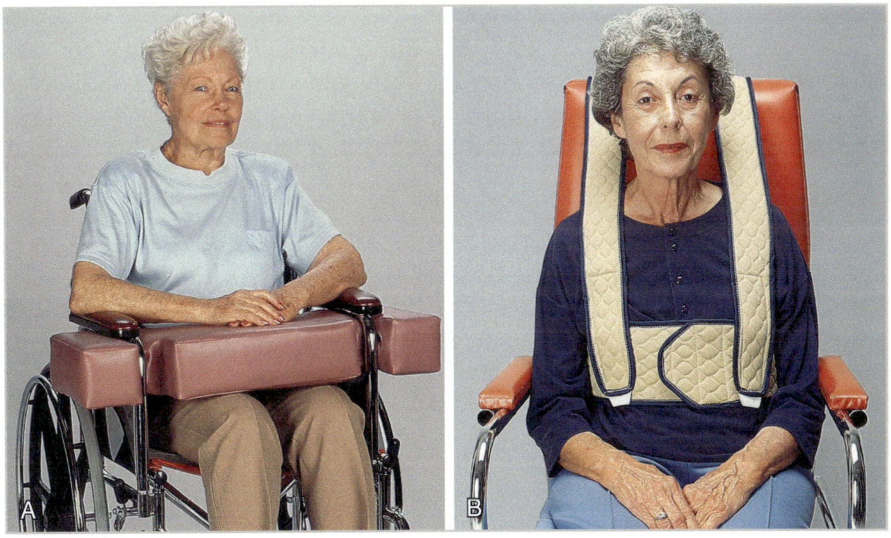

Fig. 2.45
Postural supports.
A. Pelvic holder. **B.** Torso support.

- client's feet are flat on the floor or on wheelchair footrests – never leave the feet unsupported
- backs of the knees and calves are slightly away from the edge of the seat.

The nurse may ask you to put a small pillow between the lower part of the client's back and the chair. This supports the lower back. Remember, a pillow is not used behind the back if restraints are used. Paralysed arms are positioned on pillows. Some clients have special foam positioners; these position the wrists at a slight upward angle (Fig. 2.44). Some clients require postural supports if they cannot keep their upper body erect (Fig. 2.45). Postural support helps keep the client in good body alignment. The health team selects the best product for the client's needs. The client's safety, dignity and function are considered.

INFECTION PREVENTION AND CONTROL

A **microorganism** (microbe) is a small (*micro*) living plant or animal (*organism*). It can only be seen with a microscope. Microorganisms are everywhere. They require a **reservoir** or host in which to live and grow. The human body can be a reservoir. Microorganisms are often found in the respiratory tract, the alimentary tract, the skin and on wounds. They are also found in plants, animals, the soil, food, water and other material. Microorganisms that cause infections and are harmful are called **pathogens**. Microorganisms that do not usually cause infection are called **non-pathogens**. **Normal flora** are microorganisms that live and grow in a certain area without causing harm – that is, they are non-pathogens. Specific microorganisms are found in the respiratory tract, in the intestines and on the skin. However, when a non-pathogen is transmitted from its natural site to another site or host, it can become a pathogen. For example, *Escherichia coli* occurs naturally in the human colon or bowel. If the *E. coli* enters the urinary system, which is not its natural reservoir, it will cause an infection.

Types of microorganisms

There are four main types of microorganisms:

- *Bacteria* – these organisms multiply rapidly. They consist of one cell and can cause infection in one or more body systems.
- *Fungi* – these organisms are plant and animal parasites. Mushrooms, yeasts and moulds are common fungi. Fungi can infect the mouth, vagina, skin, feet and other body areas.
- *Protozoa* – these are single-celled organisms. They can move fast and infect the blood, brain, intestines and other body areas.
- *Viruses* – these are not technically organisms but infectious agents. Viruses live and replicate inside living cells. They cause many diseases, including the common cold, herpes, human immunodeficiency virus (HIV) and hepatitis.

Requirements of microorganisms

Microorganisms require a reservoir or host to live and grow. A human can be a reservoir – microorganisms are often found in the respiratory tract, the alimentary tract, wounds or on the skin. Other reservoirs are provided by plants, animals, the soil, food, water and other material.

The microbe must get water and nourishment from the reservoir. Many microorganisms need oxygen to live, while others cannot live where there is oxygen. A warm and dark environment is usually needed. Most microorganisms grow best at body temperature.

Medication-resistant organisms

Medication-resistant organisms represent a huge problem for aged care services and all healthcare organisations. High standards of infection control are the only way to reduce the spread of these types of infections. Antibiotics are medications that can kill microorganisms. Some microorganisms can change their structure and become resistant to a specific antibiotic. This makes the microorganisms more difficult to kill and so the infection will continue. Two common organisms that are known to be medication-resistant are:

- methicillin-resistant *Staphylococcus aureus* (MRSA) – also known as golden staph. This is normally found in the nose, groin and on the skin. It causes serious wound infections and pneumonia. This microbe has become resistant to methicillin, which is a type of penicillin. The reason for this is the overuse and incorrect use of methicillin some years ago.
- vancomycin-resistant *Enterococcus* (VRE) – VRE is normally found in the intestines and can be present in faeces. It can be transmitted from one person to another by contaminated hands and equipment. When VRE is not in its natural site, it can cause infection. This microbe is resistant to many antibiotics and can cause serious illness. It is highly contagious.

INFECTION

An **infection** is a disease state resulting from the invasion and growth of microorganisms in the body (see Box 2.15). A *local infection* is in a body part, such as conjunctivitis, which is an infection of the eye. A *systemic infection* involves the whole body – examples are septicaemia and measles. **Signs** and **symptoms** of infection include:

- fever
- pain or tenderness
- redness and swelling of a body part

BOX 2.15
The older person and infections

The immune system works hard to protect us from infection and diseases. Just like other body systems, the immune system changes as we grow older. The older client who has an infection may not have signs and symptoms that are easily recognisable. There may be a slight fever but no pain, vomiting, swelling or redness. Sometimes there is confusion and delirium. This is most common in urinary tract infections of the older client. An infection can become life-threatening before the signs and symptoms are there to observe. It is important to be alert to even the most minor changes in behaviour or general condition. These observations must be reported to the registered nurse or enrolled nurse immediately.

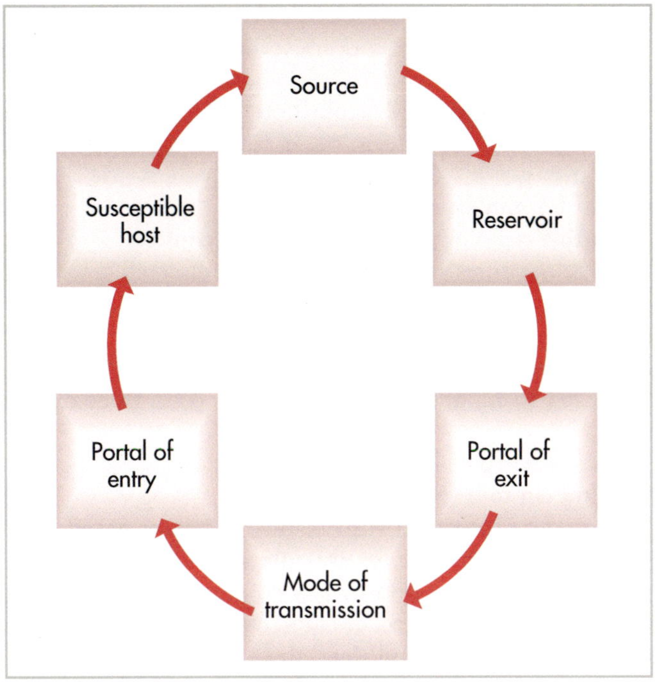

Fig. 2.46
The chain of infection.

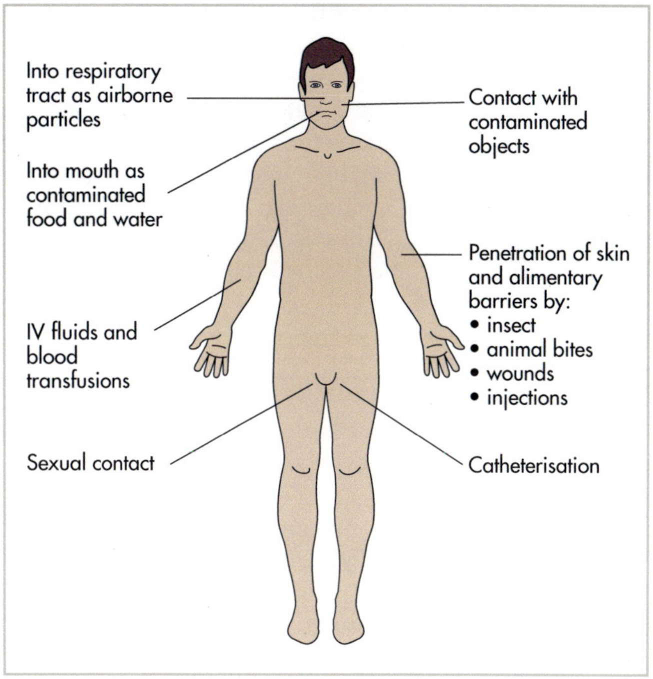

Fig. 2.47
Ways in which microorganisms enter the body.

- loss of appetite
- rash
- diarrhoea, nausea and/or vomiting
- sores in the mouth
- discharge or drainage from an affected area.

The chain of infection

The chain of infection (Fig. 2.46) is a process that requires all of the following:

- a source
- a reservoir
- a portal of exit
- a method of transmission
- a portal of entry
- a susceptible host.

Infection control is the process by which the chain of infection is broken. This is the ultimate goal for every staff member, including allied health workers, such as cleaners, catering staff and laundry staff. Infection control is achieved when all staff who deliver care ensure that pathogens are not transferred from one source to another. This includes pathogens that are present on a staff member's hands, gloves or equipment that the client comes in contact with.

As mentioned earlier, the source of infection is a pathogen, and the pathogen must have a reservoir where it can grow and multiply. If a person is acting as a reservoir for a pathogen, but does not have signs and symptoms of infection, they are known as a **carrier**. Carriers can pass on the pathogen to others. To leave the reservoir or the host, the pathogen needs a portal of exit. Exits can be the respiratory, gastrointestinal, urinary and reproductive tracts, breaks in the skin and, most importantly, blood and body fluids. After leaving the reservoir, the pathogen must be transmitted to another host. The pathogen must enter the body of the new host through a portal of entry (Fig. 2.47). Portals of entry and exit are the same. A susceptible host (a person at risk of infection) is needed for the microbe to grow and multiply.

The human body can protect itself from infection. A person's ability to resist infection depends on their age, nutritional status, stress, fatigue, immune status and general health. Certain medications can reduce a client's resistance to cross-infection. Disease and injury are also important factors.

Nosocomial infection

Clients can develop infections in healthcare settings. A **nosocomial infection** is an infection acquired after admission to a care service or a hospital (nosocomial comes from the Greek word for hospital). Nosocomial infections are caused by microorganisms transmitted to the person from another source, and these can be caused by normal flora. Remember, normal flora become pathogenic when transmitted from their natural site to another site or host. For example, *E. coli* is normally in the colon. Faeces (bowel movements) contain *E. coli*. Poor cleaning after bowel movements can cause *E. coli* to enter the urinary system. The hands can also transmit *E. coli* to other body areas. If handwashing is poor, *E. coli* can spread to any body part or anything the hands touch. It can also be transmitted to other people.

Microorganisms can enter the body through equipment used in treatments, therapies and tests. Therefore, equipment must be free of microorganisms. Staff can transfer microorganisms from one client to another and from themselves to the clients. Common sites for nosocomial infections are the urinary system, respiratory system, wounds and the bloodstream. As stated earlier, older people have a difficult time fighting infections. Therefore, the aged care team must prevent the spread of infection by breaking the chain.

INFECTION CONTROL PRECAUTIONS

Standard Precautions and additional precautions are infection control methods that apply to:

- blood
- body fluids, including secretions and saliva, regardless of whether you can actually see blood in the fluids
- non-intact skin
- mucous membranes (mouth, nose and body cavities).

Standard Precautions

Basic Standard Precautions include:

- handwashing
- environmental control – waste management
- disposal of sharps (e.g. needles and syringes or lancets)
- handling of linen and clients' clothing
- wearing of **personal protective equipment (PPE)**:
  - gloves
  - protective eye wear (not prescription glasses); glasses do not offer adequate protection against splashes to the face
  - plastic apron for protection from body fluids or hazardous chemicals; or, if necessary, a long-sleeved over gown
- staff immunisation
- routine cleaning and environmental control.

These measures are discussed in further detail below.

Additional precautions

Additional precautions are used when a client is known or suspected to be infected with a highly contagious disease that:

- is considered a significant infection risk
- is known to be highly contagious
- cannot be contained with Standard Precautions alone.

Additional precautions are intended to interrupt the transmission of infection by any combination of airborne, droplet, indirect or direct contact. Some examples of infectious or contagious conditions are:

- measles
- chickenpox
- methicillin-resistant *S. aureus*
- hepatitis infections
- HIV
- COVID-19 (Box 2.16).

Measures taken to provide additional precautions include *isolation precautions*: this means that the client is

BOX 2.16
Pandemics

A pandemic is defined as an epidemic that occurs worldwide and crosses international boundaries, affecting large numbers of people over very wide areas. This definition would seem to include seasonal epidemics such as seasonal influenza; however, seasonal epidemics are not considered pandemics because the traditional definition of a pandemic does not include the virology, disease severity or population immunity to the disease-causing pathogen. A pandemic occurs based on the rapid increase in the number of cases outside the initial outbreak zone, such as COVID-19.

COVID-19 is a disease caused by a new strain of coronavirus called SARS-CoV-2, identified late in 2019. It is transmitted through direct contact with respiratory droplets from an infected person (coughing and sneezing), but can also be transmitted through contact with a surface that has been contaminated with the virus (the individual then touches their face, nose or mouth). Common symptoms include fever, dry cough and fatigue, although symptoms may become severe to include shortness of breath, persistent pain or pressure in the chest and high temperature (above 38°C). Some individuals can continue to experience symptoms and side-effects long-term.

By September 2021, there were 237,383,711 confirmed cases of COVID-19 globally, and 4,842,716 reported deaths. Although individuals at any age can become seriously ill or die from COVID-19, people aged 60 years and over, and those with underlying health conditions such as high blood pressure, diabetes, heart and lung problems, obesity or cancer, are at higher risk of developing serious complications.

The transmission of COVID-19 can be reduced by practising physical distancing, wearing a mask (especially when distancing cannot be maintained), keeping rooms well ventilated, avoiding crowds and close contact, regularly washing and sanitising hands, coughing into a bent elbow or tissue and staying home if unwell. Individuals with symptoms should be tested and those who have been in close contact with someone who is, or may be, infected should get tested. While a person is waiting for test results, they should remain isolated from others. Testing should be prioritised for those at higher risk of infection, such as health workers, and those at higher risk of severe illness, such as the elderly and those living in aged or long-term care services.

BOX 2.16
Pandemics *continued*

Healthcare workers must adhere to precautions when providing care within the aged or community care setting to prevent transmission. It is important to follow service protocols for screening prior to providing care to clients as part of risk management planning.

To reduce the spread of COVID-19 when providing care:

- receive COVID-19 vaccination
- stay home from work if you are sick
- perform hand hygiene frequently (before and after attending clients and after contact with potentially contaminated surfaces)
- follow respiratory hygiene and cough etiquette
- ensure physical distancing from other staff and clients except when providing care
- wear gloves and a gown or apron to handle and dispose of waste and used linen in designated bags and bins
- close bags and bins and perform hand hygiene after every contact
- clean and disinfect all shared equipment.

Where a client is suspected or confirmed to have COVID-19, the following precautions must be taken when entering the client's room or living area:

- Perform hand hygiene.
- Put on a gown (fluid-resistant long-sleeved gown or apron).
- Put on a P2/N95 respirator mask.
- Check the fit of the P2/N95 respirator mask.
- Perform hand hygiene again after mask has been fitted.
- Put on eyewear then gloves.

The following precautions must be taken after care has been provided:

- Remove and dispose of gloves and gown.
- Remove eyewear and place in designated container.
- Remove and dispose of mask.
- Perform hand hygiene.

It is also important to:

- never touch the front of the mask after the fit is completed and while providing care
- change the mask when it becomes wet or dirty
- never reuse masks
- keep doors of rooms closed if possible
- change into clean clothes at work when your shift finishes and put your clothes in a plastic bag. Go straight home and shower immediately. Wash your work clothes and the clothes you wore home immediately.

Source: World Health Organisation (WHO) (2021). Coronavirus disease (COVID-19) dashboard. Online. Available: https://covid19.who.int; Australian Commission on Safety and Quality in Health Care (ACSQHC) (2020). COVID-19 precautions for staff. Online. Available: www.safetyandquality.gov.au/sites/default/files/2020-08/PPE-Aged-Care_COVID-19-Poster.pdf

removed from a shared bedroom area. In this situation, the client who has an infectious or contagious condition is cared for by one member of staff per shift and the following measures are observed:

- Hands are washed outside the room and PPE is worn when entering the room.
- Delivery of linen and supplies to the room are carried out using a separate hatched servery or by passing the linen or supplies to the carer, who receives these supplies through the doorway. In this instance, the delivery person washes their hands thoroughly once the supplies have been taken.
- Catering services are notified of the isolation precautions so that staff can observe the precautions when delivering food and fluids. Disposable equipment is not necessary in this situation. Catering staff wear clean gloves in their line of work and so they are instructed to remove the gloves once they have made their delivery to the isolated client, and to wash their hands and reapply a new set of gloves to continue their work. It is important to remember that the isolated client could be feeling quite anxious and depressed due to this type of separation from peers and the general community. It is essential to demonstrate compassion and understanding at this time. The client has to cope with the knowledge that they have a communicable condition, as well as coping with the illness itself.

Hand hygiene

Your hands are exposed to every kind of microorganism. They are easily contaminated. Most importantly, your hands are your first line of defence against infections and cross-contamination. Your hands can spread microorganisms if they are not washed correctly before and after giving care. You should take great care of your hands. Your skin must be intact when caring for your clients. If you have any breaks in the skin or any wounds on your hands, you must cover these areas with a waterproof dressing, such as a Tegaderm or Opsite.

Handwashing with soap and water is the easiest and most important way to prevent the spread of infection (Box 2.17). You must practise handwashing before and after giving care to each client. You use your hands in almost every task. They can pick up microorganisms from one person, place or item and then transfer them to other people, places or items. Hand care is, therefore, essential. You should moisturise your hands regularly to maintain the integrity of your skin.

BOX 2.17
Rules of handwashing

- Wash your hands under warm running water.
- Stand away from the sink. Do not let your hands, body or work clothes touch the sink. The sink is contaminated.
- Rub your palms together to work up a good lather. The rubbing action helps remove microorganisms and dirt.
- Pay attention to areas often missed during handwashing: pads of the thumbs, knuckles, sides of the hands, webbing in between the fingers, little fingers, around the nail cuticles and under the nails.
- Use a nail file to clean under your fingernails. Microorganisms grow easily under the fingernails.
- Wash your hands for at least 15 seconds (the time it takes to sing 'Happy Birthday'). Wash your hands longer if they are dirty or soiled with blood or body fluids. This might be the case if you are caught unprepared and have no time to put gloves on. Your first priority after settling the client is to wash your hands.
- Dry your hands starting at the fingers. Work up to your forearms. In this way, you will dry the cleanest area first.
- Use a clean paper towel for each tap to turn water off. Taps are contaminated. Using paper towels prevents clean hands from becoming contaminated again.
- Apply hand lotion or cream after handwashing. This prevents skin chapping and drying. Skin breaks can occur in chapped and dry skin. Skin breaks are portals of entry for microorganisms.

HANDWASHING PROCEDURE

1. Make sure you have soap, paper towels or nail file, and a waste bin. Collect missing items.
2. Push your watch up 10–15 cm. Also push up uniform sleeves.
3. Stand away from the sink so your clothes do not touch it. Stand so the soap and tap are easy to reach.
4. Turn on and adjust the water until it feels warm.
5. Wet your wrists and hands under running water. Keep your hands lower than your elbows (Fig. 2.48).
6. Apply about 1 teaspoon of soap to your hands.
7. Rub your palms together and interlace your fingers to work up a good lather (Fig. 2.49). This step should last at least 15 seconds.
8. Wash each hand and wrist thoroughly. Clean well between the fingers, and around the cuticles of each fingernail.
9. Clean under the fingernails by rubbing your fingertips against your palms (Fig. 2.50).
10. Clean under the fingernails with a nail file (Fig. 2.51). This step is necessary for the first handwashing of the day and when your hands are highly soiled.
11. Rinse your wrists and hands well. Water should flow from the arms to the hands.
12. Repeat steps 6 through 11, if needed.
13. Dry your wrists and hands with paper towels. Pat dry, starting at your fingertips.
14. Discard the paper towels.
15. Turn off taps with clean paper towels (Fig. 2.52). This prevents you from contaminating your hands. Use a clean paper towel for each tap.
16. Discard paper towels.

There may be occasions in the home environment when running water is not available, or the bathroom services are extremely dirty. An antimicrobial hand gel such as Microshield, which does not require water, can be used as an alternative. This is not suitable if the hands are visibly soiled. It is important that the hands are washed with running water as soon as possible.

When to wash your hands

To prevent the spread of microorganisms, wash your hands:

- before and after giving care to each client
- after a visit to the toilet
- after changing a tampon or sanitary pad
- after contact with your own or another person's blood or body fluids – this includes saliva, vomit, urine, faeces, vaginal discharge, mucus, tears, semen, wound drainage and respiratory secretions
- after coughing, sneezing or blowing your nose
- before and after handling, preparing or eating food
- after handling soiled or contaminated equipment, used linen or pets
- whenever your hands feel dirty or are visibly soiled
- before and after wearing gloves.

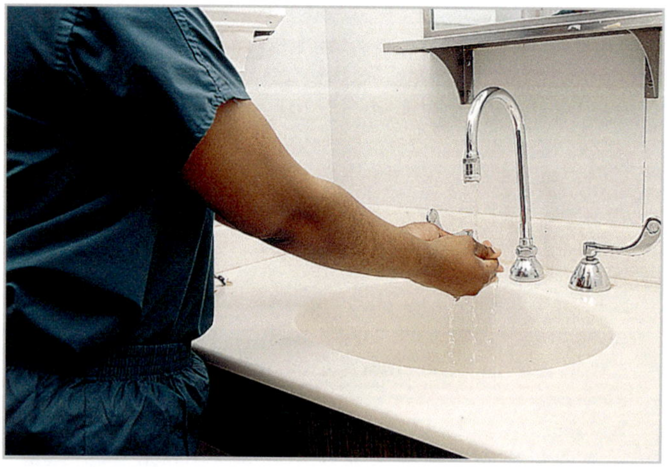

Fig. 2.48
The uniform does not touch the sink. Hands are lower than the elbows.

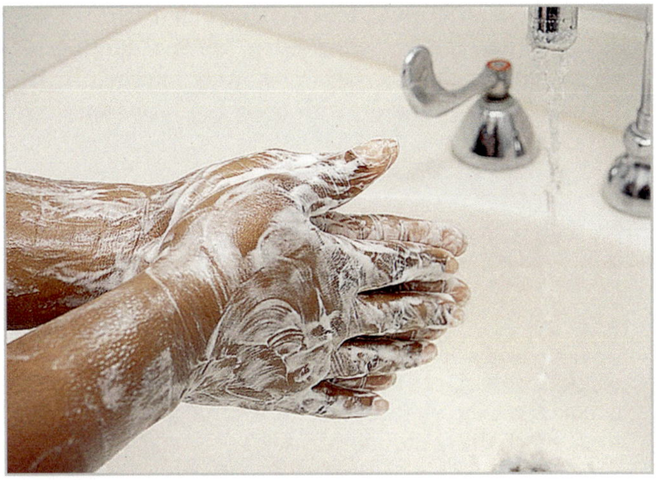

Fig. 2.49
The palms are rubbed together for a good lather.

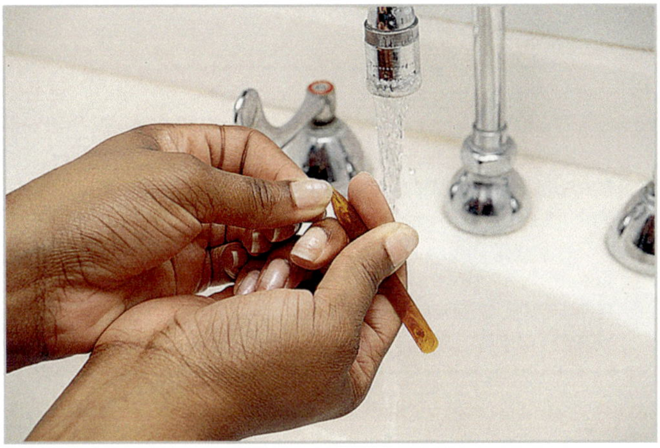

Fig. 2.51
A nail file is used to clean under the fingernails.

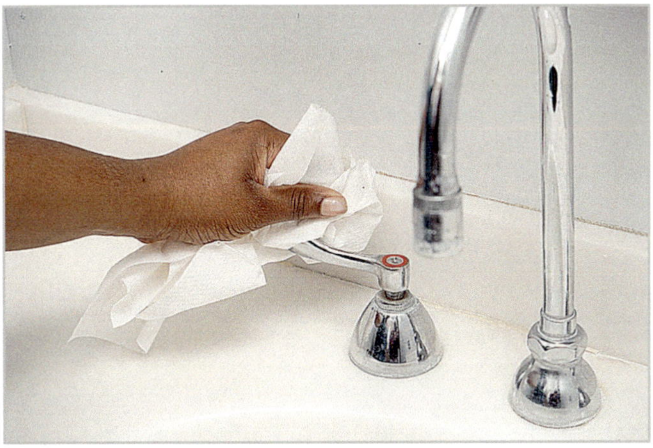

Fig. 2.52
A paper towel is used to turn off the tap.

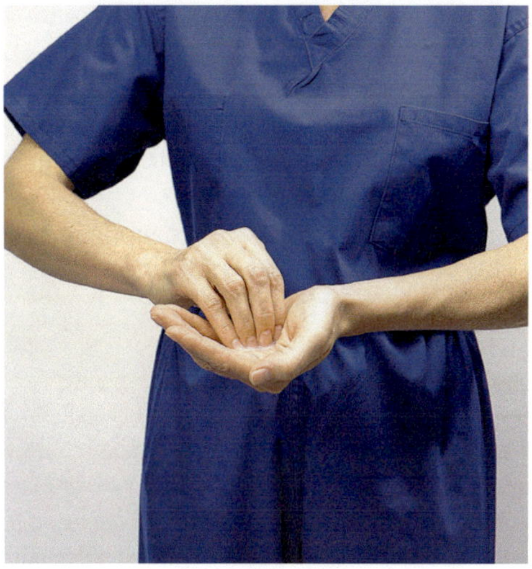

Fig. 2.50
Fingertips are rubbed against the palms to clean underneath the nails.

HANDY HINT

How long should you wash your hands for? The answer is simple and easy to remember. You should wash your hands for the same amount of time that it takes you to sing the song 'Happy Birthday to You'. This will ensure that you wash for the correct time.

Gloves

The skin is a natural barrier and helps prevent microorganisms from entering the body. Small skin breaks on the hands and fingers are common. Some are very small and hard to see. Disposable gloves give added protection if you are anticipating exposure to body fluids. Wear gloves whenever contact is likely with blood, body fluids, secretions, excretions, mucous membranes and non-intact skin. Contact may be direct, or may be with items or surfaces contaminated with blood or body fluids. Gloves should also be worn if you are:

- cleaning a client who has been incontinent of faeces or urine
- handling soiled, used linen
- handling urinals or bed pans
- handling emesis containers
- handling blood-soaked dressings.

Do not tear gloves when putting them on. Carelessness, long fingernails and rings can tear gloves. Blood and body fluids can enter the glove through the tear and contaminate the hand. When wearing gloves, remember the following:

- Put on gloves when your hands are dry.
- You need a new pair for every client.
- Remove and discard torn, cut or punctured gloves immediately – you are your hands. Then put on a new pair.
- Put on clean gloves just before touching mucous membranes or non-intact skin.

- Put on new gloves whenever gloves become contaminated with blood, body fluids, secretions or excretions. You may need more than one pair of gloves for a task.
- Make sure gloves cover your wrists.
- Remove gloves so the inside part that has been against your hand is on the outside.
- Wash your hands thoroughly after removing gloves.
- Wear gloves when you expect contact with blood or other potentially infectious materials.
- Wear gloves when handling or touching contaminated items or surfaces.
- Replace worn, punctured or contaminated gloves.
- Never wash or decontaminate disposable gloves for reuse.
- Discard utility gloves that show signs of cracking, peeling, tearing or puncturing. Utility gloves are decontaminated for reuse if the process will not ruin them. This means that they can be washed with warm soapy water and allowed to dry thoroughly on the inside and outside surfaces.
- Wear gloves once only. Discard them after use.
- It is not necessary to wear gloves when attending to a client's hygiene needs. Gloves are only required if there is risk of contamination with body fluids or secretions.

SAFETY ALERT

Gloves

Gloves are often made of latex (a rubber product). Some people are allergic to latex. It can cause skin rashes, asthma and shock. Report skin rashes and difficulty breathing to the nurse immediately.

If you have a latex allergy, you need to wear latex-free gloves. Some clients are allergic to latex. This information is on the care plan and in your client's Health History.

REMOVING GLOVES

1. Make sure that glove only touches glove. Do not let gloves touch the skin on your wrists or arms.
2. Grasp a glove just below the cuff. Grasp it on the outside (Fig. 2.53A).
3. Pull the glove down over your hand, so it is inside out (Fig. 2.53B).
4. Hold the removed glove with your other gloved hand.
5. Reach inside the other glove (Fig. 2.53C). Use the first two fingers of your ungloved hand.
6. Pull the glove down (inside out) over your hand and the other glove (Fig. 2.53D).
7. Discard the gloves into a contaminated waste receptacle or special waste bag.
8. Wash your hands.

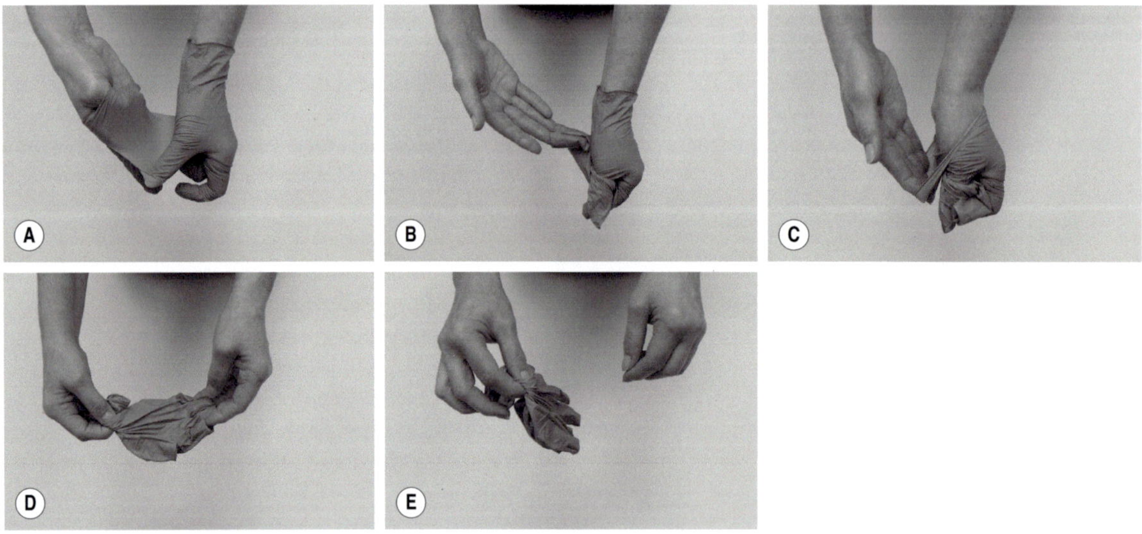

Fig. 2.53
Removing (doffing) gloves.
A. The glove is held below the cuff. **B.** The glove is pulled down over the hand. The glove is inside out. **C.** The fingers of the ungloved hand are inserted inside the other glove. **D.** The glove is pulled down and over the hand and the glove. The glove is inside out. **E.** Safe method of holding contaminated gloves. Touch only the inside surface during disposal. Hands should be washed promptly.

Face masks, eye protection, face shields, aprons

Face masks are worn for protection from airborne or droplet infection. As a carer, you should not be required to wear a face mask unless you are caring for a client who has a **communicable disease** that could be transmitted by coughing or sneezing, or you have been asked to remove a dressing from a wound or to empty a drainage bag where there is a risk of body fluid splashes.

Eye protection is worn when there is risk or a need for protection from splashes or sprays of blood or body fluids. Prescription glasses are not adequate protection. Goggles or special eye shields are supplied by the employer. However, some healthcare workers choose to purchase their own if they find themselves wearing eye protection every day.

Face shields are another form of protection similar to goggles or eye shields. A face shield is usually an all-in-one piece of protective equipment that is attached to a face mask. The mask protects against splashes around the mouth and nose. The shield is made of clear plastic and provides protection from splashes to the eyes without making it difficult for the carer to see what they are doing.

Plastic aprons are worn by carers when they are involved in the following duties:

- showering clients or bed sponging an immobile client
- cleaning and attending to spills involving body fluids or dangerous chemicals
- emptying drainage bags, such as urinary catheter bags
- cleaning duties, such as cleaning the utility, pan room, bathrooms or toilets.

WEARING A FACE MASK CORRECTLY

To wear a face mask correctly

1. Practise hand hygiene.
2. Pick up the mask by its upper ties. Do not touch the part that covers your face.
3. Place the mask over your nose and mouth (Fig. 2.54A).
4. Place the upper strings over your ears. Tie the strings at the back towards the top of your head (Fig. 2.54B).
5. Tie the lower strings at the back of your neck (Fig. 2.54C). The lower part is under your chin.
6. Pinch the metal band around your nose. The top of the mask must be snug over your nose. If you wear glasses, it must be snug under their bottom edges.
7. Decontaminate your hands.
8. Provide care. Avoid coughing, sneezing and unnecessary talking.
9. Change the mask if it becomes moist or contaminated.

Remove the mask as follows:

1. Remove the gloves. Decontaminate your hands.
2. Untie the lower strings.
3. Untie the top strings.
4. Hold the top strings. Remove the mask.
5. Bring the strings together. The inside of the mask folds together (Fig. 2.54D). Do not touch the inside of the mask.
6. Discard the mask following agency policy.
7. Decontaminate your hands.

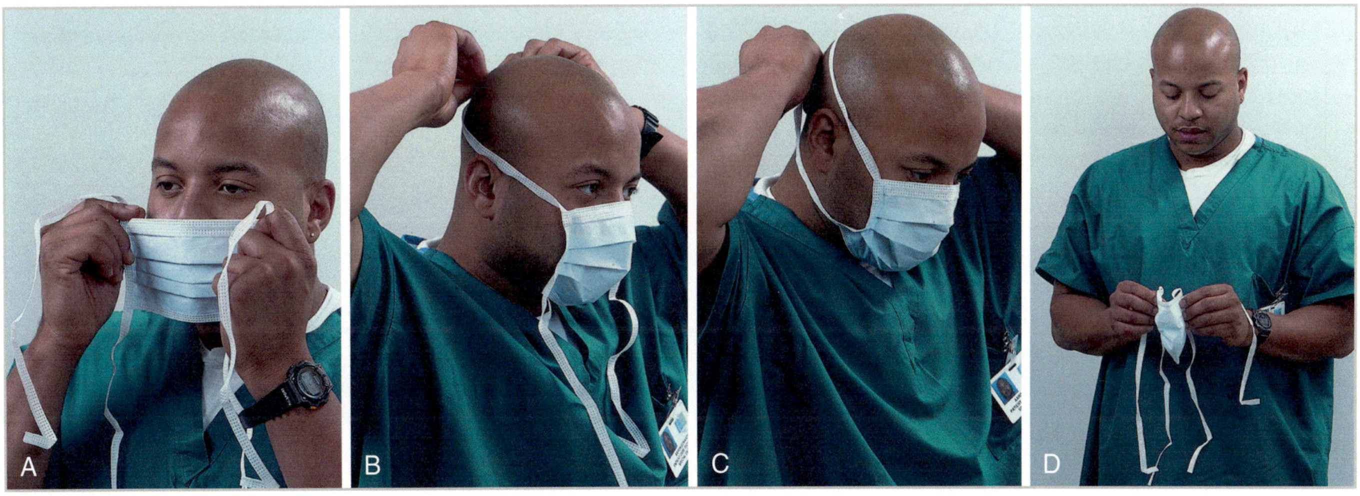

Fig. 2.54
Donning a mask.
A. The mask covers the nose and mouth. **B.** Upper strings are tied at the back of the head. **C.** Lower strings are tied at the back of the neck. **D.** The inside of the mask is folded together after removal.

ENVIRONMENTAL CONTROL AND CONTAMINATED WASTE

Good housekeeping, hygienic care and handling of laundry and correct disposal of waste are all essential elements of infection control. Waste should be segregated at the point of generation. Most healthcare services and aged care services use appropriately colour-coded and labelled containers. Waste is to be appropriately segregated as follows:

- *General waste* (usually in a container with a black or green bag) – this is waste that does not fall into any of the categories listed below. It is general waste that has not come into contact with blood or body fluids. The best examples are wrapping, packaging or paper and envelopes used for administration. Paper hand towels used for drying your hands also fall into this category, because the paper towel has only been used to dry your hands, not to mop up a body fluid spill.
- *Infectious or pathological waste* (usually yellow or red plastic bags) – often referred to as 'clinical waste'. This must be placed in bags or containers bearing the international biohazard symbol and marked 'infectious waste'. This includes: clinical waste, which means waste materials such as wound dressings or dressing sets; incontinence pads and combine pads used to soak up body fluids; tubing and devices that have been in direct contact with a client's body cavity, such as urinary catheters; and gloves used to clean up a soiled bed or a body fluid spill.
- *Sharps waste* (usually a yellow container with a red or white lid) – sharps are any object or device capable of cutting or penetrating the skin, such as: needles; syringes; broken glass; razor blades; scalpel blades or stitch cutters; lancets. All sharps must be disposed of in a sharps container that meets Australian Standard AS/NZS 4187:2014. A sharps container should be taken to the site of the sharp, for example, to the bedside of a client receiving an injection. They must not be overfilled as this increases the risk of needle-stick injury. Sharps represent one of the major causes of accidents involving potential exposure to blood-borne diseases. Therefore, it is essential that sharps be disposed of appropriately. Needles are never re-capped once they have been used to deliver medication to a client. The person using or administering a needle or syringe is responsible for its safe disposal.
- *Chemical waste* (usually purple or black container) – this includes chemical waste, solvents, alcohols and disinfectants.
- *Pharmaceutical waste* (usually black bag or container) – this includes hazardous and non-hazardous drugs, remedies, and medications partially dispensed, expired or no longer required by clients or health care services.
- *Cytotoxic waste* (usually purple bag or container) – includes medications and equipment used in chemotherapy and the treatment of cancer.

Spills management

Standard Precautions apply where there is a spill of blood or body fluids. PPE must be worn when cleaning up such a spill. It is important to deal with spills immediately and minimise traffic around the spills area until it is resolved. It is ideal to use paper towels and to have the contaminated waste bin close to where you are cleaning the spill. *Hot, soapy water* is the most effective treatment to use when dealing with spills that involve blood or body fluids (Box 2.18).

Linen and laundry services

Aged care services and organisations have documented policies regarding procedures for the collection, transport, processing and storage of linen.

- Clean linen is always kept separate from linen that is soiled or dirty.
- If used linen must be sorted, it is very important that you wear appropriate PPE to carry out this task. Aprons must be worn to carry out this task. Gloves should be of industrial quality, not the gloves worn for general care of clients. If soiled linen must be transported, it should be bagged in leak-proof plastic bags. Soiled linen should never be held close to your body. Linen skips (linen bags on wheels) should never be overfilled and should be wheeled to the place where the beds are being changed. Used laundry should never be shaken or thrown because this will disperse microorganisms in the air and create an infection risk to clients. Dirty linen should never be placed on the floor just because it is deemed dirty. This practice is contrary to current standards of infection control. Soiled linen must be placed in the correct colour-coded linen bags.
- In the home environment, soiled linen must be processed using gloves and PPE where necessary. Debulking of faecal material or blood clots into the toilet is recommended prior to cleaning the item using laundry services.
- Bath towels should never be used to soak up a body fluid spill, nor should feeding towels or clothing protectors.
- In the home environment, water temperature and detergents should be checked to ensure that they meet the appropriate standards.

BOX 2.18
Managing exposure to blood and/or body substances

- Adherence to infection control practices, including standard precautions, remains the first line of protection against occupational exposure to blood-borne viruses. If you are accidentally exposed, the following immediate actions should be taken:
  - Wash needlestick injury or cut with soap and water.
  - Spit fluid out or blow nose, then rinse with water several times.
  - Irrigate eyes with water or saline, gently and thoroughly.
  - Report the incident immediately to the nurse or manager.

- Laundries must be checked annually for pests and correction or maintenance as required.
- Washing machines should never be overfilled.
- Regular cleaning of storage areas, trolleys and vehicles is important. Clean and dirty laundry are always processed or transported in separate areas.

STAFF HEALTH AND INFECTIOUS DISEASES

Maintenance of a safe working environment for staff and clients requires coordination between management, healthcare workers and support services, so that the risk of transmission and spread of infection is minimised. Healthcare services and aged care services have an infection control officer, who is usually a registered nurse. One of the responsibilities of this position is coordination of and record keeping for staff immunisation. The infection control officer delivers education to staff and is responsible for the infection control orientation of new staff, in addition to ongoing education. It is also important for staff working in the healthcare setting to maintain personal health and hygiene by:

- getting immunised (as outlined).
- reporting any illness to the nurse or manager. Do not attend work if you are unwell.
- maintaining good health. Eat a healthy balanced diet, get plenty of sleep/rest and regular exercise.
- practising good personal hygiene. Bathe or shower daily, keep your hair clean and neat, keep nails short and clean, do not wear nail polish or false nails to work, wear a clean uniform every day and wear minimal jewellery.

Gastrointestinal infections are transmitted by contact, oral–faecal transmission or airborne transmission of viral gastrointestinal infections. Transmission is prevented by using **Standard Precautions**, personal hygiene practices and isolation precautions if necessary.

Vaccination of staff does not mean that Standard Precautions are no longer necessary. Vaccination ensures immunity. Infection control practices are vital to prevent the spread of diseases.

Hepatitis B vaccination

Hepatitis B is an inflammatory disease of the liver. It is caused by the hepatitis B virus (HBV). HBV is usually transmitted by exposure to contaminated blood – for example, when medication users share contaminated needles. It is also transmitted by sexual contact.

The hepatitis B vaccine produces immunity against hepatitis B. **Immunity** means that an individual has protection against a specific disease – that is, they will not contract or be affected by the disease. A **vaccine** is a preparation that contains dead or weakened microorganisms. The hepatitis B vaccine is recommended for all healthcare workers.

The hepatitis B vaccination involves three injections. The second injection is given 1 month after the first one. The third injection is given 6 months after the second one. The vaccination can be given before or after exposure to HBV. Some employers pay for their staff to be vaccinated.

Other vaccinations

- *Hepatitis C (HCV)* – there is no immunisation for HCV. This is a blood-borne virus transmitted by direct contact with blood. It is an inflammatory disease of the liver and is highly contagious. Transmission is prevented by using Standard Precautions. Staff who are likely to perform exposure-prone procedures have a responsibility to know their hepatitis C status.
- *Human Immunodeficiency Virus (HIV)* – active immunisation for HIV is not available. This is a blood-borne virus transmitted by direct contact with blood and body fluids. Transmission is prevented by using Standard Precautions.
- *Influenza* – the influenza vaccine is recommended for all healthcare workers. It is given annually. Many healthcare organisations offer it to their staff prior to the winter influenza season.
- *Measles, mumps, rubella and varicella (MMRV)* – these vaccinations are recommended for healthcare workers who have no history of chickenpox infection or shingles.
- *Tuberculosis (BCG)* – vaccination may be required in some instances. Discuss this with your doctor.
- *Tetanus (dT)* – vaccination is recommended for gardening and maintenance staff only. A booster of adult diphtheria and tetanus vaccine is required every 10 years.
- *COVID-19* – vaccination recommended for all staff.

CLEANING: AN ESSENTIAL ELEMENT OF INFECTION CONTROL

In providing home care it is essential to maintain high standards of cleaning. This will require some problem-solving because you may not have access to a dirty room and a clean room. Some homes will have a spacious bathroom where you can clean a wash bowl or scrub out a commode chair pan. Remember to maintain Standard Precautions at all times while cleaning these items. Your plastic apron, goggles and gloves must be worn. Wherever possible, use toilet paper to initially remove body fluids. The toilet paper can be flushed down the toilet or placed in a plastic bag for disposal. Remember to wash your hands after removing your gloves and to dispose of your plastic apron and gloves appropriately. Reusable items can be cleaned with chemical **disinfectants** or **neutral detergents**. Such items include:

- blood pressure cuffs
- commodes and the pan insert
- chairs
- bedside tabletops
- wheelchairs
- stretchers
- room furniture.

Chemical disinfectants can burn and irritate the skin. Wear utility gloves or rubber household gloves to prevent skin irritation. These gloves are waterproof. Do not wear disposable gloves when using disinfectants. Some chemical disinfectants have special measures for use or storage. Check the material safety data sheet (MSDS) before handling a disinfectant.

FOCUS ON COMMUNITY CARE

When caring for a client within their home, it is essential that a safety audit is done on the premises before the first episode of care. Many homes have areas of risk for carers; for example, loose mats are easy to pull and trip over. The water temperature is often not stable in older homes and care needs to be taken when showering the client. Electrical appliances can have frayed cords or faulty plugs, and wooden stairs and ramps can be unsteady, rotten or without handrails. If there are obvious areas of risk, they will need to be identified and rectified before delivering care.

When undertaking manual handling activities in the community, the carer must also be very careful. Often a client with a long-term disability will have specific manual handling devices, such as hoists, and their home may have been adapted to minimise manual handling risks. However, the carer will often be asked to undertake manual handling activities in situations where some risk may still be evident. For example, the height of the bed may not be able to be adjusted, or you may have to assist your client into and out of a bath. Never undertake these activities unless you have been shown a method that minimises the risk to you and your client. Always use the principles of manual handling and never attempt any activity where you may harm either yourself or your client. Always carefully check any equipment used to ensure it is working correctly. The home situation can be quite cluttered, and it may be necessary to move furniture out of the way prior to manual handling tasks.

When undertaking care tasks in the community or within a client's home, cleanliness and hygiene are essential in order to prevent infection and **contamination**. Bathroom cleaning is an important step in reducing the risk of cross-contamination in the client's home or care service. Microorganisms can flourish in any bathroom if it is dirty and if there are hair and contaminated items, such as cotton tips or used make-up pads. Essential measures to help reduce the risk of infection are as follows:

- Flush the toilet with the lid down. This prevents airborne droplets from contaminating surfaces such as door handles or sinks in the bathroom.
- Clean out sinks, bathtubs and shower recesses after each use.
- Remove hair and place it in a garbage receptacle using gloves and disposable tissue paper.
- Clean mirrors and towel racks daily with a neutral detergent.
- Clean toilet seats daily, brush the toilet bowl thoroughly and clean it with a chlorine solution.
- Occasionally, carers may be required to purchase or prepare food for clients. When grocery shopping, the following guidelines are recommended to prevent illness caused by poorly prepared or packaged foods:
  - Do not purchase produce that is bruised or damaged in any way.
  - Do not purchase processed foods that have loose or bulging lids, or cracked, dented or torn packaging.
  - Do not buy out-dated foods. Check the expiry date and do not purchase any product that has passed its expiry date, as the product may be unsafe for consumption.
  - Buy processed foods first and leave the frozen or refrigerated foods until last. This way the refrigerated foods will be more likely to maintain their low temperature, and this in turn will reduce the growth of microorganisms.
  - Collect fruit and vegetable selection bags to use as a cover for your meat purchases when you visit the butchery. Place your clear plastic bag over the packaged meat to prevent any blood or animal fluids contaminating other foods in your trolley.
  - Open egg cartons and check the eggs before buying them. Store eggs in their original carton. Use them within 3 weeks. Do not use an egg that is a strange colour or has unusual markings.
  - Store fresh, frozen and refrigerated foods promptly. Do not leave these foods in your car for lengthy periods.
  - Wash your hands before handling and preparing food. Wash your hands immediately after preparing foods such as raw meat, poultry or seafood.
  - Cutting boards should be dedicated to certain foods: a separate cutting board should be dedicated to red meat and this should be made from marble or a non-porous material.
  - Do not use cutting boards or cooking vessels with cracks or crevices, as this is where microorganisms flourish.
  - Wash cutting boards thoroughly and, if possible, place in the dishwasher for decontamination. If there is no dishwasher, use hot soapy water and scrub any food particles off the board.
  - Wash and thoroughly clean kitchen benches following food preparation.
  - Wash fresh fruit and vegetables thoroughly. Rinse them in warm water and use a scrubbing brush dedicated to this procedure if necessary.
  - Leftover foods should be used within 48 hours and should be labelled with the date and sealed correctly.
  - If a meal is not consumed immediately following cooking, it should be sealed and refrigerated within 20 minutes, to reduce the growth of harmful microorganisms.
  - Thawed foods should never be refrozen. There are no exceptions to this rule.
  - Dishcloths and tea towels should be laundered daily. It is important to wash items in a washing machine and to dry them in the sunshine if possible.
  - Kitchen sinks should be cleaned thoroughly with a scourer following each use.
  - Fatty surfaces of frying pans and baking dishes should be wiped with a paper towel prior to being cleaned in hot soapy water.
  - Garbage receptacles should be emptied daily and the receptacle itself should be washed regularly, paying special attention to the lid or surface areas at the opening of the receptacle.

QUALITY OF LIFE

Most accidents can be prevented. Promote safety by knowing the common safety hazards and causes of accidents, knowing who needs protection and using common sense. Remember that clients who are older and disabled are at great risk of accidents. Chronic illness, advanced age, disability, medications, strange surroundings and special equipment increase a client's risk of injury. Practise safety measures. Use safety devices as needed. Encourage clients to use hand rails and walkers or canes to assist them with walking. Follow the client's care plan to ensure safe care. You must identify the client before giving care. A client's life and health can be threatened if the wrong care is given or if care is omitted. Two clients in the same aged care service could have the same last name. Some may have the same first and last names.

Prevent fires by following the safety measures for smoking and electrical items. Extra measures are needed when oxygen is used. Consumers who smoke present fire safety concerns. Be sure you know where to find fire alarms, fire extinguishers and emergency exits. Also know your aged care service's procedures for dealing with a fire.

Know and follow procedures for handling hazardous substances. Physical hazards can cause fires and explosions. Exposure to some chemicals can cause acute or chronic health problems. Workplace violence is a danger in any healthcare setting. Know and practise measures to prevent and control workplace violence. Everyone must keep the aged care service safe for clients, visitors and staff.

The aged care standards require that aged care services provide care in a manner that maintains and improves each client's quality of life, health and safety. Proper manual handling and body mechanics protect the client from injuries that could affect their health and ability to function. You must protect the client's right to privacy at all times. Screen the client properly. Expose only the body part involved in the procedure. Close doors, curtains and drapes. Pull window shades as needed. The client's rights are also protected by allowing personal choice whenever possible. As long as safety is not affected, allow the client to choose such things as bed positions, where the chair or wheelchair is positioned and when to get up or go back to bed. Always check with the care plan to make sure the client's choices are safe. Also, let the client help in moving and transferring procedures to the extent possible.

The client also has the right to be free from restraint. Bed rails are considered restraints. They are used only with the client's consent. Many manual handling procedures involve raising the bed for good body mechanics and to ensure safety. Always check with the nurse and the care plan about using bed rails. If the client does not use bed rails and you need to raise the bed, you should have a co-worker help you. Your co-worker stands on the other side of the bed to protect the client from falling from that side. When you use bed rails, always explain to the client why you are using them.

CASE STUDY

Case study 1

You are caring for Margery Shaw in her home. This is your first visit there and you are required to attend to her hygiene needs and do some basic housekeeping. Her house is fairly isolated and there are not many other houses around. As you walk in the door, you notice that she has an oxygen cylinder in the lounge beside her chair. Next to her chair there is also an unemptied ashtray. When you go to tidy her kitchen, you notice that she has her cleaning products placed in the same cupboard as her breakfast cereals and biscuits. Margery has both a bath and a shower, but has considerable difficulty getting into and out of the bath. She tells you that she prefers baths.

Before you start your work, you realise that you need to advise your supervisor and speak to her about some safety issues. In consultation with Margery and your supervisor, the following plan of action is developed:

- You are to take a mobile phone with you on all occasions, and your time of arrival and departure is always known by your supervisor.
- Margery is encouraged to smoke outside the lounge only, and never when the oxygen cylinder is in use.
- Margery is to choose one high cupboard, which is to be cleared of all food items and used solely for storing cleaning products and other chemicals.
- Margery is to have showers only and is not to attempt to get into the bath.

By identifying actual and potential hazards within your workplace, you have helped to prevent serious or even fatal accidents from occurring which could harm both your client and yourself. As your workplace is also the home of a client, all hazard identification and rectifying actions were done in consultation with your client, Margery.

Case study 2

You are working in a large consumer aged care service and have noticed that one of the long-term consumers is becoming less steady when walking. Mr Olly is 84 years old, is very self-sufficient and lives in the independent living section of the service. You know he is fearful of having to move from his current unit into higher care options within the service, but you are also concerned that he may fall. After discussions with the multidisciplinary team in the aged care service, a safety audit is conducted of his unit to ensure his current needs are being met. Some additional equipment is installed into his unit and Mr Olly is assured that he is able to stay in his unit, with this additional equipment and more support from the staff. Mr Olly's safety is of prime importance, but also to ensure he retains his independence.

Case study 3

You are working a morning shift in a consumer aged care service and are assigned to care for Mr David Fabiani. Mr Fabiani is a rather tall man and he has suffered a stroke in the past few weeks. Prior to this recent stroke, he was ambulating with just one assistant and the use of a walking belt.

Morning handover included a report on Mr Fabiani which described his previous night's sleep as being quite good, with no complaints of any discomfort. Mr Fabiani's care plan indicates that two carers are required to handle client transfers and hygiene needs. Routinely, after breakfast, he is positioned to sit up on the side of the bed and then he is transferred to the standing lifter. From the standing lifter he is transferred to a shower chair and carefully wheeled into the shower.

When you and your co-worker go into Mr Fabiani's room, you notice that he is unable to bend his good leg and that he is unable to grip with one of his hands.

At this point, you go to the registered nurse on duty to ask her to check your client. The registered nurse examines Mr Fabiani and decides that he may have suffered an extension of his first stroke. After completing a set of clinical observations, she calls the doctor to come and review Mr Fabiani as soon as possible.

The action that you took was correct and demonstrated professionalism and a high standard of care. The most important message in this scenario is that the client's condition can and does change and that the care plan might then be incorrect. The care plan is valuable, but you must assess each client individually before proceeding with a manual handling procedure.

If you had continued according to the care plan and failed to observe and report the serious changes in your client's condition, there would have been a disastrous accident. The standing lifter is appropriate only for clients who can take their own weight once they are lifted to a standing position.

Case study 4

You arrive at work at the Lewisham Retirement Village to find that a new client has been admitted earlier that day. The new client, Mrs Mae Lau, has been admitted into a twin room with Mrs Xia Tran. Mrs Lau has bandages on both legs, where she has ulcers from small veins that have burst. The bandages are quite moist with wound drainage, and the nursing staff from the hospital she had been admitted from had rebandaged over them to try to contain the drainage and make Mrs Lau feel better about how her legs look.

Mrs Tran has a urinary catheter that comes out of the lower abdomen and drains her urine into a bag. The catheter site is dressed daily by the registered and enrolled nurses. The doctor who was in charge of transferring Mrs Lau from the city hospital did not mention to any of the staff members at Lewisham Retirement Village that Mrs Lau's leg wounds are being treated for a resistant organism called MRSA (methicillin-resistant *Staphylococcus aureus*).

As you have not cared for Mrs Lau before, you read her notes before starting to give care. Several weeks previously, you attended an infection control in-services program and are well aware of the additional precautions that apply to clients who have MRSA. Without making a fuss, you bring this matter to the attention of the registered nurse who has come on duty, and arrangements are made to move Mrs Lau to a single room.

Mrs Lau would have been able to share a room with another client who had the same resistant organism, but not with Mrs Tran. Mrs Tran does not have any infection present in her abdominal wound where the catheter is inserted. Her abdominal wound could have become contaminated, even if vigilant handwashing and Standard Precautions were undertaken. By using your understanding of infection control principles, you have been able to prevent Mrs Tran from acquiring a nosocomial infection.

ACCREDITATION

You are working in residential or home care and accreditors are at your service. Can you answer the following questions?

- As a carer, how, as part of the care team, do you provide input into your consumers needs, from a clinical and non-clinical perspective?
- How are relatives involved in the care of your consumers?
- What training have you attended over the past 12 months, to support you in your role?
- You find a client on the floor. What do you do?

REVIEW QUESTIONS

Circle T if the statement is true or F if the statement is false:

1 T / F Smoking is allowed where oxygen is used.

2 T / F Cleaning chemicals are kept in locked storage areas that are out of the reach of clients.

3 T / F The bathroom is a high-risk area for falls in the home.

4 T / F A communicable disease is one that does not spread.

5 T / F A pathogen can cause an infection.

6 T / F Correct handwashing will reduce the spread of infection.

7 T / F PPE stands for personal protective equipment.

8 T / F Handwashing is the single-most important infection control measure in preventing transmission of infection.

Circle the BEST answer:

9 Who provides a safe setting for clients?
  a The nursing team
  b The administrator
  c The risk manager
  d The entire aged care team

10 Which of the following statements about falls is false?
  a Meeting fluid and elimination needs helps prevent falls.
  b Call bells must be answered promptly.
  c Clients at risk of falling need to stay in their rooms.
  d Bed rails are used according to the client's care plan.

Answers to these questions are on p. 454.

Further reading

Aged Care Quality and Safety Commission (2019). Guidance and resources for providers to support the Aged Care Quality Standards. Online. Available: www.agedcarequality.gov.au/providers/standards

Australian Commission on Safety and Quality in Health Care (ACSQHC) (2020). COVID-19 precautions for staff. Online. Available: www.safetyandquality.gov.au/sites/default/files/2020-08/PPE-Aged-Care_COVID-19-Poster.pdf

Australian Commission on Safety and Quality in Health Care (ACSQHC) (2009a). Preventing falls and harm from falls in older people: Best practice guidelines for Australian community care. Online. Available: www.safetyandquality.gov.au/sites/default/files/migrated/Guidelines-COMM.pdf

Australian Commission on Safety and Quality in Health Care (ACSQHC) (2009b). Preventing falls and harm from falls in older people: Best practice guidelines for Australian hospitals. Online. Available: www.safetyandquality.gov.au/sites/default/files/migrated/Guidelines-HOSP1.pdf

Australian Commission on Safety and Quality in Health Care (ACSQHC) (2009c). Preventing falls and harm from falls in older people: Best practice guidelines for Australian consumers aged care services. Online. Available: www.safetyandquality.gov.au/sites/default/files/migrated/Guidelines-RACF.pdf

Australian Government, Department of Health (2018). Commonwealth Home Support Programme: Program manual 2018–2020. Online. Available: www.health.gov.au/sites/default/files/documents/2019/12/commonwealth-home-support-programme-chsp-manual-2018-2020.pdf

Australian Government, Federal Register of Legislation (2018). Work, Health and Safety Act. Online. Available: www.legislation.gov.au/Details/C2018C00293

Australian Nursing and Midwifery Federation (2018a). Occupational health and safety policy. Online. Available: anmf.org.au/documents/policies/P_Occupational_health_and_safety.pdf

Australian Nursing and Midwifery Federation (2018b). Safe patient handling policy. Online. Available: www.anmf.org.au/documents/policies/P_Safe_Patient_Handling.pdf

Crisp J, Douglas C, Rebeiro G, Waters D (2020). Potter and Perry's fundamentals of nursing. ANZ edn. 6th edn. Elsevier, Sydney.

Government of Western Australia: Department of Health (2020). Stay on your feet. Move, improve, remove. Home safety checklist. Online. Available: www.stayonyourfeet.com.au/over60/remove-hazards/homesafetychecklist/

National Health and Medical Research Council (2019a). Australian Guidelines for the prevention and control of infection in healthcare. Online. Available: www.nhmrc.gov.au/about-us/publications/australian-guidelines-prevention-and-control-infection-healthcare-2019#block-views-block-file-attachments-content-block-1

National Health and Medical Research Council (2019b). Clinical educators guide: Australian guidelines for the prevention and control of infection in healthcare. Online. Available: www.nhmrc.gov.au/sites/default/files/documents/attachments/Clinical-Educators-Guide-WEB.pdf

New South Wales Health (2018). Protecting people and property: NSW health policy and standards for security risk management in NSW health agencies. Online. Available: www.health.nsw.gov.au/policies/manuals/Pages/protecting-people-property.aspx

New South Wales Health (2020). Patient matters manual for public health organisations. Online. Available: www.health.nsw.gov.au/policies/manuals/Pages/patient-matters-manual.aspx

Safe Work Australia (2018). Hazardous manual tasks: Code of Practice. Online. Available: www.safeworkaustralia.gov.au/system/files/documents/1905/model-cop-hazardous-manual-tasks.pdf

Safe Work Australia (2020). Managing risks of hazardous chemicals in the workplace: Code of Practice. Online. Available: www.safeworkaustralia.gov.au/sites/default/files/2020-07/model_code_of_practice_managing_risks_of_hazardous_chemicals_in_the_workplace.pdf

Safe Work Australia (2012). National hazard exposure worker surveillance. Chemical exposure and the provision of chemical exposure control measures in Australian workplaces. Online. Available: www.safeworkaustralia.gov.au/system/files/documents/1702/nhews_chemicals_report.pdf

Safe Work Australia (2010). National hazard exposure worker surveillance: Exposure to dust, gases, vapours, smoke and fumes and the provision of controls for these airborne hazards in Australian workplaces. Online. Available: www.safeworkaustralia.gov.au/system/files/documents/1702/nhews_exposure_dust_gases_vapours_smoke_fumes_provision_contols_airborne_hazards_australian_workplac.pdf

Safe Work SA (2014). Community workers: Work health and safety guidelines, 4th edn. Online. Available: www.safework.sa.gov.au/__data/assets/pdf_file/0003/140772/Community-Workers-work-health-and-safety-guidelines.pdf

Touhy TA & Jett KF (2019). Ebersole & Hess' Toward healthy aging: Human needs and nursing response. 10th edn. Mosby, St Louis.

Workplace Health and Safety Queensland (2020). Codes of Practice. Online. Available: www.worksafe.qld.gov.au/laws-and-compliance/codes-of-practice

World Health Organisation (WHO) (2021). WHO Coronavirus (COVID-19) dashboard. Online. Available: https://covid19.who.int

CHAPTER 3
Working within a legal and ethical environment

By Tara Kent

AFTER READING THIS CHAPTER, YOU SHOULD BE ABLE TO:

- define the key terms listed in this chapter
- identify the legal structure within which you practise
- describe the legal aspects of your role as a carer
- discuss the purpose of informed consent
- recognise the signs of abuse in older people
- define ethical behaviour in the workplace
- describe ethical principles and how to apply these principles
- define an advance health directive
- discuss the rights of the client
- promote quality of life.

Key terms

abuse: Actions which lead to the mistreatment or harm of another person

accountable: Being responsible for one's actions and the actions of others who perform delegated tasks; answering questions about and explaining one's actions and the actions of others

advance health directive: A clear statement of a person's directions and wishes on medical treatment if they are no longer able to make these decisions themselves

advocacy: Providing support and/or representation on behalf of another person to ensure that their rights are upheld

assault: Intentionally attempting or threatening to touch a person's body without the person's consent

autonomy: The ability of a person to make decisions for themselves

battery: Touching a person's body without their consent

beneficence: Any action that is taken to prevent harm, done for the benefit of or to improve the situation of another

bioethics: The rights and duties of clients and healthcare professionals, including how health research is conducted

bullying: A form of harassment that consists of repeated, health-harming mistreatment of a person by one or more perpetrators

confidentiality: Entrusting others with personal and private information

criminal law: Laws concerned with offences against the public and society in general

defamation: Injuring the name and reputation of a person by making false statements to a third person

do not resuscitate: A written directive, usually within an Advance Health Directive, to provide palliative care for a person rather than resuscitating them

duty of care: The responsibility of carers to protect the health and safety of others in the workplace where reasonable and practical

elder abuse: Physical, psychological, financial, sexual or verbal abuse or neglect within a relationship with an older person

empowerment: The process by which an individual gains control over the decisions that shape their life and treatment

ethics: Knowledge of what is right and wrong conduct

harassment: To trouble, torment, offend or worry a person by one's behaviour or comments, including workplace bullying

informed consent: A client is able to refuse or accept treatment based upon the information provided by a healthcare professional, which may be either verbal or written

justice: The administration of fairness and equity

law: A rule of conduct made by a government through legislation and enacted by the court system

libel: Making false statements in print or writing, or through pictures or drawings

negligence: A situation when a person's acts or omissions result in a person not receiving a reasonable level of care, which causes harm to a person and/or their property

non-maleficence: The act of intentionally avoiding harm or injury

privacy: The state in which a person or person's actions are not observed or supervised by other people

restraint: Any type of restrictive practice that intentionally removes a person's right to freedom

restrictive practices: Any practice or intervention that has the effect of restricting the rights or freedom of movement of a care recipient

seclusion: The state of being isolated from other people; may be voluntary or involuntary

sexual harassment: Unwanted sexual behaviours by another

slander: Making false statements verbally

standard of care: The skills, care and judgement required of health team members under similar conditions

vicarious liability: A form of secondary liability in which the employer is liable for the negligent acts or omissions made by their employees

In Australia and New Zealand carers work within a system controlled by laws and regulations that govern the aged care sector and those who work within it. Along with these laws, carers work within an ethical framework that governs their practice. Legal requirements are absolute rules that must be adhered to. Ethical principles are not absolute. This chapter looks at some of the laws that affect the role of a carer, and some key ethical concepts that relate to the role of the carer.

THE LAW AND THE AGED CARE SECTOR

The current legal systems of both New Zealand and Australia are based loosely on the British legal system, although the First Nations people of both countries had customs and legal systems before European settlement. The **law** aims to reflect community values and set boundaries of acceptable behaviour, as well as to provide punishment for breaches of these community standards. The law is not stagnant but constantly changing, being updated to keep pace with changes in social values and conditions. Examples of such changes and their legal ramifications are changes in technology, such as the internet, and what that has meant for privacy, and advances in biotechnology, such as human cloning.

In New Zealand and Australia, laws are enacted by governments (in Australia, this may be federal or state) as statutes or legislation. Our everyday lives as citizens are affected by legislation on everything from ensuring food is safe to eat to punishing someone for murder.

In the aged care sector Acts of Parliament specifically affecting the work of carers include those relating to:

- workplace health and safety
- equal employment and anti-discrimination
- aged care
- health
- drugs and poisons
- freedom of information
- quality standards of practice
- disability services
- the coroner
- mental health.

There are times when a carer is required to work independently – when caring for people in their own homes, for example. It is therefore necessary for the carer to be familiar with the relevant legislation.

Negligence

Negligence is a situation where a person's acts (things they do) or omissions (things they failed to do) result in harm to another person and/or their property. The negligent person has failed to act in a reasonable and careful manner, and as a result has caused harm to the person or property of another. If found guilty of negligence, the negligent individual may have to pay damages (a sum of money) to the injured person. If the negligence is intentional, this is called *criminal negligence*, and the negligent person can be **accountable** under **criminal law**.

To prove negligence, four conditions must all be proved:

1. The client was owed a duty of care. Duty of care means that you, the carer, have a responsibility to protect the health and safety of others at the workplace where reasonable and practical.
2. There was breach of that duty – that is, your care fell below the required standard of care. For example, a carer will be taught how to shower a client in a safe and competent manner. If the carer then does something – say, leaves a client by themselves in an unsafe environment in the shower – and the client falls and is injured, then the carer has provided care below the recognised standard of care.
3. Your actions or lack of actions caused harm or damage to your client. This may be financial, psychological or physical damage.
4. The loss or damage suffered was reasonably foreseeable – for example, a nurse would know that giving a client the wrong medication might lead to harm, or leaving a person unsupervised during a shower may lead to harm.

What you do or do not do can lead to a lawsuit if harm results to the person or property of another. **Standard of care** refers to the skills, care and judgement required by health team members under similar conditions. Standards of care come from laws, textbooks and centre policies and procedures. Manufacturers' instructions for equipment use also serve as standards of care, as do job descriptions and accrediting agency standards.

Here are some examples of negligent actions:

- A nurse tells you to give a medication. State laws and your job description do not allow you to give medications. You have not been trained to give medications. However, you give the medication. In doing so, you have not followed state laws or your job description.
- A nurse asks you to apply a hot bath. You do not check the water temperature. The water is too hot and the person is burned.
- A person needs help getting to the bathroom. You do not answer the call buzzer promptly. The person gets up without help, falls and breaks a hip.
- A mechanical lift is used to transfer a client from their bed to a chair. You do not follow the manufacturer's instructions for using the lift. The client slips out of the lift and falls to the floor, breaking a hip.
- A client complains of chest pain. You do not tell the nurse. The client has a heart attack and dies.
- Two clients have the same last name. You do not identify the person before a procedure. You perform the procedure on the wrong person. In this case, both clients are harmed: one had a procedure that was not ordered, and the other did not have a needed procedure.

You are legally responsible for your own actions. The nurse is liable as your supervisor. Remember, sometimes refusing to follow the nurse's directions is your right and duty.

Defamation

To *defame* someone means to injure their name and reputation by making false statements to another person. To commit **libel** means to make false statements in print or writing, or through pictures or drawings. To **slander** someone means to make false statements orally.

As a care worker, you should never make false statements about a client, a co-worker or any other person. Be careful of passing on gossip as it is often false and you may be guilty of defamation if you do so. Examples of **defamation** include:

- implying or suggesting that a person abuses medications
- saying that a person is insane or mentally ill
- implying or suggesting that a person steals money from the staff.

Assault and battery

Assault and battery may result in civil and criminal charges. **Assault** is intentionally attempting or threatening to touch a person's body without the person's consent. The person fears bodily harm. Threatening to 'tie down' a person is an example of assault. **Battery** is touching a person's body without their consent. *Consent* is the key factor in assault and battery. The person must consent to any procedure, treatment or other act that involves touching their body. A person has the right to withdraw consent at any time.

To protect yourself from committing assault and battery, explain to the person what is to be done and obtain their consent. Consent may be verbal – 'yes' or 'okay' – or it may be a gesture – a nod, turning over for a back rub or holding out an arm for a blood pressure measurement. Never commence a procedure unless you have your client's consent. (See Informed consent, overleaf.)

Restrictive practices

Living within an environment that does not include restrictive practices is seen as a basic right for everyone. Once a client enters into a care arrangement in a residential aged care service or in their homes, or even within a community setting, these rights are not negated and must be maintained.

A **restrictive practice** is the use of any force or control that intentionally removes a person's right to freedom. These practices are often commonly referred to as **restraints.** A restrictive practice-free environment means no words, devices or actions will interfere with a person's ability to make a decision or restrict their free movement. The ultimate aim of any aged care service is to provide a restrictive practice-free environment, including physical and chemical restraint. In a long-term care service, however, restraint may be used to limit the actions of a client in circumstances where they may be at risk of injuring themselves or others. Use of a restrictive practice should only be contemplated as one of a range of possible interventions and should always be seen as a last resort.

The *Quality of Care Principles 2014* (Cth) were revised to comply with new legislation that came into effect July 2021, which identified that physical and chemical restraint can only be used as a last resort and after thorough consultation, including consent from the person and/or their decision-maker, the treating practitioner and/or nurse and that a variety of other considerations regarding safety and wellness are considered.

The Department of Health informs us that:

> The use of restraints is not only illegal without appropriate authorisation, but can also cause the client a considerable amount of distress. This may even eventuate in physical or psychological harm. All care providers have a duty of care to consider how best to avoid those situations which could potentially lead to an assumed need for restraining the client. This is also seen as best practice.

In Australia, the Australian Government Department of Health has developed two toolkits: a 'Decision-making tool: supporting a restraint-free environment in residential aged care' and 'Decision-making tool: supporting a restraint-free environment in community aged care' (see Further reading at the end of the chapter). These are designed to assist those who care for older people to think of alternative ways of dealing with client safety, using the least invasive method of restraint and only as a last resort.

All restraint must meet the legislative requirements to ensure false imprisonment, battery and/or assault are not the end result.

Restrictive practices may be divided into the following categories:

- *Physical restraint* – This involves a person using any part of their body to cease or restrain the movement of another person. This can include standing in between two people, the placement of bed rails or furniture that limits movement.
- *Environmental restraint* – This may include contained environments or planned interventions that reduce the level of social and environmental stimulation; for example, locked doors in a secure dementia unit.
- *Chemical restraint* – Medication should be the last resort and aged care services aim for no chemical restraint. Some clients may be on medications due to their medical diagnosis, and these are not considered a chemical restraint.
- *Mechanical restraint* – This is when an item is used to restrain the person. This could include using a seatbelt off a wheelchair to stop someone from moving.
  - Note: Using a seatbelt for normal safe transportation is not a restrictive practice, nor are side rails on a bed if they are used to protect someone from falling out of bed.
- *Containment* – This is when the person is locked in their residence and they are not able to leave at their discretion.
- *Seclusion* – This is when the person is both locked in their residence and isolated from other people (e.g. locked in their room).

Australian legislation also identifies that from September 2021 a Behaviour Support Plan must be completed for all care recipients which identifies if a restrictive practice is required. It is very important to remember that unauthorised use of any restraint is assault. A carer is never permitted to restrain a person if restraint has not been authorised.

AUTHORISING A RESTRICTIVE PRACTICE

Before a restrictive practice is authorised, the client should undergo a comprehensive assessment, which includes input from medical staff, nursing staff and family/whānau. Assessment should take into account the wide range of disease processes that might place the client at risk of harming themselves if they are not restrained. An example is an infection that may cause an older person to become disoriented and aggressive and hit out at other residents.

The doctor authorises the method of restraint required and can only do so in a manner that is conducive with Part 4A of the *Quality of Care Principles 2014* (Cth). Once the decision to restrain has been made by the doctor, the consumer and/or their decision-maker must provide consent. The only time restraints can be used without following this process is in situations considered to be an emergency (15F and 15G of the *Quality of Care Principles 2014* (Cth)). Consideration must also be given to the most appropriate and least restrictive method to be used. It is a legal requirement for services to document their restraint policy and ensure frequent restraint checks are made. Restraint may never be instituted by one person on their own initiative.

Monitoring restraint

A restraint record must be maintained for the duration of the restraint, containing specific instructions for the type of restraint authorised for use, as well as the signatures of the appropriate authorising people. The registered nurse is responsible for ensuring the record is maintained.

- The record must provide evidence of ongoing care during restraint. This may include, for example, 240-minute checks on the person who has been restrained and a document that is signed by the staff member who checks them at each time.
- Staff must ensure that the client comes to no harm during restraint.
- The ongoing need for restraint must be reviewed regularly by the authorising team and the consumer and/or decision-maker for the consumer. The decision-maker could be family, a friend or appointed decision-maker.
- Restraint must be taken very seriously. There have been deaths from the use of restraint; for example, people have stopped breathing when held a certain way, and/or restraint has been used when they were eating or in such a way that it affected their breathing.

Informed consent

A person has the right to decide what will be done to their body, and who can touch their body. The doctor is responsible for informing the person about all aspects of treatment. **Informed consent** is consent that is given when a person understands:

- the reason for the treatment
- what will be done
- how it will be done
- who will do it
- the expected outcomes
- other treatment options
- the effects of not having the treatment.

A person under legal age generally cannot give consent, apart from consent within the parameters of the Gillick Competence (Griffith 2015). This principle is a matter of common law which has a decision that enables young people to consent to their own health care without permission from their guardian. There are conditions regarding this consent and the manner in which the medical practitioner must acquire it. In addition to a young person, others who are unable to consent are those who have had the presumption of capacity rebutted. This usually occurs if they have a mental illness, disability or age-related illness which impairs their ability to consistently make and communicate decisions. Decision-making frameworks are stipulated in state and territory legislation, and this legislation will stipulate the process that needs to occur to rebut the presumption of capacity.

In situations where a person has impaired decision-making capacity, they will need to have someone willing and able to make decisions on their behalf or have an enduring power of attorney (EPOA) that can commence. In most states and territories of Australia, informal decision-making is supported where there is no EPOA. This means that a friend or family member can act as a decision maker for their loved one without a court/tribunal order or a power of attorney. Based on legislation in Queensland (each state and territory is slightly different), the only decisions that require the formal appointment of a guardian/attorney are those regarding money. Financial decisions usually require a formalised appointment as this allows relevant safeguards to be in place to monitor the appointment and ensure the person's finances are being used appropriately.

Consent may be given for some aspects of care when the person enters a care service. A form may be signed, giving general consent to treatment. Special consent forms are required before a person can be admitted to a secured dementia unit.

ADVANCE HEALTH DIRECTIVES AND 'DO NOT RESUSCITATE' ORDERS

An **advance health directive** is a written document which stipulates the way the person wants their healthcare to be provided, as well as any end-of-life decisions, such as resuscitation and withholding or withdrawing life-sustaining measures.

The term '**do not resuscitate**' (DNR) is a written directive, usually provided within an advance health directive, to provide palliative care rather than to resuscitate a person, and is made in the client's best interests. For example, a client with end-stage dementia or cancer may require pain management, but to provide cardiopulmonary resuscitation would not be in the best interests of the person. To make this written directive, the client, the family and the healthcare team work together to ensure that such a directive is done legally, reviewed regularly and that staff know of such a directive. This is a refusal of treatment (i.e. resuscitation) and it must be made with informed consent. If the person in question is not able to make this consent, only an approved decision-maker (e.g. enduring power of attorney, informal or appointed guardian) can do it on their behalf.

You must remember that if a 'do not resuscitate' order is organised during a visit to hospital it does not apply to a consequent visit to hospital. It is a requirement that a new order is documented for each visit to the hospital or a new service.

Duty of care

Duty of care requires everything 'reasonably practicable' to be done to protect the health and safety of clients and staff in the workplace. As an example, an employer must:
- provide a safe work environment for staff and clients
- provide equipment necessary for a carer to carry out their role
- monitor workplace conditions and workplace hazards.

Staff must comply with the occupational health and safety requirements of the workplace and report any unsafe practices.

Vicarious liability

Vicarious liability is a form of secondary liability in which the employer is liable for the negligent acts or omissions made by their employees. If you as a carer are negligent in your work activities and your client is harmed, not only may you be personally liable, but your employer may also be liable for your negligence. However, if you work outside of your scope of practice on your own accord and harm a person then it's likely that a court will not hold the employer vicariously liable for your negligence.

Abuse

Abuse is the intentional mistreatment or harm of another person. Abuse is a crime. It can occur at home or in an aged care service. Abuse has one or more of the following elements:
- wilful causing of injury
- unreasonable confinement
- intimidation (to make someone afraid by using threats of force or violence)
- punishment
- depriving the person of goods or services needed for their physical, mental or psychosocial wellbeing.

Abuse causes physical harm, pain or mental anguish. Protection against abuse extends to a person in a coma. In cases of child or elder abuse, the abuser is usually a family member or a caregiver. However, the abuser may be a friend, neighbour, property owner or another person. As a carer, you have a responsibility to report any signs of abuse.

In Australia, specific legislation makes it compulsory for the management of residential services to report suspected elder abuse. Australian staff also have to undergo federal police checks prior to working in aged care services. It is mandatory for the reporting of suspected or actual physical or sexual abuse to the police within 24 hours of becoming aware of the allegation.

ELDER ABUSE

Elder abuse can take the following forms:
- *Physical abuse* – grabbing, hitting, slapping, pushing, kicking, pinching, hair-pulling or beating. It also includes corporal punishment – punishment inflicted on the body, such as beatings, lashings or whippings. Neglect is also physical abuse. It involves depriving the person of needed medical services or treatment. Failure to provide food, clothing, hygiene and other basic needs is also neglect. In aged care services, neglect includes, but is not limited to:
  - leaving a person lying or sitting in urine or faeces
  - isolating a person in their room or other area
  - failing to answer call bells.
- *Verbal abuse* – using oral or written words or statements that speak badly of, sneer at, criticise or condemn the person. It includes unkind gestures.
- *Involuntary seclusion* – confining the person to a certain area. Older people have been locked in closets, basements, attics and other spaces.
- *Financial abuse* – the older person's money is stolen or used by another person. It also includes misusing a person's property – for example, a son sells his mother's house without her consent.
- *Mental abuse* – humiliation, harassment, ridicule and threats of being punished. It also includes being deprived of needs such as food, clothing, care, a home or a place to sleep.
- *Sexual abuse* – the person is harassed about sex or is attacked sexually. The person may be forced to perform sexual acts out of fear of punishment or physical harm.

There are many signs of elder abuse (see Box 3.1). The abused person may show only some of these signs; however, if a person displays some of these signs it does not necessarily mean they are being abused. It must be investigated by the appropriate people. If abuse is suspected, it must be reported. There is a process for investigation which the person in charge will follow. Where and how to report suspected abuse varies in each state and territory.

If you suspect that a person is being abused, discuss the problem and your observations with your supervisor. Give as much information as possible. The supervisor will then contact the appropriate people as needed.

The carer can also contact community agencies that investigate elder abuse. They will act immediately if the problem is life-threatening. Sometimes the help of police or the courts is necessary.

Care services and organisations must have and follow procedures for investigating all cases of suspected abuse. The following are examples of incidents of elder abuse:
- A person is constantly crying out for help. The person is taken to her room, and is left alone with the door closed.

BOX 3.1
Signs of elder abuse

- Living conditions are unsafe, unclean or inadequate.
- Personal hygiene is lacking. The person is unclean. Their clothes are dirty.
- Weight loss – the person shows signs of poor nutrition and inadequate fluid intake.
- Assistive devices are missing or broken – glasses, hearing aids, dentures, cane or walker.
- Frequent injuries – conditions behind the injuries are strange or seem impossible.
- Old and new injuries – bruises, welts, scars and punctures.
- The person complains of pain or itching in the genital area.
- Bleeding and bruising in the genital area.
- Burns on the feet, hands or buttocks. Cigarettes and cigars cause small circular burns.
- Pressure ulcers or contractures.
- The person seems very quiet or withdrawn.
- The person seems fearful, anxious or agitated.
- The person does not seem to want to talk or answer questions.
- The person is restrained, or is locked in a certain area for long periods of time. The person cannot reach toilet services, food and water and other necessary items.
- Private conversations are not allowed. The caregiver is present during all conversations.
- The person seems anxious to please the caregiver.
- Medications are not taken properly. Medications are not purchased. Or too much or too little of the medication is taken.
- Visits to the emergency department may be frequent.
- The person may change doctors often. Some people do not have a doctor.

- A carer tells a person to be nice because otherwise care will not be provided.
- A person cannot control her bowels. A carer calls her dirty and disgusting.
- A person is turned in a rough and hurried manner, which causes him pain and discomfort.
- A carer uses the person's telephone to call a friend.
- A person lies in a wet and soiled bed all night.
- A carer takes money from a person's wallet.
- A person uses the call bell a lot. It is taken away from him.
- A person's mouth is forced open and food is forced into their mouth.
- A person is told that her son does not visit her because she is so mean.

Helping abused older people is not always easy or possible. Often the abuse is not reported or recognised. Alternatively, the investigating agency might not be able to gain access to the person. Sometimes older people are abused by their children. A victim may want to protect their child. Some victims are embarrassed or believe the abuse is deserved. A victim may be afraid of what will happen if the abuse is revealed. They may think that the present situation is better than no care at all. Some people fear not being believed if they report the abuse themselves.

Confidentiality

Client information is private and personal. **Confidentiality** means entrusting others with personal and private information. The person's information is shared only among health team members involved in their care. Centre and co-worker information is also confidential.

To maintain confidentiality, avoid talking about clients, the service or co-workers when others are present. Share information only with the nurse. Do not talk about clients, the service or co-workers in hallways, lifts, dining areas or outside the centre, as others may overhear you. Residents and visitors are alert to comments and may think you are talking about them or their loved ones. You can easily upset the person or their family. Be very careful about what, how, when and where you say things.

Remember, not only is it professional to keep information confidential, it is also a legal requirement. For example, you may have already heard someone you have spoken to on the phone for banking ask significant questions to ascertain your identity and they may have mentioned the Privacy Act. This is part of the legislative requirements now in place to ensure confidential information is not revealed to those other than the person they directly relate to.

The *Privacy Amendment (Enhancing Privacy Protection) Act 2012 (Privacy Amendment Act)* passed through the Australian Parliament on 12 March 2014 and changes continue to be made to it. In addition, individual states and territories have a variety of legislation that affect confidentiality, including confidentiality of records.

The Office of the Australian Information Commission website contains many resources available to the public (see Further reading). There is similar information for New Zealand available from the Office of the Privacy Commissioner website (see Further reading).

Harassment

Harassment means troubling, tormenting, offending or worrying a person by one's behaviour or comments. It can be sexual or it can involve age, race, ethnic background, religion or disability. You must respect others. Do not offend others by your gestures, remarks or use of touch. Do not offend others with jokes or pictures. Harassment is illegal in the workplace.

Bullying

Bullying is a form of harassment and consists of repeated, health-harming mistreatment of a person by one or more perpetrators. It often includes:

- verbal abuse
- offensive conduct/behaviours (including non-verbal) which are threatening, humiliating or intimidating

- work interference – sabotage – which prevents work from getting done.

If you believe that you are being bullied, you need to advise the perpetrator that you consider their actions as bullying and request that they cease them. If they do not, you need to inform your supervisor and/or the human resources officer and request their support.

Sexual harassment

Sexual harassment involves unwanted sexual behaviours by another. The behaviour may be a sexual advance, or a request for a sexual favour. Some comments or touching are sexual. The behaviour affects the person's work and comfort. In extreme cases in the workplace, the person's job is threatened if sexual favours are not granted.

Victims of sexual harassment may be men or women. Men harass women or men; women harass men or women. If you feel that you are being harassed, report the matter to your supervisor and the human resources officer.

Be careful about what you say or do. Even what you perceive to be innocent remarks and behaviours can be viewed by others as harassment. If you remain respectful towards your clients, colleagues and visitors, you should avoid any difficulties.

Also, keep in mind that there are procedures in place at every workplace, so if you feel you are being harassed you need to investigate the policies and procedures for your work area and follow them.

ETHICS AND THE AGED CARE SECTOR

Ethics is about right and wrong conduct and relates to looking at the morality of any situation. **Bioethics** focuses on the rights and duties of clients and healthcare professionals, including how health research is conducted. It involves choices and judgements about what to do or what not to do. An ethical person does the right thing and does not cause a person harm. In the workplace, certain behaviours, choices and judgements are expected. Carers, like healthcare personnel, are frequently exposed to situations where ethical issues are involved.

Ethical behaviour also involves not being prejudiced or biased. Being prejudiced or biased means making judgements and having views before knowing the facts. Judgements and views are usually based on one's own personal values and standards, and one's culture, religion, education and experiences. We all have personal biases and opinions. Being aware of these will help you avoid doing anything that may be seen as biased.

A number of ethical principles are considered moral principles. Decisions within an aged care or healthcare environment can be based on these principles. Some common ethical issues in healthcare include those associated with:

- reproductive technologies
- abortion
- medical research
- euthanasia and assisted technologies
- economic rationalisation of healthcare
- refusal of treatment
- genetic technologies
- working in palliative care.

Some ethical principles that are relevant to working as a carer are described below.

Autonomy

Autonomy refers to a person's ability to make decisions for themselves (if they are adults and of sound mind). It also means their decision is respected, even if that decision may lead to harm to that person. For example, a person may have cancer but refuse medical treatment. Within this principle, that decision must be respected. If your client chooses not to have a shower, they have the right not to have a shower. You cannot make the client have one.

Non-maleficence

The principle of **non-maleficence** is: above all, 'do no harm'. In some instances, treatment can cause suffering. For example, a person may be terminally ill and have a short time to live. They may also have many pressure ulcers requiring complex and painful treatments. It is possible to do these treatments, but this may cause suffering to the person, with little chance of reversing the terminal illness. This treatment would need to be considered in the context of the person's current quality of life and the harm that the treatment may cause. Obviously, the use of effective and timely pain management to ensure procedures could be carried out without pain would be considered before the consideration of no treatment at all. However, if pain is unavoidable then serious consideration needs to be taken regarding the possibility of no treatment.

Beneficence

The principle of **beneficence** is: above all, 'do good'. Carers and healthcare professionals focus their care on this principle, which is based on empathy, compassion and doing no harm, for the benefit of others. For example, a person may become very tired and agitated as they receive rehabilitative care following a stroke. This care must be considered within the concept of helping the person in the long term, even though it may cause concerns in the short term.

Justice

Justice means fairness and equity. All clients have the same right to care. You cannot give reduced care to one person in order to give more care to another. Do not judge the person by your values or standards. Do not avoid a person just because their standards and values differ from yours. You must ensure that all clients have their rights protected and receive safe and competent care.

ETHICAL DECISION-MAKING

When faced with an ethical dilemma, consider the following questions:

- What are the facts?
- Is the act legal and consistent with organisational policy?
- Who should I ask for more information?

- Is it the right thing to do?
- What are my own biases in this matter?
- Can I justify my actions?
- Would the act stand up to public scrutiny?

Ethical problems involve making choices. You must decide what is the right thing to do. For example:

- a co-worker has been late for work 3 days this week. You find her in an empty room drinking from a cup. You also smell alcohol on her breath. She asks you not to tell anyone.
- a client has bruises all over her body. She has told the nurse that she fell. But she tells you that her son is very mean to her, and she asks you not to tell the nurse. If you are required to make a decision that poses an ethical dilemma for you, always speak to your nurse and seek advice.

Advocacy

Advocacy means that a health professional can plead a client's cause or act on behalf of a client in their care. The overall goal of advocacy is to work with the client and/or their family so that they can act on their own behalf. Advocacy is an ethical issue because the need for an advocate will depend upon the level of autonomy that a client may or may not have. Advocacy respects a client's right to:

- be informed and receive the correct information
- be involved in making decisions
- privacy and confidentiality
- dignity and respect
- freedom of religious and ethical beliefs.

The central aspects of advocacy are to inform and support. You must ensure that the client is provided with adequate and accurate information relating to their care or rights, so that the client can participate in informed decision-making. In some circumstances the client may not be able to participate in informed decision-making. You can assist by recognising and respecting the rights of the client and providing relevant assistance and access to appropriate resources. You must also provide client support in an objective manner – not conveying approval or disapproval – regarding the client's care decisions. In this way, you protect the client's basic human rights, such as autonomy.

It is important when advocating for a client that you are aware of the legal and ethical guidelines for professional practice and that you advocate within those guidelines. Nurses and carers can only provide informal advocacy support to a client and do not have any legal power to advocate for a client. Court-appointed guardians and power of attorney can act as formal advocacy avenues.

Guardianship

Sometimes in life, people lose the capacity to make decisions for themselves. The *Guardianship and Administration Act 2000* (Qld) provides a mechanism for decisions to be made on behalf of an adult if they lose capacity due to accident, illness or age. The Act enables the Queensland Civil and Administrative Tribunal (QCAT) (there are similar legislations in each of the Australian states and territories) to appoint administrators and/or guardians to make decisions on behalf of the adult. Once appointed, administrators can make financial decisions and legal decisions related to financial matters, on behalf of the adult. Guardians can make decisions on personal, health and lifestyle matters, as well as other legal matters not related to the adult's finances or property.

ENDURING POWER OF ATTORNEY

An enduring power of attorney is a legal document where a person can appoint somebody to manage their assets and financial affairs should they become unable to do so. Unlike the appointment of a legal guardian, this is undertaken while the person has full decision-making capacity to make the choice.

Empowerment

Client **empowerment** occurs when an individual is assisted in gaining control over their own lives. Empowerment increases an individual's capacity to act on issues that they define as important to themselves. The overall goal of client empowerment is to place the client at the centre of the care process so that the focus is shifted from doing things 'to' the client, to doing things 'with' the client.

Key features of client empowerment include:

- self-efficacy
- self-awareness
- confidence
- coping skills
- health literacy.

Empowering a client may involve assisting them to self-manage their own condition, gain greater control over decision-making, consider actions affecting their health or advocating for themselves.

Empowered clients tend to:

- make informed decisions about their treatment and care
- take preventive measures and seek earlier diagnosis
- be willing and able to take more responsibility for their care
- adhere more closely to their prescribed treatments
- have a better relationship with their health professionals.

Carers can assist with empowerment by ensuring that the client has access to available resources. In this way, you are assisting the client with informed decision-making and self-management. Being available and taking the time to communicate with the client about their condition, listening to their experiences and answering their questions are important features of empowerment.

Successful client empowerment involves interaction between health services, support services, community services, family, friends and care staff.

RESIDENTS' RIGHTS

All clients within care services have rights and responsibilities. Both Australia and New Zealand have their own legislation covering this aspect.

Australia

Residents of aged care services have the same legal, civil and moral rights as any other person in the community. These rights are enforceable under law. Some clients are incompetent (not able) to exercise their rights, in which case a responsible party (spouse or adult child) or legal representative does so for them. In Australia, the *Aged Care Act 1997* is an important piece of legislation and details the expectations of a client receiving care, including the right to:

- receive good quality care and services
- be treated with respect and courtesy
- have their lifestyle and cultural and personal beliefs respected
- be informed and consulted about their care
- privacy and confidentiality
- access their personal information held by the provider
- be provided with a written plan of the services they will receive
- have another person of their choice support them and advocate on their behalf
- have their comments valued
- make a complaint if they are unhappy with the services they receive
- continue to receive care and services from the provider while they are still necessary and appropriate to meet their needs.

Along with this legislation, the Charter of Care Recipients' Rights and Responsibilities (Box 3.2) is an important list of rights that carers should know and understand. Aged care services must inform clients of their rights. They must be informed orally and in writing. Such information is given before or during admission to the service. It is important to ensure that the person is able to understand their rights.

Refusing treatment

The person has the right to refuse treatment. A person who does not give consent or refuses treatment cannot be given

BOX 3.2
Charter of Care Recipients' Rights and Responsibilities

Each consumer of a residential care service has the right to:

- full and effective use of his or her personal, civil, legal and consumer rights
- quality care that is appropriate to his or her needs
- full information about his or her own state of health and about available treatments
- be treated with dignity and respect, and to live without exploitation, abuse or neglect
- live without discrimination or victimisation, and without being obliged to feel grateful to those providing his or her care and accommodation
- personal privacy
- live in a safe, secure and home-like environment, and to move freely both within and outside the residential care service without undue restriction
- be treated and accepted as an individual, and to have his or her individual preferences taken into account and treated with respect
- continue his or her cultural and religious practices and to retain the language of his or her choice, without discrimination
- select and maintain social and personal relationships with any other person without fear, criticism or restriction
- freedom of speech
- maintain his or her personal independence, which includes a recognition of personal responsibility for his or her own actions and choices, even though some actions may involve an element of risk which the consumer has the right to accept, and that should then not be used to prevent or restrict those actions
- maintain control over, and to continue making decisions about, the personal aspects of his or her daily life, financial affairs and possessions
- be involved in the activities, associations and friendships of his or her choice, both within and outside the residential care service
- have access to services and activities that are available generally in the community
- be consulted on, and choose to have input into, decisions about the living arrangements of the residential care service
- have access to information about his or her rights, care, accommodation and any other information that relates to him or her personally
- complain and take action to resolve disputes
- have access to advocates and other avenues of redress
- be free from reprisal, or a well-founded fear of reprisal, in any form for taking action to enforce his or her rights.

Each consumer of a residential care service has the responsibility to:

- respect the rights and needs of other people within the residential care service, and respect the needs of the residential care service community as a whole
- respect the rights of staff and the proprietor to work in an environment that is free from harassment
- care for his or her own health and wellbeing, as far as he or she is capable
- inform his or her medical practitioner, as far as he or she is able, about his or her relevant medical history and his or her current state of health.

Source: Department of Health, Charter of Care Recipients' Rights and Responsibilities. Aged Care Act 1997 © Commonwealth of Australia.

the treatment. The service must find out what the person is refusing and why. You should report any treatment refusal to the nurse, who may need to change the person's care plan.

Privacy and confidentiality

In addition to the privacy and confidentiality issues previously discussed, residents have the right to personal **privacy**. The person's body must not be exposed unnecessarily. Only workers directly involved in care and treatments should be present. The person must give consent for others to be present. For example, if a student wishes to observe a treatment, the person's consent is needed for the student to observe.

A person has the right to use the bathroom in private. Privacy is maintained for personal care measures as well, keeping in mind any safety precautions that may need to be taken. If a person requires assistance in the bathroom it is provided in a respectful and private manner, maintaining the person's dignity at all times.

Residents have the right to visit with others in private – in an area where others cannot see or hear them. If requested, the centre must provide private space. Offices, chapels, dining rooms and meeting rooms are used as needed. The right to visit in private also involves mail and telephone calls (Fig. 3.1). They also have the right to receive visitors in private.

Residents have the right to send and receive mail without others interfering. No one can open mail the person sends and receives without his or her consent.

Information about the person's care, treatment and condition is kept confidential. Throughout this text you are reminded to keep information about the person confidential. Providing for privacy and keeping information confidential show respect for the person, and protect the person's dignity.

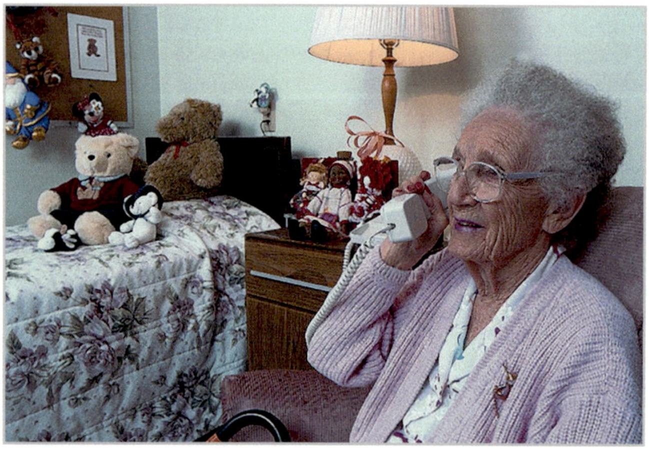

Fig. 3.1
A consumer has the right to privacy when talking on the telephone.

Personal choice

Residents can choose their own doctors. They also have the right to take part in planning their care and treatment. They have the right to choose activities, schedules and care based on their own preferences. For example, a person chooses when to get up and when to go to bed, what to wear (Fig. 3.2), how to spend time and what to eat. They also can choose to have friends and visitors inside and outside the centre.

Personal choice promotes quality of life, dignity and self-respect. You must allow personal choice whenever it is safely possible.

Disputes and grievances

Residents have the right to voice concerns, questions and complaints about their care or treatment. The problem may involve another person. It may be about treatment or care that was not given. The centre must promptly try to correct the problem. No one is entitled to punish the person in any way for voicing the dispute or grievance. All services must have documented policies and procedures regarding disputes and feedback systems. All clients, their family and staff should be aware of them.

Work

The person does not work to receive care, care items or other things or privileges. The person is not required to perform services for the centre. However, the person can

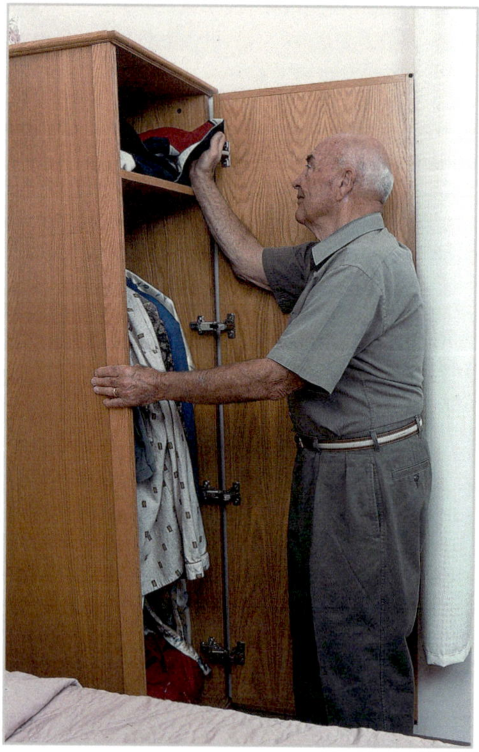

Fig. 3.2
Residents have the right to choose what clothing to wear.

work or perform services if they want to and it is safe to do so. A person may want to do gardening, repairs, building, sewing or cooking. Others may need to work for rehabilitation or activity reasons. When there is a desire or need to work, it is included in the person's care plan. A risk management plan may be required in some circumstances and any recommended actions followed and documented within the care plan.

Participation in consumers and family groups

Residents have the right to take part in client and family groups. In addition, a person's family has the right to meet with the families of other clients. They can plan activities. The group can support and comfort group members.

Residents also have the right to take part in social, religious and community activities. They have the right to assistance in getting to and from activities of their choice.

Care and security of personal possessions

Residents have the right to keep and use personal items. Available space and the health and safety of other people affects the type and amount of personal items allowed.

Treat the person's property with care and respect. The items may not have value to you, but they have meaning to the person. They also relate to personal choice, dignity and quality of life.

The centre must protect the person's property. Items are labelled with the person's name. The centre must investigate reports of lost, stolen or damaged items, and police assistance may sometimes be necessary. The person and family are advised not to keep jewellery and other costly items in the centre.

Protect yourself and the centre from being accused of stealing a person's property. Do not go through a person's closet, drawers, purse or other space without the person's knowledge and consent. A nurse may ask you to inspect closets and drawers. If so, have another worker with you and the person or legal guardian. The other worker is a witness to your activities.

Freedom from abuse, mistreatment and neglect

Residents have the right to be free from verbal, sexual, physical or mental abuse, as mentioned earlier in this chapter. They also have the right to be free from involuntary **seclusion**.

Seclusion means:

- separating the person from others against his or her will
- keeping the person confined to a certain area
- keeping the person away from their room without their consent.

If the person is incompetent, involuntary seclusion occurs against the legal guardian's consent.

No one is entitled to abuse, neglect or mistreat a client. This includes staff members, volunteers, staff from other agencies or groups, other clients, family, visitors and legal representatives. Aged care services must investigate suspected or reported cases of client abuse.

Freedom from restraint

Residents have the right not to have their body movements restricted. Restraints and certain medications can restrict body movements. Some medications can restrain the person because they affect mood, behaviour and mental function. Sometimes clients are restrained to protect them from harming themselves or others, discussed in detail earlier in this chapter. A doctor's order is required for restraint use. Restraints are not used for staff convenience, that is, the question 'whose problem is it?' should be frequently asked to ensure it is for the genuine safety of the client, not because, for example, staff find their behaviours annoying; for example, requesting extra sedation because the person gets up at 2.00 a.m. seeking a drink every night. The correct action for this is to provide the drink.

New Zealand

Code of Health and Disability Services Consumers' Rights 1996 (the Code)

The Code of Health and Disability Services Consumers' Rights 1996 (the Code) is a regulation under the *Health and Disability Commissioner Act 1994*. Every healthcare provider has obligations under the Code and, conversely, every consumer has rights that must be respected. The Code encompasses ten rights for consumers of health and disability support services, summarised as follows:

1. The right to be treated with respect – this applies whether the person is being cared for in a continuing care service or in their own home.
2. The right to freedom from discrimination, coercion, harassment and sexual, financial or other exploitation.
3. The right to dignity and independence.
4. The right to services of an appropriate standard.
5. The right to effective communication.
6. The right to be fully informed.
7. The right to make informed choice and give informed consent.
8. The right to support.
9. Rights in respect of teaching and research.
10. The right to complain.

In addition, the New Zealand Aged Care Association has published a code of residents' rights and responsibilities to guide carers in their role (see Further reading).

QUALITY OF LIFE

It is essential that when you work as a carer in a service or in the client's home you have a thorough understanding of the legal and ethical issues you may encounter. It is only by knowing and understanding the issues that you can provide safe and effective care to your clients.

All clients have the right to safe, effective and appropriate care. These rights are safeguarded by legal Acts and regulations, and policies within your workplace.

Residents have the right to be free from abuse, mistreatment and neglect. Care services have procedures for investigating all cases of suspected abuse. Be alert for signs and symptoms of abuse. If you suspect that a person is being abused, report the matter to your supervisor. Share your observations with the supervisor.

Consider the quality of life from a consumer perspective and how you would like to be cared for, whether in your own home or in a residential service. The emphasis should not be only on the physical care of a client, but also on holistic care within a legal and ethical framework.

CASE STUDY

Case study 1

When working in a residential aged care service, a carer witnesses another carer swearing at a resident and treating them roughly when taking them to the shower. The carer is new to the aged care service and is not sure what to do when this occurs. She tells her supervisor of the incident and says that she is frightened of this carer and doesn't want to get into trouble.

The director of the service speaks to the carer involved and the resident (who has felt threatened by this carer for some time, but has been too frightened to speak up). On further investigation, it appears that a number of carers have witnessed this carer bullying clients and other carers. No physical violence has been witnessed.

The director of the service has a meeting with the carer, at which a union representative is present, and details the allegations, which are extremely serious. The carer denies the allegations, but decides to resign from the service. The director also informs the carer that she has notified the police of this series of alleged incidents, as an investigation may be required.

Case study 2

You are caring for Mrs Nye, who has terminal cancer and wishes to stay at home receiving palliative care, rather than going into a healthcare service. You are one of her carers and visit her on a regular basis to assist her, and so you develop a strong professional connection with Mrs Nye and her family. As her cancer progresses, she experiences more pain and has her pain medication changed to manage this pain, but one day she tells you that she has had enough. You believe she is asking you to help her end her life. You discuss your concerns with your supervisor, who ensures the care team for Mrs Nye is informed, that Mrs Nye gets reassessed for her pain and that she is given additional psychological and emotional support. Your supervisor also discusses Mrs Nye with you and ensures that you are supported. It is important as a carer to discuss any concerns that you may have regarding a client, as well as considering your own physical and mental health, to ensure you are supported to do your job.

Case study 3

Jenny is a carer and has just put Mrs Jones in the bath when she notices she still has the hair pins of the previous resident she just finished showering in her pocket. Jenny quickly pops out of the bathroom to return them to the previous resident's room. On the way back to the bathroom another staff member sees her and asks for help to quickly get another consumer dressed. She quickly helps and then returns to Mrs Jones. On Jenny's return to the bathroom, she finds that Mrs Jones has drowned in the bath as a result of slipping under the water. Jenny is very distressed about this and does not return to work for some time, after significant counselling. The family pursue legal action and Jenny faces a negligence charge. She argues that she only left the bathroom for a brief moment and the only reason she was delayed was to help out someone else. The judge finds that Jenny owed Mrs Jones a duty of care to ensure her safety at all times. She also finds that the return of hair pins was not a priority and that Jenny should have remained with Mrs Jones. Jenny is found guilty of negligence.

ACCREDITATION

You are working in residential or home care and accreditors are at your service. Can you answer the following questions?

- You are working in a client's home and they confide in you that they are worried that one of their children is taking money from their bank account. What do you do?
- You are working in a residential aged care service, and one of your consumers has bed rails applied for their safety. Does a restraint authorisation form have to be completed with EPOA or consumer consent?

REVIEW QUESTIONS

Circle T if the statement is true or F if the statement is false:

1 T / F Legislation is a guide only. It still leaves the worker the ability to choose what they prefer.

2 T / F It is okay to leave a computer screen showing the details of a care plan for a consumers open in an area that other people, including visitors and other residents, can view it if it is in a workplace.

3 T / F Harassment is illegal in the workplace, even if the staff want to use it on a client to make them have a shower that is scheduled on the care plan.

4 T / F Negligence can still be proved if a person did not intend to cause injury.

5 T / F Residents in an aged care service still have a definite set of rights, just as people within their homes.

6 T / F Restraint is a term which relates only to those which are physically applied.

7 T / F Placing a person in a chair close to a table in order to prevent them from moving out of the chair is NOT considered restraint.

Circle the BEST answer:

8 Ethics is:
   a a set of laws
   b the policies of your service
   c knowledge of what is right and wrong conduct
   d knowledge of how to give good care

9 Which of the following is not harassment?
   a Using touch to comfort a person
   b Joking about a person's religion
   c Asking for a sexual favour
   d Imitating a person's disability

10 A document that gives instructions about a person's future health is referred to as:
   a an advance health directive
   b a will
   c a statement of intent
   d a testament

Answers to these questions are on p. 454.

Further reading

Advance Care Planning Australia (2021). Have the conversation across healthcare services. Online 28 February 2021. Available: www.advancecareplanning.org.au/for-health-and-care-workers/roles-and-responsibilities-in-healthcare

Australian Commission on Quality and Safety in Health Care (2021). Report on person-centred care organisations. Online February 28 2021. Available: Report on person-centred healthcare organisations | Australian Commission on Safety and Quality in Health Care

Australian Government (2021). Powers of Attorney: State Agencies. Online 28 February 2021. Available: www.australia.gov.au/information-and-services/family-and-community/wills-and-powers-of-attorney/powers-of-attorney

Australian Government (2021). Restrictive practices in aged care - a last resort. Available: http://www.health.gov.au/health-topics/aged-care/providing-aged-care-services/working-in-aged-care/restrictive-practices-in-aged-care-a-last-resort

Australian Government, Department of Health (2021). Charter of Care Recipients' Rights and Responsibilities – Residential Care. Online February 28 2021. Available: charter_of_care_recipients_rights_responsibilities_-_residential_care.pdf (dss.gov.au)

Australian Government, Department of Health (2021). Empowering consumers and their families and carers through participation and partnerships. Online 28 February 2021. Available: health.gov.au/internet/publications/publishing.nsf/Content/mental-pubs-p-mono-toc,mental-pubs-p-mono-inc,mental-pubs-p-mono-inc-emp

Australian Government, Department of Health (2012). Ageing and Aged Care. Decision-making tool: Supporting a restraint free environment in residential aged care. Online 28 February 2021. Available: Decision-Making Tool – Supporting a restraint-free environment.pdf (agedcarequality.gov.au)

Australian Government, Fair Work Ombudsman (2021). Bullying and harassment. Online 28 February 2021. Available: www.fairwork.gov.au/employee-entitlements/bullying-and-harassment

Australian Government, Federal Register of Legislation (2021). Privacy Act 1988. Online 28 February 2021. Available: www.legislation.gov.au/Details/C2016C00979

Australian Government, Federal Register of Legislation (2021). Privacy Amendment (Enhancing Privacy Protection) Act 2012. Online 28 February 2021. Available: www.legislation.gov.au/Details/C2012A00197

Australian Government, My Aged Care (2021). Guardianship and administration. Online 28 February 2021. Available: www.myagedcare.gov.au/legal-information/guardianship-and-administrators

Australian Government, My Aged Care (2021). Rights and responsibilities: Home Care. Online 28 February 2021. Available: www.myagedcare.gov.au/quality-and-complaints/quality-of-care-and-consumer-rights/rights-and-responsibilities-home-care
Australian Institute of Patient and Family-Centred Care (2021). Online 28 February 2021. Available: www.aipfcc.org.au/
Griffith R (2015). What is Gillick competence? Human Vaccines and Immunotherapeutics 12(1), 244–247.
Health and Disability Commissioner New Zealand (2021). The Code of Rights. Online 28 February 2021. Available: The Code and Your Rights - Health and Disability Commissioner (hdc.org.nz)
New Zealand Aged Care Association (2021). NZACA Code of Residents' Rights and Responsibilities. Online 28 February 2021. Available: nzaca.org.nz/members/rules-and-code-of-conduct/
New Zealand Health and Disability Commissioner (2021). Health and Disability Advocacy: Resources. Online 28 February 2021. Available: Resources & Publications - Health and Disability Commissioner (hdc.org.nz)
Office of the Privacy Commissioner New Zealand (2021). Codes of Practice. Online 28 February 2021. Available: www.privacy.org.nz/the-privacy-act-and-codes/codes-of-practice/
Office of the Privacy Commissioner New Zealand (2021). A thumbnail sketch of the privacy principles. Online 28 February 2021. Available: www.privacy.org.nz/the-privacy-act-and-codes/privacy-principles/
Safe Work Australia (2021). Dealing with workplace bullying – A worker's guide. Online 28 February 2021. Available: www.safeworkaustralia.gov.au/doc/dealing-workplace-bullying-workers-guide

CHAPTER 4
Workplace documentation and communication

By Ellie Kirov

AFTER READING THIS CHAPTER, YOU SHOULD BE ABLE TO:

- define the key terms listed in this chapter
- identify why care team members need to communicate
- state the rules for good communication
- state the purpose, parts and information found in the medical record
- identify the legal and ethical aspects of medical records
- discuss your role in the nursing process
- describe how information about a person is collected using the five senses
- describe the information you need to report to the registered nurse or the supervisor
- state the rules for recording and documenting
- demonstrate how to use a 24-hour clock
- describe the breakdown of medical terms and how they are constructed, and abbreviations
- discuss the use of computers and electronic networks in aged and disability care
- discuss how to protect the person's right to privacy when using computers and electronic networks
- state the rules for answering the telephone
- describe how to solve problems and deal with conflict.

Key terms

abbreviation: A shortened form of a word or phrase

admission sheet: A sheet which is completed when a person is first admitted to a facility and contains important information about the person

assessment: Collecting information about the consumer

care plan/comprehensive care plan: A written guide about the care a consumer should receive

communication: The exchange of information; a message sent is received and interpreted by the intended person

conflict: A clash between opposing interests and ideas

database: A collection of data or information that is stored electronically in a structured format

documentation: The process of creating written records of processes, care and observation; also known as written recording

effective communication: When a message sent is received and interpreted by the intended person

evaluation: A review of whether the goals in the planning step of the nursing process have been met

goal: A desired aim by a person who requires nursing care

implementation: Performing or carrying out nursing interventions in the care plan

medical diagnosis: The identification of a disease or condition by a doctor

medical record: A written account of a consumer's illness and response to the treatment and care given by the health team; chart

nursing diagnosis: A statement describing a health problem that can be treated by nursing measures

nursing intervention: An action or measure taken by the nursing team to help the consumer reach a goal

nursing process: The method used by registered nurses to plan and deliver nursing care; its five steps are assessment, nursing diagnosis, planning, implementation and evaluation

objective data: Information that can be seen, heard, felt or smelt by another person; signs; also known as factual data

observation: Using the senses of sight, hearing, touch and smell to collect information about a consumer

prefix: A word element placed at the beginning of a word that alters its meaning

progress notes: A written description of the care given and the consumer's response and progress

recording: Writing an account of care and observations

reporting: Giving an oral account of care and observations

root: A word element containing the basic meaning of the word

signs: An indication or characteristic based on physical observation, examination or treatment of a consumer; objective data

subjective data: What is reported by a consumer and cannot be observed by using the senses; symptoms; also considered as a person's opinion

suffix: A word element placed at the end of a root to change the meaning of the word

symptoms: A consumer's description of what they are experiencing

triggers: Clues for the consumer assessment

word element: A part of a word

Communication is vital in providing quality care to consumers, whether they are in hospital, community care or residential aged care services. You should already be aware of the importance of verbal and non-verbal communication strategies when communicating with these consumers to promote dignity, respect and individualised care. As such, this chapter will concentrate on the communication that occurs between members of the healthcare team to assist in high quality and consistent care of the consumers.

Communication between team members is vital for quality healthcare. Team members continually communicate with each other in order to give coordinated and effective care.

They share information about:

- what was done for the person
- what needs to be done for the person
- the person's response to treatment
- the person in general; for example, likes and dislikes, social history, family members.

As a carer, it is important for you to understand the basic aspects and rules of communication, so that you can learn ways to communicate effectively with the nursing and health teams.

The following is an example of effective communication by the care team:

> The doctor has ordered a blood test for Mrs Carter. Food affects the test results and so Mrs Carter cannot have breakfast until a blood sample has been drawn. The carer tells the kitchen staff that Mrs Carter's breakfast will be served later, in her room. She explains to Mrs Carter why her breakfast will be delayed. The pathology collector tells the carer that the blood sample has been taken. You then prepare the meal and serve Mrs Carter's tray. When she finishes eating, you remove the tray and note what she has eaten. If anything has changed, you report your observations to your supervisor and document your observations in Mrs Carter's progress notes.

In this example, the team members communicated with each other and with Mrs Carter, so her care was coordinated and effective, and Mrs Carter understood that she was not neglected or forgotten.

COMMUNICATION

Effective communication is the exchange of information: a message sent is received and interpreted by the intended person.

For good communication, follow these principles:

- Use words that mean the same thing to the sender and the receiver of the message. 'Small', 'moderate' and 'large' mean different things to different people. Is small the size of a 5-cent piece or a 50-cent piece? In healthcare, different meanings can cause serious problems. Try to avoid using words that have more than one meaning.
- Use familiar words. You will learn medical terminology. If someone uses a term that is unknown to you, ask for an explanation. You must understand the message sent to you, otherwise effective communication will not occur. Likewise, do not use terms that are unfamiliar to the person and their family.
- Be brief and concise. Do not get wordy or add unrelated or unnecessary information. Stay on the subject. Avoid wandering in thought.
- Give information in a logical and orderly manner. Organise your thoughts, then present them step-by-step.
- Give facts and be specific. The receiver should have a clear picture of exactly what you are saying. For example, reporting a pulse rate of 110 is more specific and factual than saying the 'pulse is fast'.
- Actively listen to what is being said to you. Although you may think you understand what has been said, clarify it with the person to ensure you have understood what they were saying.
- When talking with someone, make sure you are in an environment that enables communication to take place. For example, if you have to talk to a consumer who has difficulty hearing, make sure there is no or very little surrounding noise.
- Take notes. You are not expected, nor is it safe, to memorise everything you are told or times that specific events occur.

THE MEDICAL RECORD

The **medical record** is a written account of the person's condition, and their response to care and treatment. It is a way for the health team to share information about the person. The record is permanent. It can be used years later if the person's health history is needed. The record is a legal document. It can be used as evidence of the person's problems, treatment and care, including in a court of law, several years after the care was provided.

The record has many forms and is organised into sections for easy use. Each page must have the person's name, consumer record number and other identifying information. This helps prevent errors and improper placement of records. The record includes the person's:

- admission sheet
- medical history
- physical examination results
- doctor's orders
- doctor's progress notes
- aged care assessment team (ACAT) report
- progress notes
- observation sheets for vital signs, and/or blood glucose readings
- social history and lifestyle admission
- pathology results
- X-ray examination reports

- intravenous therapy record (if intravenous therapy is administered: not very common in residential aged care services)
- physiotherapy assessments and consultation sheets
- complementary therapies notes
- assessments from nursing and activities officers
- special consents.

In Australia, assessment from nursing and activities officers can include, but are not limited to, assessments of activities of daily living, behaviours, sleep, continence, nutrition and social history.

Care team members record information on forms designed by the facility for specific purposes. Other members of the team read the information. It tells of the care provided and the person's response to that care.

Facilities have policies about consumer records and who may see them. These policies address:

- who should record the information
- when to record it
- abbreviations that can be used
- how to correct errors
- what ink colour to use.

Some facilities allow carers to record observations and care and may also be involved in the extensive assessment processes. Others do not. You need to know your facility's policies.

Professional staff involved in a person's care can access the chart. Cooks, laundry and housekeeping staff and office clerks have no need to read a person's medical record. However, they may receive a separate document that explains their need as required; for example, the kitchen will receive **documentation** of special dietary requirements and preferences for beverages, but will not have access to other information about the person.

As a member of the care team, you need to read the medical record to ensure you are fully aware of what has been happening for your consumer. It is important after having days off that you read the notes to familiarise yourself with any changes. In many aged care facilities, there is a communication and/or handover book where 'out of the ordinary' events are recorded. This does not replace the use of documenting in the progress notes. This must still be done in the required detail. However, the communication book is an effective way to review changes that may have occurred during your absence as it will provide a summary of things that may have changed. In addition, refer to the consumer's notes and ask the person in charge if you are still unsure.

You have an ethical and legal duty to keep the person's information confidential. Only staff members involved in the person's care need to read the medical records. If you are not involved in that person's care you have no right to review that person's medical record. To do so is an invasion of privacy and a breach of the Privacy Act.

Many facilities let consumers see their records if they ask to do so (Fig. 4.1). In some states and territories, it is the consumer's legal right. You should know the facility's policy about consumers or their legal representatives seeing the medical record. If a consumer or a legal representative asks you for the medical record, report the request to the supervisor. The supervisor will deal with it. Parts of the medical record that relate to your work are described below.

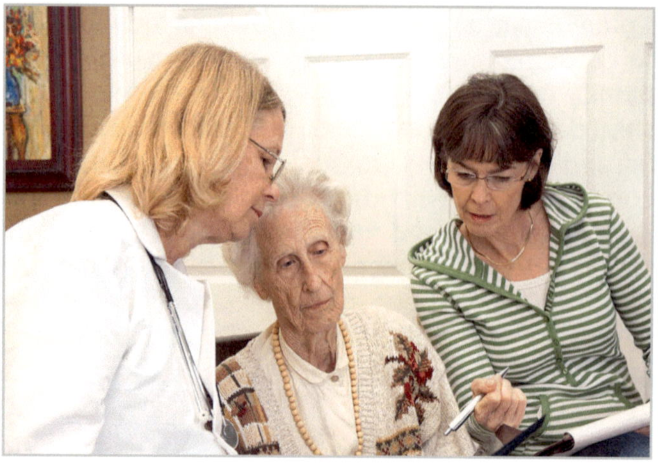

Fig. 4.1
A nurse, consumer and family member review the care plan together.

Admission sheet

The **admission sheet** is completed when the person is admitted to the facility. It contains identifying information about the person: legal name, birth date, age, gender, current address and marital status. It also has the person's Medicare and/or Social Security number. The name of the person's legal representative and next of kin are also included. Other information includes known allergies, diagnosis, date and time of admission, doctor's name, religion and church. Advance health directives may also be found here. An advance health directive is a document specifying a person's wishes for medical treatment when they can no longer make decisions for themselves, and to ensure information for healthcare professions, including about life-support measures.

An identification consumer number is given to each person, and is included on the admission sheet.

The admission sheet gives background information about a person and is used to fill out other forms that require the same information. That way, the person or legal representative does not have to answer the same questions many times.

Progress notes

The **progress notes** are a written description of the care given and the person's response (Fig. 4.2). They include:

- the person's signs and symptoms
- information about special treatments and medications
- information about consumer teaching and counselling
- procedures performed by the doctor
- visits by other health team members.

Date	Time	
19-3-22	1700	Out with family for dinner. Jane Doe, EN
	1930	Returned from outing accompanied by her son. States she had a pleasant time. Mary Smith, EN
20-3-22	0900	In bed. Complains of headache. T36.8 orally, radial pulse 72 and regular, respirations 18 and unlaboured. BP 134/84 left arm lying down. Alice Jones, RN notified of resident complaint and vital signs. Ann Adams, EN
	0910	In bed resting. States she has had a headache for about 1/2 hour. Denies nausea and dizziness. No other complaints. PRN Paracetamol given. Instructed resident to use signal light if headache worsens or other symptoms occur. Alice Jones, RN
	0945	Resting quietly. Denies headache at this time. T 36.9 orally, radial pulse 70 and regular, respirations 18 and unlaboured. BP 132/84 left arm lying down. Alice Jones, RN

Fig. 4.2
Progress notes.

Progress notes are written when there is a change in the person's condition, an unusual event or a problem. Some facilities require progress notes to be written at least once every 24 hours, others once a month or only when there is a change. Care plans may need to be reviewed each month or every 3 months, as well as when there is a change. The notes reflect the person's progress towards the goals set in the care plan. They also reflect the person's response to care. Some centres require more frequent summaries. Whether in a residential service or in a community setting, these notes form a legal record of the care given to consumers.

Care plan

The **care plan** is a guide that assists the personal care assistant in knowing what care and assistance is needed for a consumer. The plan is specifically designed to meet the consumer's needs and is individualised. The nursing process (see below) is used to plan care needs. In addition, a summary of each person's care plan may be posted in their en-suite or inside their wardrobe door to make access easier. These are usually a summary only and the carer is expected to refer to the main care plan if further information is required.

Other observation sheets

Other observation sheets are used to record frequent measurements or observations (Fig. 4.3). For example, a person's blood pressure may need to be taken twice a day, or the person may need to be weighed daily. These measurements are recorded on an observation sheet designed

WEIGHT AND VITAL SIGNS FLOWSHEET

Date	Time	Weight	T	P	R	BP				Signatures
19/10/22	0700	61 kg	36.6	72	20	142/84				Mary Smith EN
26/10/22	0715	60 kg	36.8	72	18	140/84				Jane Doe EN
2/11/22	0715	61 kg	36.0	70	18	144/82				Mary Smith EN

Fig. 4.3
Vital signs and daily weight flowsheet.

for this purpose. The fluid intake and output record is known as a fluid balance sheet.

THE NURSING PROCESS

The **nursing process** is the process used to identify and plan care for a person. This section refers to 'nurse' or 'nursing', but the implementation (intervention) is carried out by care staff, with a registered nurse (RN) doing the assessment.

Carers and nurses communicate with each other about the person's strengths, limitations, needs and care. This information is communicated through the nursing process. Nurses use the nursing process to plan and deliver nursing care. The nursing process is also used in assessing a person. The nursing process has five steps:

1. assessment
2. nursing diagnosis
3. planning
4. implementation
5. evaluation.

The process focuses on the person's nursing needs. It requires good communication between the person and the nursing team.

Each step is important. Nursing care is organised and has a purpose. All care team members do the same things for the person – they have the same goals. With consistent care the person feels safe and secure. The nursing process is ongoing and changes according to the person's needs.

Assessment

Assessment involves collecting information about the person from many sources, with the RN responsible for the assessment. For example, a nursing history tells about the person's current and past health problems. The family's health history is important. Information from the doctor is reviewed, and so are test results and the person's past medical history.

The RN assesses the person's body systems and mental status. You play a key role in the assessment, as you will make many observations while caring for and talking with the person.

Observation means using the senses of sight, hearing, touch and smell to collect information:

- Sight – you see how the person lies, sits or walks. You see flushed or pale skin. You see red and swollen body areas.
- Hearing – you listen to the person breathe, talk and cough. An RN may use a stethoscope to listen to the heartbeat and to measure blood pressure.
- Touch – through touch you feel if the skin is hot or cold, or moist or dry. You use touch to take the person's pulse.
- Smell – smell is used to detect body, wound and breath odours. You also smell odours from urine and bowel movements.

Objective data (signs) are seen, heard, felt or smelt. You can feel a pulse. You can see and smell urine. **Subjective data (symptoms)** are things a person tells you, which you cannot observe through your senses, or are based on another person's opinion. You cannot feel or see the person's pain, fear or nausea; however, the information they provide is still very important to document/record. Box 4.1 lists the basic observations you need to make and report to the nurse. Make notes to record and report your observations. Carry a notepad and pen in your pocket, so you can write your observations as you make them.

BOX 4.1
Basic observations

Ability to respond

- Is the person easy or difficult to wake up?
- Can the person give his or her name, and the time and location when asked?
- Does the person identify others accurately?
- Does the person answer questions correctly?
- Does the person speak clearly?
- Are instructions followed correctly?
- Is the person calm, restless or excited?
- Is the person conversing, quiet or talking a lot?

Movement

- Does the person have a history of falls?
- Can the person squeeze your fingers with each hand?
- Can the person move their arms and legs?
- Are the person's movements shaky or jerky?
- Does the person complain of stiff or painful joints?
- Does the person use a mobility aid?
- Does the person have trouble maintaining balance?

Pain or discomfort

- Where is the pain located? (Ask the person to point to the pain.)
- Does the pain go anywhere else?
- When did the pain begin?
- What was the person doing when the pain began?
- How long does the pain last?
- How does the person describe the pain?
  - sharp
  - severe
  - knife-like
  - dull
  - burning
  - aching
  - comes and goes
  - depends on position
- Was medication given?
- Did medication help relieve the pain? Is pain still present?
- Is the person able to sleep and rest?

BOX 4.1
Basic observations *continued*

- What does the person do to relieve the pain?
- What is the position of comfort?
- In many facilities, a pain score is used where the person is asked to rate their pain from 0 to 10. However, this is not an accurate way of measuring pain in a person with cognitive deficits, so other tools may be implemented.

Skin
- Is the skin pale or flushed?
- Is the skin cool, warm or hot?
- Is the skin moist or dry?
- What colour are the lips and nails?
- Is the skin intact? Are there broken areas? If so, where?
- Are sores or reddened areas present?
- Are bruises present?
- Where are they located?
- Does the person complain of itching?
- Does the person have a skin care regimen?

Activities of daily living
- Can the person perform personal care without help?
  - bathing?
  - brushing teeth?
  - combing and brushing hair?
  - shaving?
- Does the person use the toilet, commode, bedpan or urinal?
- Does the person feed himself or herself?
- Can the person walk?
- Does the person need assistance undressing or dressing?
- Describe the assistance needed for the above activity/ies.
- What amount and kind of assistance is needed?

Eyes, ears, nose and mouth
- Is there drainage from the eyes? What colour is the drainage?
- Are the eyelids closed?
- Are the eyes reddened?
- Does the person need bright lights when reading?
- Is the person sensitive to bright lights?
- Is there drainage from the ears? What colour is the drainage?
- Can the person hear? Is repeating necessary?
- Are questions answered appropriately?
- Is there drainage from the nose? What colour is the drainage?
- Can the person breathe through their nose?
- Is there breath odour?
- Does the person complain of bad taste in the mouth?
- Does the person have well-fitting dentures?
- Does the person complain of painful gums or teeth?
- Is the tongue moist or dry?

Respiration
- Does the person smoke?
- Do both sides of the person's chest rise and fall with respiration?
- Is breathing noisy?
- Does the person complain of difficulty breathing?
- What is the amount and colour of sputum?
- Does the person take medication for their breathing?
- What is the frequency of the person's cough? Is it dry or productive?
- Does the person become short of breath after activity, e.g. after a shower?

Bowels and bladder
- Is the abdomen firm or soft?
- Does the person take any medication for their bowels?
- Does the person complain of wind?
- What are the amount, colour and consistency of bowel movements?
- What is the frequency of bowel movements?
- Can the person control their bowel movements?
- Does the person have pain or difficulty urinating?
- What is the amount of urine?
- Does the urine have a foul smell?
- Can the person control the passage of urine?
- What is the frequency of urination?
- A continence assessment may be required, which includes time the person was toileted and times they were dry or wet. This provides the data to establish an individualised toileting program for the person.

Appetite
- Does the person have any food allergies?
- Is the person on a special diet?
- What size meal does the person usually eat?
- What are the person's food preferences?
- Can the person chew food?
- How much liquid was taken?
- What are the person's drink preferences?
- How often does the person drink liquids?
- Does the person have difficulty swallowing food and fluids?
- Does the person complain of nausea?
- Does the person have a medical condition that could affect appetite and swallowing?

Mental health
- Is there a past history of mental health issues?
- How do they perceive their mood?
- How do they perceive their self image?
- Do they have any particular worries or concerns?

The assessment step never ends. Every time you have contact with the consumer, new information is collected and new observations are made. The person shares more information. Often the family adds more information.

Behaviours

Some people in aged care facilities have behaviours that need assessments. These may include verbal behaviours, such as yelling out, crying or repetitive phrases. Physical behaviours may include agitated wandering, punching out, hitting walls and so on. In these cases, it is very important to try to identify triggers and any interventions that can assist the consumer to become less distressed. As a result, behaviour assessments may be conducted where time, place, any observable (not assumed) triggers and interventions and their results (effective or not) are recorded. This provides useful information in determining a person's care, particularly when a cognitive deficit such as dementia affects the person's ability to clearly communicate their needs.

Nursing diagnosis

The RN uses assessment information to make a nursing diagnosis. A nursing diagnosis describes a health problem that can be treated by nursing measures. The problem may exist or may develop. Nursing diagnoses and medical diagnoses are not the same. A medical diagnosis is the identification of a disease or condition by a doctor (e.g. cancer, stroke, heart attack, infection, diabetes). Doctors order medication, allied health interventions and/or surgery to cure or heal.

A person can have many nursing diagnoses. Nursing diagnoses involve the person's physical, emotional, social and spiritual needs. They may change, or new ones may be added as assessment information changes. An example might be: *Joe is prone to falls due to balance problems since his stroke.*

Planning

In the planning stage, priorities and goals for the person's care are set.

1. *Priorities* relate to what is most important for the person. Needs are arranged in order of importance – some needs are required for life and survival (oxygen, water and food), and these must be met before all other needs.
2. *Goals* are then set. A **goal** is a desired aim by a person because of nursing care. Goals are aimed at the person's highest level of wellbeing and functioning: physical, emotional, social, spiritual. Goals promote health, prevent health problems, promote rehabilitation and support the person's independence. Goals should be achievable and realistic. For example, a goal for Joe may be: *to prevent falls from occurring.*

Measures or actions are chosen to help the person meet their goals. The person, family and care team help the RN plan care.

After goals for the person's care have been set, nursing interventions are chosen. A **nursing intervention** is an action or measure taken by the nursing team to help the person reach a goal. 'Nursing intervention', 'nursing action' and 'nursing measure' all mean the same thing. A nursing intervention does not need a doctor's order. However, some nursing measures come from a doctor's order. For example, a doctor may order that a consumer walk 25 metres twice each day. The nurse would include this order in the care plan. An example for Joe could be: *Ensure call bell is within easy reach for Joe. Ensure one staff member is with Joe when ambulating and encourage Joe to use his walking stick.* You can see that at times there is more than one intervention listed to achieve one goal.

An interdisciplinary care planning conference (see below) may be required because of a person's individualised care needs or underlying issues.

The **care plan** (or **comprehensive care plan**) is a written guide about the care a person should receive. The care team develops it. The care plan includes nursing diagnoses and goals. It identifies the person's problems, goals for care and actions to take to help the person solve problems and/or issues.

The problems identified on admission give **triggers** (clues) for the consumer assessment. Information obtained during a care conference can be used to develop the person's care plan. For example:

> *Mr Samble is weak after having the flu and has been in bed for a week. The care plan shows that he cannot carry out his activities of daily living (ADLs) independently. On admission, Mr Samble was independent with his ADLs and only required assistance with buttons. Mr Samble's admission notes give information on how to increase his independence to the level he was at prior to getting the flu.*

The goal is for Mr Samble to perform his own ADLs. Staff discuss with the physiotherapist, family, consumer and doctor ways to ensure that the goals are achievable and the interventions are effective.

The interventions are as follows:

- The physiotherapy aid is to see Mr Samble 3 days per week for 30 minutes, to supervise exercises.
- Care staff are to encourage Mr Samble to walk to the dining room for all meals.
- Care staff are to set up for Mr Samble's shower and give Mr Samble lots of encouragement during the entire shower and dressing process.

The care plan also states the person's strengths. For example:

> *Mrs Jacques can walk without assistance. Therefore, she should be encouraged to walk without staff looking over her shoulder. It will also assist care staff to know that if Mrs Jacques is having difficulty walking, then this needs looking into, to find out why she is no longer independent.*

A comprehensive care plan is developed for each person. Care plan suggestions are welcomed from all team members, including personal care assistants. You use the care plan to give care. It is a communication tool. It tells what care to give and when.

Care plan forms vary in each centre. It may be in the person's medical record or a notebook. The plan must be carried out. The care plan is revised as the person's needs change.

Implementation

Implementation means to perform or carry out. The implementation step consists of performing or carrying out the interventions identified in the care plan. Care is given in this step.

Care interventions range from simple to complex. The RN or supervisor delegates interventions that are within your legal limits and job description. They may also ask you to assist with complex nursing interventions.

You report the care given to the supervisor. Some facilities allow you to record care. Reporting and recording are done *after* giving care, not before. As explained earlier, you should report or record your observations. Observing is part of assessment. If new observations change the nursing diagnoses, changes will need to be made to the care plan. To give the correct care, you need to know about any changes in the care plan. If what is required in practice is different from the care plan a new assessment may be required, which will then inform the changes required to the care plan. Sometimes the changes entered into the progress notes may be sufficient for a change in a care plan to occur; at other times a full new assessment document for the particular area of care may be required. It is not appropriate to change a care plan without documented evidence as to why this has occurred. Ultimately, it is the supervisor's role to approve the changes, but often it is the carer who observes them.

Evaluation

Evaluation means to measure. The evaluation step involves measuring whether the goals in the planning step are being met; in other words, the person's progress is evaluated. Goals may be met totally, in part or not at all. For example, for Joe an assessment may read: *No falls have occurred during the day; however, Joe has fallen out of bed at night twice when trying to get up on his own.* The assessment information (described above) is used for this step. Changes in nursing diagnoses, goals and the care plan may result. A possible change could then be the addition of further interventions: *Ensure bed is low to the floor when Joe is in the bed.* And: *Place a sensor mat on the floor next to the bed to alert staff when Joe is trying to get up unassisted* may be added to provide further safety at nighttime.

The nursing process never ends. Nurses constantly collect information about the person. Nursing diagnoses, goals and the care plan change as the person's needs change. You have a key role in the nursing process. The RN uses your observations and reports for nursing diagnoses and planning. You may help to develop the care plan. In the implementation step, you perform the care interventions in the care plan. Your observations are used for the evaluation step.

Care planning and documentation are essential for ensuring appropriate care and for funding. It is important that you receive further training in care planning if you are required to carry out this task.

CONSUMER CARE CONFERENCE

There are two types of consumer care conferences:

- The *multidisciplinary care planning (MDCP) conference* is often held regularly to review and update care plans. It is also held to develop care plans for new consumers. The RN, doctor and other care team members attend. The person and a family member also attend.
- A *problem-focused conference* is held when one problem affects a person's care. Staff directly involved in the problem attend. The person or a family member may be asked to attend.

The person has the right to take part in planning. He or she may refuse actions suggested by the care team, and this can be documented in the progress notes. Often you will attend both conferences. You should share your ideas and observations, ensuring you do so in a professional manner at all times.

Reporting and recording

Healthcare is complex and there are many policies and procedures to be followed. Communication is vital for all aspects of ensuring high quality care to consumers. At times, you may be asked to document a fall or fill in a feedback suggestion form or incident form if you witnessed the fall, but the majority of formal communication you will experience will relate directly to the care you provide to the consumers in your care. The health team communicates by reporting and recording. **Reporting** means giving an oral account of care and observations. **Recording** means writing an account of observations and care. It is often called report writing or documenting.

Reporting

You report care and observations to the RN or supervisor. When reporting, follow these rules:

- Be prompt, thorough and accurate.
- Give the person's name, room and bed number.
- Note the time your observations were made or the care was given.
- Report only what you observed or what you did yourself.
- Give reports as often as the person's condition requires. Alternatively, give them as often as the RN or supervisor asks you to.
- Report any changes from normal or changes in the person's condition. Report changes immediately.
- Use your written notes to give a specific, concise and clear report.

End-of-shift report

A report is given at the end of the shift. This is called the *end-of-shift report* or *handover*. Depending on your shift time you may be required to give your handover to the staff coming onto the new shift; however, you may be required to provide a handover to your supervisor before leaving your shift so they can provide handover on your behalf. It is important that you ensure all new information has been documented as no one else can document on your behalf (see below). The handover is given to the care team of the oncoming shift. Information is shared about the consumer care given and the care that must be given. Information about the person's condition is included.

It is important to listen carefully at handover, because this is when you can ask questions or clarify any care issues that may be raised (Fig. 4.4).

Recording/documenting

When recording on a person's chart, you must communicate clearly and thoroughly. Follow the rules in Box 4.2. The sample progress notes in Fig. 4.2 (p. 101) show how the rules apply. Anyone who reads your report should know:

- what you observed
- what you did
- the person's response
- what the outcome or follow-up was, if any
- who you are (name and position title you work under in the facility e.g. personal carer, assistant in nursing).

All written progress reports should show the date and time the report was written.

Recording time

The 24-hour clock (or military time clock) has four digits (see Fig. 4.5). The first two digits are for the hour: 0100 = 1.00 a.m.; 1300 = 1.00 p.m. The last two digits are for minutes: 0110 = 1.10 a.m. The abbreviations a.m. and p.m. are not used.

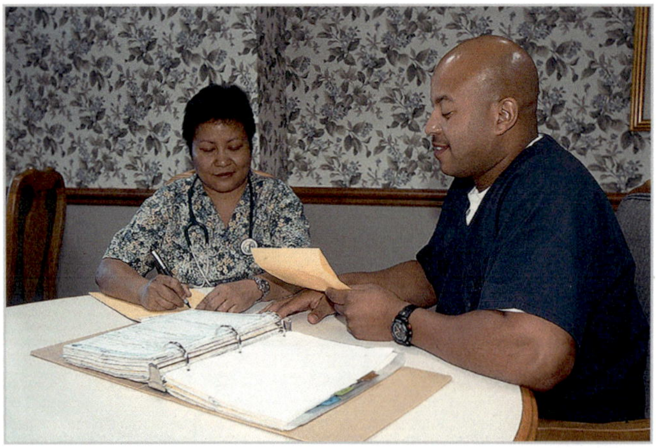

Fig. 4.4
The personal care assistant uses notes when reporting to the supervisor.

BOX 4.2
Rules for recording/documenting

- Always use ink. Use the ink colour required by the facility, usually black or dark blue.
- Include the date and the time for every recording. Use 24-hour clock time according to the facility's policy.
- Make sure your writing is legible and neat.
- Use only centre-approved abbreviations.
- Use correct spelling, grammar and punctuation.
- Never erase or use correction fluid if you make an error. Cross out the incorrect part, write 'error' or 'mistaken entry' over it and sign your initials to the mistaken entry. Rewrite the part. Follow the facility's policy for correcting errors.
- Sign all entries with your name and title as required by facility policy.
- Do not skip lines. Draw a line through the blank space of a partially completed line or to the end of a page. This prevents others from recording in a space with your signature.
- Make sure each form is stamped with the person's name and other identifying information.
- Record only what you observed and did yourself.
- Never chart a procedure or treatment until after it has been completed.
- Be accurate, concise and factual. Do not record judgements or interpretations.
- Record in a logical and sequential manner.
- Be descriptive. Avoid terms that have more than one meaning.
- Use the person's exact words whenever possible. Use quotation marks to show that the statement is a direct quote.
- Record any changes from normal or changes in the person's condition. Also record that you informed the RN or supervisor, what you told them and the time you made the report.
- Do not omit information.
- Record safety measures taken, such as placing the call button within reach, assisting a person when up or reminding someone not to get out of bed. This helps protect you if the person falls.

As Fig. 4.5 shows, the hour is the same for morning times, but 'a.m.' is not used. For p.m. (afternoon) times, add 12 to the clock hour time. For example, for 2.00 p.m., add 12 and 2 for the hour for 1400. For 8.35 p.m., add 12 and 8 for the hour and 35 for the minutes to give 2035.

MEDICAL TERMINOLOGY AND ABBREVIATIONS

Medical terminology and abbreviations are used in all areas of healthcare, including aged and disability care. If someone uses a word or phrase that you do not understand, ask

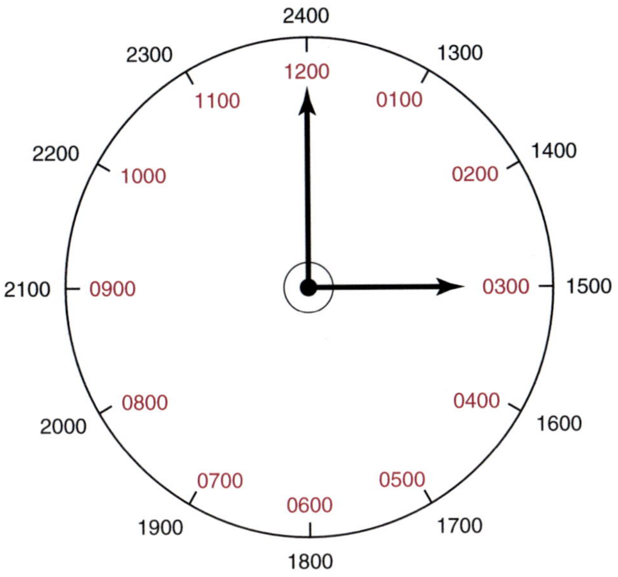

Fig. 4.5
The 24-hour clock. Instead of two 12-hour cycles, the 24-hour clock is one 24-hour time cycle.

a nurse to explain its meaning. You may also want to buy a medical dictionary so you can learn new words. Ensure it is an English, not US, version as US spelling frequently omits letters used in words in Australia and New Zealand; for example, use colour rather than color and haemoglobin, not hemoglobin.

Prefixes, roots and suffixes

Medical terms are formed by combining **word elements** – that is, prefixes, roots and suffixes (Table 4.1). Most come from Greek or Latin.

A **prefix** is placed at the beginning of a word. The prefix changes the word's meaning. As an example, the prefix *olig* (meaning 'scant', a small amount) is placed before the word *uria* (urine) to make *oliguria*, which means 'a scant amount of urine'. Prefixes are always combined with other word elements. They are never used alone.

The **root** contains the basic meaning of the word. Roots can be combined with other roots, with prefixes and with suffixes. A vowel (an 'o' or an 'i') is added when two roots are combined or when a suffix is added to a root. The vowel makes pronunciation easier.

Table 4.1
Medical terminology

Prefixes	
Prefix	**Meaning**
a-, an-	without, not, lack of
ab-	away from
ad-	to, towards, near
ante-	before, forward, in front of
anti-	against
auto-	self
bi-	double, two, twice
brady-	slow
circum-	around
contra-	against, opposite
de-	down, from
dia-	across, through, apart
dis-	apart, free from
dys-	bad, difficult, abnormal
ecto-	outer, outside
en-	in, into, within
endo-	inner, inside
epi-	over, on, upon
eryth-	red
eu-	normal, good, well, healthy
ex-	out, out of, from, away from
hemi-	half

Prefixes	
Prefix	**Meaning**
hyper-	excessive, too much, high
hypo-	under, decreased, less than normal
in-	in, into, within, not
intra-	within
inter-	between
intro-	into, within
leuk-	white
macro-	large
mal-	bad, illness, disease
mega-	large
micro-	small
mono-	one, single
neo-	new
non-	not
olig-	small, scant
para-	beside, beyond, after
per-	by, through
peri-	around
poly-	many, much
post-	after, behind
pre-	before, in front of, prior to
pro-	forwards, onwards

TABLE 4.1
Medical terminology *continued*

Prefixes		Prefixes	
Prefix	**Meaning**	**Prefix**	**Meaning**
re-	again, backward	supra-	above, over
retro-	backward, behind	tachy-	fast, rapid
semi-	half	trans-	across
sub-	under, beneath	uni-	one
super-	above, over, excess		

Roots		Roots	
Root (combining vowel)	**Meaning**	**Root (combining vowel)**	**Meaning**
abdomin (o)	abdomen	hyster (o)	uterus
aden (o)	gland	ile (o)	ileum
adren (o)	adrenal gland	laparo	abdomen, loin, flank
angi (o)	vessel	laryng (o)	larynx
arterio	artery	lith (o)	stone
arthr (o)	joint	mamm (o)	breast, mammary gland
broncho	bronchus, bronchi	mast (o)	mammary gland, breast
card, cardi (o)	heart	meno	menstruation
cephal (o)	head	my (o)	muscle
chole, chol (o)	bile	myel (o)	spinal cord, bone marrow
chondr (o)	cartilage	necro	death
colo	colon, large intestine	nephr (o)	kidney
cost (o)	rib	neur (o)	nerve
crani (o)	skull	ocul (o)	eye
cyan (o)	blue	oophor (o)	ovary
cyst (o)	bladder, cyst	ophthalm (o)	eye
cyt (o)	cell	orth (o)	straight, normal, correct
dent (o)	tooth	oste (o)	bone
derma	skin	ot (o)	ear
duoden (o)	duodenum	paed (o)	child
encephal (o)	brain	ped (o)	foot
enter (o)	intestines	pharyng (o)	pharynx
fibr (o)	fibre, fibrous	phleb (o)	vein
gastr (o)	stomach	pnoea	breathing, respiration
gloss (o)	tongue	pneum (o)	lung, air, gas
gluc (o)	sweetness, glucose	proct (o)	rectum
glyc (o)	sugar	psych (o)	mind
gyn, gynae, gynaeco	woman	pulmo	lung
haem, haema, haemo, haemat (o)	blood	rect (o)	rectum
hepat (o)	liver	rhin (o)	nose
hydr (o)	water	salping (o)	eustachian tube, uterine tube

TABLE 4.1
Medical terminology *continued*

Roots		Roots	
Root (combining vowel)	**Meaning**	**Root (combining vowel)**	**Meaning**
splen (o)	spleen	toxo	poison
sten (o)	narrow, constriction	trache (o)	trachea
stern (o)	sternum	urethr (o)	urethra
stomat (o)	mouth	urin (o)	urine
therm (o)	heat	uro	urine, urinary tract, urination
thoraco	chest	uter (o)	uterus
thromb (o)	clot, thrombus	vas (o)	blood vessel, vas deferens
thyr (o)	thyroid	ven (o)	vein
toxic (o)	poison, poisonous	vertebr (o)	spine, vertebrae
Suffixes		**Suffixes**	
Suffix	**Meaning**	**Suffix**	**Meaning**
-aemia	blood condition	-meter	measuring instrument
-asis	condition, usually abnormal	-oma	tumour
-cele	hernia, herniation, pouching	-osis	condition
-centesis	puncture and aspiration of	-pathy	disease
-coele	cavity, chamber	-penia	lack, deficiency
-cyte	cell	-phagia	to eat or consume; swallowing
-ectasis	dilation, stretching	-phasia	speaking
-ectomy	excision, removal of	-phobia	an exaggerated fear
-genesis	development, production, creation	-plasty	surgical repair or reshaping
-genic	producing, causing	-plegia	paralysis
-gram	record	-ptosis	falling, sagging, drooping, down
-graph	a diagram, a recording instrument	-rrhage, -rrhagia	excessive flow
-graphy	making a recording	-rrhaphy	stitching, suturing
-iasis	condition of	-rrhoea	profuse flow, discharge
-ism	a condition	-scope	examination instrument
-itis	inflammation	-scopy	examination using a scope
-logy	the study of	-stasis	maintenance, maintaining a constant level
-lysis	destruction of, decomposition	-tomy, -otomy	incision, cutting into
-megaly	enlargement	-uria	condition of the urine

A **suffix** is placed at the end of a root. It changes the meaning of the word. Suffixes are not used alone. When translating a medical term, begin with the suffix. For example, *nephritis* means 'inflammation of the kidney'. It was formed by combining *nephro* (kidney) and *itis* (inflammation).

Remember:

- the prefix always comes before the root. The suffix always comes after the root.
- a root can be combined with a prefix – for example, the prefix *dys* (difficult) combined with the root *pnoea*

(breathing) forms the term *dyspnoea*, which means 'difficulty in breathing'.
- a root can be combined with a suffix – for example, the root *mast* (breast) combined with the suffix *ectomy* (excision or removal) forms the term *mastectomy*, which means 'removal of a breast'.
- a root can be combined with a prefix and a suffix – for example, *endocarditis* has the prefix *endo* (inner), the root *card* (heart) and the suffix *itis* (inflammation). Endocarditis means 'inflammation of the inner part of the heart'.
- another common example that is often confused is *hypo* (means low) *glyc* (sugar) *aemia* (blood condition), so *hypoglycaemia* means low blood glucose level. This can be confused with *hyper* (high) *glyc* (sugar) *aemia* (blood condition), which means high blood glucose level. It is therefore important to clarify any terminology you hear or see being used if you are unsure, particularly as in this example the immediate treatment is very different for the person experiencing either high or low blood sugar levels.

Abbreviations

An **abbreviation** is a shortened form of a word or a phrase. Abbreviations save time and space when recording. Each facility has a list of accepted abbreviations. Obtain the list when you are hired. Use only those accepted by the facility. This is important as miscommunication can easily occur through the use of inaccurate abbreviations. For example, SOB commonly stands for Short of Breath, but SOOB can mean Sat Out of Bed: two very similar abbreviations with two very different meanings. Do not forget that you may be required to recall something you documented many years after the event. If you are unsure whether an abbreviation is acceptable, write the term out in full. This ensures accurate communication.

COMPUTERS IN HEALTHCARE

Computer systems collect, send, record and store information so it can be retrieved when needed. Many care facilities store records, charts and care plans on computer. Entering information into a computer is easier and faster than writing it by hand.

The care team uses computers to send messages and reports to other work colleagues. This reduces clerical work and telephone calls. Information is also sent with greater speed and accuracy. Some care teams use hand-held 'pilots' to assist staff in documenting changes in care needs.

Aged care facilities are increasingly using Consumer Management System (CMS) software to manage consumer records. These systems replace many paper-based forms, including charts, assessments, care plans and paper diaries. With the use of mobile devices, much documentation can be done with consumers and their families in their room or in the garden.

Computers are also used to monitor measurements such as blood pressure, temperature and heart rate. The computer detects normal and abnormal measurements. When

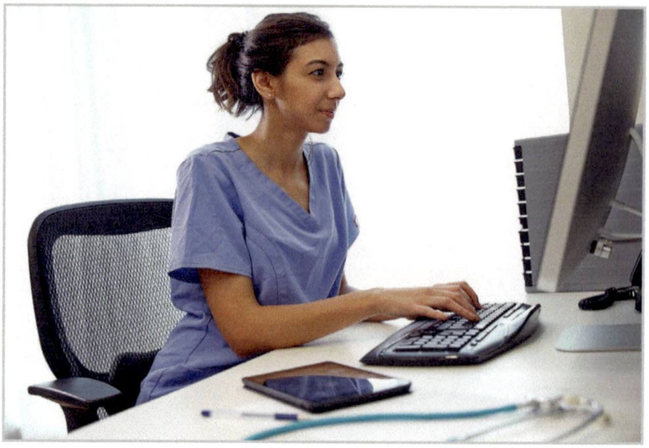

Fig. 4.6
The nurse enters information into the computer.

an abnormal reading is detected, an alarm alerts the nursing staff. Computer monitoring is common in hospitals. It also may be used in skilled nursing units (Fig. 4.6).

Computers save time, and increase the quality and safety of care. They can reduce the number of errors made in recording, and make records more complete. Staff time can be used more efficiently, as the need to document in several places is reduced.

Computers are easy to use. They contain vast amounts of information. Therefore, the right to privacy must be protected. Only certain staff use the computer. Each person has a code (password) to access computer files. If allowed access, you will learn how to use the system. You must follow the facility's policy. You should also follow the ethical and legal rules about privacy, confidentiality and defamation. Also, follow the rules in Box 4.3.

Electronic and digital technologies

Computers within a healthcare facility are generally in close proximity to one another, forming a local area network (LAN). The computers are networked so that they are linked to one another and to a wireless access point (WAP). The WAP converts information from the network into radio signals that can be captured by wireless mobile devices as part of a wi-fi system which supports mobile computing devices. Mobile computing devices may include mobile phones, laptops and tablets, but also wireless medical equipment such as blood pressure monitors. Devices that exchange information over very short distances, such as audio headsets, use Bluetooth technology where the device contains a small microchip for data transfer.

Electronic data are entered on a computer, which is linked to the wireless network. The data are entered in a database using software that may be accessed via a fixed or mobile electronic device, and stored on a server which acts as an electronic file storage system. A **database** is a collection of data or information (such as personal information, medical history, treatment, medication) that is

BOX 4.3
Using the facility's computer

- Do not tell anyone your password. If someone has your password they can access the computer under your name. It would be hard to prove that someone other than you made the entries.
- Change your password frequently.
- Do not use another person's password.
- Follow the rules for recording listed in Box 4.2.
- Enter information carefully. Double-check your entries.
- Prevent others from seeing what is on the screen.
- Do not leave the computer unattended. Log off after making an entry.
- Position equipment so that the screen cannot be seen in the hallway.
- Do not leave printouts where others can read them or pick them up.
- Destroy or shred any computer-printed worksheets used for handovers. However, do not under any circumstances destroy a record that will be filed into the person's history, e.g. completed assessments, observations sheets, etc.
- Send email and messages only to those who need the information.
- Do not use email or messages to send information that requires immediate reporting. Give the report in person. (The person might not read the email in a timely manner.)
- Do not use email or messages to report confidential information. This includes addresses, telephone numbers and pension numbers. The computer system may not be secure. Do not use the facility's computer to:
  - send personal emails or messages
  - send or receive emails or messages that are offensive, illegal or sexual
  - send or receive emails or messages for illegal activities, jokes, politics, gambling (including football and other pools), chain letters, advertising or other non-work-related activities
  - post information, opinions or comments on internet message boards
  - take part in internet discussion groups
  - upload, download or transmit material containing a copyright, trademark or patent.
- Remember that any communication may be read or heard by someone other than the intended person.
- Remember that deleted communications can be retrieved by authorised personnel.
- Remember that the facility has the right to monitor your computer use. This includes internet use.
- Do not open another person's emails or messages.

stored electronically in a structured format so that the data can be easily accessed, updated, managed and queried. In this way, specific information about a consumer can be retrieved when needed.

The information on the database is stored and retrieved via a database management system and can be accessed by any computer that is linked to the network. Data entered into the database forms part of the consumer's health record, which aids in the planning of a consumer's care and treatment.

Beyond the scope of the health facility network lies a global electronic network. This includes but is not limited to:

- email – an electronic textual method of communicating with one or more recipients, which while effective is also insecure due to interception and privacy concerns.
- World Wide Web (www) – a global electronic network service providing access to text, databases, journals, graphics, videos and audio information, where information is accessed via search engines (such as Google) and information appears in applications called browsers.
- social media – a communication platform for exchanging information about oneself, which can be valuable in fostering professional and personal networks, but can violate privacy and confidentiality.

You must follow the facility's policy where accessing these resources is concerned. You should also follow the ethical and legal rules about security and privacy (see Box 4.3).

TELEPHONE COMMUNICATIONS

You may have to answer telephones in the workplace or in the person's room. Good telephone communication skills are needed. The caller cannot see you, but you convey a lot of information by your tone of voice, how clearly you speak and your attitude. A conversation with you may be the first interaction that a family member or other person has with the facility, so it is important you make a good impression. Be professional, courteous and ethical. Follow the facility's policy and the guidelines listed in Box 4.4 when answering telephones.

DEALING WITH CONFLICT

People bring their values, attitudes, opinions, experiences and expectations to the workplace. Differences often lead to conflict. **Conflict** is a clash between opposing interests and ideas. People sometimes disagree and argue, with misunderstandings and unrest.

Conflicts can arise over issues or events, such as work schedules, absences or the amount or quality of work performed. The problems must be worked out. Otherwise, unkind words or actions may occur, the workplace may become unpleasant and care may be affected.

To resolve a conflict, you need to identify the real problem. This is part of problem solving. The problem-solving process involves these steps:

1. Define the problem. For example: *A team member ignores me.*

BOX 4.4
Guidelines for answering telephones

- Answer the call after the first ring if possible. Be sure to answer by the fourth ring.
- Do not answer the telephone in a rushed or hasty manner.
- Give a courteous greeting, identify the area and give your name and title. For example: 'Good morning. Daydream Hostel. Jeff North, personal care attendant, speaking'.
- Write down the following information when taking a message:
  - the caller's name and telephone number (include area code and extension number)
  - the date and time
  - the message.
- Repeat the message and telephone number back to the caller.
- Ask the caller to 'Please hold' if necessary. First, find out who is calling. Then ask the caller if they can hold. Do not put callers with an emergency on hold.
- Do not put the telephone down or cover the receiver with your hand when speaking to someone other than the caller. The caller may overhear confidential conversations.
- Return to a caller on hold within 30 seconds. Ask the caller if they can wait longer or if the call can be returned.
- Do not give confidential information to any caller. Consumer and employee information is confidential. Refer such calls to the supervisor.
- Transfer the call if appropriate. When transferring a call:
  - tell the caller that you are going to transfer the call
  - give the name of the department that you are transferring them to, if appropriate
  - give the caller the telephone number that you are transferring them to, in case the call gets disconnected or the line is busy.
- End the conversation politely. Thank the person for calling and say goodbye.
- If you take a message, give the message to the appropriate person.

2 Collect information. The information must be about the problem. Do not include unrelated information. For example: *The staff member does not look at me. The staff member does not talk to me. The staff member does not respond when I call her by name. The staff member does not ask me to help with tasks that require two people. The staff member talks to other staff members.*
3 Identify possible solutions. For example: *I could ignore the person, or talk to my supervisor, or talk to my co-workers about the problem. Or I could change jobs.*
4 Select the best solution. For example: *I will talk to my supervisor.*
5 Carry out the solution.
6 Evaluate the results.

Communication and good work ethics help prevent and resolve conflicts. It is important to identify and solve problems before they become major issues. The following guidelines can help you deal with conflict:

- Do not personalise the issue.
- Ask your supervisor for some time to talk privately. Explain the problem, giving facts and specific examples. Ask for advice on solving the problem.
- Issues that need follow-up need to be documented according to the facility's policies and procedures, e.g. grievance procedure (see Chapter 3).

FOCUS ON COMMUNITY CARE

Documentation within the community setting can vary considerably from the residential care setting. Most consumers will have a communication book within their homes that all carers must complete following the delivery of care. Care must be taken when writing in this book, as the consumer is within their legal rights to read all documentation written within their home. Always write objective and truthful statements. There will also be a communication book or consumer chart back at your agency's office. You may be expected to contribute to the documentation according to your organisation's guidelines and policies.

QUALITY OF LIFE

Communication among care team members is necessary for effective and coordinated care. Communication must be factual and concise, understandable and presented logically. This helps the care team provide high-quality care to consumers. False or incomplete information can harm a person.

Consumer information is personal and confidential. Always protect the person's right to privacy. Share information only with the health team members involved in the person's care. Never share it with the person's family or friends without the person's permission.

The person has the right to take part in his or her care planning. They may refuse actions suggested by the care team. Involving the person in the care planning process helps the care team to meet the person's needs. You are a key member of the team. Sharing your observations and ideas can help the team provide better care.

CASE STUDY

You are working in a high-care residential aged care service, with a large multidisciplinary team and 200 consumers. A comprehensive documentation system is in place, which all team members use and add to as required. A team meeting is held relating to the care of Mrs Jane Mettle, who has a large ulcer on her right lower leg. One of the carers in the team has raised a concern that different staff are treating the ulcer differently and that Mrs Mettle has discussed her concern that the ulcer is getting worse. Upon investigation, it has been found that the treatment for the ulcer has not been documented correctly and that staff are treating the ulcer with different wound care regimens.

The team decides on the most appropriate treatment. This is clearly documented and discussed during staff handovers. This treatment is also discussed and clarified with Mrs Mettle.

This case study demonstrates that by using appropriate oral and written communication, the best possible care can be provided to the consumer by all concerned.

ACCREDITATION

You are working in residential or home care and accreditors are at your service. Can you answer the following questions?

- How does your organisation communicate to the next of kin and/or family members about changes occurring at your service?
- As a carer, how do you document care you have provided?
- What are your responsibilities in ensuring medical records are kept confidential (may be paper-based or electronic)?

REVIEW QUESTIONS

Circle T if the statement is true or F if the statement is false:

1 T / F It is acceptable to photocopy a person's chart so you can take it home to study it further.

2 T / F Objective data is something you can observe or measure.

3 T / F It is okay to give confidential information over the telephone.

4 T / F When planning care for the person, priorities and goals are made before undertaking any interventions.

5 T / F Using medical terminology with consumers and family is a good way to demonstrate your knowledge to them.

6 T / F The medical record is a permanent legal document.

Circle the BEST answer:

7 When communicating, what should you not do?
  a Use information you have heard about the person from someone who does not work in the facility
  b Be brief and concise
  c Present information logically and in sequence
  d Give facts and be specific

8 Which of the following statements about medical records is false?
  a The record is used to communicate information about the person.
  b The record is a written account of the person's illness and response to treatment.
  c The record is a written account of care given by the health team.
  d Anyone working in the centre can read the medical record.

9 Where does the nurse describe any changes to the nursing care given?
  a In the nursing care plan
  b In progress notes
  c On a graphic sheet
  d In the medical notes

10 Which of the following statements is false?
  a The nursing process is done with the person's involvement.
  b As a carer, you are responsible for creating the nursing care plan.
  c The nursing process is used to communicate the person's care.
  d The nursing process has five steps.

Answers to these questions are on p. 454.

Further reading

Australian Commission on Safety and Quality in Health Care (2019). Clinical handover. Online. Available: www.safetyandquality.gov.au/our-work/communicating-safety/clinical-handover

Australian Commission on Safety and Quality in Health Care (2019). Patient–clinician communication. Online. Available: www.safetyandquality.gov.au/our-work/communicating-safety/patient-clinician-communication

Australian Government, Australian Digital Health Agency (2020). Resources for Healthcare Providers – Aged Care. Online. Available: www.digitalhealth.gov.au/healthcare-providers/aged-care

Australian Government, Australian Digital Health Agency (2020). Training and Support. Online. Available: www.digitalhealth.gov.au/healthcare-providers/training-and-support

Australian Government, Australian Digital Health Agency (2020). What is My Health Record? Online. Available: www.myhealthrecord.gov.au/for-healthcare-professionals

Australian Government, Federal Register of Legislation (2020). My Health Records Act 2012. Online. Available: www.legislation.gov.au/Details/C2020C00372

Australian Government, Office of the Australian Information Commissioner (2014). Data Breach Preparation and Response. Online. Available: www.oaic.gov.au/privacy/guidance-and-advice/data-breach-preparation-and-response/

Australian Government, Services Australia (2020). Your right to privacy. Online. Available: www.servicesaustralia.gov.au/individuals/privacy

Flinders University. School of Nursing and Midwifery. Clinical communication. Online. Available: https://nursing.flinders.edu.au/students/studyaids/clinicalcommunication/index.php

Health and Nursing Issues Australia (2014). The Nursing Process. Online. Available: https://agedcareact.wordpress.com/2007/02/01/the-nursing-process/

Health Information Management Association Australia (2015). HIMAA Member Principles of Professional Practice. Online. Available: https://himaa.org.au/himaa-member-principles-of-professional-practice/

NANDA International (2020). NANDA Nursing diagnosis list. Online. Available: www.nandanursingdiagnosislist.org/

Nursing and Midwifery Board of Australia (2020). Professional Standards – Codes of Conduct and Codes of Ethics. Online. Available: www.nursingmidwiferyboard.gov.au/codes-guidelines-statements/professional-standards.aspx

Nursing and Midwifery Board of Australia (2017). Enrolled nurse standards for practice. Online. Available: www.nursingmidwiferyboard.gov.au/Codes-Guidelines-Statements/Professional-standards/enrolled-nurse-standards-for-practice.aspx

Nursing and Midwifery Board of Australia (2017). Registered nurse standards for practice. Online. Available: www.nursingmidwiferyboard.gov.au/codes-guidelines-statements/professional-standards/registered-nurse-standards-for-practice.aspx

Services for Australian Rural and Remote Allied Health (n.d.). Communication in remote and rural practice. Online. Available: https://elearning.sarrah.org.au/CommunicationModule/story_html5.html

Services for Australian Rural and Remote Allied Health (n.d.). Information management. Online. Available: https://sarrah.org.au/content/information-management

CHAPTER 5
Working in the home and community sector

By Karen Scott

AFTER READING THIS CHAPTER, YOU SHOULD BE ABLE TO:

- define the key terms listed in this chapter
- explain some different types of assisted home care that exist in the community
- identify the rights of people living at home in assisted living situations and how support must be designed to facilitate acquisition of such rights
- identify what a service delivery plan is and how it is used within an assisted living situation
- identify the importance of a person's physical, emotional, medical, social, spiritual and sexual needs
- list ways in which support staff can assist people living in their own homes to meet these needs
- explain some of the workplace health and safety implications of supporting someone in their own home
- explain the importance of privacy when facilitating independence in a person's assisted living situation
- list some of the types of services that a person living at home in an assisted living situation might need to access
- promote quality of life.

Key terms

assisted living: Living in a home environment with some assistance from informal (family and friends) and/or formal (paid) support, depending on the person's needs. Most commonly used in an aged care context where the older person requires support to live safely in their own home or accommodation

care/case manager: Someone who provides individually planned and coordinated flexible packages of care to provide for the complex care needs of older people

lifestyle facilitator: Someone employed to facilitate a person's lifestyle; involves creating opportunities and taking a pragmatic, values-based approach to community development; also called a support worker

service delivery plan: A plan used by services to detail the use of funding assigned to support a person. It can include information about all facets of the person's life and the type of support required for them to continue their lifestyle

supported accommodation unit: A purpose-built unit or house where a group of people with funding packages combine their funded support to facilitate a living situation that allows them 24-hour care

Living in a person's own home environment can be extremely beneficial as they age. Even with illnesses such as dementia, familiarity plays a very large role in making the person feel calm and secure in the comfort of their surroundings. It is always best to assist a person to continue living in their home while it is safe for them and those around them to do so.

If someone is living in an **assisted living** situation (Figs 5.1, 5.2), it usually means that they want to be living independently but need some help due to age, illness and/or disability. The person may live in a house with other people who are all attempting to live as independently and cohesively as possible. It is important to constantly reinforce your acknowledgement of their abilities and remind them that you are there to 'just help out a little'. Ask them how they want you to do things – even a simple thing such as wiping a table with a particular cloth they like or folding towels in the way the person wants them folded can make a big difference. Performing household tasks in the way that the person wants them completed increases their sense of ownership of their home and lifestyle. In turn, this makes them more accepting of your assistance.

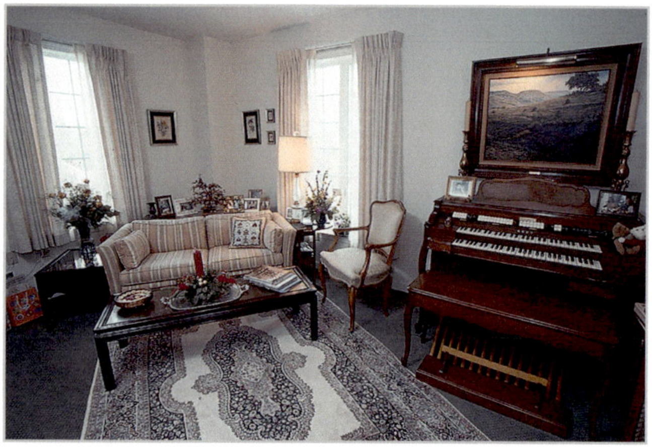

Fig. 5.1
A living area in an assisted living apartment.

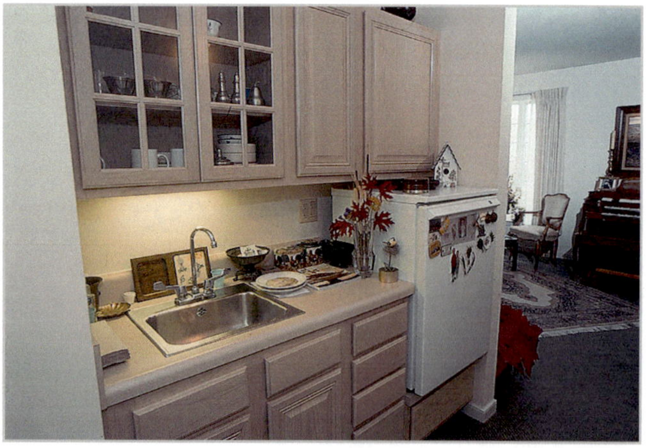

Fig. 5.2
A kitchen in an assisted living apartment.

Your responsibilities when at the person's house are to:
- carry out the task as per your position description and as per the person's care plan
- comply with all legislation (especially workplace health and safety and infection control)
- maintain your duty of care.

Many people with disabilities live in their own homes by themselves, with support from a funding package and family and friends to help. They are supported in a similar way to aged people. People with disabilities may have **lifestyle facilitators** who help them meet their needs in the way specified by them. The National Disability Insurance Scheme (NDIS) was launched in Australia by the federal government in July 2013 with the aim of providing more effective funding and services for people with disabilities between the ages of 0 and 65 years. This scheme will enable people born with a disability or who have developed a disability to access funding to provide for adequate care and equipment. If a person lives in residential aged care they continue to receive NDIS support, even when they turn 65 (NDIS must start before a person is 65).

SERVICE MODELS

Many different service models support people to live independently in the community:
- People can live in their own home or a rented house/unit in the community. Paid support people come into their residence and provide them with assistance as required (e.g. to assist with daily tasks). This is the main type of service model.
- People can live in a **supported accommodation unit**. A few people with similar interests share a house or unit and combine their separate funding packages to pay for support. Their combined funding is enough to pay for the 24-hour care that they require. This is used primarily by adults with disabilities.
- People can live in an established centre, such as a residential aged care service designed to support the diverse needs of the clients. This is usually used by those who are unable to continue living in their own homes due to illness, age or disability.

Assisted home services in Australia

An increasing number of aged care services – both Australian Government-subsidised services and those that are independent from government – help older Australians receive their care at home. However, these vary from area to area. Services for people over the age of 65 who are in need of help at home to continue to live independently are available via the Commonwealth Home Support Programme (CHSP).

Such services may include:
- community nursing and health centres
- allied health care, such as physiotherapy and dietetics
- meals and other food services
- domestic help and personal care

- home modifications and maintenance
- transport
- day therapy centres
- short-term care
- social support
- carer support
- counselling.

Community nursing and health services

Community nursing and health services provide assistance to older people in the form of a registered nurse, enrolled nurse or carer assisting the person in their own home.

A nurse may visit an older person to help:

- restore health after an illness
- ensure the older person maintains the best level of independence to enable them to remain in their own home.

Nurses and carers can also visit at home to assist with personal care, medication, continence assistance or wound care. Personal care includes showering, stoma care, application of pressure stockings or protective garments, changing incontinence pads or emptying catheter bags, applying moisturising creams or medicated ointments and assisting the person to dress in their clothing. Care can be provided regularly or occasionally as needed.

Community health centres offer a range of services to local consumers, with a focus on health promotion, disease prevention and management. Community health centres aim to improve health and wellbeing by:

- encouraging older people to actively participate in their own healthcare
- working on the needs of older people with other primary healthcare providers
- offering facilities for seniors' local community groups
- encouraging active participation in the centre's activities, including involvement in management, fundraising and volunteer work
- promoting prevention of lifestyle-related diseases and conditions
- developing healthcare programs and activities to improve social and physical environments in the community.

Community health centres offer a range of services that can help older people to remain at home by supporting them and their carers. The types of services that may be available at a health centre include:

- medical services
- physiotherapy, to help maintain flexibility, strength and movement
- podiatry, for foot and lower limb problems
- nursing, including health advice, education, counselling and monitoring
- speech pathology, to help older people to communicate more effectively should they have a speech disorder
- social workers, to help older people or carers with problems related to finances, accommodation or socialisation
- tailored programs for older people's specific dietary needs.

Many agencies now have services for people from diverse cultural or linguistically diverse (CALD) backgrounds and offer culturally sensitive care (e.g. catering to specific diets, activities, languages or spiritual needs).

Government-funded programs

The CHSP is a joint initiative of the Australian federal, state and territory governments. Its aim is to deliver high-quality, affordable and accessible services in the community that are essential to the wellbeing of eligible older Australians and their carers. Such people are supported to be more independent at home and in the community, in order to reduce the potential or inappropriate need for admission to hospital or a residential care service.

- CHSP services focus on working 'with' the person, rather than doing 'for' the person, to build on personal strengths, capacity and goals.
- The first step to access home-based services is for the person to call My Aged Care (MAC) on 1800 200 422 or contct them via their website at www.myagedcare.gov.au. This is a national online and phone service that offers assistance and information about aged care services and availability of these services. The MAC staff will ask questions about the person's current needs and circumstances and make a referral to a Regional Assessment Service (RAS) to complete an assessment.

The federal government, through the Department of Veterans' Affairs, manages the Veterans' Home Care Program to help veterans and war widows/widowers enjoy a healthier lifestyle and remain living at home longer. Its services are similar to those offered by CHSP and include help in the home, personal care, equipment, home maintenance and respite care.

The federal government also funds care 'packages'. First introduced in 2013, there are currently four levels of Home Care Packages to allow a seamless continuum of care at home:

- Level 1 – a recently introduced package to support people with basic care needs
- Level 2 – previously known as Community Aged Care Packages (CACPs), providing an alternative to low-level residential care. Services included in this package are personal care, respite, shopping and cleaning
- Level 3 – a package to support people with intermediate care needs
- Level 4 – previously known as Extended Age Care at Home (EACH), providing a higher level of support and assistance as an alternative to high-level residential aged care.

Level 3 and 4 packages provide high levels of support to assist frail older Australians to remain living in their own homes. They are individually planned, flexible and coordinated packages of care to provide for the individual complex care needs of older people. The types of services provided include:

- registered nurse care
- care by an allied health professional, such as a physiotherapist, podiatrist, dietitian, occupational therapist,

social worker, speech therapist or other type of allied healthcare
- personal care
- transport to appointments
- social support
- home help
- assistance with oxygen and/or enteral feeding
- other equipment needed to remain safely at home, such as ramps, rails, hospital beds and shower chairs
- continence aids.

In addition to these packages, a daily supplement to the value of about $16 per day is available for people who have dementia, are financially disadvantaged, live in rural and remote areas or have mental health conditions. This is to give those people the opportunity to obtain extra services that are not available within the scope of their care package.

Packages are overseen by a **care manager** or coordinator, who plans and manages the care package, tailoring it to individual needs. The packages are called Consumer Directed Care (CDC) packages as clients can choose the services they require, keeping within the funding provided for the individual package. For example, a client may choose to receive help with personal care, such as bathing and dressing; domestic assistance, such as housework and shopping; or possibly help participating in social activities. Another client may choose to have equipment supplied and domestic assistance within their package, as their personal care is provided by family members.

Need and eligibility for community aged care is assessed by Aged Care Assessment Teams (ACAT) as it is for residential aged care. This ensures the person actually requires the level of assistance delivered by the particular package. ACAT assessments are government-funded and free of charge, but a fee may apply for individual packages. Those who cannot pay the fee will not be denied a service that is needed. Packages are delivered by approved providers of aged care services. The Australian Government sets standards to ensure clients receive quality care that meets individual needs. All stakeholders have access to a complaints procedure if required.

CARER SUPPORT

Carers are those who look after frail older people or people with a disability or chronic illness in the community or in their own homes. They are usually related by family or friendship. Caring for someone full-time is both physically and emotionally demanding. Hence, carers need to be able to take breaks from their caring role from time to time. This break is called 'respite'. The Australian Government provides funding for the National Respite for Carers Program to assist carers with information, respite care and support. Respite opportunities can occur in a variety of settings and service types, such as:

- care centres, which provide respite for a half or full day. Some respite centres, particularly those catering for people with dementia, may offer overnight respite
- in-home respite services, including overnight care and personal care services
- activity programs
- respite for carers of people with dementia and challenging behaviour
- flexible respite in community settings.

Funding is also provided for Commonwealth Carer Resource Centres and Commonwealth Carer Respite Centres. These centres provide carers with information about a range of respite options and assistance to obtain respite. They also give carers support and information on how they can better manage the care needs of the person they are caring for, as well as information about other government programs that can help them. Commonwealth Carer Resource Centres can be found in each capital city.

Rights and responsibilities

On 27 February 2017 the Australian Government amended the Charter of Rights and Responsibilities for Community Care (introduced in 2009), renaming it the Charter of Care Recipients' Rights and Responsibilities – Home Care. This charter is a legal document that explains the rights of people receiving aged care services in the community, as well as their responsibilities, including towards care workers. These rights and responsibilities are outlined in Box 5.1.

Quality reporting

Services that provide community care packages and the National Respite for Carers Program are required to take part in quality reporting. This was implemented in July 2005 by the Australian Government to ensure that quality services are delivered to people through these programs.

NEW ZEALAND HOME HEALTH ASSOCIATION

The New Zealand Home Health Association, established in 1993, is the industry association for providers of home-support services. It is the national body representing providers of home healthcare services, supporting them to achieve the highest possible standards. Members are committed to meeting high standards and to working collectively to strengthen the sector.

Home healthcare encompasses a range of services available in the community for people who wish to stay living at home, but who need support to be able to do so.

Services include:

- personal care
- household management
- nursing treatment
- complex long-term care for people with serious conditions or injuries.

Services are provided by community-based agencies and companies that employ support workers, caregivers and healthcare professionals.

Generally, an assessment organised by a general practitioner will determine what government funding is available. The Accident Compensation Corporation (ACC) may fund support required because of accidents, whereas long-term

BOX 5.1
Charter of care recipients' rights and responsibilities – home care
Aged Care Act 1997, Schedule 2 User Rights Principles 2014 (amended on 27 February 2017)

1 Care recipients' rights – home care

General

1 Each care recipient has the following rights:
- a to be treated and accepted as an individual, and to have his or her individual preferences respected
- b to be treated with dignity, with his or her privacy respected
- c to receive care that is respectful of him or her, and his or her family and home
- d to receive care without being obliged to feel grateful to those providing the care
- e to full and effective use of all human, legal and consumer rights, including the right to freedom of speech regarding his or her care
- f to have access to advocates and other avenues of redress
- g to be treated without exploitation, abuse, discrimination, harassment or neglect.

Consumer Directed Care – choice and flexibility

2 Each care recipient has the following rights:
- a to be supported by the approved provider:
  - i to set goals in relation to the outcomes he or she seeks from home care
  - ii to determine the level of ongoing involvement and control that he or she wishes to have in the provision of the home care
  - iii to make decisions relating to his or her own care
  - iv to maintain his or her independence as far as possible
- b to choose the care and services that best meets his or her goals and assessed needs, within the limits of the resources available
- c to have choice and flexibility in the way the care and services are provided at home
- d to participate in making decisions that affect him or her
- e to have his or her representative participate in decisions relating to his or her care if he or she requests it or he or she does not have capacity
- f to choose the approved provider that is to provide home care to him or her, and to have flexibility to change that approved provider if he or she wishes.

Consumer Directed Care – care and services

3 Each care recipient has the following rights:
- a to receive reliable, coordinated, safe, quality care and services which are appropriate to meeting his or her goals and assessed needs
- b to be given before, or within 14 days after, he or she commences receiving home care, a written plan of the care and services that he or she expects to receive
- c to receive care and services that take account of his or her other care arrangements and preferences
- d to ongoing review of the care and services he or she receives (both periodic and in response to changes in his or her personal circumstances), and modification of the care and services as required

Consumer Directed Care – individualised budget and monthly statement of available funds and expenditure

3A Each care recipient has the following rights:
- a to receive an individualised budget for the care and services to be provided
- b to have his or her individualised budget reviewed and, if necessary, revised if:
  - i the care and services to be provided, or the costs of providing the care and services, change; or
  - ii he or she requests the approved provider to review and, if necessary, revise the individualised budget
- c to receive a monthly statement of the funds available and the expenditure in respect of the care and services provided during the month.

Personal information

4 Each care recipient has the following rights:
- a to privacy and confidentiality of his or her personal information
- b to access his or her personal information.

Communication

5 Each care recipient has the following rights:
- a to be helped to understand any information he or she is given
- b to be given a copy of this Charter
- c to be offered a written agreement that includes all agreed matters
- d to choose a person to speak on his or her behalf for any purpose.

Comments and complaints

6 Each care recipient has the following rights:
- a to be given information on how to make comments and complaints about the care and services he or she receives
- b to complain about the care and services he or she receives, without fear of losing the care or being disadvantaged in any other way
- c to have complaints investigated fairly and confidentially, and to have appropriate steps taken to resolve issues of concern.

Fees

7 Each care recipient has the following rights:
- a to have his or her fees determined in a way that is transparent, accessible and fair
- b to receive invoices that are clear and in a format that is understandable

BOX 5.1
Charter of care recipients' rights and responsibilities – home care
Aged Care Act 1997, Schedule 2 User Rights Principles 2014 (amended on 27 February 2017) *continued*

- c to have his or her fees reviewed periodically and on request when there are changes to his or her financial circumstances
- d not to be denied care and services because of his or her inability to pay a fee for reasons beyond his or her control.

2 Care recipients' responsibilities – home care

General

1 Each care recipient has the following responsibilities:

- a to respect the rights of care workers to their human, legal and workplace rights, including the right to work in a safe environment
- b to treat care workers without exploitation, abuse, discrimination or harassment.

Care and services

2 Each care recipient has the following responsibilities:

- a to abide by the terms of the written home care agreement
- b to acknowledge that his or her needs may change and to negotiate modifications of care and service when his or her care needs change
- c to accept responsibility for his or her own actions and choices even though some actions and choices may involve an element of risk.

Communication

3 Each care recipient has the following responsibilities:

- a to give information to assist the approved provider to develop, deliver and review a care plan
- b to tell the approved provider and their staff about any problems with the care and services
- c before the care recipient changes approved providers, to tell the approved provider and their staff of the day the care recipient intends to cease to receive home care services from the approved provider.

Access

4 Each care recipient has the following responsibilities:

- a to allow safe and reasonable access for care workers at the times specified in his or her care plan or otherwise by agreement
- b to provide reasonable notice if he or she does not require home care to be provided on a particular day.

Fees

5 Each care recipient has the responsibility to pay any fees as specified in the agreement or negotiate an alternative arrangement with the provider if any changes occur in his or her financial circumstances.

Source: Australian Government Department of Health (2017) Charter of Care Recipients' Rights and Responsibilities – Home Care. Aged Care Act 1997, Schedule 2 User Rights Principles 2014 (amended on 27 February 2017).

disability or health conditions may attract subsidies from the Ministry of Health. District Health Boards (DHBs) fund services for older people. Home health services may also be purchased privately (see Box 5.2).

ROLE OF THE CARER

Physical assistance

Physical assistance includes:

- support with dressing, ironing and washing clothes
- support in moving about the house and finding the least restrictive way to get housework done
- maintaining the house and all fixtures within the house. This includes contacting government departments (e.g. community housing) when necessary to organise repairs or alterations to certain parts of the house
- ensuring that the environment is safe for the person living there, along with any guests who may visit. For example, sometimes clutter can be a problem, as it makes it difficult for the client to move around. Other safety concerns are listed in Table 5.1.

It is extremely important to work with the person to help make their home a safe and happy one. This can have a profound effect on the confidence of people in assisted living situations.

Fire safety

It is extremely important to be conscious of fire safety at all times when supporting someone in their home. On many occasions, people who are aged or have an illness or disability neglect to take certain precautions that guard against fires (see Box 5.3). Therefore, it is essential that you are aware of the main principles of fire safety:

- Never use faulty, damaged or suspect equipment. Replace equipment as required.
- Not all homes have electrical safety switches installed, particularly older houses. If using an electrical device in a client's home it is a good idea to use a personal safety switch, otherwise known as a residual circuit device (RCD). This could prevent the carer receiving an electric shock from a faulty electrical device.

BOX 5.2
The future of community aged care

Australia

Australia, like most western countries, has an ageing population. This is due to vast improvements in medical technology allowing increased life expectancy, predicted to increase to 92.2 years for men and 95.0 years for women by the year 2050.

As people are living longer, the demand for health and community services is escalating. Home-based healthcare is on the increase as it is much cheaper to care for a person at home than in hospital or an aged care facility. In 2010, 70–80 per cent of healthcare in Australia was delivered in the home, with an increasing emphasis on prevention and self-management of disease.

There is a need for new healthcare workforce methods that strengthen and expand community-based primary care services.

Increasingly, complex healthcare conditions are being managed in general practice and in community settings, with rapidly emerging needs for appropriately trained case managers/coordinators of care.

New Zealand

New Zealand has signalled a major shift in direction in its health system through the development of a comprehensive primary healthcare policy and strategy. This has led to the creation of opportunities for nurses to be involved in new service delivery opportunities, the identification of barriers to effective primary health nursing practice and strategies to overcome those barriers. The development of nurses' scope of practice is extending into primary care, with nurse-led clinics and walk-in centres, and health advice by telephone where nurses increasingly substitute for general practitioners in the care of minor illness and routine management of chronic diseases.

Other countries

In Japan, the roles of nurses who work in community care have been reviewed in order that visiting nurse services are better coordinated and integrated with community health promotion.

The nursing profession in the United States responded to the changing healthcare environment in the early 2000s with a fundamental shift in education and nursing practice to meet healthcare needs, integrating health promotion and disease prevention into curricula and practice to prepare nurses for changing healthcare environments.

Major issues

In the Australian context, the major issues about primary and community care nursing that have been identified are:

- the impact and effectiveness of primary and community care nursing on patient health outcomes compared with doctor-led care or usual care
- funding for community nurse/practice nurse roles
- education models and policy frameworks that support career pathways and enhance recruitment and retention of nurses.

Nurses in primary healthcare, in Australia, New Zealand and other countries, are increasingly working with multidisciplinary teams, with their practice aligned to key primary health directions.

Table 5.1
Managing dangerous situations

Potentially dangerous situation	Danger/injuries possible	Management strategy
Clutter around the house	Slips and falls	Speak to the person about finding places for the clutter. Suggest some alternatives that are conducive to their current method of organisation.
Slippery floor tiles	Slips and falls	Speak to the person about getting a non-slip coating put over some of the tiles, particularly in the bathroom.
Frayed cord on a toaster	Electrocution	Speak to the person about replacing the appliance.
Slippery outdoor path	Slips and falls	Speak to the person about putting a non-slip coating on the path or having it pressure cleaned to make it less slippery.
Faulty kettle that doesn't switch off properly	Electrocution	Speak to the person about purchasing another one. Explain the danger.
Sharp edges on cupboards	Grazes and bruising	Speak to the person about applying protective corners or just being careful when moving about the house.

Table 5.1
Managing dangerous situations *continued*

Potentially dangerous situation	Danger/injuries possible	Management strategy
Poorly labelled or decanted chemicals (i.e. chemicals that have been poured into a different container)	Poisoning	Speak to the person about the high level of danger. Explain the laws regarding decanting and the likelihood of poisoning.
Barred windows that are locked, without any visible keys close by	Unable to escape fire, inadequate ventilation	Advise the person to place a key next to each window, so in the instance of a fire there is ready access to the outside.

BOX 5.3
Disability considerations

For someone using a wheelchair or walking aid, a fire is an even more hazardous situation, because it is more difficult for the person to escape the fire quickly. It is essential that any mobility aid a person uses is placed in the person's room at night, and that excess clutter is moved from the exit pathway so the person has easy access to the necessary exits in case of a fire.

- If you notice that any equipment is in need of repair, speak to the person you are supporting about this immediately. Document all reports of this nature.
- Smoke alarms save lives. The best types are those that are hard-wired to the electrical system. If battery operated, it is important that batteries are renewed annually. There are some government agencies, such as the Home Assist Program, that will install smoke alarms.
- Always make sure that you and the person you are supporting are aware of the fire evacuation procedure.
- Make sure the evacuation path is free from clutter or objects that might hinder a fast exit. If the person uses a walking aid, make sure it is always kept close to them at night, so a fast exit is possible.
- Ensure keys are left in door and window locks to expedite a quick exit.
- Ensure you know how to operate all necessary fire equipment.

It is also essential to remember your childhood rhymes regarding fire safety. For example:

'Get down low and go, go, go.'
'Stop, drop and roll.'

Remind the person that you are supportive of these principles, so that you can both be conscientious and safe regarding fires. In a house fire, most deaths occur from carbon monoxide poisoning rather than actually being burned by flames.

PROCEDURE
USING FIRE BLANKETS AND FIRE EXTINGUISHERS

To use a fire blanket

1. Turn off the power source.
2. Pull the tabs of the blanket and remove it from its covering.
3. Lower the blanket gently over the flames, ensuring your hands are protected by the blanket.
4. Leave the blanket there to cool.
5. Hot oil can take over an hour to cool down. Don't lift the blanket until it is entirely cool as the introduction of oxygen can cause the fire to reignite.
6. Dispose of the blanket. It cannot be reused, so ensure a new one is purchased.

To operate a fire extinguisher, use the PASSword, as follows:

1. **P**ull the ring pull.
2. **A**im the nozzle at the base of the fire.
3. **S**queeze the lever and handle.
4. **S**weep the nozzle from side to side.

Operate the extinguisher at a distance of 2 metres from the fire. Ensure you remain between the exit and the fire, so you don't get trapped if the fire becomes uncontrollable.

You should attend any fire safety training offered by your organisation. Fire safety training may seem tedious at the time, but it is an essential skill that should be kept refreshed. When offered training, ensure that you attend and take all information on board, because it is important and potentially lifesaving.

SAFETY ALERT

Switching off

It is common for someone with an illness, who is aged or who has a disability, to leave things like irons, electric blankets and heaters on when they go out. This is a major safety concern as these appliances can lead to fires. It may be necessary to brainstorm some methods to assist the person to remember to switch off these devices at the wall each morning or when they have finished using them. It is good practice to get the person into the habit of switching off all electrical equipment at the wall prior to leaving the house, as this can prevent power surges doing damage and/or starting fires.

Health needs

One of the many personal tasks that a person needs assistance with is the management of their health needs (see Box 5.4). Health needs include:

- appointments with the doctor
- getting prescriptions filled
- managing minor injuries and first aid requirements
- personal hygiene
- skin management
- monitoring minor illnesses, such as colds and gastro-intestinal upsets
- following through with specialist appointments, getting X-rays, blood tests as required
- storing medication in the correct way, as per the instructions
- not eating contaminated food, discarding used items appropriately
- reheating and defrosting food in a safe manner
- following the doctor's advice about nutrition and general health, where possible.

BOX 5.4
Understanding health needs

The best person to manage someone's health is themselves! You need to acknowledge the important role that the person you are supporting should take in the management of their health and wellbeing. Ask questions about how they are feeling and how that compares with normal. Even though some people can exaggerate symptoms when describing their health, never dismiss concerns they have or refuse to accept their voiced problems.

The best indicator of a health problem is uncharacteristic behaviour. If someone is acting differently from normal, ask them questions to determine the reason for this different behaviour. Ensure you document everything.

Emotional needs

Most people have a close personal bond with their home, and this needs to be acknowledged and accepted by support staff at all times. Things that make up this bond include:

- children who were born and raised in the house
- partners or friends who have passed away, who used to frequent the house
- pets the person has or had
- major life experiences that occurred in the house or while the person was living in the house (e.g. marriages, divorces, births)
- feelings of security or safety linked to the house
- neighbours and friends close by
- the independence they feel, because of being able to manage life within the familiar confines of their house.

Be careful how you speak about the person's home. Do not make any derogatory comments. Remember that you are a guest in their home and treat it with as much respect as you would your own.

Medication handling, storage and administration

The handling, storage and administration of medication is an essential part of assisted living. One of the leading causes for hospital admission of older people is medication non-compliance. Increasingly these days, people rely on prescription and non-prescription medication. Vitamins and natural remedies advised by non-health professionals are more popular than ever.

The term 'medication' is no longer limited to prescription medications. It can also include things like:

- vitamin C tablets
- cough syrups
- cold and flu remedies
- laxatives
- indigestion remedies
- herbal ointments
- paracetamol
- aspirin.

Regardless of its scheduling, medication can be harmful for people if administered unnecessarily or incorrectly. We must treat all medication in the same way and take specific precautions to guard against an incident occurring.

Medication can be presented in a number of different ways, including:

- inhaler
- suppository
- injection
- capsules
- elixir
- tablet
- ointment
- nebule
- patch.

You should be aware of the medication that the person you support uses and how to assist them to take it safely. When assisting a client with their medication, it is important to be aware of the following information:

- the correct way to administer the medication
- the reason for the medication
- possible side-effects
- the expected results.

If the person has difficulty in taking their medication, they may benefit from having a dosing aid. Most pharmacies offer to package medications in blister packs, so the person presses the medications out of the appropriate blister. This is particularly beneficial for people with arthritis who find it difficult to unscrew medicine bottles, or those who take a large number of different medications.

Sometimes the person you are supporting will need assistance in storing the medication. It is common for people with dementia and other associated health problems to store medication incorrectly. You need to be aware of the correct way to store the medication.

When considering how to correctly store the person's medication, ask:

- Does the medication need to be stored at a certain temperature?
- Are there people/children in the house who may tamper with or attempt to digest the medication?
- Is it past the expiry date?

Always ensure that you have considered the above points. If there are children in the house, the medication should be kept in a high place or locked in a cupboard. Medications that are past the expiry date may not work correctly, so advise the person to obtain new medication.

Check the medication bottle or packet for instructions regarding appropriate temperature for the medication. If unsure about how best to store medication, consult the label on the medication, or telephone the pharmacist.

Food handling

As a support worker, it is common to be required to prepare and cook meals for those we support. In handling and preparing food, you have a duty of care at all times.

Personal hygiene

The following points should assist you to maintain a high standard of personal hygiene:

- Wash your hands before and after preparing food in any form. Wash your hands in between preparation of meats and vegetables. If you touch any part of your body (e.g. nose, pimple, mouth), you need to rewash your hands, as they may be contaminated.
- After handling garbage or garbage bins, wash your hands.
- After touching pets, wash your hands.
- Do not go to the toilet with food residue on your hands. Also wash them after using the toilet.
- If you have a sticking plaster or bandage on your hand/s, cover it with a plastic or latex glove to prevent contamination.
- Keep jewellery to a minimum.
- Long hair should be tied back.
- Cover your mouth and nose with a tissue if you sneeze or cough. Remember to wash your hands straight away. If you have a severe cold, or vomiting or diarrhoea, do not prepare food.

CARING ABOUT CULTURE

Of the 26 million people in Australia, more than 6 million were born outside of Australia. People from other cultural backgrounds have different customs and practices that must be respected when providing care in their home. It is important not to stereotype people, as not everyone from a particular cultural group will follow the same customs. Take time to learn about the beliefs of other cultures. If in doubt, ask what is appropriate.

In some cultures, such as Japanese, Chinese, Muslim and Hindu, it is polite to remove your shoes at the front door prior to entering the house. You may be provided with indoor shoes to be worn while attending to your duties. As long as workplace health and safety principles are maintained, this is acceptable. Also be mindful to wear modest dress, as scanty clothing can be unsuitable to some cultural groups.

Gender must be considered. For some cultural groups it is not appropriate for women to be cared for by a male. It may also be necessary to approach the head of the household to ask questions or make changes to care provision.

There are also cultural differences regarding food. Hindus believe that cows are sacred and therefore do not eat beef. For members of the Islamic faith, pork and alcohol are prohibited. Their meat must be halal, which means it is slaughtered with a sharp knife on the name of their god Allah. When preparing food in the home of a Jewish person, there are many cultural aspects to consider. Pork and shellfish are not eaten, and some foods need to be prepared in a special way or blessed prior to consumption.

Whatever the culture or religion, it is important to be mindful and accepting of the beliefs of others, even though they may differ greatly from your own.

Food poisoning

There are three sources of food poisoning:

- *chemical* – this can be from pesticides or storing food in containers made of certain materials, such as zinc
- *biological* – this includes natural toxins produced by living things (e.g. green potatoes, certain mushrooms and seafood)
- *bacterial* – this is the most common source. There are two ways in which bacteria can cause poisoning:
  - *food-borne infection* – bacteria in food or water enter the body

- *food-borne intoxication* – poisonous toxins produced by bacteria enter the body. Bacteria can be destroyed by cooking, but the toxins they produce are not destroyed.

Thawing and storage of foods

Food should always be stored below 5° Celsius or over 65° Celsius. A bacterium grows fastest at a 'warm' temperature: 7–45° Celsius. Food should be stored according to the following categories:

- *Cold* items (e.g. butter, milk, cheese) should be stored in a refrigerator.
- *Frozen items* (e.g. frozen vegetables, ice cream) should be stored in a freezer.
- *Dry* items (e.g. flour, cereal, biscuits) should be stored in an airtight container.

Frozen food should *not* be thawed on the bench. To thaw frozen food, place it in the refrigerator on the lowest shelf for 24 hours. A microwave oven can be used to thaw out frozen foods, but you must take care when doing it this way. The food should be cooked immediately after thawing. It should not be refrozen if it has not been cooked.

Cross-contamination

Cross-contamination is when microorganisms from contaminated people, food, equipment and/or areas cross over into food.

To prevent cross-contamination:

- use separate cutting boards for raw meats, cooked meats, vegetables and dairy food. If this is not possible, wash the board thoroughly and dry it between each use
- wash fruits and vegetables before consumption to reduce microbes and remove soil, insects and residue, such as insecticides
- clean knives or other implements between contact with raw meats, cooked meats, vegetables and dairy food
- dishwashing cloths, sponges and tea towels must be changed daily as these are a common source of contamination
- use paper towels, not a cloth hand towel, to dry your hands
- keep raw food on the bottom shelf of the refrigerator to prevent leakage into other foods
- cover food with waterproof wrapping or store it in sealed containers
- before storing tinned food in the refrigerator, transfer it into a sealed container.

Expiration of foods and spoilage

Always check for expiration dates on food before using or consuming them. If foods have passed their expiration date, they should be disposed of. When assisting a person to shop for groceries, remind them to check the expiration dates on all foods.

Food is spoiled when it is past its expiration date, or if:

- meat is smelly or slimy
- bread is mouldy
- vegetables or fruit are brown and/or soft
- cheese is stale, mouldy or dried out
- butter is rancid and smells
- dried food has pests (e.g. weevils) in it.

If food displays any or all of the above, it should not be consumed.

Social needs

One of the key benefits of a person staying in their own home is that they can continue with their social life, uninterrupted. Friends and others are more likely to drop in, and this can increase the person's comfort considerably.

It is important to respect the person's privacy and need for space in their home. You can further support a person's social life by asking what tasks they would like assistance with prior to people coming over or them going out. They may want to put out some flowers or some help cooking something special. These little touches can increase the person's sense of ownership of their life and help maintain their self-esteem and feelings of empowerment and confidence.

Spiritual needs

The needs of a person extend past eating, drinking and taking medication. We need to feel nurtured, respected and empowered, and we all need something to hold sacred and value. Many people meet these personal needs through spirituality. There are many ways to demonstrate spirituality, and people find many different outlets for this need, such as:

- attending a church, synagogue, mosque, temple or other religious institution
- being involved in bible studies, or reading the bible or other religious writings
- meditating
- praying and speaking with God
- using natural therapies, such as yoga and/or Pilates, to relax the mind, body and soul
- performing community services
- attending retreats or relaxation seminars.

A person's spirituality is a very personal thing. We cannot tell someone how they should demonstrate their spirituality, but it is important to acknowledge their right and need to do so.

Sexual needs

When providing support for a person in their own home it is important to be conscious of a person's sexual needs. Support workers need to ensure that the person is given privacy and respect at all times.

There may be times when a person in an assisted living situation wishes to have someone come over and visit. It is not important to know the reason for this visit. Just be polite and ask if there is any assistance they require to prepare for the visitor.

SUPPORT STAFF

Although it is the person's home that you are working in, there are certain laws and advisory standards that regulate and stipulate how that work must be carried out. We must remember first that this is not our house. Any alterations to the physical environment or the way we provide support must be done with the person's involvement and approval where possible. However, it is imperative that the law be met. Sometimes it is necessary to do this in a way that the person may not necessarily agree with. The best way to manage such situations is to involve the person in all parts of the decision. Let them understand the reason for the changes, including the underpinning legislation.

The support worker in an assisted living situation needs to consider:

- appropriate clothing for the environment
- risk assessment
- documentation management and completing reports.

When you are working in the houses of those you support it is often easy to forget that you are still employed and have the same types of responsibilities that you would have anywhere else. Things like wearing the right clothing and being well rested are still extremely important (see Chapter 2).

The right clothing to wear is:

- nothing too revealing (such as short skirts and shorts or a top with a low neckline)
- shoes with a closed toe, heel support and maximum grip
- nothing too excessive or flowing that will be likely to catch on things
- no excessive jewellery.

The home environment is not always easy to negotiate from a safety perspective. Use risk assessment to identify hazards and manage them accordingly. Legislation stipulates that the workplace must be safe and that workers must use equipment to facilitate this safety, when provided by the employer. If you identify any potential or actual hazards within the home you are working in that could affect your ability to work safely, it is your duty to inform your supervisor.

Documentation

Documentation management is another important component of supporting someone in their own home. It is important, especially when you are not the only person providing support, to correctly document the assistance you provide. The person may have specific forms to record certain details of their support, or they may be included in the service delivery plan. Some of the types of information that might need to be recorded include:

- housework completed
- meals prepared
- medication assistance given
- groceries purchased
- general maintenance performed.

Service delivery plan

The **service delivery plan** is the personalised plan that sets out how the service will be delivered to the client. It details the way in which the funding will be used to meet the person's needs. Included in the plan are details about:

- the type and number of staff the person requires and will have
- the types of jobs the staff need to focus on
- the goals, needs and wishes of the person
- other networked services that will be included in the service delivery
- medical needs of the person that are to be met by the service
- details about the living situation, including the status of the residence – whether it is a housing commission house, or is owned or rented by the client
- the spiritual needs of the person and how they are to be met with service delivery
- any allied health professionals involved in service delivery
- the health and nutritional needs of the person
- the social and recreational needs of the person.

The service delivery plan is designed with participation from the service user, their family and friends, representatives from the service and any allied health professionals involved in the person's life. It is essential that the service delivery plan is designed to comprehensively meet the person's needs. This is the main document that all service needs are highlighted in.

QUALITY OF LIFE

The context in which we care for our clients will vary considerably. While some are in facilities, others will stay within their own homes to receive care.

People choose assisted living for many reasons. Most need some help, but want to live independently with dignity and respect. You can help them by following their service plans and assisting them as needed. Be sure that the care you give reflects the person's right to privacy, dignity and personal choice.

CASE STUDY

Marisa Algernon is 81 years old, lives alone and had a fall several months ago, which resulted in a broken hip. She now has difficulty mobilising and tending to her household chores and personal needs. Her doctor got in touch with the Aged Care Assessment Team and she now has a Level 2 package, which allows her to continue living in her own home with support. She has lived in the same house for 50 years and wants to stay in it for as long as she can. She has many memories attached to the house and knows her neighbourhood well. Her family live a few streets away, and her doctor lives in the adjoining suburb. She has a small dog who is 10 years old and is her faithful companion. She knows that if she had to leave her home, she would lose many treasured memories and her canine companion. Marisa's carer comes into her home twice per week and assists her with bathing and basic household chores. She has meals on wheels delivered Monday to Friday.

Assisting people to stay within their homes for as long as possible has many benefits for the person – not only physical benefits, but also social and emotional ones.

ACCREDITATION

You are working in home care and accreditors are visiting your service. Can you answer the following questions?

- How do you ensure the privacy and dignity of the clients you are caring for, when you are in their home?
- You suspect that a family member of one of your clients is stealing from your client's bank account. What do you do?
- As a carer, how do you feedback to nursing staff when you think a client needs more help in their home (could be help with activities of daily living or cleaning around the home)?

REVIEW QUESTIONS

Circle the BEST answer:

1 Which is not a service for care available via the Commonwealth Home Support Programme (CHSP)?
  - a Allied health care
  - b Domestic help and personal care
  - c Home modification and maintenance
  - d Long-term residential care

2 A nurse may not visit an older person to help:
  - a restore health after an illness
  - b allow him/her to maintain the best level of independence
  - c assess what needs have changed
  - d organise finances

3 The types of services that may be available at a community health centre do not include:
  - a physiotherapy to help maintain flexibility, strength and movement
  - b podiatry for foot and lower limb problems
  - c speech pathology to help older people to communicate more effectively should they have a speech disorder
  - d hairdressing

4 The aim of the CHSP program is to:
  - a support people to be more independent at home and in the community
  - b reduce the need for admission to a residential care service
  - c alert the health professionals when their assistance is required
  - d both A and B

5 Which of the following services is not included in a Home Care Package?
  - a Nursing care
  - b Housing
  - c Help with activities of daily living
  - d Support services

6 Which statement is least likely? Many older people who have mobilisation problems need help with:
  - a bathing, dressing, elimination and eating
  - b ambulation and transfer
  - c infection control and taking medications
  - d communication

7 Which of the following statements about Home Care Packages is false?
   a There is no assessment necessary to obtain a package
   b They do not include household chores
   c There is sometimes a small fee to pay
   d A care manager is allocated to manage each package

8 Which of the following statements about Level 3 and 4 Home Care Packages is incorrect?
   a They provide high levels of support to assist older people.
   b They allow frail older people to remain living in their own home.
   c They are generic and not planned for the individual.
   d They are flexible and designed to help with individual care needs.

9 Which of the following statements is incorrect? Quality reporting ensures that quality services:
   a are delivered to the people who have been assessed as requiring them
   b are assumed to be delivered when service providers say they are
   c are regulated to ensure care standards are adequate
   d are managed with systems and processes to ensure quality results

10 Which of the following is NOT correct procedure for using a fire blanket?
   a Turn off the power source.
   b Pull the tabs and remove the blanket.
   c Gently lower the blanket over the fire.
   d After 5 minutes raise the blanket to check if the fire is out.

Answers to these questions are on p. 454.

Further reading

Australian Government, Department of Health (2017). Charter of Care Recipients' Rights and Responsibilities – Home Care. Aged Care Act 1997, Schedule 2 User Rights Principles 2014 (amended on 27 February 2017).

Bain H, Chilton S (2017). A textbook of community nursing, 2nd edn. Taylor & Francis.

CHAPTER 6
Working with Australian Aboriginal and Torres Strait Islander Elders

By Odette Best, Ali Drummond and Melanie Robinson

AFTER READING THIS CHAPTER, YOU SHOULD BE ABLE TO:

- briefly describe the pre-invasion health status of Aboriginal Australians
- describe the current health status of Aboriginal Australians
- differentiate between Aboriginal and Torres Strait Islander Australians
- identify eras of management of Aboriginal Australians and describe some of the effects
- show some insight into the historical impacts on the Torres Strait Islander people, their culture and their health
- describe the role change of Torres Strait Islander Elders from pre-invasion to the present day
- know how to promote quality of life.

Key terms

Aboriginal Australians: The original inhabitants of the Australian continent and nearby islands, excluding the Torres Strait Islands

country/nation: Interchangeable terms used to identify the land of ancestral origin

culture: The behaviours, beliefs and characteristics of particular social and ethnic groups

customs: Traditions passed from one generation to the next

Elders: Highly regarded keepers of knowledge, including lore, language, customs, beliefs and creation stories, among Torres Strait Islander and Aboriginal communities

Indigenous Australians: The original inhabitants of the Australian continent and nearby islands, and these peoples' descendants; Indigenous Australians are distinguished as either Aboriginal Australians or Torres Strait Islanders

mob: Colloquial term used by many Aboriginal peoples to define their country or family of origin

pouri-pouri: Traditional form of Indigenous black magic; involves supernatural concepts of spirits, mostly bad spirits; although it was forced into secrecy by the church, *pouri-pouri* is still practised today

terra nullius: A Latin expression deriving from Roman law meaning 'land belonging to no one' (or 'no man's land'), which is used in international law to describe territory that has never been subject to the sovereignty of any state, or over which any prior sovereign has expressly or implicitly relinquished sovereignty; sovereignty over territory that is *terra nullius* may be acquired through occupation

Torres Strait Islanders: The original inhabitants of the Torres Strait Islands

This chapter has been written by two writers providing separate insights into their culture and knowledge base. The text that focuses on Aboriginal Elders was written by Odette Best, an Aboriginal registered nurse, a Boonthamurra/Goreng Goreng woman. The text that focuses on Torres Strait Islander Elders was written by Ali Drummond, a Torres Strait Islander registered nurse, a Dauareb/Wutha-thi man.

INTRODUCTION

In order to provide exceptional care to Aboriginal and Torres Strait Islander Elders, one must first gain an understanding of the life that many of them, including their parents and grandparents, have experienced. This chapter will provide you with a brief outline of the major foreign impacts on the Indigenous Australians, the Aboriginal and Torres Strait Islander people; it will also account for some significant milestones achieved. The extent of historical impacts on a particular country correlate with the current health of the country's culture, which differs from country to country. The health of the culture reflects the lifestyle and health status of the people. Be mindful that this chapter can only provide a brief insight into historical impacts, with intentions to nurture sound knowledge and empathy for the Aboriginal and Torres Strait Islander Elders who will be in your care.

SETTING THE SCENE

Across Australia there are hundreds of different Aboriginal **nations**. Queensland is unique within Australia as it not only includes many Aboriginal nations but also encompasses the Torres Strait Islands, with its own Indigenous population, within the geographical parameters.

It is important to remember that **Aboriginal Australians** and **Torres Strait Islanders** are very different and unique. While there are cultural similarities, in a number of ways their differences are remarkable and call for different care within your caring role.

Aboriginal Elders

Within the Aboriginal cultures, since the time before colonisation, there has been the respect of Elders. Often this has meant that history and **culture** is learnt from the Elders. This knowledge is passed on orally. The **Elders** teach **customs**, lore, healing practices, languages and creation stories. The Elders are seen as carriers of old knowledge. This is why you may hear Aboriginal Australians refer to older Indigenous people as Aunty or Uncle. While there is no 'bloodline' that may connect them, it is about paying respect to their knowledge and the legacy they have lived. Elders are well respected and well treated by the broader Indigenous community.

Due to there being such a diminished number of Elders within the Aboriginal community, they are particularly well looked after. The history that the Elders have also lived under is particularly taken into account for the younger Aboriginal community.

Torres Strait Islander Elders

In the Torres Strait Islander culture, Elders are considered the centre of the society, the keepers of ancient knowledge and true custodians of the land and sea. However, the role of the Elders in Torres Strait Islander society today has changed in definition and function due to the numerous events that have affected Torres Strait Islander culture.

The knowledge possessed by the Elders, once held at the highest value, has been shrouded by the impact of colonisation. Elders have found it difficult to share their knowledge about the intimate relationship Torres Strait Islander peoples once shared with the environment. This is a result of such knowledge being forced into secrecy as a response to religious demands and government policies. The Western mindset conflicts with the values held by the Torres Strait Islanders – ideas around industrialisation and exploitation of natural resources are perfect examples; however, history has shown that those who chose to challenge the new order were alienated.

PRE-INVASION HEALTH STATUS

It is now indisputable that **Indigenous Australians** were, at the time of colonisation, a fit and healthy race of people. The Indigenous oral tradition of passing on history tells us uniformly that it was a functional community, one that was full of physical exercise that took many forms – hunting and gathering, preparation of food and also ceremonial activities – not only within individual clans, but also at larger gatherings of several thousand Aboriginal peoples.

The colonisers also noted this level of physical fitness:

> The health status of Aboriginal people before colonisation is difficult to assess in ways comparable to current data. However, there is strong evidence that a number of infectious diseases (such as measles, flu and smallpox) were not present before the invasion. It also appears that 'life style' diseases (such as diabetes, high blood pressure, ischaemic heart disease) were unknown. Early descriptions of Aborigines painted a picture of a lean, athletic, robust and dignified people.
>
> (Bartlett 1995, p. 10)

While Aboriginal health was not perfect, the style of living was more in tune with the environment in which people lived. Diets were good, bush tucker was plentiful and people lived on their **country** and accepted the responsibility of caring for their country, protecting waterholes and sacred sites. People lived in harmony with their environment, accessing the land's resources in ways that protected each resource. Waste disposal was not a major issue due to the nomadic lifestyle and the lack of non-biodegradable products.

Prior to invasion, Indigenous people had control over every aspect of their life. In today's terminology, this has been called a holistic approach to health, but in Indigenous society prior to 1788 this was perceived as the norm. Every aspect of the person was equally regarded; this being the biological, psychological, sociological, spiritual and communal aspects. The National Aboriginal Health Strategy (NAHS) identifies health for Indigenous peoples as:

> … not just the physical well-being of the individual but also the social, emotional and cultural wellbeing of the whole community. This is a whole of life view and it includes the cyclical concept of life–death–life.
>
> (National Aboriginal Health Strategy Working Party 1989)

Traditional medicines and healing practices

Before colonisation Indigenous communities had their own traditional medicinal practices, which were effectively administered and valued for generations. As part of the colonisation process, these treatments and practices were often quashed by traditional Western medical practices.

The havoc wrought on Indigenous society through the destruction of traditional medical practices also proved profoundly damaging to Indigenous health. Indigenous peoples themselves saw the introduction of disease and the decline of their health as 'white man's' poisons or diseases, and were ill-equipped to combat them. The establishment of missions (mostly by religious organisations) and the incarceration of entire communities led, to a large extent, to the demise of traditional medical practices. These practices were forbidden on the missions, being seen as 'witchcraft'.

However, when traditional Indigenous practices were tested within Western means, they were often deemed effective. For instance:

> Lawson Holman found confirmation of the effectiveness of a particular traditional treatment. Patients with lacerations and compound fractures occasionally arrived at the hospital with 'antbed' plasters on their wounds, made from material obtained from specific types of anthills. These were usually promptly replaced with a conventional dressing. Having noticed that there seemed to be more problems with infection following removal, Holman opted in certain cases to leave the antbed plaster on, with good results. Subsequent testing demonstrated antimicrobial properties.
>
> (Hunter 1993, p. 55)

However, after years of colonisation, the reality is that Australian Indigenous health status has been radically and irreparably altered; Indigenous Australians are no longer fit and healthy peoples as they were pre-invasion. It is now well recognised by many health authorities that these health statistics are the result of invasion and colonisation, which has led to dysfunctional families and communities.

CARING ABOUT CULTURE

While many traditional medicinal practices have been lost, there are still traditional practices that have continued unbroken for many thousands of years. These medicines are real to many Indigenous peoples who use them and are part of self-identified healing practices. While these may not comply with Western practices, they are still a vital part of the lives of many older Indigenous peoples.

Some examples include: within the Torres Strait Islands, pawpaw leaves which are used for bathing and treating the symptoms of chickenpox; across Australia, many different Aboriginal nations rub witchetty grubs on the gums of teething babies as a mild anaesthetic.

THE ONSLAUGHT AND EFFECTS OF COLONISATION

The Aboriginal experience

For Indigenous Australians, it is not merely a question of having the poorest health status of any identifiable group within Australia, but also about struggling with the ongoing effects of the colonisation process.

Since colonisation, the health of non-Indigenous Australia has flourished while that of Indigenous Australia has diminished. Indigenous Australians felt the effects of colonisation almost immediately. Diseases that Indigenous peoples had no immunity against had devastating effects. As the frontier between the colonists and the Indigenous Australians expanded over decades, the pattern of degeneration in health continued.

The Aboriginal perspective is that it is the initial loss of land that has changed Aboriginal Australia forever. It is essential to understand the importance of Aboriginal people's link to the land. The 1989 report of the National Aboriginal Health Strategy (NAHS) Working Party identifies that 'Aboriginal people were totally dependent on the land and on all it could provide. To cope with this, they developed a social organisation that would enable them to use their natural environment successfully' (p. ix).

Further to this, the Governor-General stated in August 1996:

> The present plight, in terms of health, employment, education, living conditions and self-esteem, of so many Aborigines must be acknowledged as largely flowing from what happened in the past. The dispossession, the destruction of hunting fields and the devastation of lives were all related. The new diseases, the alcohol and the new pressures of living were all introduced. True acknowledgement cannot stop short of recognition of the extent to which present disadvantage flows from past injustice and oppression.
>
> (Couzos & Murray 1999, p. 1)

Table 6.1 outlines the interaction between the history of colonisation and legislation directed towards Aboriginal people and the impact that these have had.

Anecdotally, Aboriginal registered nurses and midwives will openly discuss the very palpable effects of removal that they feel when providing health service provision to Aboriginal people. In discussions with many Aboriginal people, they expressed the grief and loss they felt over many issues. However, one issue that remained constant was the effects that removal had not only on themselves, but also on their immediate family members. Not surprisingly, as the Human Rights and Equal Opportunity Commission Report, *Bringing Them Home*, states:

> Grief and loss are the predominant themes of this report … the histories we trace are complex and pervasive. Most significantly, the actions of the past resonate in the present and will continue to do so in the future. The laws, policies and practices that separate Indigenous children from their families have contributed directly to the alienation of Indigenous societies today. For individuals, their removal as children and the abuse they experienced at the hands of the authorities or their delegates have permanently scarred their lives. The harm continues in later generations, affecting their children and grandchildren.
>
> (Australian Human Rights Commission 1997, p. 3).

Torres Strait Islander experience

The Torres Strait Islanders also experienced an invasion from foreigners, although this differed from their mainland counterparts. The Islanders suffered great loss and hardship; however, many Islanders were able to maintain the connection with their homeland and practise and pass down culture, at times in secret. This was because the Torres Strait Islands were not deemed valuable land resources for mass agricultural and pastoral development. The value of the Torres Strait Islands lay beneath their waters: the resource-rich seabeds, abundant in trochus and mother-of-pearl shell and trepang (*beche-de-mer* or sea cucumber).

Seabed resources exploitation

In the 17th century, fishermen from Indonesia, Macassan trepangers, traded peacefully with the Torres Strait Islanders and Northern Aboriginal nations. Cloth, rice, alcohol and tobacco were traded for rights to fish in their waters and sometimes to recruit crew. In the 1860s the trepang industry boomed, with stations built on a number of the Torres Strait Islands. The Europeans boats, often crewed by South Sea Islanders (i.e. Fijians, Solomon Islanders or Samoan Islanders), exploited the Torres Strait seabed. There are documented accounts of some fruitful relations between the Islanders and the foreigners; however, mostly they were grim. The Islanders had to defend themselves against hordes of armed men, who essentially took what they wanted, including the women.

Coming of the 'light'

On 1 July 1871 the London Missionary Society (LMS) landed on Erub (or Darnley) Island, with the intention of converting Torres Strait Islanders to Christianity. Darnley Island, an eastern island, was suggested as a base by an experienced explorer, as he believed the locals had a milder demeanour compared to the other Islanders. Additionally, Darnley Island already had an established trepang station, with a number of crew members and a depleting Islander population. Once established, Christianity spread quite easily throughout the Torres Strait Islands.

The LMS had both positive and negative impacts on the Torres Strait Islanders. They brought Western order to the Torres Strait which made life safer for the Torres Strait Islanders from neighbouring islands and foreigners. However, the LMS demanded the surrender of any traditional acts, including language, dance and ***pouri-pouri*** (black magic). There are accounts of severe penalties delivered by the missionaries as a result of disobedience. The LMS also hand-picked Islanders who they thought had potential of spreading and maintaining the 'light' in the Torres Strait Islands. The initial contact with the LMS is now an annual celebration called 'The Coming of the Light', celebrated on 1 July by Torres Strait Islanders Australia-wide.

CARING ABOUT CULTURE

Christianity has embedded itself well within the Torres Strait Islander culture and it is not rare to nurse a Torres Strait Islander Elder who is a devout Christian. Often, the head of a family and community leaders will have strong associations with the church.

Pouri-pouri, or black magic, is a concept that is very real to Torres Strait Islanders, especially those dwelling on traditional land. Many still associate illness with *pouri-pouri*, despite what a modern health practitioner may suggest.

Table 6.1
Interaction between the history of colonisation and legislation directed towards Aboriginal people

Historical facts	European justification	Aboriginal action
1 European settlement (1788–1880s)		
• Taking the land • Extermination poisoning/shooting • Hopelessness, soul destroying	• Aboriginal people = 'the missing link' • No culture – no morality • No humanity	• Retaliation • Defeat • Resignation to white domination • Sickness/loss of heart, loss of land, leadership, traditions, language
2 Segregation (1890s–1950s)		
'Era of protection': • Missions, government reserves • Poor housing, health, employment	• 'Smoothing the dying pillow' • 'Civilise the savages' • 'Bearing the white man's burden' • Heavy influence from the church	• Rejection of domination • Passive resistance • Endurance of many missionary ideals • Distrust of/caution towards other Aboriginal people • Negative self-image • Endurance of bad housing, health, employment • Continued struggle for equality
3 Assimilation (1950s–60s)		
Policies to elevate standards: • Housing • Health • Education	Aboriginal people were to be educated for full citizenship, without distinction, either among themselves or between them and white people. They were to be given equal opportunity whenever possible progressively through training and welfare	• Distrust, suspicion • Passive resistance, endurance – growing anger at society and its discrimination • Development of Federal Council for the Advancement of Aborigines and Torres Strait Islanders (FCAATSI) as a national pressure group
4 Integration (1967–72)		
Emphasis on positive relations, chance for Aboriginal people to say what they want (choice)	Pressure to make up for some past mistakes – internal, as well as overseas (e.g. infant mortality rates rivalled those of many Asian and African countries)	• Distrust of Europeans • Efforts to achieve • Growing movement pressing for self-determination • Growth of Black Power movement, National Tribal Council
5 Self-determination (1972–75)		
Aboriginal people are/should be in charge of their own affairs – financial help, technical skills, socioeconomic support	Recognition of multicultural society, cultural diversity/difference, some rights, etc.	• Growing awareness of making own decisions • Tent Embassy • Strong pressure to become self-reliant, but still subject to 'We'll help you to do what we want you to do' • Development of National Aboriginal Consultative Committee (NACC)
6 Self-management stage I (1975–88)		
Aboriginal people must be held accountable for their decisions and management of finance	Some white backlash Government review of NACC, reshaped into National Aboriginal Conference (NAC) and its eventual disbandment Attempts to introduce national land rights abandoned	• Heavy push for land rights, separate legal, health, housing services • Development of NAC 'Makarrata': 'resumption of normal relations following a period of hostility' • Recognition of prior ownership of Australia: land rights; cash compensation; reserved seats for Aboriginal people in parliament

Table 6.1
Interaction between the history of colonisation and legislation directed towards Aboriginal people *continued*

Historical facts	European justification	Aboriginal action
7 Self-management stage II (1988–96)		
Aboriginal affairs reorganised under the Aboriginal and Torres Strait Islander Commission (ATSIC): emphasis on welfare issues (e.g. housing, health, employment, education)	Aboriginal decision-making in Aboriginal affairs recognised: pressure to 'normalise' relationships via a compact or Treaty of Reconciliation	Some hope for change but some suspicion – continued stress on global issues (e.g. land rights, compensation, etc.)
The Royal Commission into Aboriginal Deaths in Custody (RCIADIC) set up to investigate 'suicides' in custody	Acceptance that the legal system does not provide adequately for Aboriginal people	Renewed vigilance and suspicion of the agents of the law
Native Title legislation	High Court judgement that Aboriginal and Torres Strait Islander people have prior ownership rights to Australia	Hope for change, respect and recognition; enormous activities in all communities to develop Native Title claims
8 Reconciliation or economic rationalism? (1996–2007)		
Inquiry into the Stolen Generations	Government reluctant to accept the history of colonisation	Anger and anguish; formation of community-based support groups
The Wik Decision, which extends Native Title rights, and the Ten-Point Plan, which limits Native Title rights	Government reluctant to proceed with Native Title; pressure from pastoralists to water down legislation	Anger and despair; conflicts within some communities about who are the traditional owners of land, disputes about borders
Council for Reconciliation established	Government unable to apologise, wants 'practical reconciliation' rather than 'black armband' approach to history	Anger
	Grassroots movement, Australians for Native Title and Reconciliation (ANTaR)	Some Aboriginal people join the Australians for Native Title and Reconciliation (ANTaR) movement, others support it tacitly, still others are suspicious of 'Aboriginal' reconciliation and want to establish true Native Title and compensation before beginning discussions about what reconciliation means
ATSIC abolished in 2004 and a National Indigenous Council (NIC) appointed by the federal government	Government argues that ATSIC is inefficient and corrupt, and does not represent Aboriginal people. The NIC will advise the government, and its members are chosen because of their expertise rather than their representativeness	Ambivalence towards ATSIC, but deep suspicion towards the NIC
A growth in dysfunction in Aboriginal communities documented by a range of reports, such as *Violence in Indigenous Communities* (2001), *Indigenous Education 2005–2008* (2006), *The Little Children Are Sacred Report* (2007)	• Belief that dysfunction is due to Aboriginal parents' neglect • Some argument that 'this' (i.e. child sexual exploitation and family violence) is a 'cultural matter'	• General condemnation of male perpetrators and demands for stronger action against them • Some shame and demands that Aboriginal people not be labelled • Demands for better access to appropriate infrastructure
Increased media attention on child abuse and family violence, particularly in remote Aboriginal communities	Debate about the reasons for such dysfunction fills the newspapers; strong call for government action and intervention	Some Aboriginal people call for government action, others call for governments to face their responsibilities in providing access to services and infrastructure

Table 6.1
Interaction between the history of colonisation and legislation directed towards Aboriginal people *continued*

Historical facts	European justification	Aboriginal action
Introduction of the Northern Territory Emergency Response (NTER) aka 'the Intervention' on 21 June 2007	Government believes that level of child sexual abuse and family violence is of epidemic proportions and 'something' has to be done quickly to improve the safety and wellbeing of children and to lay the basis for a sustainable and better future for residents of remote communities in the Northern Territory	Confusion and fear about government intervention and labelling of communities
Most controversial radical action in 73 specific communities: • child health checks (at first to be compulsory, but changed to voluntary) • income management, without mechanisms for review or appeal • abolition of Community Development Employment Projects (CDEP) • resumption of Aboriginal lands in the 73 communities on a 5-year lease • abolition of the permit system for entry to Aboriginal lands • suspension of the *Racial Discrimination Act 1975 (Clth)* (RDA), and the *NT Anti-Discrimination Act* to accommodate the processes and practices of the Intervention	• Belief among many politicians and some of the public that Aboriginal people are a 'problem' that has to be solved because they are not capable of solving the problems themselves • Agreement that 'something' has to be done, but heated debate about what should be done, the time frame and the philosophy underlying the Intervention • Deep concern about the suspension of the RDA and its ramifications • Concern that the real issues of poor housing, education, health and inadequate infrastructure are not being addressed	• Many Aboriginal people feel belittled, shamed and humiliated by being singled out on the basis of 'race' and not worthy of protective legislation, particularly in relation to the compulsory acquisition of land and the blanket application of income management without access to review • A great deal of confusion about the new regulations and extent of the Intervention • Condemnation of the government for acting without extensive planning and coordination • Condemnation of the government for annexing Aboriginal lands in 73 communities without compensation • Condemnation of government for revoking the permit system, which gives Aboriginal people control over who accesses their lands
9 A new beginning? 2008 and beyond		
Labor wins the election in November 2007	The majority of Australians reject the Coalition's conservative politics	Some hope for the future
NIC is disbanded January 2008	The NIC does not represent Indigenous people	Some hope that there will be appropriate consultation and a new representative body
Labor retains the Intervention with amendments (e.g. CDEP is reinstated and compensation is paid for annexed lands)	• Belief that the 'problem' is so huge that the government cannot step back from its responsibilities • Concern that the government will never commit enough funds to reverse the years of neglect in remote communities • Continued concern about the abolition of the RDA and its consequences of generating policies according to 'race'	• Continued concern about the level of racism inherent in the Intervention • Support for the reintroduction of CDEP and its new component of compulsory training for permanent jobs • Acknowledgement of the government's compensation as right and a move towards a more respectful relationship between governments and communities
PM Rudd (2008) makes a formal apology, on behalf of the government and the Australian people, to the Aboriginal people for the wrongs of the past	• Acceptance by the majority of Australians that the past has to be acknowledged and atoned • Formalisation of 'Sorry Day', the unofficial response by ANTaR and others to former PM Howard's resolve never to apologise for the past	• Pride in their struggle for recognition and justice • Hope for the future • Expectation that future relationships will be marked by respect, trust and partnership
The government sets up consultative committees to advise on the creation of a National Indigenous Representative Committee (NIRC)	Acknowledgment that Aboriginal people must have representation at the highest level to ensure Indigenous policies and practices are appropriate	Support for a new era in government/Aboriginal interaction, negotiation and Aboriginal self-determination

Source: Adapted from A-K Eckermann, T Dowd, M Martin et al. (2010), Binan Goonj: Bridging cultures in Aboriginal health, 3rd edn. Sydney: Elsevier, pp. 22–25.

Torres Strait treaty

The trepang was of great value to the Chinese market as it was prized for its flavour-enhancing, medicinal and aphrodisiac qualities. The trochus and mother-of-pearl shell were used for buttons and other ornaments worldwide. Their abundance in the Torres Strait attracted more fishing boats to the islands. At the time, the northernmost point of a governing officer in Queensland was Somerset, on the tip of Cape York. The Queensland Government decided to expand its grasp on the seafood and shell industry, thus encompassing the Torres Strait Islands under its control.

In 1978, the Australian and Papua New Guinean governments signed the Torres Strait Treaty. The Treaty endeavoured to achieve cooperation between the two states, in areas of conservation, management and sharing of fisheries resources, the last being the most valuable. The issues of sovereignty include marine boundaries, seabed mineral resource development and marine environment protections. The Treaty deems the Torres Strait Islands to be a protected zone, recognising the traditional fishing practised by the Torres Strait Islanders, and the traditional trading between Torres Strait Islanders and people from Papua New Guinea's southern coastal villages. Australia's borders and fishing boundaries have changed numerous times since the development of the Treaty. The Torres Strait Treaty also permits commercial fishing in the area; however, this is another issue that has been heavily opposed by the Torres Strait Islanders for a number of years.

Caste system

The mix of races in the Torres Strait around the turn of the 20th century nurtured a caste system, with Europeans at the top, the black-skinned people at the very bottom and the other races ranked in the middle according to their skin colour. There was even a hierarchical system among the black-skinned people, with the Torres Strait Islanders ranked superior to the Papua New Guinean and Aboriginal people. This system was encouraged by government policy and the marine industry structure, where it was evident in wages and ranked position on fishing boats.

CARING ABOUT CULTURE

Torres Strait Islanders can be offended if they are mistaken for being of Aboriginal or Papua New Guinean origin. Do not assume the origins of your patient. Ask politely where they are from or who their people are.

The caste system has since become redundant; however, you will quite often hear Torres Strait Islanders refer to fairer skinned Islanders as 'half-castes', which has become a part of the Torres Strait Islander Creole vocabulary.

Please note carefully that this is unique to the Torres Strait Islanders. Many Aboriginal people take offence at being called 'half-castes', owing to the fact that this was part of the reason behind the removal of Aboriginal children from their families.

Living under the Act

Early in the 20th century the Queensland Government decided to strengthen compliance with national policy by ceasing interaction between the different hierarchical levels. Regulations were imposed that excluded Torres Strait Islanders from Thursday Island, which by then had become the main port in the Torres Strait. Pearling luggers with Islander crew that docked at Thursday Island had to comply with a curfew that required Islander crew to return to their boats before sunset. Interracial relationships were made illegal, and marriage required the Protector's permission. Families resulting from an interracial communion were relocated to missions on the outer islands, and were placed under the Aboriginal Act.

CARING ABOUT CULTURE

Many Torres Strait Islanders are from 'mixed' background. This means that many Torres Strait Islanders do not have strong Melanesian physical qualities. Do not judge someone's connection to their land and culture by their skin colour.

Maritime strike and the Torres Strait Islander Act

The late 1930s brought about great changes for the Torres Strait Islanders in governance and acquiring equality. Driven by the pearl divers, the Islanders demanded better control over their personal affairs and wages; this led to the *Torres Strait Islander Act*. The Act gave Islanders more power over governing the Islands. Each populated island was given the ability to elect its own council, usually a chairperson and two councillors. However, the elected chairperson was still strongly influenced by white government administrators, most likely the local schoolmasters, and rules were often aligned with White Australia Policy.

World War II involvement

The Torres Strait was one of the priority defence areas during World War II. As the Japanese forces pushed south towards Australia, the government sent many troops to the Torres Strait in anticipation of an assault. Many Torres Strait Islanders were recruited and contributed to the defence of Australia and of their home islands. Some men were obliged to join 'Man Power', an all-male construction organisation that developed roads, airstrips, forts and cannon foundations. Many Islanders joined the Torres Strait Defence Force, which was based in the Torres Strait.

Their involvement in the War gave many Islanders a sense of competence and an expectation that they would benefit from entitlements equal to their non-Indigenous comrades. However, their contribution was not recognised and entitlements were not granted.

It was not until 1967 that Torres Strait Islanders were bestowed equal rights in Australia, and not until 1986 that Torres Strait Islander returned servicemen received their full entitlements.

> **OF INTEREST**
>
> In 1999, a ceremony was held on Thursday Island to recognise some of the Islanders who contributed to Australia's defence during World War II. The grandfather of Ali Drummond received the Civilian Services Medal (1939–1945) for his work with the Civilian Construction Corporation.

The 1980s and the Torres Strait Islander Land Rights Movement

The late Eddie 'Koiki' Mabo, a Torres Strait Islander and a Meriam (i.e. a native of Mer, or Murray, Island), began his battle for land rights in 1981, when he spoke out publicly for the first time in Townsville. He proved to have a strong sense of cultural identity, evident in his knowledge of traditional laws and customs. He was aware of his birthright, taught to him by his father; however, this contrasted with Australian law.

On its discovery, Australia was deemed ***terra nullius***, a Latin term meaning 'land belonging to no one'. This deemed the land vacant for the colonisers, leaving the Indigenous people without rights to access and use the land that they had maintained and lived on for many thousands of years.

This conflicted with Meriam lore and, once discovered by Koiki, became the beginning of a long battle between the Meriam people and the Queensland and Commonwealth governments. Alongside Koiki, a number of Meriam plaintiffs argued for their personal property, achieving a result that would benefit all Indigenous Australians.

On 3 June 1992, the High Court in Canberra passed judgement that deemed the Meriam people as the Native Title holders of the land. This date is commemorated annually as Mabo Day. Indigenous people nationwide celebrate the victory that Koiki led. Despite being refused his personal claims, he continued to fight for the cause.

In contrast to many mainland counterparts, Torres Strait Islanders were, for the most part, kept on their traditional islands. Arguably, their link to the land and sea has not been severed. However, despite the maintenance of the relationship to land and sea, health disparities are still evident between Torres Strait Islander populations and non-Indigenous Australians. The lack of health data that is specific to Torres Strait Islanders makes it impossible to measure the health disparities compared with the Aboriginal population and non-Indigenous Australians.

PRESENT-DAY FACTS AND FIGURES

There are just over half a million Aboriginal and Torres Strait Islander people in Australia today, comprising 2.5 per cent of the Australian population. Although many Indigenous Australians have access to life opportunities and a good standard of living, too many Indigenous Australians experience unacceptable levels of disadvantage in living standards, life expectancy, education, health and employment. Current data shows a significant gap in these critical areas between the Indigenous and non-Indigenous population.

The Australian Bureau of Statistics 2016 Census data show some important differences between the Indigenous population and other Australians. The life expectancy for Indigenous Australians was approximately 10 years less than for the total population in 2015–17 (Figure 6.1):

- for Indigenous males, 71.6 years compared with 81.2 years in the non-Indigenous population
- for Indigenous females, 75.6 years compared with 83.4 years (AIHW 2020).

The following figures illustrate the poor health experiences of Aboriginal and Torres Strait Islander people in 2016:

- the median age of the Indigenous population is 23 years (38 years for non-Indigenous)
- 34 per cent of Indigenous people are under the age of 15 (18.3 per cent for non-Indigenous)

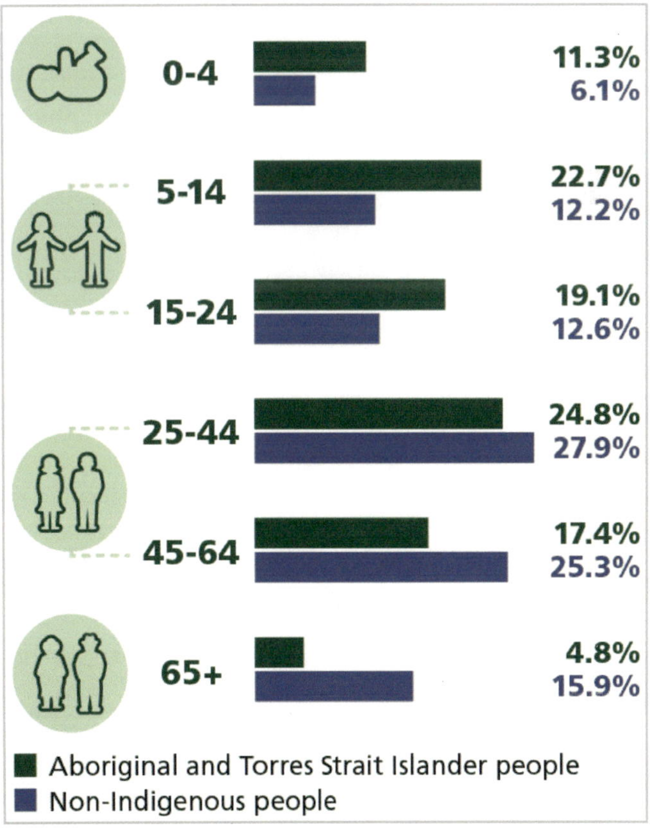

Fig. 6.1
Age distribution of the Australian Indigenous and non-Indigenous population as at 2016.

- only 4.8 per cent of Indigenous people are aged over 65 (16 per cent for non-Indigenous) (ABS 2017a, 2017b).

Fig. 6.1 illustrates the differences in the age profile between the Indigenous and non-Indigenous populations. This figure provides a clear picture of the small number of aged Indigenous Australians in the population. This is the exact opposite for non-Indigenous Australians, of which there is a large ageing population. This disparity is due to the diminished life expectancy of Indigenous Australians. The lack of separate data for the Torres Strait Islanders is also obvious from this graph.

OTHER PIECES OF THE PUZZLE

Men's and women's business

Another issue that needs to be considered in the provision of care for Aboriginal and Torres Strait Islander Elders is the fairly strict adherence to what is called 'women's and men's business' in many Aboriginal and Torres Strait Islander communities, from the very remote communities to the very urban setting.

What does this mean? For many communities different knowledge is held in regard to differing issues that impact on women or men. Men's issues are dealt with by men, and women's issues are dealt with by women.

Aboriginal female nurses should not be expected to shower older Aboriginal men or talk to them about issues that affect their genitalia and sexuality. This is not such an issue among many non-Indigenous peoples, so you need to be mindful when showering or bathing older Aboriginal and Torres Strait Islander peoples that gender-specific care may be needed. To illustrate this further, very few Indigenous male nurses attain qualifications for midwifery as this is seen purely as women's business.

Kinship and families

Traditional Indigenous society practised a complex kinship system, which governs communication and relationship within one's **mob** and between multiple nations. The kinship system provided the rules for communication, interactions with other nations and even interactions with one's in-laws. The kinship system also nurtured a tight bond within families and extended families.

The period of the Stolen Generations dramatically affected this system. The forced removal of children meant that family ties were broken and sometimes customs were forgotten. However, the tight bond associated with the kinship system proved harder to break. Family is highly valued by Indigenous people, and the term 'family' extends beyond the immediate family.

It is common practice when being introduced to another Indigenous person that an explanation of one's family genealogy occurs, including the recital of one's parents, grandparents and sometimes great-grandparents. It is also worth noting the contrasting constructs that define family from an Indigenous perspective. To illustrate this construct, in non-Indigenous culture the sister of one's grandmother is identified as a 'Great Aunty'; however, in Indigenous culture, one's grandmother's sisters are respected and addressed as 'Grandmother'. Within Indigenous communities there may be multiple grandmothers and grandfathers, who are the sisters and brothers of one's 'bloodline' grandmother or grandfather. The rule also applies to the cousins of one's parents, who are respected and addressed as one's 'Aunty' or 'Uncle'.

It is common when an elderly person is hospitalised that you would expect family to visit. It is no surprise when Indigenous people are hospitalised that a significant number of family members will visit. Family will travel considerable distances to visit a sick family member and in great numbers.

CARING ABOUT CULTURE

Be prepared for a number of visitors if you are nursing an Indigenous Elder. The number of visitors is likely to escalate if a death is imminent for an Indigenous Elder.

Sometimes visitors may arrive during non-visiting hours or breach the limit of the allowable number of visitors at one time. Adhere to your facility procedures and policy; however, be mindful about the distance that the family may have travelled and their concerns. Clearly explain the situation and provide them with information on the appropriate visiting hours and numbers. Suggest that the family meet with your Elder patient at a reasonable time during visiting hours outside where there is room for a visiting crowd.

Indigenous Liaison Officers

Most major hospitals in Australia employ at least one Indigenous Liaison Officer (ILO). An ILO should be your first point of contact if an Indigenous patient is admitted, as long as you have the patient's permission. The ILO is your local expert on Indigenous customs and protocols. If you have any queries or require an interpreter, or maybe someone to assist with difficult situations, contact your facility's ILO for assistance.

Provision of care

Many Indigenous Elders who you may be caring for have lived under a destructive legacy of Australian policies. Many have distressing histories of being removed from their family or having had children removed from them, living on missions, traditional knowledge being forced to extinction and not receiving wages for work. For many of them, this may be a part of their history that they do not want to discuss or acknowledge.

The provision of physical healthcare via services for Aboriginal and Torres Strait Islander Elders is essentially the same as for non-Indigenous Australians. However, be mindful that the Indigenous construct of health is not just the physical element alone. For many Indigenous peoples, health includes spiritual, social, community and psychological wellbeing. Hence, Indigenous-specific health services have been developed to address the holistic healthcare needs of Indigenous people.

The Aboriginal and Islander Community Health Service sector

The Aboriginal Medical Service was set up in the 1970s. The first service was established in Redfern, Sydney, in 1971 to counteract the poor access to healthcare and racism experienced by many Aboriginal people in the mainstream health services. The Aboriginal community was in need of appropriate healthcare that nurtured and understood its culture. One of the very first doctors attached to Redfern was the late Professor Fred Hollows, who donated his time for free to this clinic and encouraged a number of doctors within Sydney to do the same. The service did not receive any government funding at the time.

There are now over 100 Aboriginal Medical Services across Australia. Within Queensland, these services also extend to Torres Strait community members. For example, the service in Brisbane is called the Aboriginal and Torres Strait Islander Community Health Service (ATSICHS).

An Aboriginal (and Islander) Community Controlled Health Service must be:

- an incorporated Aboriginal organisation
- initiated by a local Aboriginal community
- based in a local Aboriginal community
- governed by a body that is elected by the local Aboriginal community
- delivering a holistic and culturally appropriate health service to the community, which controls it.

The National Aboriginal Community Controlled Health Organisation (NACCHO) has this further to say about community control:

> … that each independent and autonomous health service is controlled by the community it serves, in order to provide that community with health care delivery to meet its health needs, as defined by that community. The solution to each community's health needs is in the hands of that community. Therefore, it cannot be said that there is strict uniformity in all Aboriginal Medical Services as different regions and communities face different health problems, or the same health problems but to varying degrees. However, what is uniform in all of the Aboriginal Medical Services is that they all operate under the philosophy of community control.
>
> (NACCHO 2017).

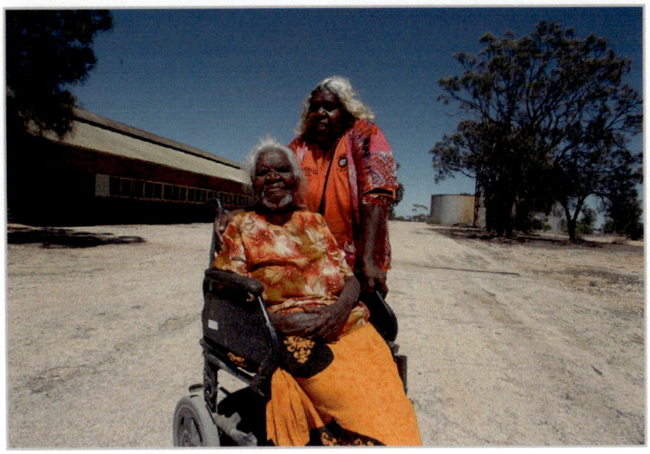

Fig. 6.2
Indigenous-specific health services address holistic healthcare needs.

Aged care facilities can be found within some Aboriginal and Torres Strait Islander Community Health Services. For example, the Brisbane ATSICHS operates the Jimbelunga Nursing Centre, which means 'A place of friendship'. Jimbelunga was established to meet the cultural and spiritual needs of Aboriginal and Torres Strait Islander people (Fig. 6.2).

REVIEW QUESTIONS

Circle T if the statement is true or F if the statement if false:

1 T / F The health of Indigenous Australians is worse than it was 200 years ago.

2 T / F Indigenous Australians have a long history of traditional medicine.

3 T / F The Stolen Generations occurred over a 10-year period.

4 T / F *Pouri-pouri* is practised in the Torres Strait Islands.

5 T / F The term 'half-caste' is offensive to many Indigenous Australians.

6 T / F The Torres Strait community played a key role in the defence of northern Australia.

7 T / F *Terra nullius* was the concept overturned with the Mabo judgement.

8 T / F The average life expectancy for Indigenous Australians is 5 years lower than for non-Indigenous Australians.

9 T / F It is inappropriate for a female health worker to talk to a male Indigenous man about sexual health issues.

10 T / F Elders are less respected in Indigenous culture.

Answers to these questions are on p. 454.

Further reading

Australian Bureau of Statistics (ABS) (2017a). Census of Population and Housing: Reflecting Australian stories from the Census, 2016. Aboriginal and Torres Strait Islander population 2016 Census data summary. Australian Government. Online 11 Dec 2017. www.abs.gov.au/ausstats/abs@.nsf/Lookup/by%20Subject/2071.0~2016~Main%20Features~Aboriginal%20and%20Torres%20Strait%20Islander%20Population%20Data%20Summary~10.

Australian Indigenous Health InfoNet (2017). Online 7 Dec 2017. Available: www.healthinfonet.ecu.edu.au/.

Pascoe B (2014). Dark Emu Black Seeds: agriculture or accident? Magabala Books, Broome WA.

References

Australian Bureau of Statistics (ABS) (2017a). Census of Population and Housing: Reflecting Australian stories from the Census, 2016. Aboriginal and Torres Strait Islander population 2016 Census data summary. Australian Government. Online 11 Dec 2017. www.abs.gov.au/ausstats/abs

Australian Bureau of Statistics (2017b). Media Release. 2016 Census shows growing Aboriginal and Torres Strait Islander population. www.abs.gov.au/ausstats/abs@.nsf/MediaRealesesByCatalogue/02D50FAA9987D6B7CA25814800087E03?OpenDocument.

Australian Human Rights Commission (1997). Bringing Them Home: Report of the National Inquiry into the separation of Aboriginal and Torres Strait Islander Children from their families. AGPS, Canberra.

Australian Institute of Health and Welfare (AIHW) (2020). Indigenous life expectancy and deaths. Online 6 September 2021. Available: www.aihw.gov.au/reports/australias-health/indigenous-life-expectancy-and-deaths

Bartlett, B. (1995). An Aboriginal Health Worker's guide to family, community and public health. Central Australian Aboriginal Congress Publication, Alice Springs.

Couzos, S. & Murray, R. (1999). Aboriginal primary healthcare: An evidence-based approach. Kimberley Aboriginal Medical Services Council, WA.

Eckermann A-K, Dowd T, Martin M et al. (2010). Binan Goonj: Bridging cultures in Aboriginal health, 3rd edn. Elsevier, Sydney.

Hunter, E. (1993). Aboriginal health and history: Power and prejudice in remote Australia. Cambridge Press, Hong Kong.

National Aboriginal Community Controlled Health Organisation (NACCHO) (2017). Online 7 Dec 2017. Available: www.naccho.org.au.

National Aboriginal Health Strategy Working Party (1989). National Aboriginal Health Strategy Working Party Report. Canberra: AGPS.

CHAPTER 7
Working with the older Māori – kaumātua and aged care

By Mihi Ratima, Will Edwards and Rangimahora Reddy

AFTER THIS CHAPTER, YOU SHOULD BE ABLE TO:

- define the key terms listed in this chapter
- appreciate the relevance of the Treaty of Waitangi
- broadly understand the impacts of colonisation
- describe Māori development phases
- understand the concept of Māori identity
- appreciate Māori understandings of health
- describe the circumstances of older Māori in New Zealand society
- show insight into the impact of determinants of health on the wellbeing of older Māori
- describe roles of older Māori within Māori society
- appreciate distinctive Māori perspectives on ageing
- appreciate key issues in the provision of aged care for older Māori.

Key terms

cultural competence: The ability to interact effectively with people of different cultures and backgrounds

hapū: Sub-tribe

health literacy: For individuals, health literacy is the ability to obtain and understand basic health information and services required to make informed and appropriate health decisions. Health literacy for those who work in health fields is about their ability to convey health information and to support those they work with to build their skills and knowledge.

iwi: Tribe

kapa haka: Māori performing arts

karakia: Ritual chant or prayer

karanga: Ceremonial call

kaumātua: Male elders (koroua) and female elders (kuia)

kaupapa Māori: Provision within a Māori worldview and in a Māori way, e.g. kaupapa Māori health services

kōhanga reo: Māori culture and language immersion early childhood programmes

korowai: Traditional cloak

kura kaupapa Māori: Māori medium schools at the primary and secondary levels of provision

marae: Customary Māori community centres

mirimiri: Massage

papakāinga: Māori co-housing which may be on ancestral lands

raranga: Weaving

rongoā: Māori traditional healing system that includes the use of plant-based remedies

tino rangatiratanga/rangatiratanga: Self-determination

tohunga: Māori experts or specialists in a range of areas who are leaders in their fields

waiata: Song

waka ama: Outrigger canoeing

whaikōrero: Formal speech-making

whakapapa: Genealogy or lines of descent from ancestors

whānau: Extended family

The purpose of this chapter is to provide an overview of the context for aged care for kaumātua in New Zealand, and to discuss a number of key cultural issues in the provision of care. To understand this better and to be able to provide high quality care (including care that is culturally appropriate) you will need a basic understanding of the social, economic, cultural, political and environmental determinants or drivers of the wellbeing of kaumātua in New Zealand. The chapter is relevant to the provision of care for older Māori in Australia.

MĀORI AS INDIGENOUS PEOPLES

Despite the many differences between Indigenous peoples around the world, there are five factors many of these groups have in common that help to understand what it means to be Indigenous peoples. These are:

- having occupied a specific land area earlier than others
- attachment to a particular land area, demonstrated in the special nature of their relationship to their lands
- the choice to maintain a unique cultural identity
- self-identification and being recognised by others as a distinct group
- an experience of being oppressed and powerless, stripped of their lands and other possessions, excluded or discriminated against (Daes 1996).

These factors are characteristic of Māori. Māori are recognised as the Indigenous peoples of New Zealand, and were the first people to occupy New Zealand around 1000 years ago. The impacts of British colonisation have been devastating for Māori, with Māori society oppressed and marginalised, robbed of their lands and subject to enduring racism. Despite this, the special nature of the relationship between Māori and their lands remains important as a source of identity.

In 2020, the total population of New Zealand was estimated at close to 5.1 million, including around 816,500 Māori. Māori are a young population, so that while one in six New Zealanders are Māori, among those aged under 25 years one in four are Māori (Stats NZ 2021).

TREATY OF WAITANGI

The Treaty of Waitangi was signed in 1840 between Māori chiefs and the British Crown. It is one mechanism through which Māori have sought to have their unique rights addressed as Treaty partners (and alongside Indigenous rights). There were three original intentions of the Treaty – to protect Māori, to promote British settler interests and to give strategic advantages for the British Crown. It is the founding document of New Zealand and is part of New Zealand's Constitution.

The Treaty principles of partnership, participation and active protection were identified by the Royal Commission on Social Policy and have guided the way the Treaty is applied in the health, aged care and other sectors (Royal Commission on Social Policy 1988). Partnership refers to a relationship of equals between Māori and the Crown. Participation requires Māori involvement and input at all levels on matters relevant to their own development. The principle of protection implies a Māori right to good health and care.

CARING ABOUT CULTURE

The Treaty of Waitangi and the Declaration on the Rights of Indigenous Peoples (an international human rights instrument) provide ways through which Māori have sought to have their unique rights to health as Treaty partners and Indigenous peoples met. Culturally responsive aged care is a way in which carers and the aged care sector can do their bit to address Treaty and Indigenous rights (Palmer 2008).

MĀORI DEVELOPMENT

To understand the context for aged care for **kaumātua**, we need to think about the mix of historical, social, economic, political and cultural factors that have shaped Māori development. This section is mainly about the post-European contact period (i.e. post-colonisation), as during that time a national Māori identity emerged (before that, identity was tribally based) and Māori faced the greatest threat to their survival as a group (see Edwards 2010 for further detail).

Pre-1900: Adaptation for survival

Following the initial migration from wider Polynesia to New Zealand, the main challenges to Māori survival were about adapting to the new environment (Durie 1999). Some centuries later, British settler colonisation became the greatest threat to Māori survival (Durie 1999). In 1769, the Māori population was around 100,000 (Pool 1991). By the late 1830s organised colonisation was well underway. The 1840 signing of the Treaty of Waitangi provided a structure for the relationship between Māori and the British settlers. Continued European colonisation led to the emergence of a national Māori identity in 1935, when the Declaration of Independence was signed by 34 Māori chiefs and the British Crown, recognising Māori sovereignty. Up until then, Māori society was firmly tribal in nature. The impact of pākehā (New Zealanders of European extraction) settlement was catastrophic for Māori, due to, among other things, the introduction of guns (which made warfare more deadly), new infectious diseases and land alienation.

Large land conflicts between Māori and pākehā from 1845 to 1870 had devastating effects (Belich 1986). Vast tracts of land were taken through state-sponsored land alienation. From almost 30 million hectares of land in Māori ownership in 1840, Māori land holdings reduced to less than 5 million hectares by 1891 (Durie 1998). Land alienation meant the loss of the economic, social, spiritual and cultural foundations of Māori society. Māori population decline at the end of the 19th century can be linked to land alienation (Kunitz 1994; Pool 1991).

1900–1950: Re-emerging Māori leadership

Customary Māori leadership was severely undermined by colonisation at the start of the 20th century (Walker 1990). The *Tohunga Suppression Act 1907*, for example, made it illegal to practise as a **tohunga** or traditional expert and leader in fields such as healing. Māori leadership then took a new form involving Western-trained professionals who were Māori, culturally skilled and connected to Māori communities (Durie 1998). The approach to Māori development during this period was to fully exploit Western tools while maintaining Māori cultural values. Unfortunately, this was difficult to sustain.

Consolidation of land was also a key strategy to avoid further loss of land and to provide for the economic wellbeing of Māori as a group rather than the interests of individuals (Walker 2001).

1950–1975: Urbanisation and protest

Within a 25-year period around 80 per cent of Māori moved from their tribal homelands to cities; this was due to poverty (as a result of land loss) in rural areas where most Māori lived, industrialisation and the need for a workforce for a growing capitalist society and World War II (Durie 1998). Impacts on Māori included:

- undermining of tribal identity for many and reducing whānau unity because people lived too far away to maintain active links; challenges in Māori–pākehā relations as urbanisation meant greater contact between the two groups, and Māori marginalisation and lack of authority in cities.
- Māori political activism, which grew in the 1960s and '70s due to discontent among urban Māori. Activism was largely about increasing Māori control of their own development. The most high-profile protests were the 1975 Land March against land alienation, the 1977–78 Bastion Point protest, which was also about land issues, and the Waitangi Day protests calling for the New Zealand Government to honour the Treaty of Waitangi (Durie 1998; Walker 1990).

1976–2000: Treaty of Waitangi claims, language revitalisation, strengthened Māori development, addressing disparities

Following the 1975 Land March, Parliament passed the *Treaty of Waitangi Act*, which established the Waitangi Tribunal. The Tribunal's role was to make recommendations on claims made by Māori where the Crown was alleged not to have fulfilled its Treaty obligations. The establishment of the Waitangi Tribunal provided a forum for Māori claims regarding Crown breaches of the Treaty to be heard. Māori were particularly preoccupied with the claims process and expended huge resources preparing and contesting claims and subsequent settlements. While the process distracted Māori from other development options, much was achieved, including the Tribunal's 1986 *Te Reo Māori Report*, which recommended that the government take an active role to protect Māori language. It resulted in far greater support for Māori language revitalisation.

The 1984 Hui Taumata (the Māori Economic Summit), held at Parliament, foreshadowed the decade of Māori development (1984–94). The key elements of Māori development were:

- positive advancement (i.e. improving the position of Māori in New Zealand society)
- increased freedom from external control and greater independence
- fair sharing of the benefits of society
- that economic development was not to be at the cost of social, cultural and ecological (e.g. the natural environment) concerns.

Between 1984 and the late 1990s, political and economic policies that increased income inequality had a major negative impact on Māori life. Benefit cuts, growing poverty and worsening employment conditions are factors that impacted to a greater extent on Māori than non-Māori. By the late 1990s the then Labour Government had recognised the need to address the major socioeconomic differences between Māori and non-Māori. The government introduced its 'Closing the Gaps' strategy to address inequalities.

2001 onwards: inequities, Whānau Ora, post-settlement, planetary health

Labour-led coalition governments embraced 'Third Way' policies (i.e. an attempt to reconcile right-wing and left-wing approaches) from 1999 to 2008, and tried to reduce inequities between Māori and non-Māori. However, wide inequalities across the board remained.

Following the 2008 general elections, a National-led centre-right coalition government was formed which included the Māori Party. Within the context of the international recession, the government moved to reduce the role of the state, including in service provision (a similar approach from 1984 through to the 1990s led to increased inequities for Māori). At the same time, however, pushed by the Māori Party, Whānau Ora found political support (Ministry of Social Development 2010). Whānau Ora is about supporting families to achieve their potential.

The Whānau Ora philosophy:

- recognises whānau as a collective entity
- endorses a group capacity for self-management and self-determination

- has a lifecourse and intergenerational dimension
- builds on a Māori cultural foundation
- asserts a positive role for whānau within society
- can be applied across a wide range of social and economic sectors.

Efforts continue to embed this philosophy across sectors, including aged care, in order to advance the wellbeing of whānau through implementation of a whānau-centred approach to core business.

A major shift in the Māori political landscape is the move to a post-settlement environment, as increasingly **iwi** reach Treaty of Waitangi settlements with the Crown. For many years iwi focus and capacity has been tied up in the settlements process. Achieving settlement enables iwi to refocus on those things at the heart of the concerns of their members and to use settlement resources for their benefit.

Perhaps what most defines the 21st century is the extent to which Māori have more opportunities to express Māori values in everyday life. In education (e.g. Māori culture and language immersion education – **kōhanga reo**, **kura kaupapa Māori**), sports (e.g. **waka ama** outrigger canoeing and other Māori dominated sports like touch rugby) and cultural events (e.g. **kapa haka** festivals), media (e.g. Māori television and radio) and accessing **kaupapa Māori** service options (e.g. kaupapa Māori health services). Despite some ongoing tensions, there is increasing acceptance within New Zealand society of the rights of Māori to live as Māori, speaking the Māori language and expressing Māori beliefs and values in everyday life.

CARING ABOUT CULTURE

- Being aware of the effects of historical, social, political, economic and cultural factors linked to health and wellbeing on the lives of older Māori helps carers to have a greater understanding and empathy when working with them. This is a foundation for developing rapport and trust, and therefore better communication and cooperation.
- An understanding of the historical context, such as how Māori have fought over many years for Māori language revitalisation, helps carers appreciate the importance of getting the basics right, like the correct pronunciation of people's names.

MĀORI IDENTITY

An understanding of Māori identity is important in being able to deliver culturally appropriate aged care. One way in which Māori identity can be understood is as a mix of personal perceptions, cultural heritage and access to Māori institutions (Durie 1995). However, Māori should not be stereotyped as they are a diverse group and people express their cultural identity in different ways.

Personal perceptions

The basis for Māori identity is **whakapapa** to Māori ancestors and self-identification as Māori. A secure Māori identity also relies on knowledge of, or access to, things Māori, and on 'living it' and expressing Māori beliefs and values through attitudes and behaviours (Durie 1995).

Cultural heritage

Cultural heritage encompasses those things that are inherited from the ancestors. That does not mean they are necessarily unchanging, but that their origins go back in time. Key elements of Māori heritage include:

- distinctly Māori beliefs and values
- links to the natural environment
- Māori process and protocols
- genealogy and other forms of Māori knowledge
- the Māori language (Durie 1995).

The range of concepts that express the beliefs and values underpinning a Māori experience of the world include:

- ***tino rangatiratanga*** – self-determination or Māori control over their own affairs
- *kaitiakitanga* – guardianship and protection of cultural resources, such as the Māori language and the natural environment, and caring for people (Edwards 2010)
- *manaakitanga* – a combination of caring, respect, hospitality and generosity. Can be applied in terms of the respect shown for Māori individuals and whānau, and for Māori cultural beliefs, values and practices
- *mana* – a form of authority, power and prestige, which can be applied to individuals and groups
- *whanaungatanga* – concerned mainly with strengthening relationships, extended family cohesion and the reinforcement of whānau obligations and commitment (Ratima et al 2001). Implies that family cohesion is of high worth and that some priority should be given to involvement with whānau
- *tapu* and *noa* – tapu refers to a special state in which restrictions are imposed, as opposed to noa, which is a state free of restrictions. For example, the head is a body part that is tapu
- *whakapapa* – the world is described in terms of genealogical connections. Individuals may identify themselves in relation to other Māori people, Māori institutions (e.g. marae, hapū and iwi), the natural environment (e.g. ancestral land) and the supernatural.

Importantly, the land and the wider environment are considered by Māori to be fundamental sources of identity. Māori personified prominent geographical features, such as lakes, rivers and mountains, and these features were then used to symbolise tribal groups.

Māori institutions

Māori institutions are Māori-controlled bodies that operate in ways consistent with Māori protocol, and include iwi, hapū, whānau and marae (Durie 1995). Customary Māori society was built on descent lines that dictated membership within a kinship-based hierarchy. The **whānau** was the basic unit of this social structure. A grouping of whānau collectively formed the **hapū**, the level at which everyday life functioned. The iwi was comprised of a number of hapū, and was the largest social and political group in customary Māori society. **Marae** are customary Māori community centres.

Some Māori are alienated from their tribal base. In the 2013 Census, 80% of Māori stated their affiliation with one or more iwi, however, 17% said they did not know their iwi (Stats NZ 2014). Nevertheless, all Māori have these connections and for many who have maintained their tribal links it is their relationship to whānau, hapū, iwi and marae that is central to their identity. These institutions provide environments where Māori heritage may be given full expression and where 'being Māori' is normalised.

MĀORI CONCEPTS OF HEALTH

Te Whare Tapa Whā is the most widely known model of Māori health (Durie 1998). The model is holistic and likens health to the four walls of a house; it proposes that good health is the balance between four interacting dimensions that are necessary to ensure the house is stable.

- *te taha wairua* – spirituality; for many kaumātua spiritual awareness is essential to wellbeing, and in particular the connection between people and the natural environment. Spirituality may be expressed in different ways, such as in relationships with the environment and enjoying being outside, formal religion, karakia, etc. Kaumātua should be supported to express their spirituality in whatever ways are important to them. A need to expand caregiver training in order to support recognition of, and respond to, the spiritual needs of those in aged care in New Zealand has been identified (Hardie 2014).
- *te taha hinengaro* – thoughts and feelings; this is the mental dimension and is about being able to communicate (verbally and non-verbally), think and feel. For support workers it may be about taking the time to talk with kaumātua about how they are feeling, having a cup of tea with them and giving them some attention and encouragement so that they feel good.
- *te taha tinana* – the physical aspects of wellbeing.
- *te taha whānau* – the importance of the link between good health of kaumātua and being connected with their whānau. Carers can help kaumātua to rebuild or maintain their connections with whānau, for example, by helping them to use technology such as Zoom.

CARING ABOUT CULTURE

- Spirituality is important to many Māori, during life and after death. Cultural processes that link the material and spiritual worlds may be profoundly important to kaumātua and their whānau, and must be respected, such as the use of karakia during important times, including when a kaumātua is dying.
- Whānau are often a vital support for kaumātua. Aged care providers need to accommodate the role whānau may wish to take in providing support and care for kaumātua, particularly if the kaumātua is dying. This will have implications for service policies, carers' cultural competence and communication. For example, policies and strategies may need to be in place to allow for large numbers of visiting whānau, for example, in regard to physical space and visiting times.

OLDER MĀORI – DEFINITION AND ROLES

Older people are generally understood in New Zealand to be those aged 65 years and over, which is the stated retirement age. While Māori make up around 15% of the New Zealand population, they account for only 6% of the population aged over 65 years. This is largely due to shorter life expectancy (around seven years less than non-Māori) and higher premature mortality compared to non-Māori.

A definition of the aged population based solely on age is biased towards those groups with a longer life expectancy, especially where age is a criteria for access to services. It would be fairer to define the aged population either as a percentage of the population (e.g. the oldest 10% of Māori) or in relation to the health and disability experience of the population (e.g. age at onset of disability). Either definition would mean that Māori would be included as part of the aged population at an earlier age. This would be appropriate given that Māori experience many of the issues associated with old age before age 65. It has been suggested that needs assessments for the aged should be available to Māori at age 55, as opposed to age 65 for the general population (New Zealand Guidelines Group 2003).

While overall the Māori population is young, Māori have an ageing population structure. By 2038, it is projected that the Māori population aged 65-plus will more than double from 48,500 to 126,000 and grow to make up 10% of those aged over 65 years.

Māori use a number of terms when speaking about older Māori people, such as kaumātua, kuia or koroua. These terms often imply a certain status as an older person, and the expectation that older people will have the experience and knowledge to fill cultural roles (Durie 1999). Generally ageing is thought of in a strength-based way as a positive part of life, as opposed to a view that focuses on dependency, vulnerability, isolation and limitations.

THE CIRCUMSTANCES OF OLDER MĀORI

Wide and longstanding inequities

Positive ageing is a lifelong process that begins early in life and continues through until the end of life. There are many factors that influence the ageing process through the life course of individuals (Edwards et al 2018). These factors can advantage or disadvantage people, and build up over people's lives, eventually leading to big differences in health and wellbeing, and ultimately in life expectancy (Health Quality and Safety Commission New Zealand 2019).

Some of these factors are historical; they have their roots in the past but continue to impact on the lives of people today. An important example is colonisation and how it continues to act through the health system and health services. The health system and most health services are designed and run by non-Māori. The system and these services provide better support for non-Māori to be healthier and live longer than for Māori (Health Quality and Safety Commission New Zealand 2019).

Research demonstrates that health services are less accessible for Māori. For example, older Māori with disabilities are more likely to have unmet needs for specialist equipment compared to non-Māori. Further, Māori receive lower quality services and treatment than non-Māori. It is known that following a hip fracture from a fall, it is important to have an operation as soon as possible. For non-Māori the percentage of those receiving an operation for their hip fracture on the same or next day of admission consistently increased over the period 2013–16, while for Māori the percentage steadily decreased. As well, there is a much higher rate of inappropriate prescribing of a combination of medicines for older Māori (Health Quality and Safety Commission New Zealand 2019). There is also evidence that work to improve health service quality does not always lead to improvements in equity for Māori (Health Quality and Safety Commission New Zealand 2019). In terms of outcomes, there are wide and longstanding differences in health between Māori and non-Māori in almost all major health conditions, including heart disease, stroke, diabetes and cancer. These differences can be seen through measuring risk factors, hospitalisation, disability and mortality. Diseases that are associated with older age are experienced earlier in Māori and there is also an earlier age of onset of disability compared to non-Māori (Health Quality and Safety Commission New Zealand 2019).

There are other factors (social, political, environmental and economic) that are outside the control of individuals, but shape their lives, the choices they are able to make and cause differences in health outcomes between Māori and non-Māori. This is most obvious in the unfair sharing of socioeconomic resources (e.g. good education, employment opportunities, secure housing, high income) within New Zealand. Māori of all ages are much more likely to live in the most deprived areas, and non-Māori are much more likely to live in the wealthiest areas (Ministry of Health 2015). Research findings indicate that older Māori experience a high level of disadvantage, poverty and material hardship; around three or four times that of non-Māori. Māori have lower incomes, levels of savings and assets and home ownership. One in seven older Māori face some financial difficulty (15 per cent compared to 10 per cent of the older population generally), and an additional one in five face severe financial difficulties (20 per cent compared to 6 per cent of the older population generally) (Ministry of Social Development 2017).

Māori also have greater exposure throughout life to negative factors like racism, which add further disadvantages (Edwards et al 2018). This helps to explain a recent finding that for New Zealanders aged 61–81 years, non-Māori receive greater health benefits from higher childhood socio-economic status and education than Māori (Stephens et al 2020).

Culture

Research indicates that Māori individuals' satisfaction with their Māori language fluency is linked to feelings of wellbeing, contentment in life and wider cultural involvement. There also appears to be a link between marae involvement and wellbeing, with low levels of involvement linked to low levels of health. LiLACS NZ, a longitudinal study of life and living in advanced age (age 80–90 years for Māori participants), found that almost all Māori participants had been to marae in the previous year (Kerse & LiLACS NZ 2014). Increasing visits to marae and other places of cultural significance were associated with better physical health-related quality of life (Dyall et al 2014). The study also found that Māori language and cultural engagement are linked to a higher quality of life, and that just over half of the 417 participants used the Māori language for everyday conversation (Dyall et al 2014).

The implication for those providing aged care is that they should respect and enable kaumātua to express their Māori identity in their everyday life. Aged care should not contribute to the racism and discrimination that many kaumātua have experienced throughout their lives.

Social connectedness

Kukutai (2006) described wellbeing of older Māori (as Māori) as the achievement of a balance between participation and achievement in te ao Māori/the Māori world (including whānau) and te ao whanui/wider society. This view of wellbeing recognises the following:

- Older Māori are living in both worlds at the same time, and the extent and quality of their involvement in the Māori world and wider society directly affects their wellbeing.
- Older Māori generally place a high value on extended family relationships and this should be taken into account.
- Relationships with whānau are two-way and, while often close, may be both rewarding and demanding. A high degree of reciprocity provides a sense of satisfaction for kaumātua and promotes intergenerational understanding. Research indicates that older Māori include reciprocity and their role in caring for others are part of what makes for a good life (Allport et al 2018; Butcher 2012).

- The types of assistance older Māori provide to whānau include cultural support and encouragement to pursue education and leadership in relation to the Māori language. In turn, whānau provide financial assistance, transport and support during illness.
- Older Māori are carriers of culture within their whānau and communities, and are leaders in Māori cultural contexts.
- The cultural strength of the Māori community and opportunities for the transfer of cultural knowledge from older to younger generations rely upon the active involvement of culturally skilled older Māori. Further, the standing of an iwi relies upon the visible presence and authority of elders (for more detail, see Edwards 2010).

CARING ABOUT CULTURE

- Taking into account the capacities of older Māori, care provided for kaumātua should support them to fulfil roles within their whānau and the wider Māori community if they wish. Those providing care should understand that the role-based expectations on older Māori and their priorities may be quite different and wider from those of non-Māori. Further, the roles and status of older Māori within Māori communities (e.g. as carriers of culture and language leaders) are often not the same as the roles and status they may hold in the wider community.
- Differences in the circumstances of kaumātua compared to non-Māori older people are mostly due to the unfair distribution of social, economic and other resources between Māori and non-Māori. For kaumātua, these differences have grown and impacted over lifetimes resulting in poorer health, more limited resources to call on in times of need and shorter lives than non-Māori. Aged care workers need to keep this wider context in mind and avoid victim blaming and racism that may further add to discrimination experienced by kaumātua.

AGED CARE PROVISION FOR MĀORI

Māori health providers

Increasingly, Māori expect that services will be clinically and culturally safe and responsive. There have been growing numbers of providers of kaupapa Māori health and other services. Kaupapa Māori health services are owned and governed by Māori and provide services mainly to Māori. They work within Māori cultural frameworks, emphasise whānau ora and focus on improving Māori health and reducing inequalities through the provision of affordable and acceptable services for Māori. However, they are part of the existing health system that does not work equally well for Māori and they are constrained by the limitations of that system. In 2015–16 there were around 280 Māori health providers, receiving just under 2% of the government's Vote Health funding (Ministry of Health 2017).

Generally there are three types of Māori providers:

- Small and specialised providers that focus on one type of health service, such as mental health.
- Comprehensive providers that deliver a mix of personal and public health services (which may include general practice, primary health care and **rongoā**.
- Integrated providers delivering a range of health and social support services.

Māori providers have a number of distinctive features (Ministry of Health 2009):

- kaupapa Māori-inspired and Māori-led
- culturally authentic and responsive
- dedicated to achieving whānau ora – supporting Māori families to achieve their maximum health and wellbeing
- committed to fostering, building and maintaining trusting relationships with service users and their whānau
- holistic in their approach to the assessment, monitoring and treatment of patients (e.g. being inclusive of whānau and taking into account the wider circumstances of kaumātua)
- using multidisciplinary teams with a mix of clinical, non-clinical and community workers
- employing Māori where possible and committed to growing the Māori health workforce
- investing in professional development opportunities for all staff, including supporting non-Māori staff to understand and practise Māori cultural values
- committed to community buy-in and involvement in the design, development and implementation of services.

Some Māori health providers also work with rongoā, the traditional Māori health system which incorporates the use of plant-based remedies, physical therapies and spiritual healing. Rongoā is practised by tohunga (specialists). Some providers are contracted to provide rongoā services, which are often used concurrently with Western medicine. Rongoā treatments that may be used by kaumātua include plant remedies, massage, prayer or incantation (bpac NZ Better Medicine 2017). The treatments may be used for a range of aspects of health, such as spiritual, psychological, emotional, cultural, social, environmental, whānau and physical dimensions. As an example, a plant commonly used in rongoā is kawakawa (Māori pepper tree). Kawakawa may be boiled and used in the treatment of boils, arthritis and as a diuretic. Developing positive and respectful relationships with kaumātua will encourage them to speak freely about their use of rongoā. It is the role of clinicians to discuss with kaumātua any potential interactions between rongoā and their other medications.

Aged care for kaumātua

Many Māori health providers hold one or more contracts to deliver services for kaumātua as part of their overall service portfolio, and as well they are able to refer kaumātua and their whānau to a range of 'mainstream' and other services. There are very limited numbers of small providers that specialise in aged care for kaumātua. The Rauawaawa Kaumātua Charitable Trust (the Trust) is one such organisation, set up in 1997 as a response to the needs identified by a group of kaumātua for culturally focused, appropriate and accessible health, social and community-based activities and services (Rauawaawa Charitable Trust 2017). Based in Hamilton, New Zealand, the service provides whānau-oriented programs, activities and services aimed at enhancing the quality of life for kaumātua. The service is kaumātua-led and governed. Rauawaawa provides health, social and educational services for those aged 55 years and over, including health clinics and advocacy for registered nurses, **mirimiri**, transport, and social service support and advocacy with government agencies. The Trust is involved in running community classes (e.g. computing, performing arts, waiata and **whaikōrero**, healthy cooking, Māori language, Māori crafts such as making **korowai**), socialisation days and events (e.g. Kaumātua Olympics, Kaumātua Triathlon). Over 600 kaumātua are registered with the organisation.

While many Māori health providers include a focus on kaumātua support, and some Māori providers specialise in this area, most older Māori will receive aged care through 'mainstream' provision. Quality aged care for kaumātua therefore relies on the **cultural competence** of the range of service providers and support workers.

Cultural safety and cultural competence

Cultural safety in aged care for Māori is about providing effective care when working with kaumātua and their whānau. It involves the carer working through a process of reflecting on their own identity and recognising how their own personal culture influences how they provide care. The effectiveness of care is judged by the kaumātua and their whānau.

While cultural safety is mostly about the experiences of kaumātua and their whānau, cultural competence is about the ability of aged care workers to improve the health and wellbeing of kaumātua by incorporating Māori culture into the aged care setting. Cultural competence involves:

- recognising your own values and how they influence the way you provide care
- awareness that Māori are not all the same and that Māori have a unique place in New Zealand as Treaty partners and Indigenous peoples
- working respectfully and effectively with people from different cultural backgrounds to your own
- working to reduce unfair differences in health
- having the knowledge, attitudes and skills to meet cultural competencies identified by relevant authorities; and showing in the way you provide care that you are able to meet those agreed standards.

Māori culture and ways of doing things should be respected and seen as normal in aged care settings such as homes and rest homes. This involves, for example, respecting the use of **karakia** and **waiata** by kaumātua and their whānau or the wishes of whānau to be involved in providing care for dying kaumātua. Cultural preferences must be respected in the everyday things that carers do. For example, the head is tapu and therefore pillows used for the head should not be used interchangeably with those used for other body parts like the feet.

It is very important when working with kaumātua to develop a positive, meaningful and productive relationship. Based on the experience of the Rauawaawa Kaumātua Charitable Trust Team, key actions are listed below that make it easier for kaumātua and support workers to develop positive relationships.

- *Easy identification* – If you are working in the community there will always be an initial visit when you and the kaumātua first meet. Easy identification is important. If you are going into their home, wearing a uniform will help them to identify who you are and what group you work with. Wearing name badges or carrying business cards that identify your name and organisation also help. These types of measures are especially worthwhile if the person lives alone or has dementia.
- *Showing respect* – From the moment you walk in the door of a home you can show your respect for the cultural values of kaumātua by removing your shoes. A kaumātua may say don't worry, come in with them on. The key is you have shown respect for them, their home and their culture. If you are not Māori it shows them that you have bothered to learn about their culture and are aware of what to do. It is equally important to understand what you must never do (e.g. sit on the table, use their face cloth on their feet etc.), so you avoid disrespecting their culture and maintain respect in the relationship. When you show cultural respect, you lay the groundwork for a positive relationship with kaumātua.
- *Introductions* – For kaumātua and support workers the first meeting will often set the scene for the relationship, so making ample time for introductions on both sides is important for developing a positive relationship. If the person has a Māori name, ask them or their whānau how to pronounce it to help you get it right, and if you have difficulty check with them if it is okay for them to help you to keep working on your pronunciation to get it right. Share information about yourself, your family and extended family and where you are from, and show interest when they talk not only about themselves, but about their whānau and where they are from. This form of introduction is normal among Māori when meeting for the first time.
- *Showing you care* – There are many ways in your everyday work with kaumātua to show them that you care and that they are valued and not a burden: being really present; talking with them and actively listening; showing interest in them and their whānau and where they are from; not being on your phone or other devices all the time; walking beside them and not way ahead or behind; ensuring they feel safe at all times. For example, a blind kuia should be seated securely if the support worker needs to go to another room or park a car.
- *Help them remember* – Reinforce messages and keep them consistent. If they have appointments, set up a reminder system so they can feel on top of things. If you are visiting them in their home, a reminder call the day

before or in the morning can help them to be ready for you on time and thereby feel more in control. If possible, keep the schedule for activities much the same so it is easier for them to remember. For example, Friday mornings at 9 a.m. is pick-up time.

- *Empower them to lead their healthcare* – Ask them how they want to be supported, who they want involved (e.g. their whānau or experts in Māori cultural practices), when they want things done, what activities they may want to take part in (e.g. Māori community events) and enable them to lead their own care pathway. It is easy to explain what things may have to be done differently if their wishes cannot be met, but not asking and assuming you know what is best for them is inexcusable.

KEY ISSUES IN THE PROVISION OF AGED CARE FOR KAUMĀTUA MĀORI

Kaumātua and their whānau share many of the concerns of other New Zealanders with regard to aged care. However, there are issues specific to Māori (e.g. Māori cultural factors in assessment and processes of care), which are made worse because of inequities or unfair differences between Māori and non-Māori health and in other areas. The accessibility of care is a key issue for kaumātua; in particular:

- cultural barriers (e.g. institutional racism, the cultural competence of services and carers and a lack of understanding of the cultural needs of kaumātua and their whānau)
- financial barriers (e.g. material wellbeing and cost for high standards of supported housing and other care)
- physical barriers (e.g. cost of transport and physical distance to services).

In-depth workforce training and education to support the development and strengthening of cultural competence and **health literacy** skills (e.g. communication) among those providing residential and home-based support is important, including for new immigrants working in aged care. This is particularly the case for those providing palliative care. Carers should take every opportunity to learn about the cultural beliefs, values and practices of kaumātua, so that they can provide the best possible care. There will also be courses that may not be specifically about Māori or kaumātua, but will be relevant. For example, Hospice New Zealand runs the Fundamentals of Palliative Care education programme at a very low cost to participants, targeting support workers and others. Palliative care takes a holistic approach, consistent with Māori understandings, and the program includes an education session on spiritual care and discusses Māori concepts of health.

There are many gaps in service provision for kaumātua. This includes the need for affordable community-based kaumātua housing that is village-style (such as **papakāinga** housing at marae), warm and secure, and designed to support those with mobility issues and maintain links with community (including locations close to facilities and centres of Māori community activity such as kōhanga reo and kura kaupapa). Further measures to reduce isolation, exclusion and loneliness and to enhance positive engagement could include actively promoting and normalising the involvement of whānau in services (especially at important appointments) and kaumātua-focused comprehensive services. One provider may be the access point to comprehensive services, which may include health, welfare, housing, recreation and lifelong learning initiatives (e.g. in **karanga**, whaikōrero, **raranga**, korowai, and so on). Care for kaumātua can also be facilitated through the use of information technology systems and streamlined referral, assessment and exit processes. This would better enable information sharing and safe transitions and care of kaumātua within the primary, secondary and tertiary health care sectors, as well as across sectors.

Overall, a key message in this chapter is that it is necessary for carers to meet both the basic cultural expectations of kaumātua and the general care standards in their daily work in order to provide high-quality care for kaumātua. Carers who are committed to the highest possible standards of quality care for all people will commit to ensuring they develop their cultural competencies.

CARING ABOUT CULTURE

- Like other groups, Māori are diverse, so it is important not to stereotype or make generalisations about the cultural preferences of individual kaumātua and their whānau.
- Carers must meet basic cultural expectations in order to best ensure cooperation, avoid insult and for the comfort of the kaumātua and their whānau. Key Māori concepts should inform how care is provided. Examples of how the concepts of tapu and whakawhanaungatanga may guide care are given below.

Tapu (prohibited, sacred or restricted)

- Food trays and urinals should be placed on appropriate surfaces. For example, food is not to be placed on chairs, which are for the body, but on tables, and urinals should not be placed on eating surfaces such as tables.
- Carers should ask permission to touch areas of the body considered tapu (such as the head), and explain what is to be done and why.
- The body is to be cleaned with appropriate materials. For example, cloths that are used to clean the face and head should not be used on other parts of the body.
- Māori may request the return of an amputated limb for cultural processes and burial.

Whakawhanaungatanga (strengthening relationships)

- All of those providing care to a kaumātua and whānau, including those observing, should take the time to introduce themselves at the first point of contact.
- Carers should talk with, rather than about, patients.
- Carers should take time to establish relationships.
- Carers should show an interest in individual patients and their whānau.

QUALITY OF LIFE

The cultural competence of carers is critical to the provision of quality care for kaumātua. Quality care for kaumātua is not only about physical, emotional and psychological needs; it is also about ensuring that care does not compromise the cultural and spiritual wellbeing of older Māori. Ideally, care for kaumātua should reinforce or enhance cultural and spiritual wellbeing. In order to promote the quality of life of kaumātua, those providing care need to be given opportunities to build cultural competence through appropriate training and education. Most importantly, cultural competence learnings should be integrated into daily practice in areas such as communication with kaumātua and whānau (i.e. supporting health literacy), routine processes of care and during more demanding situations (such as care of a dying person). Importantly, culturally competent care should be supported by aged care facilities that demonstrate cultural responsiveness to Māori in organisational structures, policies, guidelines and expectations.

CASE STUDY

The manager of the aged care facility in which you work has received a written complaint about the cultural competence of medical staff and other carers from family members of a resident, Tane, a Māori man aged 75, who passed away at the facility earlier in the year. Tane had many health problems, unexplained weight loss and loss of appetite, and he and his whānau had made the decision he was not for investigation or resuscitation. The manager wants to discuss the case with you as you were one of Tane's carers and there are several other Māori men and women currently in the facility. The letter raises the following concerns:

1. Although Tane lived in the facility for 2 years, and despite the issue being raised with individual staff members over that time, staff still mispronounced his name.
2. His whānau were unhappy that the cloths used to clean the face and head were the same cloths used on other parts of the body (i.e. only one type of flannel is used in the facility) and pillows were used for the head and for other parts of the body (such as for raising the feet).
3. Some of the ways in which Tane was treated were inappropriate, particularly given his status within the Māori community as a renowned leader of hapū and iwi affairs. The letter gave an example of a well-intentioned young nurse saying to him, 'What are we going to do with you today, honey?' and patting him on the head.
4. When Tane was dying some staff objected to the number of whānau visiting. They did not want whānau to be involved in his personal care and were resistant to the use of rongoā. His whānau were told that karakia and waiata disturbed others and the tohunga who had supported Tane and the whānau was treated dismissively.
5. Whānau said that they were not fully aware of the palliative care options for Tane and did not understand the palliative care that was provided to him.

Identify the problem in each of the examples. What should be done to fix each problem? How will you approach the other Māori men and women you provide care for in the future?

Model answers

1. Ongoing mispronunciation of Tane's name is disrespectful. Those providing care should receive cultural competence training that includes emphasis on the importance of correct Māori language pronunciation, particularly of people's names. All personnel in New Zealand should be required to participate in basic Māori language pronunciation training and there should also be support for wider Māori language learning for those staff who have an interest. Those in Australia should also have access to support to help them pronounce Māori names correctly. Simple resources should be made available as a reminder to guide Māori language pronunciation, such as a cultural competence wall flip chart that includes a page on Māori pronunciation.

   By taking part in basic Māori language pronunciation training I will learn how to correctly pronounce Māori names. On first meeting a kaumātua I will provide care for, if they have a Māori name I will check with them and/or their whānau that my pronunciation of their name is correct. If available, I will also refer to a wall flip chart and check with the kaumātua and their whānau from time to time to make sure that I continue to pronounce names correctly.
2. Carers were not respecting Māori beliefs and values relating to tapu (sacredness and restriction). Routine cultural competence training for staff should include processes of care that are appropriate for Māori and meet basic cultural expectations. This should be supported by practical measures within the aged care facility. For example, white cloths may be used for cleaning the face (the head is tapu), and blue cloths for other body parts (which are not tapu). Similarly, pillows within the facility may be blue or white, with matching pillow cases. White pillows are used for the head only, while blue pillows are used with other body parts (e.g. raising the feet). The placement of urinals as containers for body excrement on food surfaces is also culturally inappropriate. Small flip

charts that support cultural competence learnings may be hung in areas such as nursing stations to provide quick reminders.

When I work with other Māori men and women I will ensure that the same cloths and pillows are not used for the head and other parts of the body. I will also avoid placing urinals on tables or other food surfaces. If available, I will refer to cultural competence flip charts as a reminder of the practical things I can do to provide culturally appropriate care.

3 A young person patting a respected elder on the head is disrespectful, and because the head is tapu it should not be touched in this way. Cultural competence training is required for staff. Cultural competence training includes learning about the historical, social, economic, cultural, political and environmental factors that influence Māori health, so that staff are able to contextualise the way they interact with kaumātua. For example, by understanding the impacts of colonisation on Māori society, staff may better appreciate the high value that Māori communities place on culturally skilled kaumātua as carriers of cultural knowledge and the respect that young people are expected to demonstrate with elders. Further, training should also include understandings of Māori beliefs and values, such as the concept of tapu and its implications for practice.

In approaching other kaumātua for whom I am providing care I will be aware of the need to respect elders and ensure that my actions are not condescending, and that the head is tapu and should only be touched as necessary and with agreement from the kaumātua.

4 Staff were resistant to the integration of culture into Tane's palliative care. That is, the involvement of whānau and tohunga and the use of rongoā (including karakia and waiata). Cultural competence training related to working with whānau to facilitate their involvement in care, beliefs and values regarding care for the dying (e.g. the importance of karakia and waiata and the roles of whānau at that time) should support staff to provide quality palliative care for kaumātua. This will also rely on support from the aged care facility, such as ready access for staff to cultural advisers (e.g. formal kaumātua support positions so cultural experts are in place), physical space available to accommodate whānau visitors, and policies that provide clear guidance for staff with regard to issues such as supporting the use of rongoā and the role of tohunga.

My approach to providing care for dying kaumātua will be to support whānau involvement in personal care and be accepting of the use of rongoā, given that any discussions about the use of rongoā alongside other treatments will be carried out with appropriate clinicians. As well, I will be respectful of tohunga as specialists in rongoā who have been asked by kaumātua and whānau to provide support.

5 There was a lack of clear communication by those providing care to kaumātua with the whānau. Cultural competence training should include health literacy and the important role of health professionals and others involved in care in the two-way communication process with whānau.

When I am providing care to dying kaumātua as appropriate I will explain in plain language what I am doing and why, and invite them to ask me any questions.

REVIEW QUESTIONS

Circle T if the statement is true or F if the statement if false:

1 T / F Since colonisation, and including modern times, Māori have experienced marginalisation, dispossession and discrimination.

2 T / F The Treaty of Waitangi is a constitutional document in New Zealand (i.e. is part of New Zealand's Constitution).

3 T / F An implication of the Whānau Ora policy for aged care is that aged care facilities and carers will recognise that interactions with whānau are important for the wellbeing of kaumātua and enable whānau involvement in care.

4 T / F There are wide and unfair differences in the health and material circumstances of older Māori and older non-Māori that are shaped by systems and structures in New Zealand society.

5 T / F The current definition of the aged population (65 years and over) is biased towards those populations with a long life expectancy, particularly where the definition is used as a criterion for access to resources (e.g. superannuation payments).

6 T / F All older Māori people share the same or very similar cultural beliefs and values, and therefore want to be cared for in the same way.

7 T / F Culturally competent care enhances communication, cooperation and understanding between carers and kaumātua and their whānau.

8 T / F Māori and non-Māori have similar life expectancies as a result of the fair distribution of resources within society, such as access to education, warm and dry housing and quality health services.

9 T / F Carers who are committed to quality care for all people will commit to developing their cultural competencies.

10 T / F Much more could be done within the aged care sector generally, and by aged care facilities and carers to strengthen the sector's cultural competence in providing services for kaumātua and their whānau.

Answers to these questions are on p. 454.

Further reading

Bycroft C, Reid G, McNally J et al (2016). Identifying Māori populations using administrative data: A comparison with the census. Online 9 March 2021. Available: www.stats.govt.nz/assets/Research/Identifying-Maori-populations-using-administrative-data-A-comparison-with-the-census/Identifying-Maori-populations-using-administrative-data-a-comparison-with-the-census.pdf

Ministry of Health (2011). Tatau kura tangata: Health of older Māori chart book 2011. Ministry of Health, Wellington.

References

Allport T, Martin G & White H (2018). Kaumātuatanga: The needs and wellbeing of older Māori. Te Whānau o Waipareira Trust, Auckland.

Belich J (1986). The New Zealand wars. Auckland University Press, Auckland.

bpac NZ Better Medicine (2017). Demystifying Rongoā Māori: Traditional Māori healing. Online 8 March 2021. Available: www.bpac.org.nz/BPJ/2008/May/rongoa.aspx

Butcher E (2012). This is my ideal life: The importance of place for how Māori elders understand a good life. Masters thesis, Psychology. Massey University, Palmerston North. Online 9 March 2021. Available: https://mro.massey.ac.nz/handle/10179/3937

Daes E (1996). Working paper on the concept of 'indigenous people': United Nations Sub-commission on Prevention of Discrimination and Protection of Minorities. Working Group on Indigenous Populations. United Nations, Geneva.

Durie M (1999). Whānau development and Māori survival: The challenge of time te uru mai o te motu, the 1999 Millennium Lecture. Massey University, Palmerston North.

Durie M (1998). Whaiora: Māori health development. 2nd edn. Oxford University Press, Melbourne.

Durie M (1995). Nga matatini Māori: Diverse Maori realities. A paper prepared for the Ministry of Health. Massey University, Palmerston North.

Dyall L, Kepa M, Teh R et al (2014). Cultural and social factors and quality of life of Māori in advanced age. Te puawaitanga o nga tapuwae kia ora tonu – Life and living in advanced age: a cohort study in New Zealand (LiLACS NZ). New Zealand Medical Journal, 127(1393):62–79. Online. 4 March 2021. Available: http://europepmc.org/abstract/med/24816957

Edwards W (2010). Taupaenui: Māori positive ageing. PhD thesis, Public Health. Massey University, Palmerston North. Online 4 March 2021. Available: mro.massey.ac.nz/handle/10179/1331

Edwards W, Theodore R, Ratima M et al (2018). Māori positive ageing. New Zealand Medical Journal, 131(1484):10–12. Online 2 March 2021. Available: www.nzma.org.nz/journal-articles/maori-positive-ageing

Hardie J (2014). Hear to care: the role of caregivers in the spiritual care of residents in New Zealand Rest Homes. Unpublished masters thesis, Arts. Victoria University of Wellington, Wellington. Online 9 March 2021. Available: http://researcharchive.vuw.ac.nz/xmlui/handle/10063/3269

Health Quality & Safety Commission (2019). He matapihi ki te kounga o ngā manaakitanga ā-hauora o Aotearoa 2019. A window on the quality of Aotearoa New Zealand's health care 2019. Health Quality & Safety Commission, Wellington. Online 9 March 2021. Available: www.hqsc.govt.nz/assets/Health-Quality-Evaluation/PR/Window_2019_web_final.pdf

Kerse N & LiLACS NZ (2014). Participation in Māori society in advanced age: Findings from LiLACS NZ. Auckland. School of Population Health, The University of Auckland.

Kukutai T (2006). Elder or merely older? Enhancing wellbeing of older Māori in an ageing Māori population. Population Studies Centre, University of Waikato, Hamilton.

Kunitz S (ed.) (1994). Disease and social diversity. Oxford University Press, New York.

Ministry of Health (2017). Annual Report for the year ended 30 June 2017 – Ministry of Health. Ministry of Health, Wellington.

Ministry of Health (2015). Neighbourhood deprivation. Online 9 March 2021. Available: www.health.govt.nz/our-work/populations/maori-health/tatau-kahukura-maori-health-statistics/nga-awe-o-te-hauora-socioeconomic-determinants-health/neighbourhood-deprivation

Ministry of Health (2009). Te toi hauora-nui: Achieving excellence through innovative Māori health service delivery. Ministry of Health, Hamilton.

Ministry of Social Development (2017). Living standards research. Online 4 March 2021. Available: www.msd.govt.nz/about-msd-and-our-work/publications-resources/monitoring/living-standards/index.html

Ministry of Social Development (2010). Whānau-centred initiatives. Whānau Ora: Report of the Taskforce on Whānau-centred Initiatives. Wellington.

New Zealand Guidelines Group (2003). Assessment of older Māori. New Zealand Guidelines Group. Ministry of Health, Wellington.

Palmer M (2008). The Treaty of Waitangi in New Zealand's law and constitution. Victoria University Press, Wellington.

Pool I (1991). Te iwi Māori: A New Zealand population past, present & projected. Auckland University Press, Auckland.

Ratima M (2001). Kia uruuru mai a hauora being healthy, being Maori: Conceptualising Maori health promotion. Unpublished doctoral thesis. Department of Public Health. University of Otago: Dunedin.

Rauawaawa Kaumātua Charitable Trust (2017). Online 2 March 2021. Available: www.rauawaawa.co.nz/

Royal Commission on Social Policy (1988). The April Report: Report of the Royal Commission on Social Policy. Royal Commission on Social Policy, Wellington.

Stephens C, Szabo A & Breheny M (2020). Life course socioeconomic predictors of healthy ageing in Aotearoa/New Zealand: Differences by Māori ethnicity and gender. Ageing & Society. Online 9 March 2021. Available: https://doi.org/10.1017/S0144686X20001130

Stats NZ (2021). Maori population estimates: Mean year ended 31 December 2020. Online 3 September 2021. Available: https://www.stats.govt.nz/topics/population.

Stats NZ (2014). 2013 Census iwi grouping profiles. Online 7 September 2021. Available: www.stats.govt.nz/reports/2013-census-iwi-grouping-profiles

Walker R (2001). He tipua: The life and times of Sir Apirana Ngata. Penguin Books, Auckland.

Walker R (1990). Ka whawhai tonu matou: Struggle without end. Penguin Books, Auckland.

CHAPTER 8
Working with older people from diverse cultural backgrounds

By Margaret Webb

AFTER READING THIS CHAPTER, YOU SHOULD BE ABLE TO:

- define the key terms listed in this chapter
- briefly describe the history of multicultural migration into Australia and New Zealand
- demonstrate a basic understanding of government migration policy
- identify factors that contribute to an individual's cultural make-up
- demonstrate a basic understanding of some non-Christian religions
- identify some of the factors required to give culturally sensitive care
- explain how culture and religion influence health and illness
- identify services available to support the older client
- know how to promote quality of life.

Key terms

biculturalism: The existence of two distinct cultural groups within the one nation

Buddhism: A religion and philosophy founded in India by Siddhartha Gautama, called the Buddha

CALD: Culturally and linguistically diverse

colloquial language: Informal language that should not be used in formal situations

cultural awareness: A basic understanding of the differences between cultures

cultural safety: Safe care provided to those of all cultures as defined by the recipients of that care

cultural sensitivity: An understanding of your own cultural values and perceptions and how these have shaped your opinions of other cultures

culture: The characteristics of a group of people – language, values, beliefs, habits, likes, dislikes

customs: Traditions passed from one generation to the next

ethnicity: A sense of peoplehood or nationhood in which a person or group's ethnic background is reflected in their identity, history, language, nationality and religion

Islam: A monotheistic religion that originated with the teachings of the prophet Muhammad, having the same roots as Christianity and Judaism; its revelatory scripture is the Koran (Qur'an); its followers are called Muslims

lexical gap: The absence of a word form in a particular language

multiculturalism: The acceptance of multiple ethnic cultures into one nation

race: Group of persons belonging to the same genetic group

religion: Spiritual beliefs, needs and practices

You would have heard and read frequently that Australia is referred to as a multicultural country and that New Zealand is a rapidly emerging multicultural society. Multiculturalism basically means many different racial groups with their own cultures living in the one nation. Both the Australian and the New Zealand populations include many people from different cultures and ethnic backgrounds, including Indigenous and migrant cultures, besides those of European origins. All these cultures engage with the world differently.

The current Australian population derives from more than 100 different country origins. According to Australian Bureau of Statistics (ABS) (ABS 2021) estimates, 29.8% of all Australians were born overseas as of 30 June 2020. The largest number of migrants come from England (3.8 per cent), followed by India (2.8 per cent), followed by China (2.5 per cent), New Zealand (2.2 per cent), and then the Philippines (1.2 per cent) and Vietnam (1.1 per cent) (ABS 2021). No other country accounts for more than 1 per cent of the Australian population. Western Australia had the highest number of overseas-born population in 2016 with 35% born overseas (ABS 2021).

The 2018 NZ census identified that 27% of New Zealand's population of 5 million were born overseas (Stats NZ Tatauranga Aotearoa 2020). Approximately 10 per cent of the New Zealand population identify with an ethnic minority other than Māori or Pacific Islander peoples.

HISTORY OF MULTICULTURALISM IN AUSTRALIA

The original people in Australia are the Aboriginal and Torres Strait Islander peoples. Following the introduction of British colonisation in the 18th century, mostly European settlers travelled to Australia to settle. While many of the early settlers were convicts transported from the United Kingdom to live out their sentences, many free people also came to Australia to find a better life for their family, many establishing farms and working on the land.

For many years Australia was seen as an English-speaking, British-based nation. However, this began to change as economic and other conditions changed within Australia and overseas. When gold was found in Australia in the 1800s, people from other countries started to come to Australia to work within the goldfields and associated industries. A considerable number of these were Chinese. In the 1880s, Australian plantation owners encouraged the recruitment of labourers from Melanesia to work on their plantations and, during the second half of the 19th century, Afghani, Pakistani and Turkish camel handlers played an important role in allowing people to travel throughout Australia, by assisting with the construction of telegraph and railway lines.

Australia was also beginning to be seen as a prospective home for migrants who needed to escape from harsh or difficult conditions within their homelands. In the 1840s, many Irish migrants arrived to escape the Irish famine. Following the end of World War II, there was an increase in people migrating from Europe. This resulted from agreements made with the United Kingdom, some European countries and the International Refugee Organisation, to encourage migrants, including displaced persons from post-war Europe, to come to Australia. By 1950, almost 200,000 people had arrived.

Migration policy

Australians have many different views about the benefits and drawbacks of having a culturally diverse population. In 1901, the government of the time (supported by the Opposition) introduced the *Immigration Restriction Act 1901*. This became the basis of the White Australia Policy and effectively limited the migration of non-white migrants into Australia. Although we now view this as a racist policy, at the time it was believed that Australia wanted to remain a country of white people who lived by British customs. Trade unions were also keen to prevent labour competition from Chinese and Pacific Islander migrants, whom they feared would undercut wages. However, this policy has since been amended by the introduction of the *Migration Act 1958* (which regulates the entry into Australia of non-citizens). Although in 1986 further amendments were introduced allowing an increase in selected non-European migration, it was not until 1993 that all racial qualifications for immigration were removed from government policy.

In the 1990s Asian peoples were the fastest growing group of migrants to Australia. An average of 8500 people from Asia have settled in Australia each year. At 30 June 2020, 29.8% of Australian consumers were born overseas (7.5 million persons) (ABS 2021).

Today's migration

According to the Australian Government's Department of Home Affairs, Australia's Migration program has four primary programs: Skill Stream, Family Stream, Special Eligibility migrants and Child.

The planning level for the 2020–21 Migration Program was set at 160,000 places (Department of Home Affairs 2021) in 2020. Of these places, 79,600 places for the Skills stream, 77,300 for the Family stream, 100 for Special Eligibility and 3000 for child.

- The Skills Stream component is mainly aimed at those persons who are able to provide skilled labour and who wish to live permanently in Australia.
- The Family Stream is predominantly made up of Partner visas, enabling Australians to reunite with family members from overseas and provide them with pathways to citizenship.
- The Special Eligibility stream is for those who have close ties with Australia, have distinguished talent or are

former consumers wishing to return to Australia. The numbers of migrants entering Australia on this stream are minimal.

Australia also has a Humanitarian program – for refugees and others in humanitarian need. The Humanitarian program provides permanent visas for refugees and others in humanitarian need. This is split into two components: offshore and onshore. The number of places allocated varies and has remained at around 12,000–13,750. Although in 2012–13 the numbers rose to nearly 20,000, in 2018–19 the quota was set at 18,750 places (Refugee Council of Australia 2021) (see Box 8.1).

In March 2020 it was estimated that there were 2,172,648 temporary visa holders in Australia. A temporary entry visa allows people to enter Australia to undertake specific work or business, or to entertain, play sport, have a working holiday or study (Parliament of Australia 2020).

BOX 8.1
The current asylum seeker debate

You will often find references to asylum seekers in the media, especially in relation to those who arrive by boats. Asylum seekers are people who are seeking a safe place where they can find protection until they are able to return safely to their countries of origin, to their own homes. The United Nations High Commissioner for Refugees (UNHCR) estimates that there were 65.6 million forcibly displaced people worldwide in 2017. Of these, 22.5 million were refugees. Australia, as part of the international community, shares some responsibility for protecting these refugees, and asylum seekers.

Asylum seekers are not illegal immigrants as long as they declare their asylum seeker status on arrival and make a claim for refugee status. Once this claim has been lodged it will be processed and either proven or disallowed. This process is set by international guidelines and Australia follows these to decide who should be considered a refugee and who should not.

In recent years, a considerable number of refugees have sought entry into Australia from a number of countries: Somalia, Sri Lanka, Iran and Iraq, Afghanistan and other Middle Eastern areas. Asylum seekers often undertake very difficult and perilous journeys to reach Australia to seek asylum, often at great personal cost to themselves and their families.

However, this is a highly controversial topic and some people have very strong opinions in relation to this issue. As you may be caring for somebody who identifies with some of the asylum seeker nationalities or has strong views linked to this issue, it is best not to express your personal viewpoints.

Source: Refugee Council of Australia (2017). Australia's Refugee and Humanitarian Program 2017–18.

HISTORY OF MULTICULTURALISM IN NEW ZEALAND

Approximately 1000 years ago the Māori people arrived and established their communities in New Zealand. This was followed by the arrival and settlement of European settlers in the first half of the 19th century. Although many were from Ireland and England, there were also large numbers of French and especially Dutch settlers in the 1950s. Following the discovery of gold in the 1880s, a considerable number of Chinese came to New Zealand to take part in the Otago Gold Rush. In the 1980s a new wave of migration developed with the arrival of people from the Pacific Islands, with approximately half of the Pacific Island migrants identifying themselves as coming from Samoa. Since then, there has been an increasing number of migrants from countries such as Thailand, China and India (Box 8.2).

In the 2001 Census, 10 per cent of the New Zealand population identified with a minority ethnic group other than Māori or the Pacific Islands. In the 2018 Census, this number had increased, with 27.4 per cent of New Zealanders being born overseas. While there has been a slight decrease in consumers born in Europe, there have been significant increases in people born in Africa, the Middle East and Asia.

CULTURE, RACE AND ETHNICITY

Culture, race and ethnicity are often seen as the same thing, but they are not. They have quite different meanings.

Culture

Culture is the characteristics of a group of people – their language, values, beliefs, habits, likes, dislikes and **customs**. These characteristics are passed on from one generation to the next. The person's culture influences their health beliefs and practices. Not everyone knows everything about their own culture. Culture also influences the person's behaviour during illness and in residential care services.

For example, in Australia and New Zealand we believe that we have a cultural norm of 'fair go' and mateship, whereby we see it as a common value that we help each other when needed and that we stand by our mates when they need our help. Australia also has a culture that embraces backyard traditions. Owning a barbecue and playing

BOX 8.2
A bicultural nation

Biculturalism is the existence of two distinct cultural groups within the one nation. New Zealand has worked hard to develop itself as a bicultural nation, and both the Māori culture and predominant European culture are accepted as cultural norms in New Zealand. As such, the concept of multiculturalism in relation to migrants does not apply to the Māori culture.

ball games in the backyard of our homes is very much part of Australian culture.

People come from many cultures, races and nationalities. Their family practices and food choices may differ from yours, as may their hygiene habits and clothing styles. Some speak a foreign language. Some cultures have beliefs about what causes and cures illness. Many have beliefs and rituals about death and dying.

Race

Race is a term that is applied only to the genetic group that a person belongs to. It does not include the way we think or act or even speak. It is used only to identify who we are based on the way we look and from our genetic heritage. There is no such thing as a person belonging to the Australian or New Zealand race. A person living in Melbourne could identify with being Australian culturally but also as being from the Polynesian race.

Ethnicity

Ethnicity is a sense of belonging and identity. Identity is not limited to only sharing the same characteristics, such as country of origin, language, religion, ancestry and culture, but also realising that one's thoughts, perceptions, feelings and behaviours are consistent with those of other members of the ethnic group. For example, groups throughout the world who practise **Islam** identify with each other, although they come from an extreme range of cultural and racial groups.

CULTURAL AWARENESS AND CULTURAL SENSITIVITY

We all have personal values and perceptions based on our own cultural backgrounds. In order to be able to give culturally appropriate care (i.e. care that is appropriate within the culture of your client), you need to have **cultural awareness**. This involves having **cultural sensitivity** – an understanding of what your own cultural values and perceptions are and how you have shaped your opinions of other cultures. It is also essential for you to recognise or be sensitive to the fact that everyone has a cultural identity and that your clients' cultural beliefs and values may be quite different from your own. It is important not to stereotype your client by commonly held beliefs about their culture. Not all that you may have heard or believe about specific cultures may be true. Likewise, not all people within the same culture hold exactly the same beliefs or have the same behaviours. For example, it is a widely held belief that the Australian culture includes a love of the beach. However, we know that while many Australians do love the beach, there is a considerable number of them who do not go to the beach and prefer to undertake other outdoor activities. Therefore, to presume that all Australians want to go to the beach would be wrong.

Your client has the right to be given culturally safe care. **Cultural safety** is care that respects and safeguards the specific cultural needs of clients. To be able to provide cultural safety, you need to understand that culture is a major aspect of most people's lives and that, as a carer, you are obliged to assist your client in a way that is culturally appropriate for them. If you are asked to attend to the needs of a client and you feel that you would not be able to give them culturally appropriate care, you need to ask to be relieved of caring for that client. For example, it would be culturally highly inappropriate for a male carer to attend to the hygiene needs of an older Muslim woman. Her cultural safety would be severely compromised.

Cultural safety and the carer

Although this chapter discusses caring for the client in a culturally appropriate manner, consideration must also be given to the cultural safety of the carer. If you are asked to care for a client and undertake any activities that you believe will compromise your cultural safety, you have a right to refuse to undertake them. For example, an Aboriginal woman carer should not be asked to shower an elderly Aboriginal male as it would place her cultural values at risk. A Muslim or Jewish carer should not be expected to prepare or handle food containing pork products.

Attitudes to ageing

Attitudes to ageing vary across cultures. Many migrant groups also have views and practices that may differ from your own. In some cultures, a person who is older will be given more respect and status, whereas in other cultures youth is revered and old age is seen as merely the end-stage of life. For example, the North American culture places a very high value on youth. In contrast, Chinese culture is very respectful of seniors. They are valued for their knowledge and experience. They believe that age brings wisdom. When you provide care for somebody who comes from a different ethnic group to yours, ensure that you are aware of their specific cultural attitudes. For example, an older Asian man may be offended if you are too casual in your approach to him.

Addressing the older person

Always check with your client about how they wish to be addressed. In some cultures, such as Indian, older people are never addressed by their first names. Their first names are always followed by the term 'aunty' or 'uncle', whether they are related to you or not. For example, a man named Aashish Singh would be addressed as 'Aashish Uncle'. It is also expected that some people who have had positions of authority in their working life are still addressed as Sir or Ma'am. Always ask your client what they wish to be called. If you are doubtful at all, ask their relatives or check with your supervisor.

CARING ABOUT CULTURE

Cultural safety is a concept that extends beyond cultural awareness and sensitivity. Cultural safety means that the person's values, attitudes and beliefs are supported by the organisational culture and structure. Unsafe cultural practices are made up of any actions that diminish or disempower the wellbeing of an individual (see Box 8.3).

Some Indigenous Australians find residential care very distressing. When removed from their family and friends, they can experience a profound sense of isolation and loneliness. Many older Indigenous Australians have experienced family separation due to previous government policies and practices. This has left a legacy of fear towards health services and services.

Muslims believe that pain and suffering are a way of life and may be a way of atoning for sins, but are encouraged to seek treatment and care. Illness may be viewed not as an enemy to be overcome, but as an opportunity to cleanse, purify and obtain balance or forgiveness (Islamic Council of Victoria 2021).

Touching

Some cultures have rules about touching and you need to be aware of these before attending to care (Fig. 8.1). As noted above, it is inappropriate for an Aboriginal female carer to attend to the personal care of a male Aboriginal elder. So, too, many Asian and Middle Eastern cultural groups expressly disapprove of men touching women and women touching men. This may even include simple handshakes. Although hugging members of the opposite sex is not appropriate, often members of the same sex will embrace or shake hands. In Indian culture, deliberately touching somebody from the opposite sex, even in a friendly gesture, will often make them feel uncomfortable.

BOX 8.3
Making decisions

As carers, we always ensure that our client is part of the decision-making processes in determining care. We consult with them and their families and they are always seen as essential for any decision making. However, in some cultures, the role of the healthcare provider is seen as the 'expert' and the client is seen as a passive participant. To offer too many choices to such clients can result not only in the client becoming confused, but also in the client and family viewing you as incompetent and not knowing what to do.

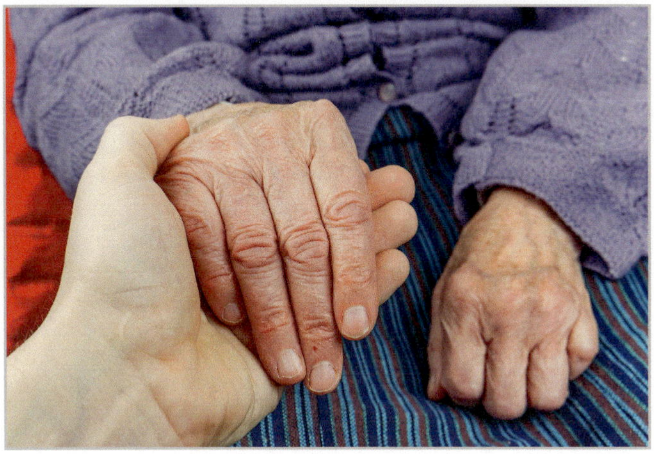

Fig. 8.1
In some cultures it is inappropriate to touch members of the opposite sex.

Family attitudes

Many cultural groups hold strong beliefs in caring for the older person. The idea of admitting an older relative into an aged care facility or employing a non-family member to enter the home to attend to care can be seen as shameful. They could even see this as their own failure to provide appropriately for their relative. Always be mindful of this when giving care or communicating with relatives. This can result in the family or your client appearing to be angry or shameful, or even to appear not to listen to what you are saying. Be aware of this possibility. Always be patient and consider how they must feel. Try and reassure them that they have made the appropriate choice in ensuring that their relative receives support and care.

Language

Approximately 240 languages are spoken within Australia (not including the many Aboriginal and Torres Strait Islander languages). In Australia, approximately 1 million migrants cannot speak English, and some 3 million consumers (around 12 per cent of the population) speak a language other than English at home. In 2016, 72.7 per cent of Australians aged 5 years and over spoke only English at home, while 2 per cent spoke no English at all (ABS 2020). The most common languages spoken at home (other than English) were Mandarin (2.5 per cent), Italian (1.2 per cent), Arabic (1.4 per cent), Cantonese (1.2 per cent) and Vietnamese (1.2 per cent) (ABS 2020). In New Zealand, approximately one in five people speak a language other than English at home, and one in 50 people cannot speak English (Statistics New Zealand 2020). In Australia, approximately 85 per cent of all non-English speaking migrants live in Sydney or Melbourne. Two-thirds of all Asian migrants in New Zealand live in the greater Auckland area. Hence, a number of older migrants may not have a good understanding of English, especially **colloquial language**.

As some people age, there is, on occasion, some loss of language skills. This is especially true in persons developing dementia. Generally speaking, the last language learnt is often the first language lost. For example, if a migrant grew up in Lebanon and their first languages were Lebanese and Arabic, with English being learnt on arrival in Australia or New Zealand, then it will be their English words and grammar that will be lost first. Often when speaking English, if they cannot remember a particular word (a **lexical gap**) they will replace it with a word from one of their other languages or a word with a similar meaning.

CARING ABOUT CULTURE

When communicating with people from other cultures:

- find out about the beliefs and values of the person's culture. Learn as much as you can
- do not judge the person by your own attitudes, values, beliefs and ideas
- follow the person's care plan. It includes the person's cultural beliefs and customs.

Do the following when communicating with foreign-speaking clients:

- Convey comfort by your tone of voice and body language.
- Do not speak loudly or shout. It will not help the person understand.
- Speak slowly and distinctly.
- Keep messages short and simple.
- Be alert for words the person seems to understand.
- Use gestures and pictures.
- Repeat the message in different ways.
- Do not use medical terms and abbreviations.
- Be alert for signs that the person is pretending to understand. Nodding and answering 'yes' to all questions are signs that the person does not understand what you are saying.

All languages develop colloquial or casual ways of speaking. In Australia, we tend to shorten our words and add suffixes such as 'o' or 'ie' on to them. For example, a fisher becomes a 'fisho', a cigarette break becomes a 'smoko' and a barbecue becomes a 'barbie'. A number of words that are peculiar to Australians may be unfamiliar to older migrants. For example, a can of beer is called a 'tinnie', but 'tinnie' can also be used to describe a small aluminium boat. When caring for an older person who comes from a non-English-speaking background, be aware of your client's ability to speak and understand English and use your language accordingly. Try to avoid colloquial language or casual speech.

It is good practice to set up a chart for your client if there are any concerns with their understanding of English. On this chart, clearly write in English the words and phrases they may require and alongside those words the corresponding words and phrases in their native language. It may help at times to add graphics to further clarify the meaning. This can be used by your client and you. It is especially helpful to ask the family to assist you with this so that you can incorporate any special phrases or needs your client may like to use or have. Table 8.1 is an example of a sample language chart.

Dress

Many cultural groups have specific dress codes that must be followed (Fig. 8.2). Always ensure your client is dressed as per their individual dress code, even though this may, at times, conflict with what you may consider to be good dress practices. For example, an Italian woman may insist on covering her legs with stockings, wearing a long dress with long sleeves on a hot day and may even cover her hair. Do not try and dissuade her if this is her personal preference as she is likely to become offended. Make sure that she is in the shade, offer her frequent drinks and generally try to keep her physical environment as cool as possible. If you believe that her personal dress preferences will endanger her health, speak to your supervisor and seek direction. If your client wears clothing that you are unfamiliar with, such as a sari, ask your client or their family to demonstrate the correct way of arranging the clothing.

Diet

Your client may be used to a diet that is different from what is generally considered normal within mainstream Australian and New Zealand society. Personal likes and dislikes are often linked to cultural preferences and, at times, religious requirements. For example, people from Asia may be more accustomed to eating rice several times a day and more vegetables than meat (Fig. 8.3). Sometimes, families will bring in special foods for your client. Make sure that this food is refrigerated if required and clearly labelled.

If you are caring for your client at home and are required to prepare a meal, make sure that you know exactly how your client likes their food to taste and how it should be prepared.

Some of your clients may need to have special foods brought in or prepared in certain ways before they can be eaten. Islamic and Jewish clients are very specific about the types of foods that they are not able to eat and have extremely prescriptive guidelines on how to prepare these foods. Foods permitted to be eaten are referred to as *halal* by Muslims and *kosher* by the Jewish community. If you have any concerns about meeting your client's specific dietary needs appropriately, always speak to your client, the family or your supervisor for advice.

Religion

Religion relates to spiritual beliefs, needs and practices. Religion is a highly personal issue and within a culturally diverse country a number of religions will be practised. It is important that you recognise the importance of your client's religious practices and assist them to observe these

Table 8.1
Sample language translation chart

English	Chinese (simplified)	Hindi	Tagalot (Filipino)	Te Reo Māori	Samoan
Hello Good morning	Wèi, ni hao, zao shang hao	Namaste	Hello Magandang Umaga	Kia ora	talofa
Goodbye	Zàai jiàn	Namaste	Paalam	Ka kite	tofa
How are you?	Nìn hao ma?	Aap kaisay hain?	Kamusta ka?	Tēnā koe e pēhea ana koe	'o a mai oe'
My name is	Wo de mìng zhì shì	Mera naam hai	Gutom ka ba	Ko taku ingoa	o lo'u igoa 'o'
Are you hungry?	Ni e ma?	Tuma ho bhukha?	Sigurado ka gutom?	E matekai ana koe?	ua e te fia ai?
Are you thirsty?	Ni ke ma?	Aap ko piyas hai?	Ikaw ba ay nauuhaw?	Kai te hiahia koe?	o e fia inu?
Do you want to go to the toilet?	Ni yao shang ce suo ma?	Kya aap bathroom main jana chahtay hain?	Gusto mo bang pumunta sa banyo?	Me haere tonu ki te whare paku?	e te fia alu i le fale taua?
Are you tired?	Ni lei ma?	Aap thaak ga'e ho?	Pagod ka ba?	Kua ngenge koe?	ua e vaivai?
Do you have pain?	Ni you teng tong ma?	Aap ko dard ho raha hai?	Mayron kabang masakit?	He mamae koe?	e iai sou tiga?
Are you comfortable?	Ni shu fu ma?	Aap ko araam hai?	Komportabli ka ba?	He hāneanea?	e te lagolelei?
Yes	shi	haan	oo	āe	ioe
No	bu shi de	nahin	hindi	kāore	lēai
Please	qing	kr paya—	paki/pakisuyo	tēnā koa	fa'amolemo
Thank you	xie xie nǐ	dhanayavad	salamat	Ngā mihi	fa'afetai
I want	Wo xiang	Main chahta hun	Gusto ko	hiahia	'ou te mana'o
I want to call my family	Wo xiang qing wo de jia ren or Wo yao da dian hua gei wo de jia ren	Main apane parivara ko phon karana chahta hoon	Gusto kung tumawag sa aking pamilyar	e hiahia ana ahau ki te waea atu ki taku whānau	'ou te fia valaau i lo'u aiga
Food	shǐ wu	bhojana/ Khaana	pagkain	kai	meaai
Water	shui	pānī	tubig	wai	vai
Tea	cha	chai	tsaa	tī	lauti
Sleep	shul jiao	sona	matulog	moe	moe
One	yige	ek	isa	kotahi	tasi
Two	er	do	dalawa	e rua	lua
Three	san	teen	tatlo	toru	tolu
Four	si	chaar	apat	e wha	fa
Five	wu	panch	lima	rima	lima
Six	liu	cha	anim	e ono	ono
Seven	qi	saat	pito	whitu	fitu
Eight	ba	aath	walo	waru	valu
Nine	jiu	no	siyam	iwa	iva
Ten	shǐ	dus	sampu	tekau	sefulu

Table 8.1
Sample language translation chart *continued*

English	Chinese (simplified)	Hindi	Tagalot (Filipino)	Te Reo Māori	Samoan
Twenty	er-shi	bees	dalawang po	rua tekau	luasefulu
Bed	chuang	bistaar	kama	moenga	moega
Chair	yi zi	kursi	upuan	tūru	nofoa
Table	zhuo zi	meza	mesa	ripanga	siata
Head	tou	sir	ulo	upoko	ulu
Arm	sh⍰ubi	bahna	braso	ringa	lima
Leg	tui	paira/taang	binti	waewae	vae
Body	shen ti	sarira	katawan	tinana	tino
Foot	jiao	pair	paa	waewae	vae
Hand	shou	haath	kamay	ringa	lima

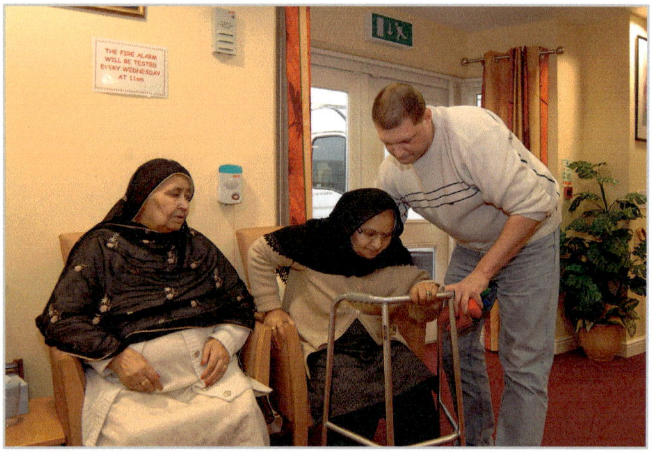

Fig. 8.2
Cultural groups often have specific dress codes.

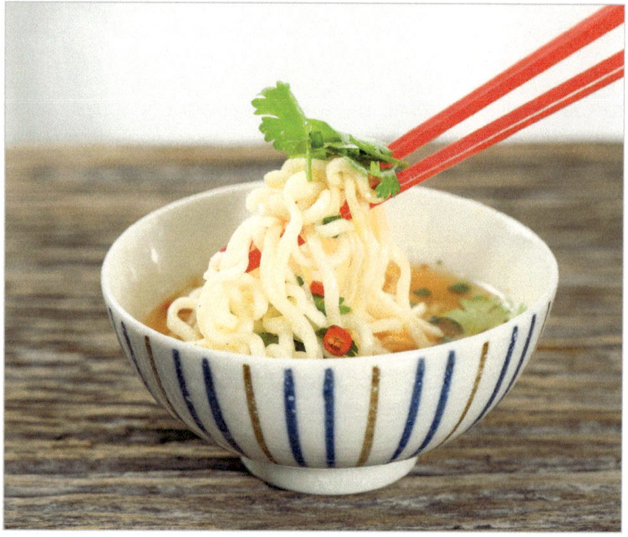

Fig. 8.3
A traditional Asian diet includes more vegetables than meat, and noodles and rice.

practices. As the culturally diverse populations of Australia and New Zealand are now becoming older, it is highly probable that you will need to care for people who practise religions that you may be unfamiliar with. If you are caring for a client whose religion you do not understand, ask your client for advice. If your client is unable to provide you with advice, ask your supervisor or consult the client's family. It is far better to ask for help than to unintentionally offend somebody by failing to observe or even contravening a religious practice.

Your client has a right to observe their own religious practices (Fig. 8.4). This includes attending their own spiritual place of worship or displaying their personal religious artefacts (objects). Please ensure that you do not touch or handle religious texts and objects unless permitted and only then with considerable respect. For example, within the Islamic religion, the holy book the Koran is extremely important. Failure to treat the book with respect is seen as showing extreme disrespect to your client's religious beliefs.

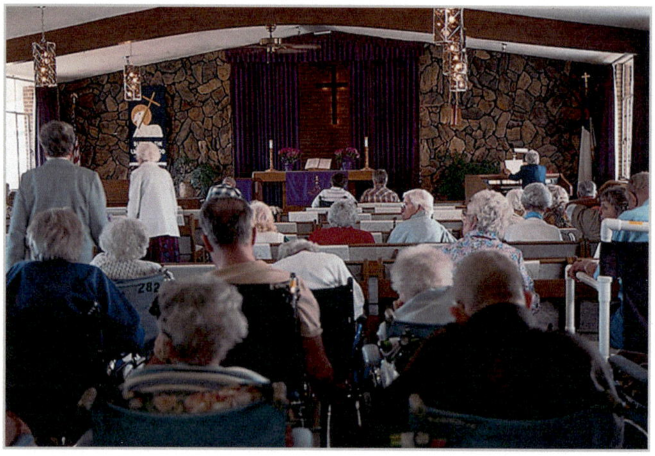

Fig. 8.4
Consumers attend a religious service at a residential care service.

If your client wishes to spend time with their spiritual adviser, ask the family to arrange this as they will be familiar with your client's preferences, or contact a representative of the appropriate local religious body. A pastoral care adviser is often available within many aged care services. They will be able to assist your client to make contact with the appropriate people and attend to their spiritual needs.

Christianity is the predominant religion in both Australia and New Zealand. Tables 8.2 and 8.3 outline the main religions practised in both countries.

Table 8.2
Religions practised in Australia, 2016

Religion	Number of people	Percentage of population
Christianity	12 205 000	52.1
Buddhism	563 600	2.4
Islam	604 000	2.6
Hindu	440 200	1.9
Jewish	97 300	0.5
Other non-Christian religions	143 000	0.9
No religion	7 000 000	29.9

Source: ABS 2017 Census of population and housing: Australia revealed 2016 cat. no. 2024.0

Table 8.3
Religions practised in New Zealand

Religion	Number of people	Percentage of population
Christianity	2 000 000	55.6
Buddhism	41 834	1.0
Islam	23 831	0.5
Hindu	39 898	0.9
Spiritualism	18 082	0.4

Source: Stats NZ and licensed by Stats NZ for re-use under the Creative Commons Attribution 4.0 International License.

FOCUS ON ISLAM

Muslims across the world differ in their interpretation of religious belief and in the way certain rituals are performed. These differences are influenced by the cultures and customs of the countries and regions in which Muslims live or have roots and traditions, and by the different types of Islam that are followed (e.g. Sunni or Shia). Nevertheless, the basic fundamentals of the Islamic faith remain the same across all countries and regions. These basic fundamentals are called the 'Five Pillars of Islam':

1. **Faith and belief in oneness of God and finality of the prophethood of Mohammad (*Tawheed*):** 'There is no God but One God and Muhammad is the last messenger of God'. This declaration of faith is called the *Shahadah*. It is through this declaration of faith that one becomes a Muslim. An important point to mention here is that, unlike with Catholicism or other Christian religions, no hierarchy exists in Islam. Anyone can be a priest and everyone can be close to God without having to pass through 'intermediaries'.
2. **Daily prayers – five times (*Salat*):** Praying is a daily ritual that is performed five times a day after certain cleansing rituals. Prayers are given at dawn, midday, late afternoon, sunset and nightfall, and are always given when facing Mecca. During prayer, various verses from the Koran are recited. There are special types of prayer used during the month of Ramadan and for other purposes. The most important prayers are used before burial.
3. **Charity (*Zakat*):** In Islam, the giving of charity and sharing of wealth is highly emphasised. The amount of annual charity individual Muslims are expected to give is based on income and assets, but can range from a minimum of 2.5 per cent up to 8.5 per cent of net assets held over a year.
4. **Fasting (*Ramadan*):** Every year during the month of Ramadan all Muslims are expected to fast from sunrise to sunset, abstaining from food, drink and sexual relations. Fasting is mainly a method of self-purification and showing self-restraint. By cutting oneself off from worldly comforts, even for a short time, a fasting person focuses on his or her purpose in life by constantly being aware of the presence of God. The last 10 days of Ramadan are considered one of the holiest periods. Eid Fitr, a three-day festive period, celebrates the end of Ramadan.
5. **The Pilgrimage (*Hajj*):** The pilgrimage to Mecca is an obligation that Muslims are expected to undertake once in a lifetime. The essence of the Hajj is to reinforce the sense of equality among all Muslims and to enable them to meet one another. The Hajj begins in the twelfth month of the Islamic year (which is lunar, not solar). Pilgrims are expected to wear special clothes. Men are expected to dress in two separate (i.e. not sewn) pieces of white cloth. This is the same clothing in which Muslims are buried.

The rites of the Hajj are of Abrahamic origin. These include going around the Ka'bah seven times, and passing seven times between the hills of Safa and Marwa. The pilgrims later stand together on the wide plains of Arafat (a large expanse of desert outside Mecca) and join in prayer for God's forgiveness, in what is often thought of as a preview of the Day of Judgement. The close of the Hajj is marked by a festival, the Eid al Adha, which is celebrated with prayers and the exchange of gifts in Muslim communities everywhere. During this festival, there are also ritual animal sacrifices, after which meat is distributed to the poor.

Islamic (Sharia) law

In most of the Middle East, Islamic (*Sharia*) law is the basic criteria for many decisions and local clergy will have a strong influence. Local religious censor boards may review new products and services to see how well they comply with Sharia. For several types of products/services, particularly new ones, it is vital to secure certificates of Islamic compliance. Sharia boards may also be asked to give their opinions if there is some kind of doubt about the product itself. For example, the introduction of television in the 1950s had to be approved by this type of committee. Many Muslims attend a mosque, which is a place of worship for followers of Islam (Fig. 8.5).

There are four sources from which Islamic rules are derived. The hierarchy is strictly followed.

Koran: The Koran is the divine book and the word of God delivered to Mohammad. It is the principal source of all Islamic laws.

Hadith and Sunnah: The Sunnah refers to the sayings, actions, approvals and disapprovals of Mohammad. The Sunnah is collected in books separate from the Koran, which are known as Hadith books. Not every Hadith is authentic and Muslim scholars have classified them into various categories according to their level of authenticity.

Fiqh: Where there are no clear guidelines found in the Koran or Sunnah, Muslims look at traditional jurisprudence. For example, in the Koran there is no mention of whether cannabis is allowed. Jurists have used statements referring to alcohol (such as 'do not come under the effect of the substance that distorts the judgement') to rule that cannabis is illegal. Similarly, the same applies to the use of animal gelatine in food products. As pork is prohibited, so animal gelatine is prohibited.

Fatwa: A Fatwa is an Islamic ruling as issued by a Mufti (i.e. a religious wise man similar to Rabbis in Judaism) based upon his own interpretation of the holy texts. A Fatwa ruling is not a legal obligation and may be followed or not followed depending upon the perceived legitimacy of the Mufti issuing the Fatwa.

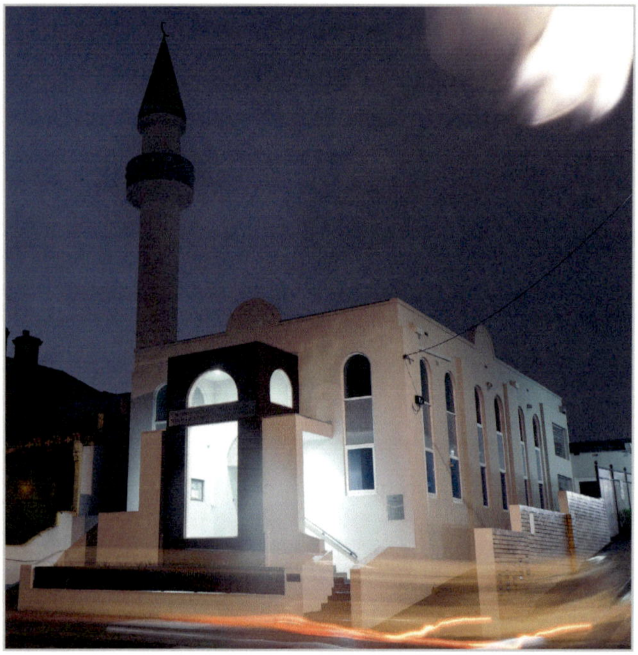

Fig. 8.5
This Islamic mosque is in Mareeba, on the Atherton Tablelands in Queensland.

Services available

When you care for a client from a culturally and linguistically diverse **(CALD)** background, a number of organisations and services can assist you to provide appropriate care. These include:

- telephone interpreter services
- internet services
- printed and online fact sheets written by both government and non-government organisations (NGOs)
- multicultural advisory committees available in all states and territories
- multicultural community centres
- state or territory government websites, which have links to a multicultural resource directory
- specific cultural group organisations.

FOCUS ON BUDDHISM

Buddhism is a religion and philosophy that has between 200 million and 500 million followers throughout the world, most of whom reside in Asia. Buddhism is based on the teachings of the Buddha, who lived in Nepal. A Buddhist is a person who reveres the Buddha as the highest spiritual guide and strives to live according to his teachings.

The basic doctrines of early Buddhism, which remain common to all Buddhists, include the 'four noble truths': existence is suffering (*dukh ka*); suffering has a cause, namely craving and attachment (*trishna*); there is a cessation of suffering; and there is a path to the cessation of suffering – the 'eightfold path' of right views, right resolve, right speech, right action, right livelihood, right effort, right mindfulness and right concentration.

The Buddhists have four sacred days in a month, which are observed as days of fasting. These days are the new moon, full moon and the two quarter moon days, and are called *Uposatha* (*Roya* in Sri Lanka) (i.e. fast day). On the Uposatha days, the devout Buddhist follows the eight precepts (*Atthanga Sila*) and abstains from worldly pleasures. They visit *viharas* (Buddhist monasteries) and offer *dana* (offerings) to the Bhikkhus, a fully ordained male Buddhist monk, and Bhikkhuni, female monk.

The most sacred and the most important festival for all Buddhists is Vaisakha Purnima, known in India as Buddha Purnima or Buddha Jayanti. It is fixed by the full-moon day of Vaisakha, which falls in May. This day is the 'Thrice Blessed' day as Lord Buddha was born, attained enlightenment and entered into *Mahaparinirvana* on this day.

A Buddhist temple is the place of worship for Buddhists (Fig. 8.6). It includes a number of structures that may vary according to the region in which the temple is situated.

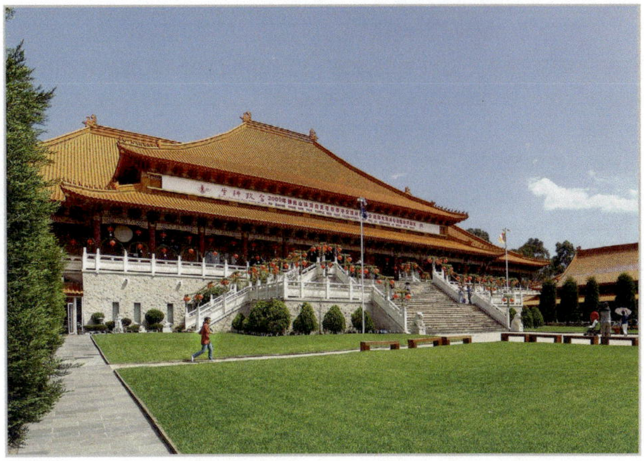

Fig. 8.6
The Nan Tien Temple, which means 'paradise of the south', is located just south of Wollongong and is the largest Buddhist temple in the southern hemisphere.

CASE STUDY

You are currently working within an aged care facility and have been rostered to care for Mrs Deeba Khan. Mrs Khan has been a consumer for almost a year and is a Muslim woman who originally came from Pakistan. While she does understand some English, she has difficulties speaking it at times and will often ask her relatives to translate for her. With the assistance of her family, a communication chart has been set up for her with words in English and Urdu that could be used when her family are not there. When she was first admitted, her family were invited to instruct all staff members on the basis of her religion and how to manage her Islamic practices. A safe place by her bed was found for her to keep her copy of the Koran and careful consideration was given when assisting her with eating. Her diet was discussed with the dietitian and special measures were commenced to ensure that she was given only halal (approved) food. A scarf was kept with her at all times to cover her hair and shoulders.

While her family expressed considerable concern and guilt at Mrs Khan being admitted for care, over time they have come to feel less guilty about the decision and willingly participated in making decisions relating to their mother. By understanding Mrs Khan's cultural needs, you have been able to ensure that she receives good culturally safe care.

CRITICAL THINKING ACTIVITY

You are a carer working for a community agency on the outskirts of a city. You have been assigned the care of Mrs Angha Patel. Mrs Patel is a southern Indian migrant and a practising Hindu. She has only recently started receiving care after she had a fall at home and required surgery for a fractured hip. You are required to prepare a meal for her, wash and vacuum the tiled floors, vacuum all carpets, clean the bathroom and toilet and hang out her washing. You are also required to assist her with her shower and dressing. All carers who have cared for Mrs Patel have reported that she shouts at them in Hindi, speaks minimal English only, gets angry with them very quickly and often cries. When she does speak of her family, it is very derogatory and she blames them for why she is not getting better quickly. She often does not eat the meals that you prepare.

Questions

1. Considering her cultural background, what do you believe could be some of the reasons why Mrs Patel is behaving this way?
2. What steps could you take to try and assist Mrs Patel without her becoming angry?
3. What could you do to ensure that she eats the prepared meals?
4. Who would you ask for advice to better understand Mrs Patel?
5. What government and non-government organisations and services are available in your local area to assist you?
6. Once you have completed questions 2–5, develop a care plan for Mrs Patel that all carers could use when assisting her.

ACCREDITATION

You are working in residential or home care and accreditors are at your service. Can you answer the following questions?

- As a carer, how would you treat a consumer with dignity and respect if they are from a different culture than you?
- What would you consider discrimination in care delivery within a service?
- How can you support a person's identity when providing care?

REVIEW QUESTIONS

Circle T if the statement is true or F if the statement if false:

1 T / F Australia has a White Australia migration policy.

2 T / F According to the ABS, in 2020 29.8 per cent of all Australians were born overseas.

3 T / F Asylum seekers are illegal immigrants.

4 T / F Culture, race and ethnicity are the same thing.

5 T / F All cultures consider their elders to be wise.

6 T / F In some cultures it is inappropriate to hug a person of the opposite sex.

Circle the BEST answer:

7 The current Australia population comes from approximately how many countries?

a 50
b 100
c 200
d 240

8 There are approximately how many different languages spoken in Australia (excluding Indigenous languages)?

a 50
b 100
c 200
d 240

9 The major religions in Australia are:

a Christianity, Hinduism and Buddhism
b Christianity, Islam and Buddhism
c Christianity, Buddhism and Islam
d Christianity, Shintoism and Islam

10 The basic fundamentals of Islam are called:

a The Five Pillars of Islam
b The Four Cornerstones of Islam
c The Five Rules of Islam
d The Five Cornerstones of Islam

Answers to these questions are on p. 454.

Further reading

Aged Care Quality and Safety Commission (2019). Guidance and resources for providers to support the Aged Care Quality Standards. Online 10 Setpember 2021. Available: https://agedcare.royalcommission.gov.au/system/files/2020-06/CTH.0001.4000.4927.pdf

Doutrich D, Arcus K, Dekker L et al (2012). Cultural safety in New Zealand and the United States: looking at a way forward together, Journal of Transcultural Nursing, 23(2):143.

Nursing Council of New Zealand (2011). Guidelines for Cultural Safety, the Treaty of Waitangi and Māori Health in Nursing and Midwifery Practice.

Raukawa-Tait M (2012). Cultural safety an issue for all NZ's elderly. The Daily Post (Rotorua). 1 May, A8.

References

Australian Bureau of Statistics (ABS) (2021). Migration Australia. Online 10 September 2021. Available: www.abs.gov.au/statistics/people/population/migration-australia/latest-release

Australian Government, Department of Home Affairs (2021). Migration program planning levels. Online 10 September 2021. Available: https://immi.homeaffairs.gov.au/what-we-do/migration-program-planning-levels

Islamic Council of Victoria (2021). Taking care of Muslim patients. Online 10 September 2021. Available: www.icv.org.au/media/icv-policy-research/taking-care-of-muslim-patients/

Parliament of Australia (2020). Temporary migration figures: the quarter before COVID-19 hit June 2020. Available: www.aph.gov.au

Refugee Council of Australia (2021). How do refugees come to Australia under its Refugee and Humanitarian program? Online 10 September 2021. Available: www.refugeecouncil.org.au/coming-to-australia/

Stats NZ Tatauranga Aotearoa (2020). New Zealand's population passes 5 million. Online 18 May 2020. Available: www.stats.govt.nz/news/new-zealands-population-passes-5-million

CHAPTER 9
Interpersonal communication and care

By Margaret Webb

AFTER READING THIS CHAPTER, YOU SHOULD BE ABLE TO:

- define the key terms listed in this chapter
- identify the parts that make up the whole person
- list the basic needs for life identified by Abraham Maslow
- discuss the psychological and social effects of illness
- identify the types of people cared for in residential care service
- list the elements needed for effective communication
- explain how verbal and non-verbal communication are used
- discuss the methods of, and barriers to, effective communication
- explain how to communicate with the angry person, the person with a disability and the person who is comatose
- understand why family and visitors are important to the person
- identify the courtesies given to the person and visitors
- know how to promote quality of life.

Key terms

body language: Messages sent through facial expressions, gestures, posture and body movements; non-verbal communication

comatose: Being unable to respond to verbal stimuli

communication barriers: Barriers that prevent us from sending and receiving messages effectively, such as using unfamiliar language, acknowledging cultural differences and failing to listen

culture: The behaviours, beliefs and characteristics of particular social and ethnic groups

disability: A lost, absent or impaired physical or mental function

esteem: The worth, value or opinion one has of another person

holism: A concept that considers the whole person; that each person has physical, social, psychological, emotional and spiritual parts that are woven together and cannot be separated

need: Something necessary or desirable for maintaining life and mental wellbeing

non-verbal communication: Communication that does not involve words

optimal level of functioning: A person's highest potential for mental and physical performance

paraphrasing: Restating a message in your own words

self-actualisation: Reaching one's full potential

self-esteem: Thinking well of oneself, seeing oneself as useful and being well thought of by others

verbal communication: Communication that can involve the spoken and written word

written communication: Communication that can be read

The client is the most important person in the aged care sector. Age, religion, culture and nationality are some of the factors that make each person unique, along with education, occupation and lifestyle. Each person is someone who thinks, acts, feels and makes decisions.

Every person you support or care for has fears, needs and rights. When a person has reached a stage when they require support or assistance to undertake activities of daily living (ADLs) they will have experienced some losses. These may include loss of a home, family, friends, physical function and independence. Family and community roles may have been lost too.

All these aspects of life will affect the way that the person communicates to you and others, and the way that your communication styles will be interpreted by your client. Your communication techniques and styles within your practice must reflect and accommodate these unique differences between individuals.

COMMUNICATING WITH CLIENTS

You communicate with clients every time you give care. You give information to the person and the person gives information to you. Your body sends messages all the time – at the bedside, in the hallway, in the dining room and everywhere else. The person and family are aware of what you say and what you do. You communicate not only by what you say, but also by how and when you say things. Good work ethics and an understanding of the person are needed for good communication.

The communication process

The process of communication begins with a sender who establishes a message to convey to the receiver. On occasion, the message – be it written, verbal or non-verbal – is not sent or received as intended. This is referred to as interference. Interference may be a result of the sender not conveying the message accurately or it may be a fault of the receiver's interpretation of the message conveyed. There may be multiple causes of interference, which will be discussed in this chapter.

Effective communication

For effective communication between you and the client, you must:

- follow the rules of communication
- understand and respect the client as a person
- view the person as a physical, psychological, social and spiritual human being
- appreciate the person's problems and frustrations
- respect the person's rights
- respect the person's religion and culture
- give the person time to process (understand) the information that you give
- ask questions to see if the person has understood you. Repeat information as often as needed. Repeat exactly what you said. Do not give the person a new message to process. This is very important for people with hearing problems.
- be patient. People with memory problems may ask the same question many times. Do not say that you are repeating information; memory loss is not a choice.

Messages are sent by what you say and do. You communicate verbally and non-verbally with the person. You must use both methods well.

Verbal communication

Verbal communication means using words. The words can be spoken or written. Verbal communication is used to talk with people. It is used to find out how they are feeling and to share information with them. Most communication involves the spoken word. When speaking with a client, follow these rules:

- Face the person.
- Control the loudness and tone of your voice.
- Speak clearly, slowly and distinctly.
- Avoid using slang or vulgar words.
- Repeat information as needed.
- Ask one question at a time. Wait for an answer.
- Do not shout, whisper or mumble.

Written communication

Written communication with a client is used when the person cannot speak or hear, but can read (Fig. 9.1). The nurse and the care plan can tell you how to communicate with the person. Write messages to those who are deaf or have severe hearing problems. Clients who are deaf may also use sign language (Fig. 9.2).

Besides hearing problems, some people also have poor vision. If you need to write messages to them, use a black felt-tipped pen on white paper and print in large letters. Make sure the room is well lit and that you are standing near the person.

Some people can hear, but cannot speak or read. Ask questions that can be answered 'yes' or 'no' with nods, blinks or other gestures. A picture board may be helpful (Fig. 9.3).

Your communication with the person should be kind, courteous and friendly. This may be hard when they are not courteous in return. Remember, clients who are hard to deal with probably need your understanding the most.

Non-verbal communication

Non-verbal communication (body language) does not use words. Messages are sent through gestures, facial expressions, posture, body movements, touch and smell. Non-verbal messages more accurately reflect a person's feelings than words do. They are usually involuntary and can

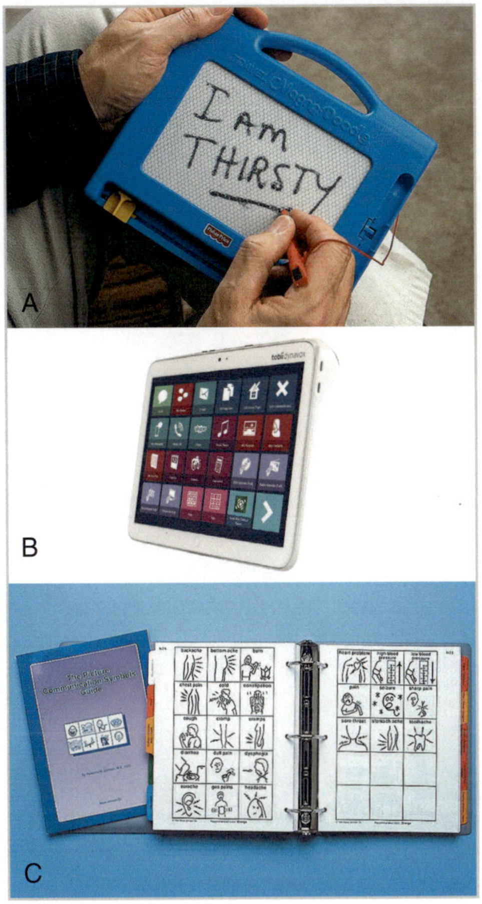

Fig. 9.1
Communication aids. **A.** Magic slate. **B.** Electronic talking aid. **C.** Communication board.

be hard to control. A person may say one thing but act another way. You need to watch the person's eyes, hand movements, gestures, posture and other actions. These can tell you more than words. You also need to be aware of your own non-verbal communication.

Touch

Touch is a very important form of non-verbal communication. It conveys comfort, caring, love, affection and reassurance. Touch means different things to different people. The meaning depends on the person's age, gender (male or female), experiences and culture. Always be aware that within some cultures there are specific rules and taboos in terms of touching (see Chapter 8).

Some people do not like to be touched. However, touch can show caring and warmth. Often, holding hands or touching forearms is more comforting than words. Touch should be gentle. It should not be hurried, rough or sexual.

Body language

People send messages through their body language. **Body language** includes:

- posture
- gait (how a person walks)

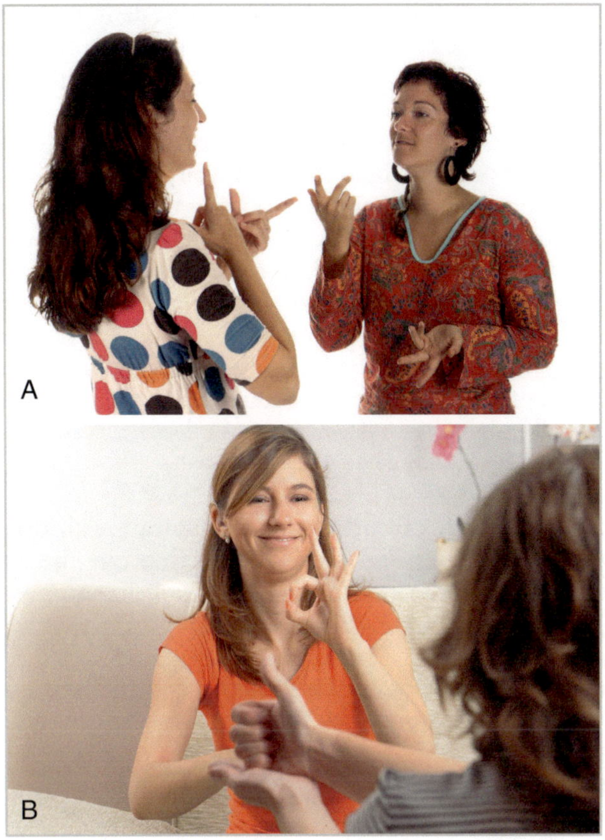

Fig. 9.2
Sign language is another way to communicate.

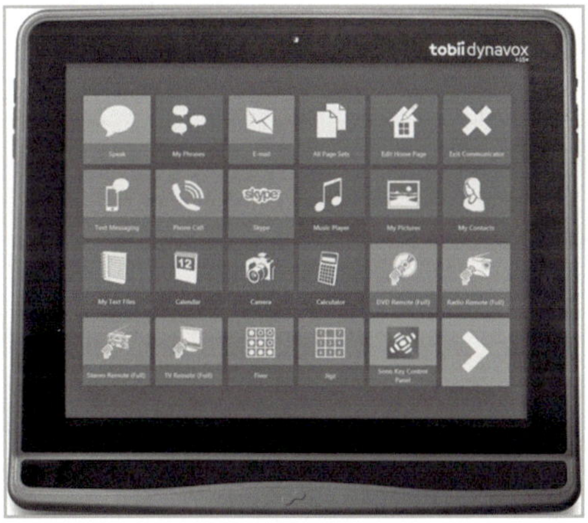

Fig. 9.3
A picture board is used to communicate.

- facial expressions
- eye contact
- hand movements
- gestures
- body movements
- appearance (dress, hygiene and adornments, such as jewellery, perfume and cosmetics).

Consumers send messages with their body language. For example, slumped posture may mean the person is not happy or not feeling well. A person may deny pain, but protect the affected body part by standing, lying or sitting in a certain way. Many other messages are sent with body language.

Your actions and movements also send messages that are often more powerful than the words you speak. Your facial expressions send messages, as does how you stand, sit, walk and look at a person. Your body language should show enthusiasm; it should also show caring and respect for the person. Often you will need to control your body language. You should also control your reactions to odours from excretions or the person's body. Many odours are beyond the person's control. The person's embarrassment and humiliation will only increase if you react to odours.

COMMUNICATION METHODS

Certain methods can help you communicate with others and will result in better relationships. They can also help you to obtain more information for the nursing process.

Listening

Listening means focusing on the person's verbal and non-verbal communication. You use sight, hearing, touch and smell. You focus on what the person is saying (Fig. 9.4). You observe non-verbal clues. These clues can support what the person is saying, or they can indicate other feelings. For example: Mr Hardt says, 'I want to stay here. That way my daughter won't have to care for me', but you see tears and he looks away from you. His verbal communication says he is happy, but his non-verbal communication shows sadness. Listening shows that you care and have interest.

To listen effectively:

- face the person
- maintain good eye contact with the person (if this is culturally appropriate)
- lean towards the person. Do not sit back with your arms crossed
- respond to the person. Nod your head. Say 'Uh huh', 'Mmm' and 'I see'. Repeat what the person says and ask questions
- avoid communication barriers.

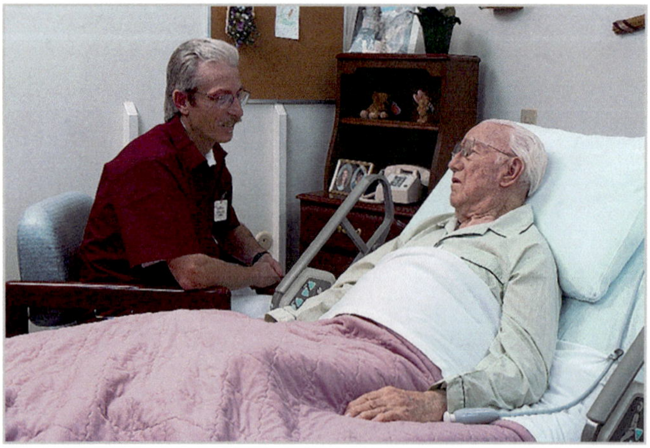

Fig. 9.4
The carer shows they are listening by facing the client, having good eye contact and leaning towards the client.

Paraphrasing

Paraphrasing is restating a person's message in your own words. You use fewer words than the person did to send the message. Paraphrasing:

- shows you are listening
- lets the person see whether you have understood the message sent
- promotes further communication.

The person will usually respond to your statement. For example:

Mr Hardt:	My wife was crying after she spoke with the doctor. I don't know what he said to her.
You:	You don't know why your wife was crying.
Mr Hardt:	He must have told her that I have a tumour.

Direct questions

Direct questions focus on certain information. You ask the person something you need to know. Some direct questions have a 'yes' or 'no' answer. Others require the person to give more information. For example:

You:	Mr Hardt, do you want to shave this morning?
Mr Hardt:	Yes.
You:	When would you like to do that?
Mr Hardt:	Could we start in about 15 minutes? I'd like to call my son first.
You:	Yes, we can start in 15 minutes. Did you have a bowel movement today, Mr Hardt?
Mr Hardt:	No.
You:	You said you didn't eat well this morning. Can you tell me what you ate?
Mr Hardt:	I only had toast and coffee. I just don't feel like eating this morning.

Direct questions are especially useful when communicating with dementia clients. Simple yes/no questions may be easier for them to process and therefore respond to than complicated questions.

Open-ended questions

Open-ended questions lead or invite the person to share their thoughts, feelings or ideas. The person chooses how to respond and what to talk about. He or she controls what is talked about and the information given. Answers require more than a 'yes' or 'no'. For example:

'What do you like about living with your daughter?'
'Tell me about your grandson.'

'What was your wife like?'

'What do you like about being retired?'

Responses to open-ended questions are generally longer and give more information than direct questions.

Clarifying

Clarifying ensures that you understand the message. You can ask the person to repeat the message, say you do not understand or restate the message. For example:

'Could you say that again?'

'I'm sorry, Mr Hardt. I don't understand what you mean.'

'Are you saying that you want to go home?'

Focusing

Focusing means dealing with a specific topic. It is useful when a person rambles or wanders in thought. For example: Mr Hardt talks at length about foods and places to eat. You need to know why he did not eat much breakfast. To focus the conversation on breakfast, you say, 'Let's talk about today's breakfast. You said you didn't feel like eating.'

Silence

Silence is a very powerful way to communicate. Sometimes, especially at sad times, you do not need to say anything. Just being there shows you care. At other times silence gives you time to think, organise thoughts or choose words. Silence is useful when making hard decisions. It is also useful when the person is upset and needs to regain control. Silence on your part shows caring and respect for the person's situation and feelings.

Sometimes pauses or long silences are uncomfortable. But do not think you need to talk when a person is silent. The person may need silence. Dealing with silence gets easier as you gain experience in your role.

COMMUNICATION BARRIERS

Communication barriers prevent us from sending and receiving messages effectively. When this happens, communication fails. You need to be aware of these barriers. Some common barriers to communication include:

- using unfamiliar language – you and the person must use and understand the same language. If not, messages between you are not accurately interpreted.
- cultural differences – the person may attach different meanings to verbal and non-verbal communication than you do.
- changing the subject – a person may change the subject when the topic is uncomfortable. Avoid changing the subject whenever possible.
- giving your opinion – opinions involve judging values, behaviour or feelings. Let others express their feelings and concerns without adding your opinion. Do not make judgements.
- talking a lot when others are silent – talking too much is usually due to nervousness and discomfort with silence. Silences have meaning. They can show acceptance, rejection or fear. They can also show the person's need for quiet and time to think.
- failing to listen – do not just pretend to listen, as this shows lack of interest and caring. It causes poor responses. If you do not listen, you can miss important complaints of pain, discomfort or other symptoms that must be reported to the nurse.
- giving insincere or 'pat' answers – such as 'Don't worry', 'Everything will be okay', 'Your doctor knows best'. These block communication because they make the person feel that you do not care about their concerns, feelings and fears.
- illness and disability – some disorders affect speech, hearing, vision, cognitive function and body movements. Temporary or permanent disabilities can affect verbal or non-verbal communication.

CARING FOR THE PERSON

Communication is not just how you speak with a person, *it is conveyed in all the care practices* that you do. Your communication must reflect who they are. For care to be truly effective, you must consider the whole person. **Holism** means treating something or someone as a 'whole'. The whole person has physical, social, psychological, emotional and spiritual parts (Fig. 9.5). These parts are woven together and cannot be separated. How you care for a person holistically is an important aspect of communication.

Each part relates to and depends on the other parts. As a social being, a person speaks and communicates these parts and needs with others. Physically, the brain, mouth, tongue, lips and throat must function for speech. Communication is also psychological; it involves thinking and reasoning.

To consider only the physical part is to ignore the person's ability to think, make decisions and interact with others. It also ignores the person's experiences, lifestyle,

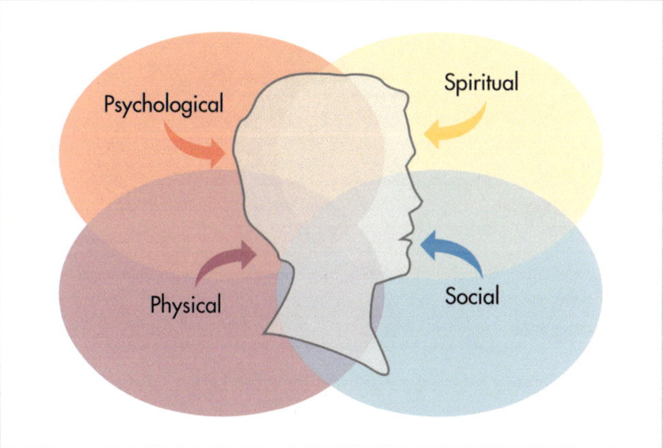

Fig. 9.5
A person is a physical, psychological, social, emotional and spiritual being. The parts overlap and cannot be separated.

culture, emotions and needs. When you ignore these aspects of a person's experiences, you are communicating to them that they are not important.

Disability and illness affect the whole person. For example: Mr Lund has had a stroke and needs help with his physical needs. He has had to leave his home. His relationships with his wife and children have changed. He may be angry with God for letting this happen to him. The health team plans care to help him deal with his problems and to encourage his independence and optimal level of functioning.

You must know and respect the whole person, to provide effective, quality care. Too often, a person is referred to as a room number. For example, '12A needs to go to the toilet', rather than 'Mrs Martinez in 12A needs to go to the toilet'. This strips the person of his or her identity. It reduces the person to a thing, or a task to be performed. Clients are often denied the dignity and respect of being called by their titles – Mrs Tan, Mr Singh, Miss Turner. Instead, they are called Rita, Ramesh or Mia. Some have even been called Grandma, Papa or Sweetheart. Never call a person by his or her first name or any other name unless they ask you to do so or before asking that person if it is okay. Clients are not things, your relatives or children. They are complex, adult human beings who think and feel. Your communication with clients must always convey respect.

NEEDS

A **need** is something necessary or desirable for maintaining life and mental wellbeing. According to psychologist Abraham Maslow, for a person to survive and function at their optimum, their basic needs must be met. These needs are arranged in order of importance (Fig. 9.6). Lower-level needs are generally met before higher-level needs. These basic needs, listed in order from the lowest level to the highest, are:

- physiological or physical needs
- safety and security needs
- love and belonging needs
- self-esteem needs
- the need for self-actualisation.

People normally meet their own needs. When they cannot, it is usually because of disease, illness, injury or advanced age. A person's needs will change according to their situation. They are not static, nor do they stay the same throughout life.

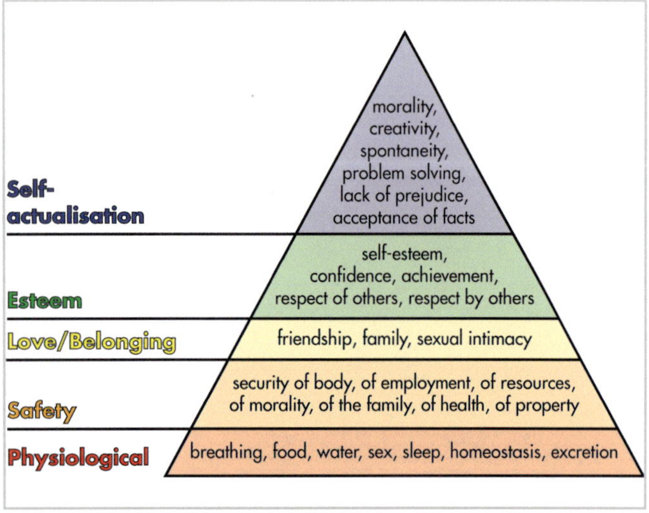

Fig. 9.6
The basic needs for life as described by Maslow, in order from the lowest to the highest level. Maslow's hierarchy of needs. Created by J. Finkelstein.

Physical needs

Oxygen, food, water, elimination, rest and shelter are needed for life. Without oxygen a person will die within minutes. Without food or water a person will feel weak and ill within a few hours. The kidneys and intestines must function normally; otherwise poisonous toxins build up in the blood and can cause death. Without enough rest and sleep, a person becomes very tired, irritable and may function in a manner that is unsafe. Without shelter, a person is exposed to extremes of heat and cold, which can be life-threatening.

You will be helping people meet their physical needs and you need to truly understand the importance of these needs. How do you feel when you are choking? How do you feel when you are thirsty or hungry? How do you react without enough sleep? How do you feel when you do not have a bathroom to use? How would you feel if you needed to use the bathroom urgently and were told to wait?

The need for safety and security

Safety and security needs relate to feeling safe from harm, danger and fear. Many people are afraid of residential care services. Some care involves strange equipment. Some care causes the fear of pain or discomfort or loss of control over one's environment. People feel safer and more secure if they know what is going to happen. For every procedure, even a simple bath, the person should know:

- why it is needed
- who will do it
- how it will be done
- when it will be done
- what sensations or feelings to expect.

Many people do not feel safe and secure when admitted to a residential care service. They are not in their usual, secure home setting and may well require time to adjust to their new surroundings. They are in a strange place with strange routines, where strangers care for them. Some people become frightened and confused. Be kind and understanding and take the time to explain all routines and procedures. Show the person their new setting and listen to their concerns. You may have to repeat explanations and directions many times. Sometimes they need repeating for many days or weeks until the person feels safe and unafraid.

Be patient. Remember that many of your clients may have been working hard to maintain their independence to stay at home and that to be admitted to residential care will be seen by them as their failure. They may demonstrate this by showing anger.

When working in a residential care service, remember that you are working in someone else's home and you should show the clients the same respect that you would if you were a visitor in their house. In community care settings this is even more the case, as you are a visitor and guest in someone's home. For residential aged care consumers, assist the client to view the service as their home. Allow them to choose where their belongings will go, or to make other choices that will allow them to tailor their surroundings to their personal tastes. Knock on their door and ask permission before entering their room. People feel safer and more secure when they have control over their own environment.

The need for love and belonging

Love and belonging needs relate to love, closeness and affection. They also involve meaningful relationships with others. There are many cases in which people have become weaker or died because they lacked love and belonging. This is especially true in some Indigenous societies. It may be seen in older people who have outlived their families and friends.

Family, friends and the health team can meet love and belonging needs. The service is the person's home. You must help the person feel loved and accepted. Remind the person that you are there to help him or her. Encourage them to maintain communication with friends and family outside the service.

Self-esteem

Esteem means the worth, value or opinion one has of a person. **Self-esteem** means to think well of oneself, seeing oneself as useful and being well thought of by others. Sometimes people lose some portion of their self-esteem following loss of a body function or when they become ill.

For example: an older man once built his own home and worked a farm. He supported and raised a family. Now he cannot dress or feed himself. How might he feel about himself? Cancer treatments have caused a woman to lose her hair. She feels unattractive and less than whole. People with slow, crippling diseases may feel less than whole, as might those who have lost an arm or leg. You must treat all clients with respect and understanding. Although it takes more time, encourage clients to do as much for themselves as possible and encourage individual choice. A positive attitude to maintaining a person's maximum function and freedom of choice will create a climate of mutual respect and foster independence. This also focuses on what people can do for themselves, rather than highlighting areas of dependence. This helps to increase self-esteem.

The need for self-actualisation

Self-actualisation means fulfilling one's potential. It involves learning, understanding and creating to the limit of a person's capacity. This is the highest need. It is rarely, if ever, totally met. Rather, it is an ongoing process. Most people constantly try to learn and understand more. This need can be postponed and life will continue. The need for self-actualisation is a lifelong need – it never ends. Many older people are investigating new ways to realise their potential and enrol in community or university courses, or participate in volunteer work. In residential aged care services, care workers need to help clients find appropriate avenues to meet this need. This may include providing reading materials, access to television/DVD players or the internet. Never presume that just because a person needs your support and care that they do not have the capability to further develop themselves.

CULTURE AND RELIGION

Culture is the characteristics of a group of people – their language, values, beliefs, habits, likes, dislikes and customs. Culture is highly important in communication and you will need to learn how to communicate respectfully with people from many different backgrounds. You will find more details about caring for persons from other cultures in Chapter 8.

A person's religion influences their health and illness practices. It may affect their beliefs and practices about diet, healing, days of worship, birth and death.

Many people find comfort and strength in religion during illness. They may want to pray and observe religious practices. Residential care services may offer religious services. Assist clients in attending the services if they wish, or to contact spiritual leaders outside the service to arrange a visit. Some may wish to leave the service to attend religious services.

If a person wants a spiritual leader or adviser to visit, report this request to your supervisor or the nurse in charge. Make sure the room is neat and in order. Have a chair ready for the spiritual advisor. The person and the adviser should be allowed privacy during the visit.

The care plan should always reflect the person's culture and religion. You need to respect and accept the person's culture and religion. You will meet people from cultures or religions other than your own. Take time to learn about their beliefs and practices. This will help you to understand the person and provide better care.

A person may not follow all the beliefs and practices of his or her culture or religion. Some people do not practise a religion. Each person is unique. Do not judge the person by your personal standards or beliefs.

CARING ABOUT CULTURE

In some Australian cultures, for many people, eye contact signals a good self-concept. It also shows openness, interest in others, attention, honesty and warmth. Lack of eye contact is often considered to indicate feelings such as:

- shyness
- lack of interest
- humility
- guilt
- embarrassment
- low self-esteem
- dishonesty.

In some Asian and Indigenous cultures, however, eye contact is considered to be impolite. It can also be an invasion of privacy. In certain Indian cultures, eye contact is avoided with people of higher or lower socioeconomic class. It can also have a special sexual meaning.

Direct eye contact is practised in Poland and Russia, but it is considered rude in Mexican and Vietnamese cultures. In the United Kingdom, staring is a part of good listening.

Blinking also has meaning. In Vietnam, it means that a message has been received. In the United Kingdom, it indicates understanding.

EFFECTS OF ILLNESS AND DISABILITY ON COMMUNICATION

People will often communicate to you how they feel about things by their behaviours and emotions. People do not choose to be sick or have disabilities. A **disability** is a lost, absent or impaired physical or mental function. Illness and injury have physical, psychological and social effects. Normal ADLs – work, driving, fixing meals, gardening and hobbies – may be difficult or impossible. Daily activities bring pleasure, worth and contact with others. When unable to perform them, people often feel angry, upset and useless. These feelings may increase if others must perform routine functions for them.

Some people feel alone and isolated after outliving their family and friends. Those who have disabilities or chronic illnesses may have many fears and concerns about residential care services. They may feel lonely and abandoned by family and friends. They may fear being dependent on strangers. Many may fear increasing loss of function. While some express their fears, others do not or cannot.

Anger is a common response to illness and disability and may be an indication of a stage of grief. Although the person may direct their anger at you, it is in fact the situation that they are angry at. Do not take that direction of anger personally. Always remember that the person may have very limited ways in which to display their anger and that the person who gives their care may be at times their only outlet for expression. You might have problems dealing with a person's anger. If the situation upsets you, ask your supervisor for help. Anger should be assessed by a qualified health professional to determine how best to assist the client in resolving the issues that are causing them to feel angry.

You can help the person feel safe, secure and loved. Take an extra minute to 'visit', to hold a hand or to give a hug, if that is culturally appropriate. Show that you are willing to help with personal needs. Respond promptly. Treat each person with respect and dignity. This is an essential component of holistic communication.

Sometimes the health team cannot prevent increasing loss of function. However, clients can be helped to maintain their optimal level of functioning. This is a person's highest potential for mental and physical performance. Encourage and support the person to be as independent as possible. Sometimes this is difficult as it takes more time, but it is vital in helping the client to maintain their self-esteem. Use initiative when managing your time. For example, allow a client to shower independently on a shower chair near their nurse call button, while you prepare their clothes for the day and gather equipment ready for the next task at hand. Instruct them to press the nurse call button when they are done. This will help to prevent you from falling behind in your workload and maintaining client independence. However, be mindful that safety comes first. Remember to always focus on the person's abilities, not their disabilities.

Older clients with a disability

A person may acquire a disability at any time from birth through to old age. Disease and injury are common causes. For example, children can develop hearing problems from ear infections. Head injuries from accidents can impair cognitive function. Spinal cord injuries can affect a person's movements. Loud noise from music and machinery is linked to hearing loss. The cause of disability or the age at onset does not matter. A person does not choose to have a disability. The person has to adjust to the disability. For many people, this can be long and hard. You will care for many people with disabilities. Your attitude is important for effective communication. People with disabilities have the same basic needs as you and everyone else. They feel joy, sorrow, happiness, sadness and other emotions, just like you and everyone else. They laugh, cry, have families, go to school, work, get married and pay bills like you and everyone else and they have the right to be treated with dignity and respect, just like you and everyone else.

Communicating with people who have certain disabilities is discussed in Chapter 15. However, common courtesies and manners (etiquette) apply to any person with a disability. Basic guidelines for communicating with people with disabilities and their families are outlined in Box 9.1.

BOX 9.1
Disability etiquette

Disability Etiquette List

- Treat adults as adults
- Ask if and what assistance may be needed.
- Hand grocery or other receipts to the individual who is paying the bill.
- Only ask questions about the person's disability if you know that person.
- Ask questions of the person with a disability and not of his/her companions.
- If help is required in a given situation, do not assist without asking first.
- Always respect the person's dignity, individuality and desire for independence.
- Refer to adults with a disability in the same way you would refer to any other adult.
- Never assume you know what assistance, if any, a person with a disability requires.
- Treat a person with a disability in the same manner and with the same respect and courtesy as you would anyone else.
- Speak directly to the person rather than through the companion, attendant or sign-language interpreter who may also be present.
- Never speak about the person as if they are invisible, can't understand what is being said or that they can't speak for themselves.
- Do not put people with a disability on a pedestal or talk to them in patronising terms as if their performance of normal, everyday activities was exceptional.
- Don't discourage children from asking questions about disabilities. Most people are not offended by questions children ask them about their disabilities or wheelchairs.

Do not assume:

- that a person with a disability is easily offended.
- that rejection of aid is meant as a personal affront.
- that a person with a disability either wants or requires assistance.
- a person who appears to have one kind of disability also has others.
- a disabled person is dissatisfied with his/her quality of life and is thus seeking pity.
- companions accompanying a person with a disability are there strictly to render service.
- upon acceptance of your help, that you know, without being told, what service to perform.
- that a person with a disability will be receptive to personal questions, particularly in a public setting.
- that when a person with a disability is in a public place, that they are being escorted by a caretaker, instead of travelling alone.
- that a person who does not appear disabled, or who uses assistive devices intermittently instead of all of the time, is faking or imagining their disability.

Disabled World (2021). Disability etiquette and awareness information. Online 14 September 2021. Available: www.disabled-world.com/disability/awareness/etiquette.php

CONSUMERS AND CLIENTS

Consumers of care services have often been treated as sick, dependent people. Promoting this 'sick role' in residential care reduces quality of life and creates dependency. The aged care team's focus is on improving the person's quality of life. You must help each person regain or maintain as much physical and mental function as possible. Ageing, like giving birth, is a normal process and not something that can be cured. Therefore, clients in aged care services are not 'patients' in a hospital, but aged people in their own homes. Care needs to be directed at maintaining optimal function in all clients.

Some clients with disabilities may have challenges communicating to you their needs. Never forget that there will always be some way to communicate appropriately with a person with a disability. If you find the communication process difficult ask for assistance.

Most clients are older. Some are alert and oriented. Often, they have chronic problems that prevent them from living alone or with their family and are related to mobility. Some are confused and disoriented and cannot care for themselves. Some clients are terminally ill (dying). They need special care to maintain comfort and make their last days as peaceful as possible. The manner in which they communicate to you their needs and the way that you interpret this communication will differ considerably between each group.

Confused and disoriented consumers

Some clients are mildly to severely confused and/or disoriented. Some simply have trouble finding the dining room or knowing the month and year. Others have more severe problems. For example, a man may think he is waiting for a train. The most severely disoriented clients do not know who they are.

Sometimes confusion and disorientation are temporary. This is especially true for new clients. Some will have Alzheimer's disease and other dementias. A person who has some confusion or dementia may become more confused and disoriented when moving into a residential care unit. It is essential that you use patience and remain calm until they settle in. Confusion can be caused by many things, some of which are reversible. Because of this, confusion needs to be assessed by healthcare professionals experienced in dealing with confusion and dementia. Do not accept that confusion is 'normal' without investigating other possibilities. Some other causes of confusion can be illness, medication interactions and urinary tract infections. Communicating with clients who have dementia requires considerable patience and skills. Refer to Chapter 14 for more detail on communicating with clients with dementia.

High care clients

Some people have very high care needs and may require assistance with all their activities of daily living (Fig. 9.7). They may also be confused and disoriented. Therefore, they cannot meet many or any of their own needs and may not

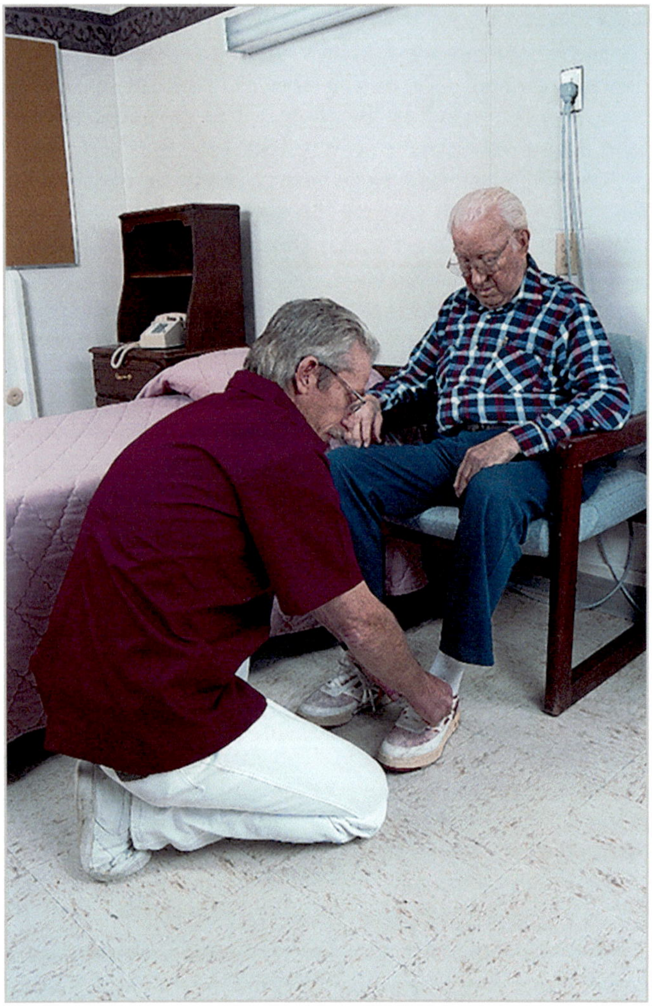

Fig. 9.7
This older man needs the services of a residential care service.

be able to verbally express what they need or want. Never assume that because a client cannot communicate with you, they do not understand what is being said. The health team must keep them clean, safe and comfortable. You must treat the person with respect and compassion. Touch, massage, music and television may provide comfort and ease their loneliness and are also important communication tools.

Clients with mental illnesses

Some people have problems coping or adjusting to stress. Their behaviour and functioning are affected. In severe cases, self-care and independent living are impaired. Some have physical and mental illnesses. If you are unsure what the person is trying to get you to understand, ask your supervisor or more experienced colleague for help. You will find more details about caring for a person with a mental illness in Chapter 16.

Clients who are terminally ill

A terminally ill person is in the final stages of their life. They may have advanced cancer, or liver, kidney, respiratory or heart disease. Care of terminally ill people is called *palliative care*. Palliative care is aimed at maintaining quality of their life. The care provided will depend on the illness and must be based on individual needs. Some people are alert and oriented; others are comatose. **Comatose** means being unable to respond to verbal stimuli. More details of working and communicating with a comatose person are included later in this chapter.

COMMUNICATION AND CHALLENGING BEHAVIOURS

Historically, many people have accepted illness and loss of physical function as part of normal ageing. However, in residential care services, a large proportion of the clients will be adapting to changes in their life that may be difficult for them to accept. They may demonstrate some of the behaviours discussed below. These behaviours may be new, or they may be a part of the client's personality. Behaviours will often convey something the person wishes to communicate.

Anger

Anger is a common emotion. Causes include fear, pain, dying and death, loss of function and losing control of one's health and life. Anger may be a symptom of underlying behavioural or physical problems. Some people are generally angry. Anger is communicated verbally and non-verbally. Verbal outbursts, shouting, raised voices and rapid speech are common. Some people are silent, while others are uncooperative. They may refuse to answer questions. Non-verbal signs include rapid movements, pacing, distressed facial expressions, clenched fists and a reddened face. Glaring and getting close to you when speaking are other signs. Violent behaviours can occur as a result of anger and aggression management may need to be implemented in such cases.

Demanding behaviour

Some clients will demand much of your time and will seem to be always seeking your attention. Efforts to please the person may be met with criticism – nothing seems to please the person. Often people develop demanding behaviours as a result of loss of independence and control over their life and health. When people have needs that are not met, they may learn that demanding is one way of getting their needs met.

Sometimes a person wants care at a certain time and in a certain way. That, in itself, is not demanding behaviour. Clients have the right to express their care choices. However, there may be times when the caregiver is unable to provide the client with the care they request. Explain to the client why you are unable to meet their request and communicate their request to your supervisor or nurse to see if the request can be met at a future time.

Self-centred behaviour

People who are ill have with a disability may sometimes focus all their attention on their own needs. They may ignore the needs of others. Frequent demands for time and attention are made. They may become impatient if their needs are not met first.

Aggressive behaviour

A person may swear, bite, hit, pinch, scratch or kick. Causes of this behaviour include fear, anger, pain and dementia. Most aggressive behaviours can be minimised by the carer's behaviour. You need to protect the person, others and yourself from harm.

Withdrawal

When a person withdraws, they choose to have little or no contact with their family, friends and staff. They may spend most of the time in their room, not involved in social events or group activities. Withdrawal may signal physical illness or depression. Some people are generally not social and simply prefer to be alone.

Inappropriate sexual behaviour

Some people make inappropriate sexual remarks or may touch other clients or staff. Some disrobe or masturbate in public. These behaviours may be deliberate, or may be due to disease, confusion, dementia or the side effects of medications.

Although a person's behaviour may be unpleasant, you should not avoid the person or lose control. What you can do is attempt to understand why the person is behaving in this manner and implement strategies to minimise these behaviours. Good communication is important between the client and nursing staff, as well as between members of the healthcare team. Inappropriate behaviour should be addressed in the care plan (Box 9.2).

BOX 9.2
Dealing with behaviour issues

- Recognise situations that are frustrating and frightening for the client. Put yourself in their position. How would you feel? How would you want to be treated?
- Treat the person with dignity and respect.
- Answer questions clearly and thoroughly. Ask the nurse to answer questions you cannot answer.
- Keep the person informed. Tell them what you are going to do and when.
- Do not keep the person waiting. Answer nurse call buzzers promptly. If you tell the person that you will do something, do it promptly.
- Explain the reason for long waits. Ask if you can get or do something to increase the person's comfort.
- Stay calm and professional if the person is angry or hostile. Often the person is not angry at you, but is angry with another person or with the situation.
- Do not argue with the person.
- Listen and use silence. The person may feel better if able to express his or her feelings.
- Protect yourself from violent behaviour.
- Report the person's behaviour to the nurse. Discuss how you should deal with the person.

The client who is comatose

The client who is comatose is unconscious. They cannot respond to others, but often they can hear and feel touch and pain. Often pain is shown by grimacing or groaning. Promptly report any sign of discomfort to the nurse. Medications for pain relief are important, as is the care you give. Turning and positioning, gentle back rubs and touch may promote comfort and peace. You must always assume that the person hears and understands what you are saying. You need to use touch and give care gently. You will be communicating to a comatose client through your care activities. Make sure that you treat them with respect and dignity and speak to them during their care. Practise the following measures to communicate and care for people who are comatose:

- Knock before entering the person's room.
- Tell the person your name, the time and the place every time you enter the room.
- Follow the care plan to give care on the same schedule every day.
- Explain to the person what you are going to do.
- Explain care measures step-by-step as you are doing them.
- Tell the person when you are finishing care.
- Use touch to communicate care, concern and comfort.
- Tell the person what time you will be back to check on him or her.
- Tell the person when you are leaving the room.

Remember that you may also be caring for the client's family and friends, and that they may need to be included in planning the client's care. Many centres work with hospice programs. The goal is to provide quality care to those who are dying.

FAMILY AND FRIENDS

Communication does not stop with the person you are caring for. You need to ensure that you communicate well with their family and friends. Their knowledge of the person will often help communicate to you a number of specific care needs. Family and friends can help meet the person's safety and security, love and belonging and self-esteem needs. They can offer support and comfort and can lessen loneliness. Some also help with the person's care. This helps both the family and the person. The family know they are doing something to help the person and the person's physical and emotional needs are met. The presence or absence of family members or friends affects the person's quality of life.

The person has the right to visit with family and friends in private and without unnecessary interruptions (Fig. 9.8). If you need to give care while visitors are present, protect the person's right to privacy. Do not expose their body in front of visitors. Politely ask the visitors to leave the room and show them where to wait. Politely tell them when they can return. A partner or close family member may want to help you. If the client consents, you may allow that person to stay.

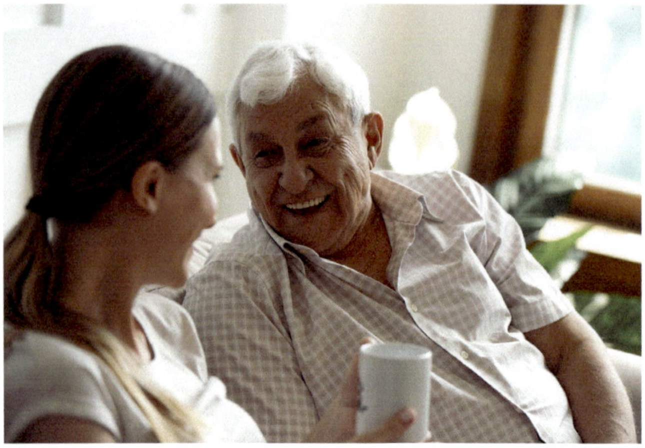

Fig. 9.8
A client is visited by a member of his family.

Treat family and visitors with courtesy and respect. They may have concerns about the person's condition and care. They need support and understanding. However, do not discuss the person's condition with them. Refer any questions to the nurse.

FOCUS ON COMPLEMENTARY THERAPIES

Many services are beginning to recognise the positive effects that music and aromatherapy have on reducing stress levels. Relaxing or peaceful music has been proven to reduce stress and to help avoid aggressive behaviours. Some services may even employ a qualified aromatherapist. This person will then make up a blend of essential oils that is used in massage and/or as an inhalation, which helps meet the needs of the individual.

QUALITY OF LIFE

The client is the most important person in the residential care service. Each person has physical, psychological, social, emotional and spiritual needs. To provide quality care, you must know and respect the whole person. You will care for people from different cultures and religions. Learn as much as you can about a person's religious and cultural beliefs and practices. This will help you to understand the person and give the best possible care. Illness and disability affect quality of life. Normal tasks and activities that bring pleasure and contact with others may be difficult or impossible. People often feel angry, frustrated and useless. You can help by treating each person with dignity and respect. You can also help each person reach or maintain his or her optimal level of functioning. Always focus on the person's abilities. Do not focus on disabilities. Family and visitors are important to the person. They can offer support and comfort and enhance the person's quality of life. Always treat them with respect.

CASE STUDY

Within a dementia unit, it is common to have clients who speak a number of languages. A common problem for clients with English as their second or third language is that, as dementia symptoms progress, the person loses their understanding of English. This does not just occur for immigrants, but also for Indigenous Australians, who may speak a number of languages other than English. Within one centre, staff were having some communication problems with Mrs Dimitri, who emigrated to Australia at the end of World War II from Russia with her husband. Mrs Dimitri was becoming increasingly agitated and aggressive towards staff. To help Mrs Dimitri, staff introduced a number of strategies:

- They obtained a list of key Russian terms written phonetically for staff to use.
- With the support of Mrs Dimitri's family, they introduced items from Mrs Dimitri's younger life to trigger memories.
- Visits from family and friends were increased, particularly those who spoke Russian.
- When the staff used communication skills relevant to Mrs Dimitri's needs, she became more settled and her care improved considerably.

ACCREDITATION

You are working in residential or home care and accreditors are at your service. Can you answer the following questions?

- What strategies do you use to communicate with a consumer with diverse needs, such as a person from a non-English speaking background, or a client with dementia that has cognitive impairment?
- You are caring for a consumer with a hearing and/or vision impairment. How would you ensure clear communication with this consumer?
- What are some communication aids that might be of help in your role as a carer?

REVIEW QUESTIONS

Circle the BEST answer:

1 Which of the following are forms of communication?
  a Touch
  b Speech
  c Writing
  d All of the above

2 The communication process involves which of the following?
  a A sender, a message and a receiver
  b A sender, an interpreter and a receiver
  c A message, writing implements and a carrier
  d None of the above

3 When assisting someone with a disability, which of the following should you do?
  a Always check with any caregiver present what you should do
  b Offer assistance based on your observations and assessment
  c Ask the person with the disability how you can assist them
  d Give the assistance you believe is needed regardless of what the person with a disability says

4 Holism refers to which of the following?
  a Understanding that the person has a hole or gap in their needs
  b Considering the person as a complete being, even if they have lost a body part
  c Considering that the person is complete despite requiring complex care
  d Understanding that the person has physical, social, psychological, emotional and spiritual parts

5 A need is described best as which of the following, according to Maslow?
  a something that a person really wants
  b a desire
  c an essential aspect for maintaining life and wellbeing
  d an essential aspect for staying alive physiologically

6 You should let a family member stay with you when attending care if:
  a they are trained health professionals
  b the client gives consent
  c you need assistance with caring
  d they are women

7 Which of the following are barriers to communication?
  a Cultural differences
  b Giving your opinion
  c Illness or disability
  d All of the above

Circle T if the statement is true or F if the statement if false:

8 T / F An open-ended question requires more than a 'yes' or 'no' answer

9 T / F The body language of the person speaking is not important

10 T / F A comatose or unconscious person is usually unable to hear what is happening

Answers to these questions are on p. 454.

Further reading

Agingcare (2020). 10 tips for communicating with a senior. Online April 2020. Available: www.agingcare.com

Disabled World (2021). Disability etiquette and awareness information. Online 14 September 2021. Available: www.disabled-world.com/disability/awareness/etiquette.php

Office for Disability Issues (NZ) (n.d.). Disability Etiquette. Online 14 September 2021. Available: www.odi.govt.nz/assets/uploads/Disability-Etiquette-in-Word.pdf

Simply Psychology (2021). Maslow's Hierarchy of Needs. Online 13 March 2021. Available: www.simplypsychology.org/maslow.html

ThoughtCo (2021). The basic elements of the communication process. Online 13 March 2021. Available: www.thoughtco.com/what-is-communication-process-1689767

CHAPTER 10
The human body in health and disease

By Karen Scott

AFTER READING THIS CHAPTER, YOU SHOULD BE ABLE TO:

- define the key terms listed in this chapter
- define some common anatomical terms
- describe the basic structure of a cell and how cells divide
- list four types of tissue
- identify the key structures of each body system
- list the functions of each body system
- identify the changes in each system as it ages
- identify the common condition for each system and how it impacts on each of these systems.

Key terms

abducted: To draw away from the midline of the body

aphasia: The inability (*a*) to speak (*phasia*)

arteries: Blood vessels that carry blood away from the heart

arthritis: Joint (*arthr*) inflammation (*itis*)

atelectasis: A complete or partial collapse of a lung or lobe of a lung

Braille: A tactile writing and reading system that uses raised dots; used by blind and vision-impaired people

capillaries: Tiny blood vessels; food, oxygen and other substances pass from the capillaries to the cells

cell: The basic unit of body structure

central nervous system (CNS): Part of the nervous system, which controls, directs and coordinates body functions; consists of the brain and spinal cord

chromosomes: Thread-like structures within a cell that carry genes and transmit hereditary information

closed fracture (simple fracture): When a bone is broken but the skin remains intact

digestion: The process of physically and chemically breaking down food so that it can be absorbed for use by the cells

dysphagia: Difficulty swallowing

dyspnoea: When difficult, laboured or painful breathing occurs with activity

expressive aphasia: Difficulty expressing or sending out thoughts; thinking is clear

expressive–receptive aphasia: To have both expressive and receptive aphasia – difficulty expressing thoughts and receiving information

Fowler's position (high Fowler's): The head of the bed or chair is raised to 45–60 degrees; the patient sits in an upright position with knees slightly elevated

fracture: A broken bone. Tissues around the fracture (muscles, blood vessels, nerves and tendons) are injured

gangrene: A condition in which there is death of tissue, caused by infection, injuries and circulatory disorders

haemoglobin: The substance in red blood cells that carries oxygen and gives blood its colour

hemiplegia: Paralysis on one side of the body

hormone: A chemical substance secreted by the glands into the bloodstream

hyperglycaemia: High (*hyper*) sugar (*glyc*) in the blood (*aemia*)

hypoglycaemia: Low (*hypo*) sugar (*glyc*) in the blood (*aemia*)

immunity: Protection against a certain disease

metabolism: The burning of food for heat and energy by the cells

open fracture (compound fracture): When a broken bone has come through the skin

organ: A group of tissues with the same function

organelles: Tiny structures in the cell that perform specialised functions

paraplegia: Paralysis from the waist down; cervical injuries cause loss of function to the arms, chest and below the chest

peripheral nervous system: Part of the nervous system that controls, directs and coordinates body functions; involves nerves throughout the body

peristalsis: Involuntary muscle contractions in the digestive system that move food through the alimentary canal

presbyopia: Age-related far-sightedness

receptive aphasia: Difficulty receiving information; the person has trouble understanding what is said or read

respiration: The process of supplying the cells with oxygen and removing carbon dioxide from them

rheumatoid arthritis (RA): An inflammatory disease that causes joint pain, swelling and stiffness

semi-Fowler's position (semi-upright): The head of the bed is raised to 30–45 degrees; the patient reclines with knees either straight or slightly bent

stroke: A cardiovascular disease affecting the blood vessels that supply blood to the brain

system: Organs that work together to perform special functions

tetraplegia: (formerly quadriplegia) Paralysis of both arms and legs

tinnitus: Ringing in the ears

tissue: A group of cells with similar functions

vein: A blood vessel that carries blood back to the heart

vertigo: Dizziness

This chapter will cover the basic anatomy and physiology of the ten systems, together with the ageing processes that occur within each system. The systems covered in this chapter include integumentary, nervous, musculoskeletal, cardiovascular, respiratory, digestive, urinary, reproductive, endocrine and immune systems. Selected conditions that affect each of the systems will be covered, together with the caring considerations required for these conditions.

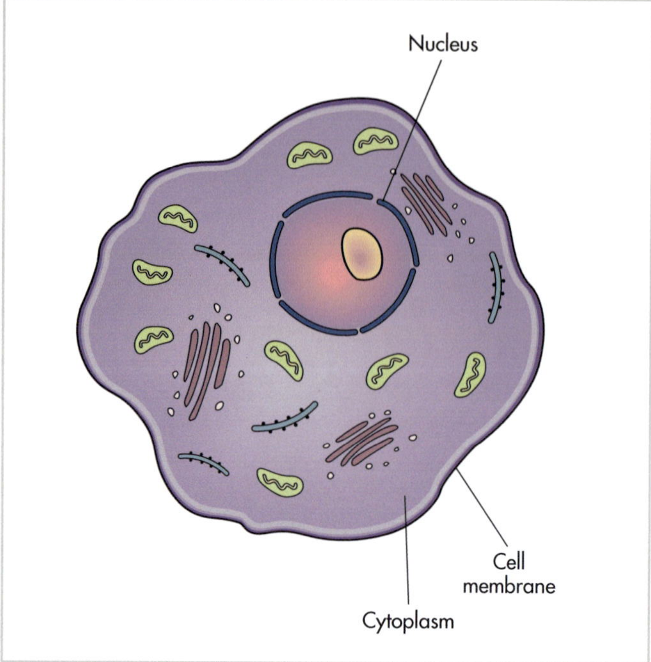

Fig. 10.1
Parts of a cell.

INTRODUCTION: CELLS, TISSUE AND ORGANS

When working with people, whether young or old, you need a basic understanding of the structure of the human body and how it works. By understanding the body's normal functions, from the smallest cell in the body to the body as a whole, you can begin to understand what happens to the human body during illness, disease or injury. This knowledge can then be used to promote comfort, provide education and work within the healthcare team to provide holistic support and care. It will also help you to understand signs, symptoms and the reasons for care and procedures.

The human body can be classified into six different levels of organisation. These include the chemical, cellular, tissue, organ, organ system and whole body systems.

The chemical level

The chemical level of organisation of the human body is the chemistry that makes up the different components that contribute to the cellular level. This level of organisation involves the elements and compounds that make up the cells. Four basic elements make up the cell: carbon (C), hydrogen (H), oxygen (O) and nitrogen (N).

The cellular level

The **cell** is the smallest living unit within the human body. Each cell has the same basic structure: a cell membrane, cytoplasm, nucleus and **organelles**. The function, size and shape of cells differ within different tissue types of the human body. The structure of the cell is related to the functional characteristics of that cell (for example, ciliated respiratory cells contain cilia to help remove debris; red blood cells contain a large amount of haemoglobin and are doughnut shaped – this allows for the transport of oxygen around the body). Cells are so small that a microscope is needed to view them. Cells need nutrients, water and oxygen to live and perform their functions.

The cell and its structures are shown in Fig. 10.1. The *cell membrane* is the outer covering that encloses the cell and helps it hold its shape. The *nucleus* is the control centre of the cell and directs cellular activity. The *cytoplasm* surrounds the nucleus and contains many smaller structures called organelles that perform several different functions within the cell and are essential to its survival. Protoplasm means 'living substance'. It refers to all the structures, substances and water within the cell. Protoplasm is a semiliquid substance much like the white of an egg.

Chromosomes are thread-like structures within the nucleus. Each human cell has 46 chromosomes. Chromosomes contain genes. Genes control the physical and chemical traits inherited by children from their parents, including height, eye colour and skin colour.

The nucleus controls cell reproduction. Each cell reproduces by duplicating all its genetic material, organelles and membrane structures, and then divides into two daughter cells. The process of cell division is called mitosis, which is important for growth and repair of body tissues (Fig. 10.2). Before mitosis begins, the genetic material is duplicated. As the cells enter mitosis, the chromosomes arrange themselves into pairs, and as the cell begins to divide into two, the chromosomes are pulled in half and each cell gets each half of the genetic material, so the two new daughter cells are identical. Each of the new daughter cells contains all of the genetic material, membranes and organelles as the original parent cell from which it was produced. Mistakes can happen during cell division, resulting in congenital abnormalities. Inherited problems can also make humans susceptible to disease. This is an area in which much medical research is occurring, with the potential to cure many diseases in the future.

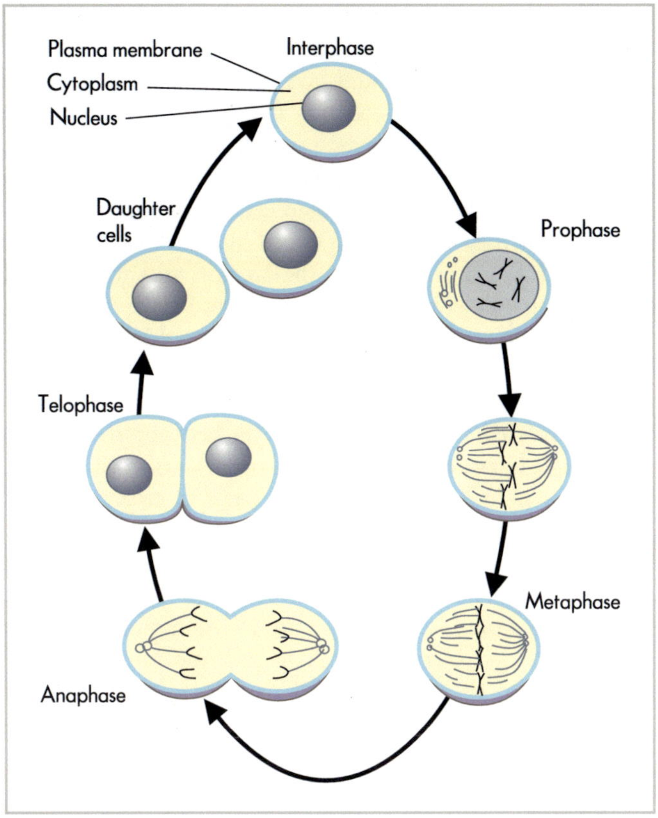

Fig. 10.2
Cell division.

The main goal of cell division is to produce two daughter cells that are identical to the one parent (starting) cell. This process is quite complex and involves a number of steps:

1 Interphase: DNA is replicated and doubled to start the process of creating two new cells.
2 Prophase: DNA molecules condense and the nuclear membrane starts to disappear.
3 Metaphase: Chromosomes are attached to specialised fibres (called spindle fibres) and are arranged along the centre of the cell in preparation for splitting the DNA material into two daughter cells.
4 Anaphase: The DNA starts to be separated to either end of the cell for preparation into two cells.
5 Telophase: Chromosomes are at either side of the cells, a nucleus membrane forms around both sets of genetic material. It is the first point in mitosis where the development of two new cells can be seen.
6 New daughter cells: The plasma membranes form around the two cells and then separate into two identical daughter cells.

There are other important organelles located in the cytoplasm of the cell; these include the mitochondria and the ribosomes. The mitochondria play an important role in producing adenosine triphosphate (ATP), an important energy molecule; ribosomes are important for synthesising (forming) proteins.

Tissues

Cells are the body's building blocks. Groups of cells with similar functions combine to form **tissues**. The body has four basic types of tissue:

1 *Epithelial tissue* – covers internal and external body surfaces. This tissue helps with protection, absorption, excretion, secretion and filtration. Tissue that lines the nose, mouth, respiratory tract, stomach and intestines is epithelial tissue. So are the skin, hair, nails and glands.
2 *Connective tissue* – anchors, connects and supports other body tissues and is the most abundant tissue in the body. This tissue supports, protects, binds and insulates the body, as well as transports substances around the body. Connective tissue is found in every part of the body. Bones, tendons, ligaments and cartilage are connective tissue. Blood is a form of connective tissue.
3 *Muscle tissue* – allows the body to move by stretching and contracting. The three types of muscle – skeletal, smooth and cardiac – are vital to the body's movement.
4 *Nerve tissue* – receives and carries impulses to the brain and back to body parts. Tissue includes the brain and nerves throughout the body.

Organs

Groups of tissues form **organs**. Organs perform numerous different biological functions. Examples of organs are the heart, brain, liver, lungs and kidneys. An organ will usually function together with organ systems to carry out important biological processes that keep the body in a constant homeostatic environment.

Organ system

Systems are formed by groups of organs working together to perform special functions (Fig. 10.3). For example, the heart – an organ – is part of the cardiovascular system.

WHOLE BODY SYSTEM

This chapter will examine:

- the basic anatomy and physiology of the 12 different organ systems of the human body
- the impact of ageing on each of the organ systems
- the basic diseases/conditions that impact on the system in the older population
- specific considerations when caring for an individual with the disease.

THE INTEGUMENTARY SYSTEM

The integumentary system consists of the skin, hair and nails, and is the largest body system. *Integument* means 'covering'. The skin is the body's natural covering and is critical to protecting the body against infection. Skin is made up of epithelial, connective and nerve tissue. It also

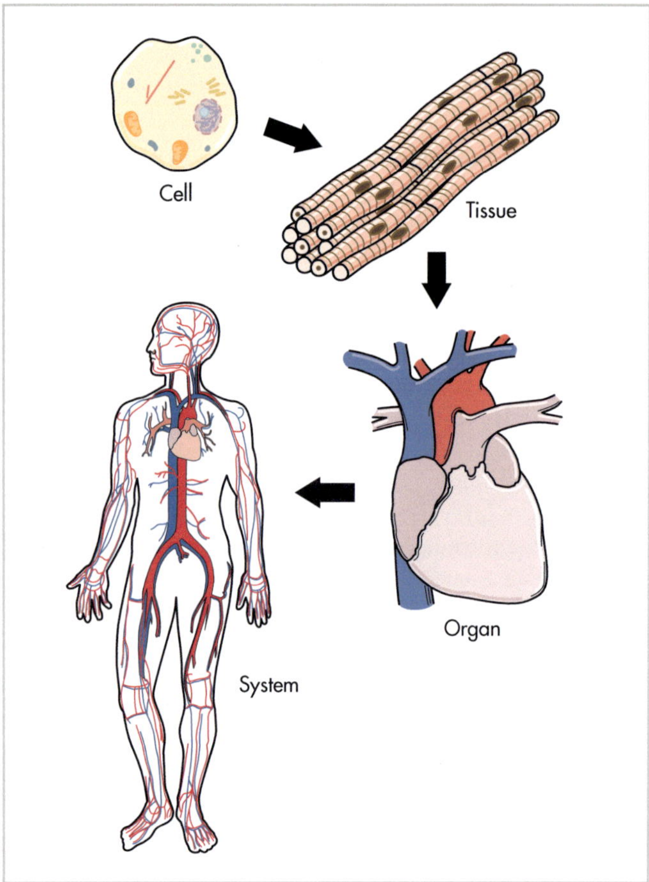

Fig. 10.3
Organisation of the body.

has oil and sweat glands. There are three skin layers: the epidermis, dermis and hypodermis.

- The *epidermis* is the outer layer and is composed of five individual layers (including the germinative or base layer, *stratum spinulosum*, *stratum granulosum*, *stratum lucidum* and *stratum corneum*) (Fig. 10.4). It contains living and dead cells. The dead cells were once deeper in the epidermis. They were pushed outwards as other cells divided. Dead cells constantly flake off and are replaced by living cells. Living cells also die and flake off. Living cells of the epidermis contain pigment which gives skin its colour. The epidermis has no blood vessels and few nerve endings.
- The *dermis* is the intermediate layer between the epidermis and hypodermis. It is made up of connective tissue, which includes blood vessels, nerves, sweat and oil glands, and hair roots are found in the dermis.
- The *hypodermis* (*subcutaneous fatty tissue*) is the thickest layer of the skin and is composed of adipose tissue, which is stored with triglycerides. The hypodermis acts as an energy reserve, as well as an important structural mechanism by anchoring the dermis. It also conserves body heat by insulating the body and helps protect the organs.

Important cells and structures of the integumentary system

There are several specialised cells in the integumentary system, including keratinocytes, melanocytes and Langerhans cells.

- *Keratinocytes:* Ninety per cent of the cell types in the epidermis are keratinocytes. They are found in the basal

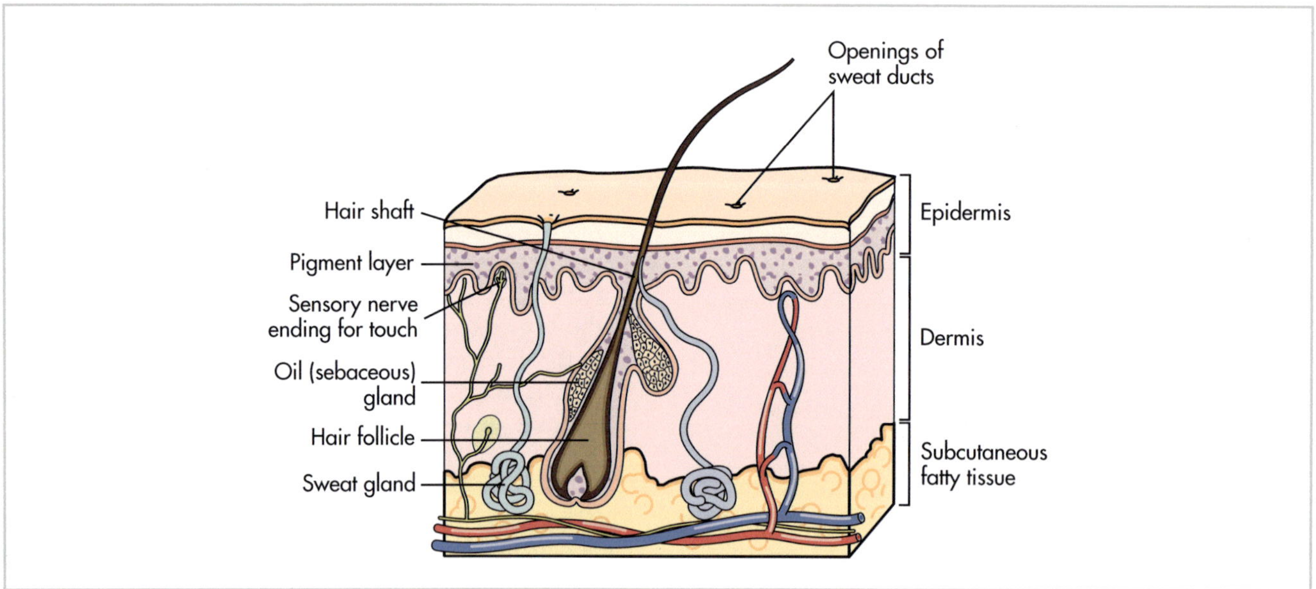

Fig. 10.4
Layers of the skin.

cell layer. The primary function of these cells is to form a protective barrier against the invasion of microorganisms such as bacteria, viruses, fungi and parasites.

- *Melanocytes:* Melanin-producing cells located at the bottom of the skin's (basal layer) epidermis; responsible for skin colour. These cells make up 5–10 per cent of the cells of the epidermis. Melanin production in these cells is stimulated by sunlight and acts as a protective agent by converting the UV radiation to heat – thus preventing damage caused by UV radiation.
- *Langerhans cells:* Specialised cells that are a part of the immune system. These are found in all layers of the integumentary system and mucosa. They are usually found in the spinulosum layer of the epidermis, as they are located close to the external surface of the epidermis.

Oil and sweat glands, hair and nails are skin appendages: The entire body, except for the palms of the hands and soles of the feet, is covered with hair. Hair in the nose, eyes and ears protects these organs from dust, insects and other foreign objects. Nails protect the tips of fingers and toes and help fingers pick up and handle small objects.

Sweat glands help the body regulate temperature. Sweat consists of water, salt and a small amount of wastes and is secreted through pores in the skin. As sweat evaporates, this cools the body. Sebaceous glands lie near hair shafts and secrete an oily substance, sebum (composed of triglycerides, oils, wax and squalene), into the space near the hair shaft. Sebum travels to the skin surface, where it prevents the hair from drying out and becoming damaged. This gives hair its shiny appearance. It also helps keep the skin moist and provides an antimicrobial function.

Summary of skin function

- It is the protective covering of the body.
- It prevents bacteria and other substances from entering the body.
- It prevents excessive amounts of water from leaving the body.
- It helps to synthesise vitamin D.
- It removes waste through sweat.
- It protects the organs from injury.
- Nerve endings in the skin sense both pleasant and unpleasant stimulation. There are nerve endings over the entire body. The body senses cold, pain, touch and pressure to protect the body from injury.
- It helps regulate body temperature. Blood vessels dilate (widen) when the temperature outside the body is high. More blood is brought to the body surface for cooling during evaporation. When blood vessels constrict (narrow), the body retains heat because less blood reaches the skin.

AGEING OF THE INTEGUMENTARY SYSTEM

Ageing affects all aspects of the integumentary system. The changes in cellular function, activity and number of cells all contribute to the changes in the integumentary system as an individual gets older. The following section summarises the major changes in the integumentary system as it matures, and briefly describes the observed effects due to the ageing processes.

- *Germinative cell (base layer of the epidermis) activity declines:* The decline in activity of these cells means that the connection between the epidermis and dermis becomes weakened. This contributes to the increased likelihood of skin tears and infections. As the germinative layer is not replenishing the outer layer of the epidermis, it does not provide physical protection.
- *Langerhans cells decrease:* The number of immune cells present in the skin decreases by about 50 per cent. This decreases the ability of the immune system to detect pathogens, which makes the body more susceptible to infection and further skin damage.
- *Melanocyte activity declines:* Since the role of melanocytes are to protect the body from UV damage, a decline in the function of these cells leads to a greater risk of sunburn and skin cancer.
- *Glandular activity declines:* The amount of sebum produced declines, which contributes to the skin becoming dry and scaly. The activity of sweat glands decreases; thus, the body has reduced perspiration and cannot lose heat as it once could. This leaves the older person at greater risk of overheating in hot climates.
- *Fibroblast cell activity declines:* These cells are responsible for the production and distribution of collagen and elastin, which give skin its strength and elasticity and contribute to the structural integrity and appearance of the skin. As the activity of these cells decline, the amount and quality of collagen and elastin decreases. This contributes to the physical signs of ageing: skin thinning, sagging, folds, lines and wrinkles.
- *Vitamin D_3 production decreases:* The amount of vitamin D_3 synthesised by the integumentary system declines by 75 per cent as the individual ages. Vitamin D_3 plays an important role in maintaining blood levels of calcium and phosphorus, critical for bone strength and muscle function. A decline in these minerals leads to loss of bone strength and muscle weakness.
- *Blood flow and sensory nerves in the dermis decline:* Reduced blood flow to the skin makes the integumentary system feel cold; this in turn stimulates the thermoreceptors in the skin, making the person feel cold, even though the external environment may be very hot. The body is therefore receiving confused signals from the integumentary system about the external temperature. In addition to this effect, the impaired sweat function also reduces the person's ability to lose body heat. If they are in a hot environment where they are unable to lose body heat and have the sensation of cold when it is in fact hot, their body temperature can become dangerously high.
- *Hair follicles decline:* The follicles stop functioning or produce hairs that have a thinner or finer appearance. In

conjunction with this effect, the reduced melanocyte activity gives the hairs a grey or white coloured appearance – it is the melanin that gives hair its colour.

- *Dermis size decreases:* The elastic fibre network decreases in size, thus contributing to weaker, less resilient, sagging and wrinkling skin. The physical changes are more pronounced in areas that have been exposed to ultraviolet radiation from the sun. The loss of fatty tissue in the dermis also makes the person more sensitive to cold environments.
- *Skin repair declines:* The repair process in the skin declines, which increases the risk of recurring infection. This is also in part due to reduced blood flow to the skin and decline in activity of the Langerhans cells. Brown spots appear on the skin. These are called 'age spots' or 'liver spots'. They are common on the wrists and hands.

CARING FOR AN AGEING INTEGUMENTARY SYSTEM

There are several factors to be considered when caring for the skin of an older person:

- Loss of the skin's fatty layer makes the person more sensitive to cold, so they should be protected from draughts and extreme cold. Methods include jumpers, lap blankets and adjustment of air conditioning or heater systems to the client's comfort.
- Dry skin causes itching and is easily damaged. A shower or bath twice a week is usually enough for hygiene. Partial baths are taken at other times. Soap-free cleanser or pH neutral soaps are used, with soaps best avoided as they may dry the skin. Lotions, oils and creams can prevent drying and itching. Powder is not recommended. Deodorants are not usually needed, as sweat gland secretion is decreased.
- The nails become thick and tough, and the feet usually have poor circulation. A nick or cut can cause a serious infection. For diabetics, a podiatrist will usually be in charge of ensuring safe care of the feet.
- Thinning of hair occurs on the head, in the pubic area and under the arms. Women and men may choose to wear wigs, or may colour their hair to cover the greying. The hair becomes drier because of reduced scalp oil. Brushing the hair promotes circulation and oil production. Frequency of shampooing will depend on personal choice, although usually it decreases with age. It is done as needed for hygiene and comfort.

Skin disorders

Skin disorders increase with age due to a decline in Langerhans cell, fibroblast and melanocyte activity. They rarely cause death if treated early; however, it is important to note that the risk of skin cancers increases as the individual ages; this is most likely due to a decline in melanocyte activity (cells that product us from UV damage) and decline of Langerhans cell activity (the cells that detect and destroy pathogens in the integumentary system).

The following section explores several common conditions that impact on the integumentary system.

- *Seborrhoeic keratosis* is a wart type of lesion of the skin. The lesion looks like a greasy, yellowish or brownish wart. (*Seborrhoeic* comes from *sebum*, which means 'sweat'. *Kerat* means 'horny', *osis* means 'condition of'.)
- *Senile (or solar) keratosis* is a premalignant condition of thick, scaly or crusty patches of skin (Fig. 10.5).

Psoriasis

Psoriasis is a chronic condition characterised by red patches covered with thick, dry, silvery scales (Fig. 10.6). The lesions can occur anywhere on the body, but most commonly appear on the elbow, knees and scalp. The condition may be *exacerbated* (made worse) by stress, infection, dryness and some medications. Infection and dryness of the integumentary system increase with age, so it is common for this

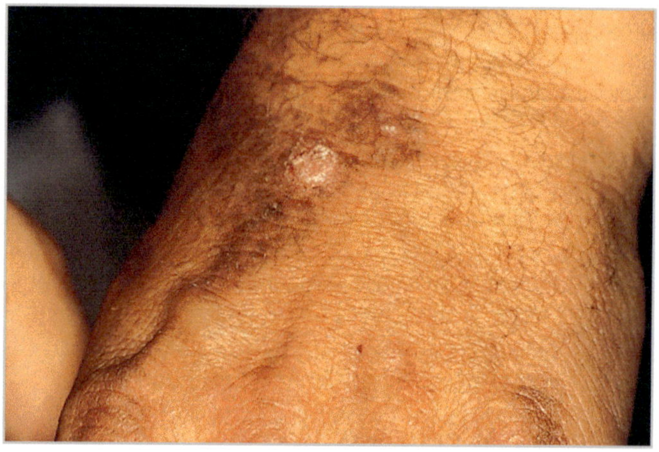

Fig. 10.5
Senile or solar keratosis.
Shows the thick, scaly or crusty patches of skin.

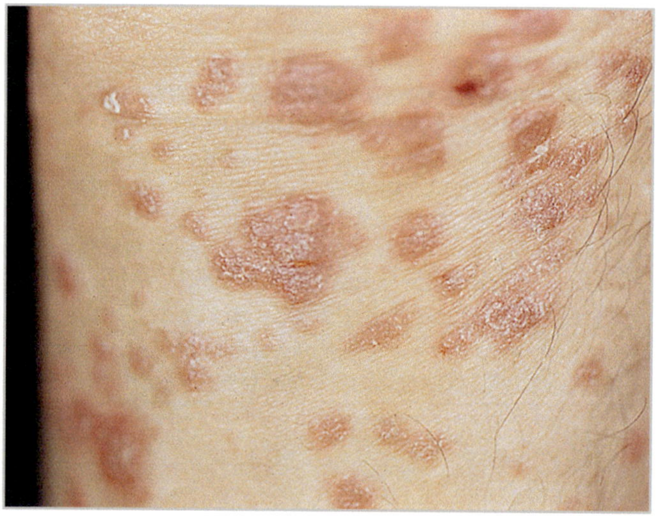

Fig. 10.6
Psoriasis lesions.

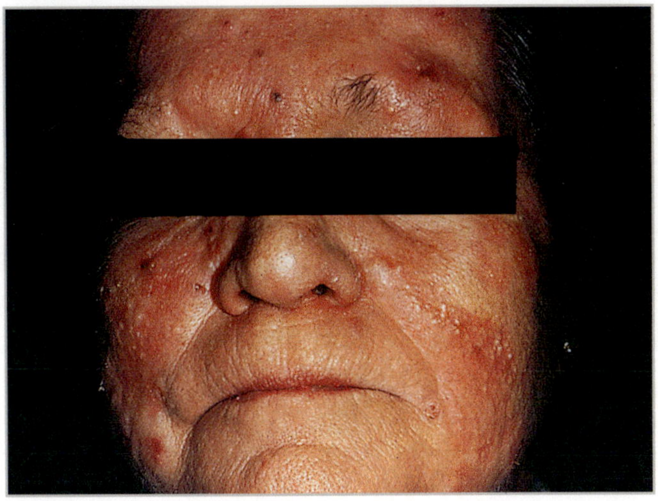

Fig. 10.7
Rosacea.

condition to get worse as the individual ages. Treatment is difficult but aims to slow down the growth of cells. Topical *corticosteroid therapies* are used and it is also important to keep the skin moist and prevent it from becoming dry.

Rosacea

Rosacea is a chronic skin disorder that commonly affects the forehead, nose, cheekbones and chin (Fig. 10.7). The capillaries at the surface of the skin are involved and because they become weaker with age, they can cause blotchy red skin with small bumps and sometimes pimples. The redness that takes place in rosacea can come and go, but it may be permanent if the blood vessels dilate. This flushing is caused by increased blood flow to the surface due to temporary dilation of the capillary blood vessels. As the condition progresses, the flushing can spread across the face. This may take several years. Treatment involves identifying the underlying triggers of the condition and avoiding them if possible. There can be many triggers, including hot and cold temperatures, wind, hot drinks, caffeine, exercise, spicy foods, alcohol and medications that cause flushing.

THE MUSCULOSKELETAL SYSTEM

The musculoskeletal system provides the framework for the body. It allows the body to move, provides protection and provides it with its shape.

Bones

The human body has 206 bones (Fig. 10.8). There are four types of bones:

- *Long bones* bear the weight of the body; for example, leg bones.
- *Short bones* allow skill and ease in movement; for example, bones in the wrists, fingers, ankles and toes.
- *Flat bones* protect the organs. Such bones include the ribs, skull, pelvic bones and shoulder blades.

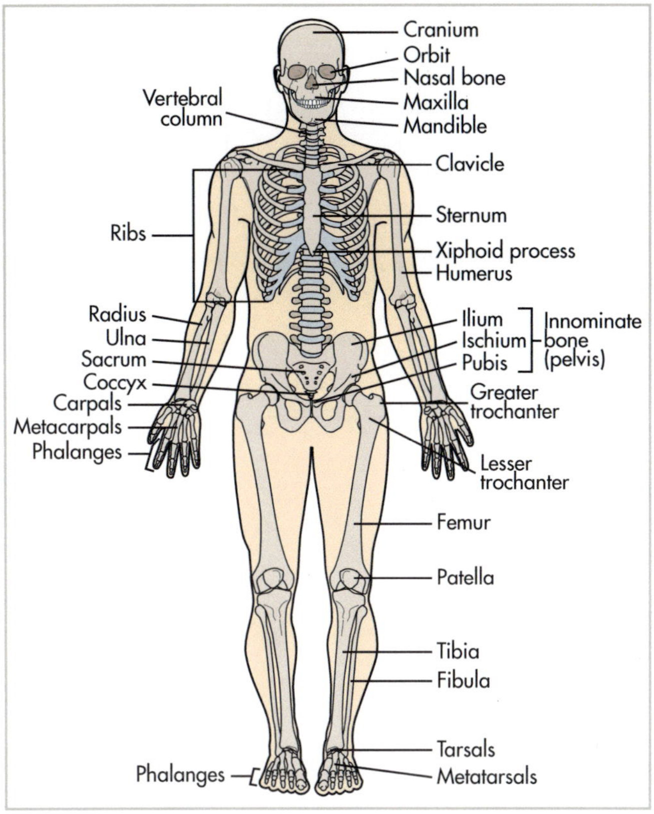

Fig. 10.8
Bones of the body.

- *Irregular bones* are the vertebrae in the spinal column. They allow various degrees of movement and flexibility.

Bones are hard, rigid structures made up of living cells. They are covered by a membrane called the *periosteum*. The periosteum contains blood vessels that supply bone cells with oxygen and food. Inside the hollow centres of bones is a substance called *bone marrow*. Blood cells are manufactured in the bone marrow.

Bones have several functions:

- *support* – bones provide a framework that supports the body and protects the body's soft organs
- *protection* – bones protect body organs, such as the heart, lungs and brain
- movement – skeletal muscles and bones work together to allow us to walk and move in different ways
- *storage* – bones store minerals, such as calcium, which can be released into the body when needed
- *blood cell formation* – most blood cells are created in the bone marrow.

Joints

A *joint* is the point at which two or more bones meet. Joints allow for movement to occur. *Cartilage* is the connective tissue at the ends of long bones; it cushions the joint so the bone ends do not rub together. The *synovial membrane* lines the joints, which secretes *synovial fluid.* This fluid acts as a lubricant so the joint can move smoothly.

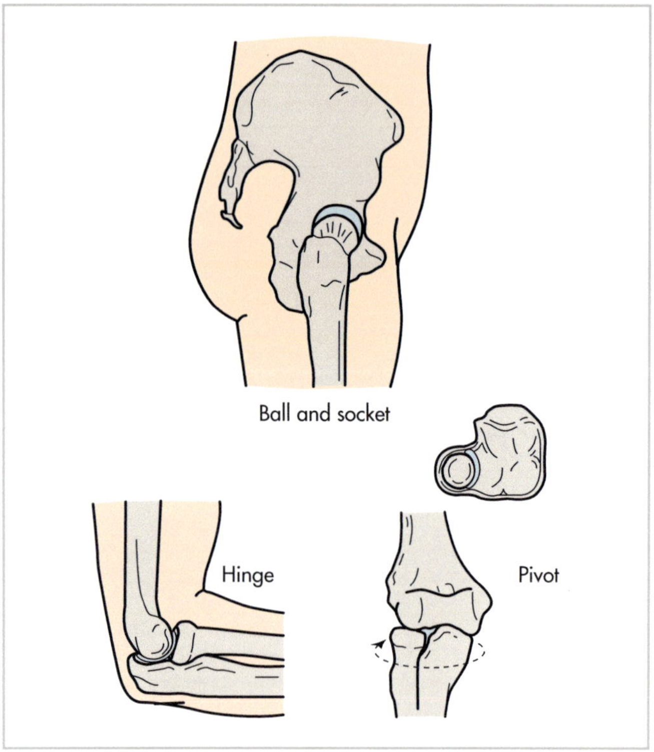

Fig. 10.9
Types of joints.

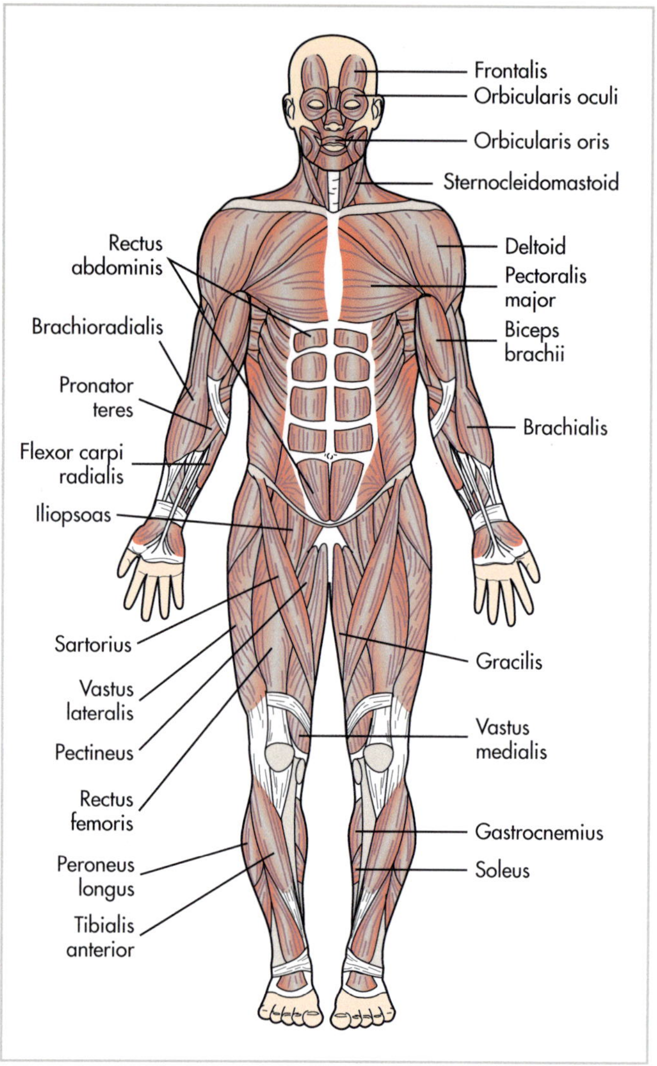

Fig. 10.10
Anterior view of the muscles of the body.

Bones are held together at the joint by strong bands of connective tissue called *ligaments*.

There are three types of joints (Fig. 10.9):

- *Ball-and-socket joint* – allows movement in all directions. It is made up of the rounded end of one bone and the hollow end of another bone. The rounded end of one fits into the hollow end of the other. The joints of the hips and shoulders are ball-and-socket joints.
- *Hinge joint* – allows movement in one direction. The elbow is a hinge joint.
- *Pivot joint* – allows turning from side to side. The skull is connected to the spine by a pivot joint.

Muscles

The human body has more than 500 muscles (Figs 10.10, 10.11). Some muscles are voluntary and others are involuntary.

- *Voluntary muscles* can be consciously controlled. Muscles attached to bones (skeletal muscles) are voluntary. Your arm muscles do not work unless you move your arm; likewise, for leg muscles. Skeletal muscles are striated – that is, they look striped or streaked.
- *Involuntary muscles* work automatically and cannot be consciously controlled. Involuntary muscles control the action of the stomach, intestines, blood vessels and other body organs. Involuntary muscles are also called smooth muscles. They look smooth – not streaked or striped.
- *Cardiac muscle* is in the heart. Although it is an involuntary muscle, it appears striated like skeletal muscle.

Muscles perform four important body functions:

1. movement of body parts
2. maintenance of posture
3. production of body heat
4. stabilising joints.

Strong, tough connective tissues, called tendons, connect muscles to bones. When muscles contract (shorten), the tendons at each end of the muscle cause the bone to move. The body has many tendons. The Achilles tendon is shown in Fig. 10.11. Some muscles constantly contract to maintain the body's posture. When muscles contract, they burn food for energy and heat is produced. The more muscle activity, the greater the amount of heat produced. Shivering is how the body produces heat when exposed to cold. The shivering sensation is from rapid, general muscle contractions.

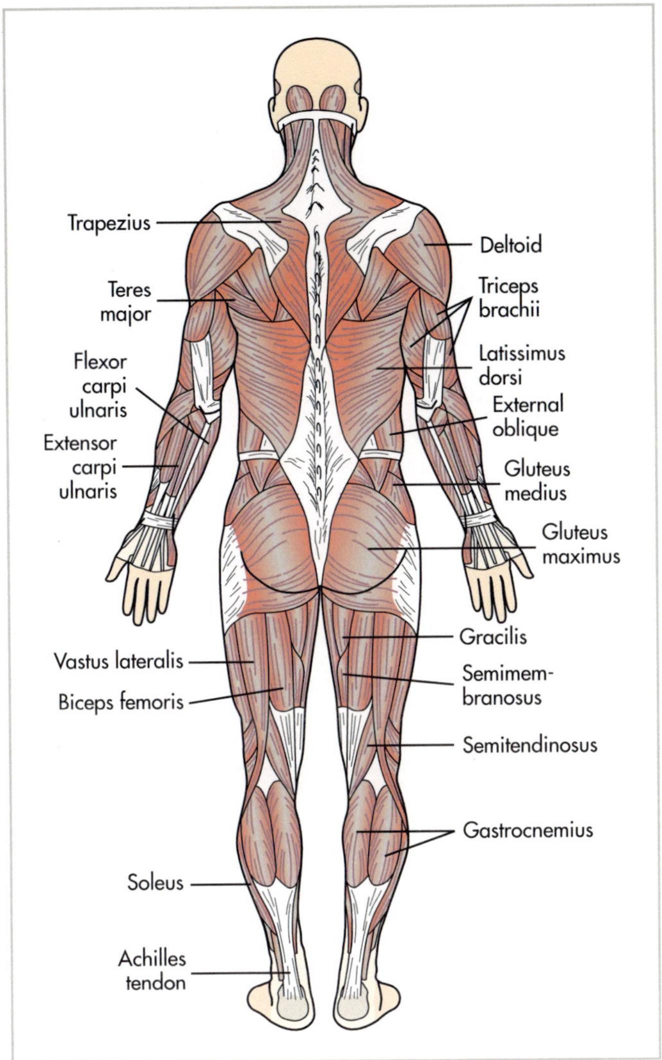

Fig. 10.11
Posterior view of the muscles of the body.

AGEING OF THE MUSCULOSKELETAL SYSTEM

Ageing affects all aspects of the musculoskeletal system. The changes in cellular function, activity and number of cells all contribute to the changes in the musculoskeletal system as an individual ages.

The musculoskeletal system changes as it matures. Effects due to the ageing process include:

- *a decline in the size of skeletal muscle fibres:* The number of muscle cells decrease in muscle as the person ages. The muscle also has reduced levels of adenosine triphosphate (the main energy molecule of the body) and glycogen reserves (sugar molecules are stored as glycogen and required for muscle to do its work) and less myoglobin. The overall effect of this is reduced skeletal muscle size, reduced strength and endurance and a tendency for fatigue to develop rapidly.
- *skeletal muscles become less elastic:* As the ageing process continues, the skeletal muscles undergo a fibrosis, which is an increase in the amount of the fibrous connective tissue. This makes the muscles less flexible with the collagen fibres restricting movement and circulation.
- *exercise tolerance decreases:* As the person ages, the level of tolerance during exercise decreases, in part due to the structural (reduced size of muscle) and metabolic changes to muscle (reduced myoglobin and ATP). The ability to lose heat also lowers tolerance and increases the likelihood of fatigue. These changes in heat regulation are also seen in the integumentary system described above.
- *reduced ability to recover from muscle injury:* The satellite cells respond to muscle injury and are actively involved in the repairing of muscle tissue. However, as ageing progresses the number of these cells decreases, thus reducing injury recovery capabilities.
- *bony matrix decrease:* There is a reduction in the mineral content in bone (calcium and phosphorus), thus increasing the risk of osteoporosis (described below).
- *bone markings reduce in size and increase in roughness:* Bone markings attach muscles, ligaments and tendons and are also where blood vessels and nerves pass through bone or between bones. As the individual ages, these markings reduce in size and increase in roughness, thus contributing to decreased muscular strength and mass.

MUSCULOSKELETAL CONDITIONS

Musculoskeletal disorders can affect movement, with injury and age-related changes being the common causes.

Arthritis

Arthritis means joint (*arthr*) inflammation (*itis*). It is the most common joint disease. Pain and decreased mobility occur in affected joints. There are two basic types of arthritis: osteoarthritis and rheumatoid arthritis. Fig. 10.12 shows the major regions in the human body where they occur.

Osteoarthritis (degenerative joint disease)

Osteoarthritis occurs with ageing, joint injury and obesity. Finger and thumb joints are often affected. Bony growths are common in the fingers (Fig. 10.13). The disease also occurs in the hips, knees and spine, as these joints bear the body's weight. Fig. 10.14 highlights the changes in the pathology of osteoarthritis as the condition progresses. The amount of available cartilage decreases as the condition progresses. The number of bone spurs increases, protruding into the soft tissue and causing further irritation and inflammation.

Signs and symptoms are joint stiffness, pain and swelling or tenderness. Joint stiffness occurs with rest and lack of motion. Pain occurs with weight-bearing and joint motion.

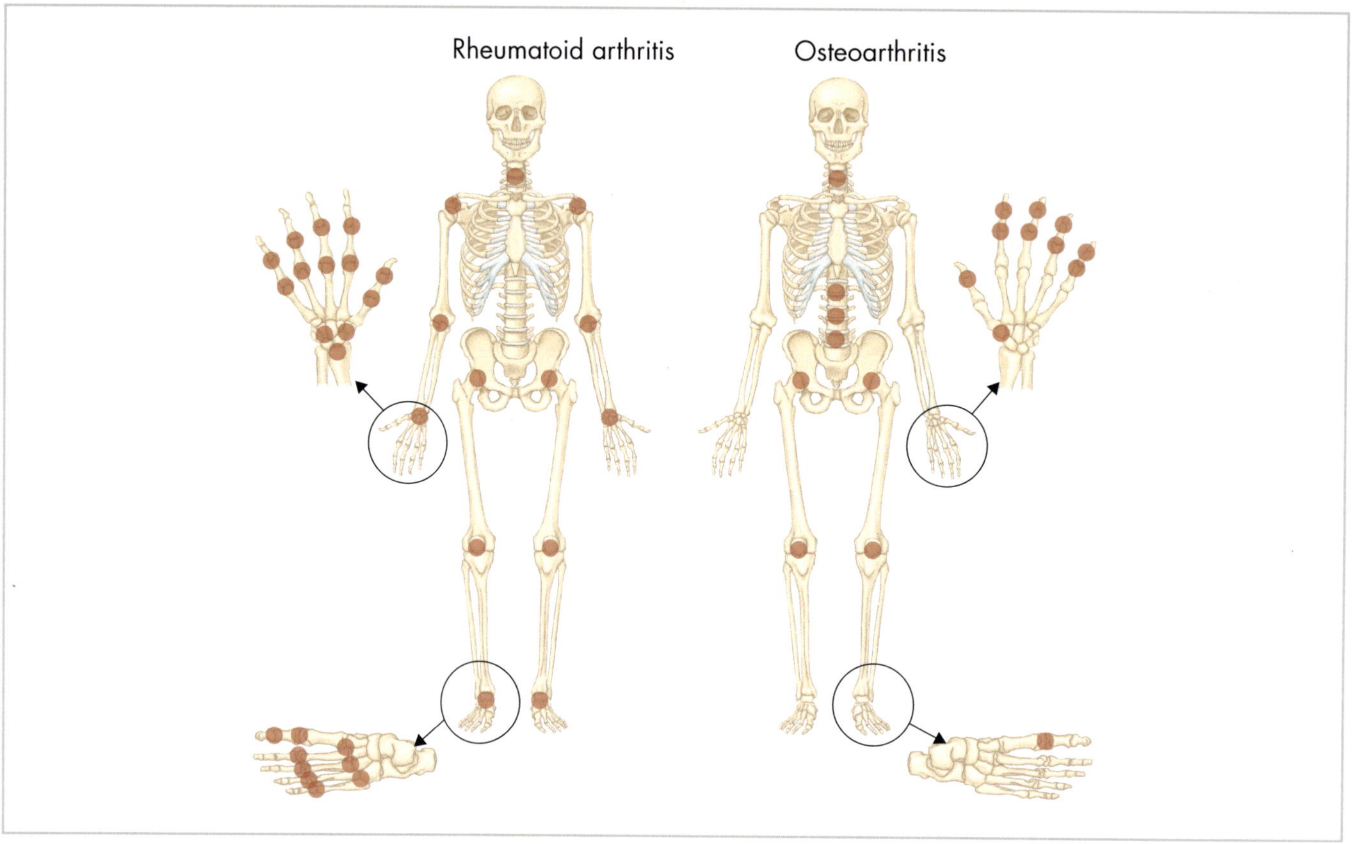

Fig. 10.12
Joints involved in rheumatoid arthritis and osteoarthritis.

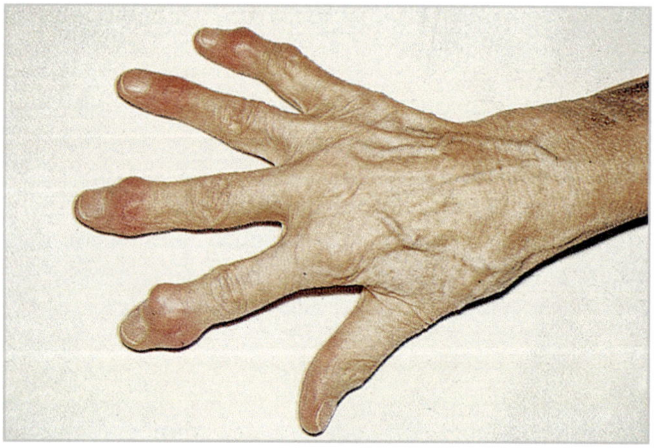

Fig. 10.13
Bony growths called Heberden's nodes occur in the finger joints.

Severe pain affects rest, sleep and mobility. Cold weather and dampness seem to increase symptoms.

Currently there is no cure for osteoarthritis, with treatment focused on the management of symptoms.

Treatment may involve several different approaches, including:

- *pain relief* – medications decrease swelling and relieve pain. Heat applications, warm baths or showers and water therapy in heated pools can be used to relieve pain and stiffness. Cold applications can be used to relieve pain or numb the area.
- *exercise* – decreases pain, increases flexibility and improves blood flow. It helps with weight control, promotes fitness and improves mental wellbeing.
- *rest and joint care* – regular rest protects joints from overuse. Relaxation methods are helpful. Canes and walkers also provide additional support. Splints support weak joints and keep joints in alignment.
- *weight control* – weight loss is stressed for obese persons. It reduces stress on weight-bearing joints and helps prevent further injury.
- *healthy lifestyle* – arthritis support programs can help the person develop a good outlook. Abilities and strengths are stressed. The focus also is on fitness, exercise, rest, managing stress and good nutrition.

The person's care plan includes measures to prevent falls. Assistance with activities of daily living (ADLs) is given as needed. Elevated toilet seats are helpful when hip and knee motion is limited. Some people may need joint replacement surgery. Arthroplasty is the surgical replacement (*plasty*) of a joint (*arthro*). Ankle, knee, hip, shoulder, wrist, finger and toe joints can be replaced. The diseased joint is removed and replaced with a prosthesis (Fig. 10.15). The surgery relieves pain and restores joint motion.

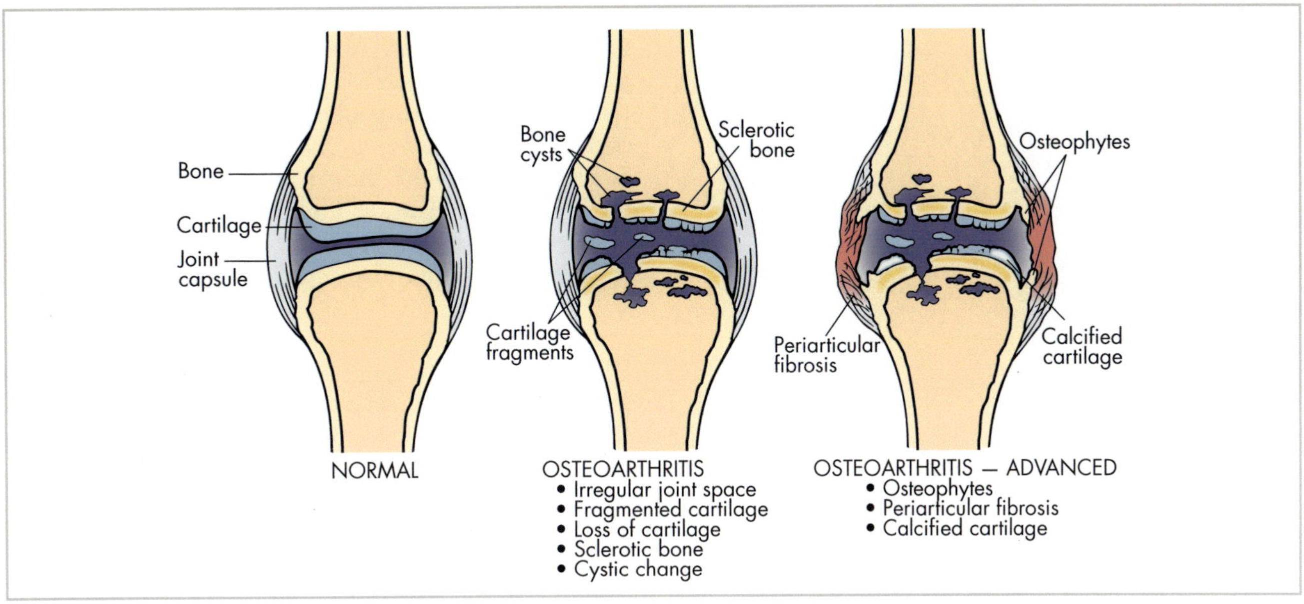

Fig. 10.14
Diagrammatic representation of the pathology in osteoarthritis.

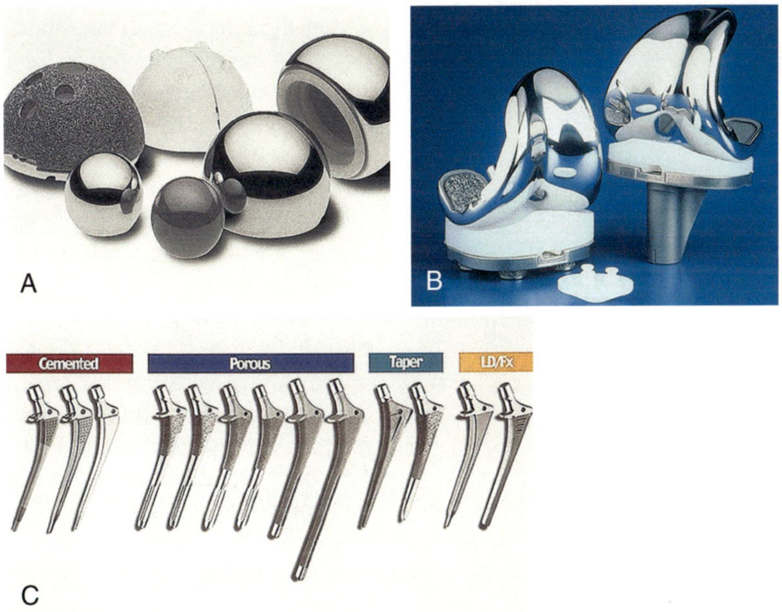

Fig. 10.15
A. Hip replacement prostheses. **B.** Knee replacement prostheses. **C.** Hip replacement prosthesis stems.

Rheumatoid arthritis

Rheumatoid arthritis (RA) is an inflammatory disease that causes joint pain, swelling and stiffness. It is more common in women and occurs at any age. RA occurs on both sides of the body. For example, if the right wrist is involved, so is the left wrist. The wrist and finger joints closest to the hand are most commonly affected. Fig. 10.16 clearly shows the deformities that take place due to RA. RA can also affect other body regions, including the neck, shoulders, elbows, hips, knees, ankles and feet joints. Common symptoms of rheumatoid arthritis include tender joints that are warm and swollen. Fatigue and fever are common and the person may not feel well, with symptoms lasting for years.

Care considerations for rheumatoid arthritis

RA varies from person to person. Some people have flare-ups and then feel better. In others, the disease is active most of the time. Treatment goals are to relieve pain, reduce inflammation and slow down the progression or stop the

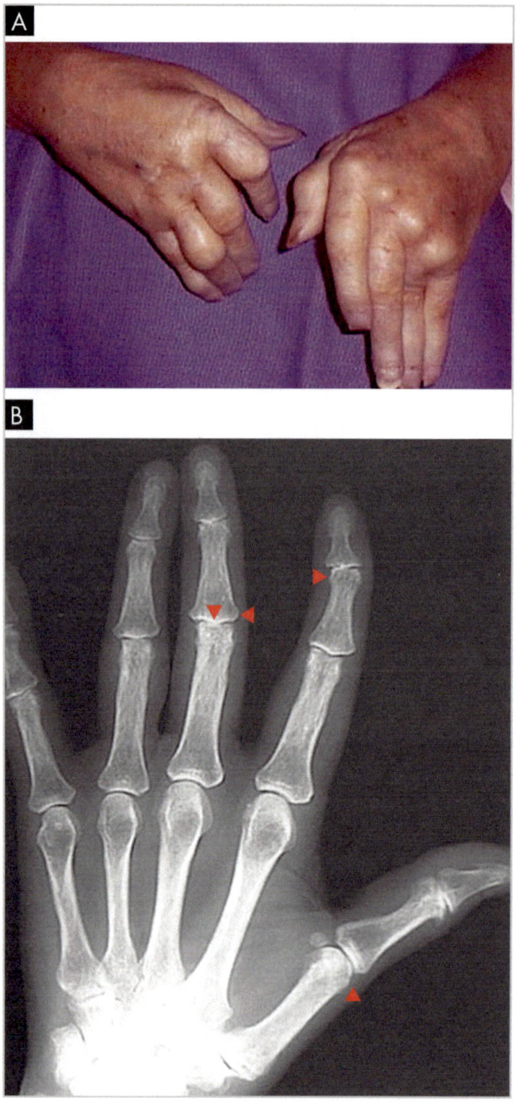

Fig. 10.16
Rheumatoid arthritis in the finger joints.

joint damage. Improved wellbeing and function are other goals. The person's care plan may include:

- rest, balanced with exercise – more rest is needed when the RA is active; more exercise is needed when it is not
- turning and repositioning every 2 hours during rest
- good body alignment
- positioning to prevent contractures and deformities – bed boards, a bed cradle, trochanter rolls and pillows are used
- 10–11 hours of sleep each night – morning and afternoon rest periods are needed
- an exercise program
- walking aids and self-help devices as needed
- splints to support affected joints – they also reduce pain and swelling
- safety measures to prevent falls
- measures to reduce stress.

Medications are ordered for pain relief and to reduce inflammation. Heat or cold applications may also be used to help reduce inflammation and pain. In some instances, some individuals may require joint replacement surgery. Emotional and counselling support may be needed during this period, as it can be quite stressful, although a positive outlook is very important. The person needs to stay as active as possible, since this creates independence and improves the individual's quality of life. While caring for a person in this situation it is always important to give encouragement and praise and listen when the person needs to talk.

Osteoporosis

With *osteoporosis*, the bone (*osteo*) becomes porous and brittle (*porosis*). Bones are fragile and break easily with spine, hip and wrist fractures common. Over 2.2 million Australians have osteoporosis. Older people and women after menopause are most at risk. As the ovaries do not produce oestrogen after menopause, bone changes start to develop. Large spaces develop within the bone matrix, contributing to the fragility and increased risk of breaks. Low levels of dietary calcium, vitamin D and reduced levels of oestrogen in women can also increase the risk of osteoporosis developing.

People of European or Asian descent are at greater risk and a family history of the disease is also a critical risk factor. Other lifestyle factors contribute to an increased risk in the development of osteoporosis, including tobacco use, alcoholism, lack of exercise, bed rest and immobility. As the condition progresses the person will experience increased back pain, a gradual loss of height and develop a stooped posture. In severe cases, simple activities such as turning over in bed, getting up from a chair or coughing can cause a fracture. The risk of fractures from falls and accidents is high. It is estimated in Australia that over 60 per cent of women and 30 per cent of men over the age of 60 will sustain an osteoporotic fracture (Healthy Bones Australia 2021).

Prevention is important and, where possible, preventive strategies should be implemented; for example, a diet must contain enough calcium and vitamin D to help ensure that optimal bone strength and health can be maintained. Often doctors order calcium and vitamin supplements. Oestrogen is often ordered for women after menopause. Exercise should be included as a preventive strategy, since weight-bearing (walking, jogging, stair climbing, etc) and strength training (lifting weights) can reduce the risk of osteoporosis. Smoking and alcohol should be avoided and caffeine intake should be limited. Good posture is also important and some people may wear back braces or corsets to help enforce appropriate posture. Others need walking aids to help protect them from falls and accidents.

Fractures

A **fracture** is a broken bone. Tissues around the fracture (muscles, blood vessels, nerves and tendons) are injured. While there can be many different types of bone fractures (Fig. 10.17), the main categories of bone fractures are open or closed (Fig. 10.18):

- **closed fracture (simple fracture)** – the bone is broken but the skin is intact

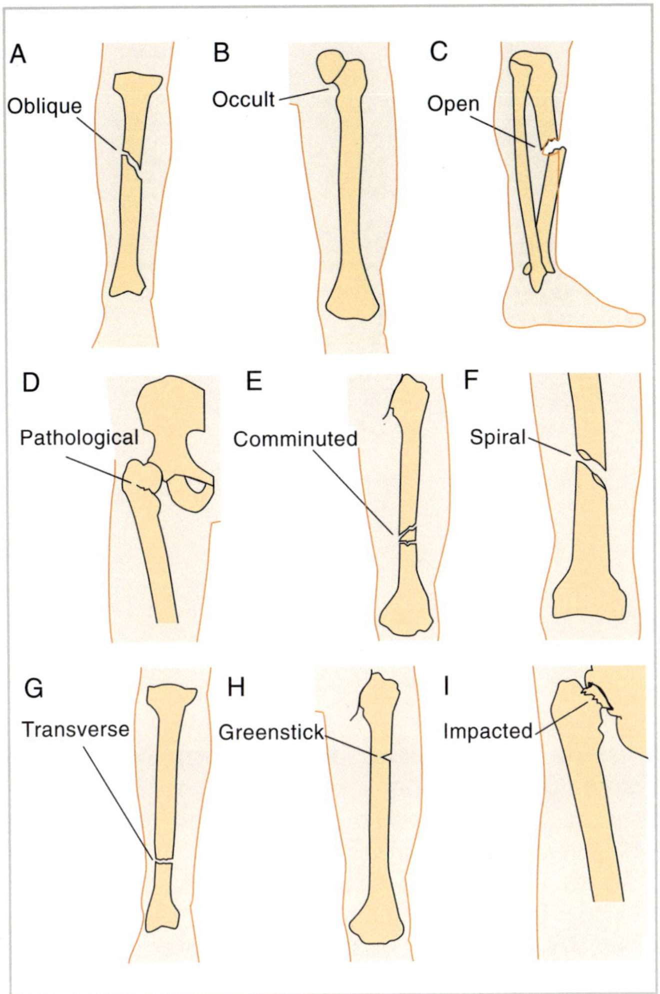

Fig. 10.17

Examples of bone fractures.

A. Oblique fracture at oblique angle across both cortices. Cause: direct or indirect energy, with angulation and some compression. **B.** Occult: fracture that is hidden or not readily discernible. Cause: minor force or energy. **C.** Open: Skin broken over fracture; possible soft tissue trauma. Cause: moderate-to-severe energy that is continuous and exceeds tissue tolerances. **D.** Pathological: transverse, oblique or spiral fracture of bone weakened by tumour pressure or presence. Cause: minor energy or forces, which may be direct or indirect. **E.** Comminuted: fracture with two or more pieces or segments. Cause: direct or indirect moderate-to-severe force. **F.** Spiral: fracture that curves around cortices and may become displaced by twist. Cause: direct or indirect twisting energy or force with distal part held or unable to move. **G.** Transverse: horizontal break through bone. Cause: direct or indirect energy towards bone. **H.** Greenstick: break in only one cortex of the bone. Cause: minor direct or indirect energy. **I.** Impacted. Fracture with one end wedged into opposite end of inside fractured fragment. Cause: compressive axial energy or force directly to distal fragment.

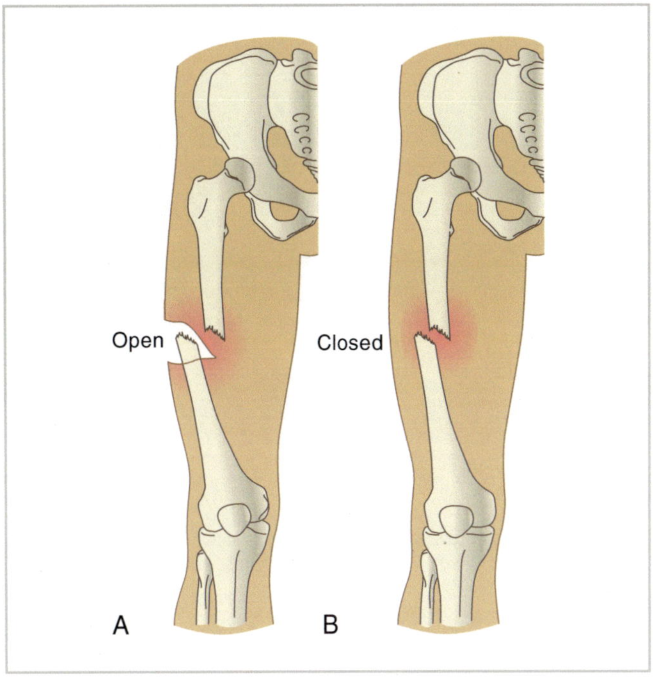

Fig. 10.18

A. Open fracture. **B.** Closed fracture.

- **open fracture (compound fracture)** – the broken bone has come through the skin.

Falls and accidents can cause fractures. It is well known that older adults are more likely to suffer falls. In combination with brittle bones (see above section on osteoporosis) and other age-related changes to the skeletal system, this means an increased risk of fractures for that age group. Bone tumours, metastatic cancer and osteoporosis are other causes that may increase the risk of fractures to bones occurring.

The signs and symptoms of a fracture are:

- pain and tenderness
- swelling
- limited movement
- loss of function
- deformity (the part is in an abnormal position)
- bruising and skin colour changes at the fracture site
- bleeding (internal or external).

For healing, the bone ends are brought into normal position. This is called *reduction*.

- *Closed reduction* involves moving the bone back into place. The skin is not opened.
- *Open reduction* involves surgery. The bone is exposed and brought into alignment. Nails, rods, pins, screws, plates or wires keep the bone in place (Fig. 10.19).

After reduction, movement of the bone ends is prevented by means of a cast or traction. Other devices, such as splints, walking boots and external fixation devices, are also used (Fig. 10.20).

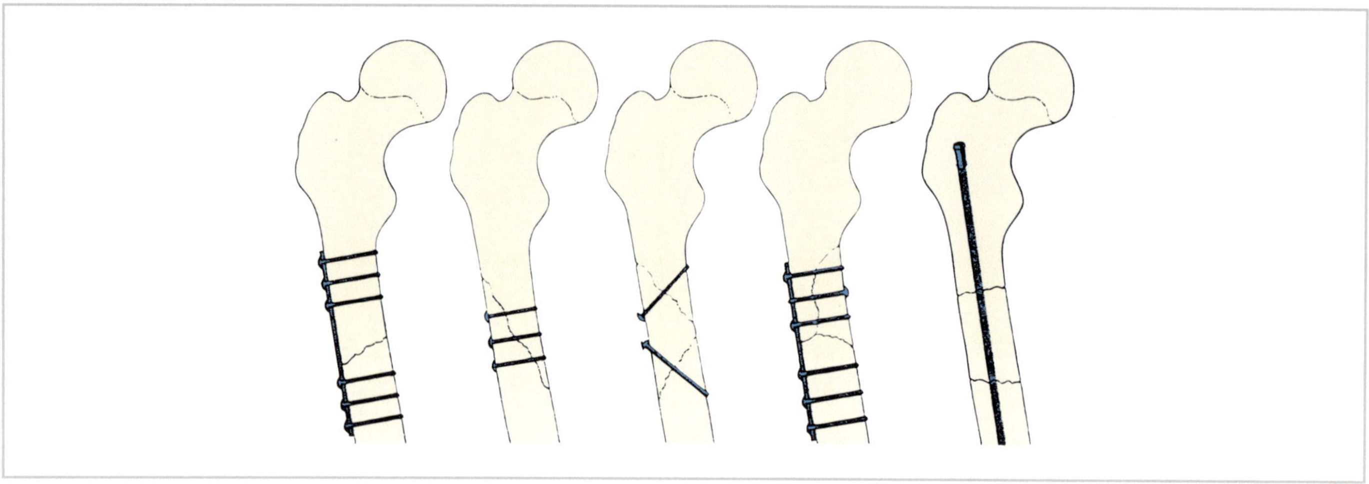

Fig. 10.19
Devices used to reduce a fracture.

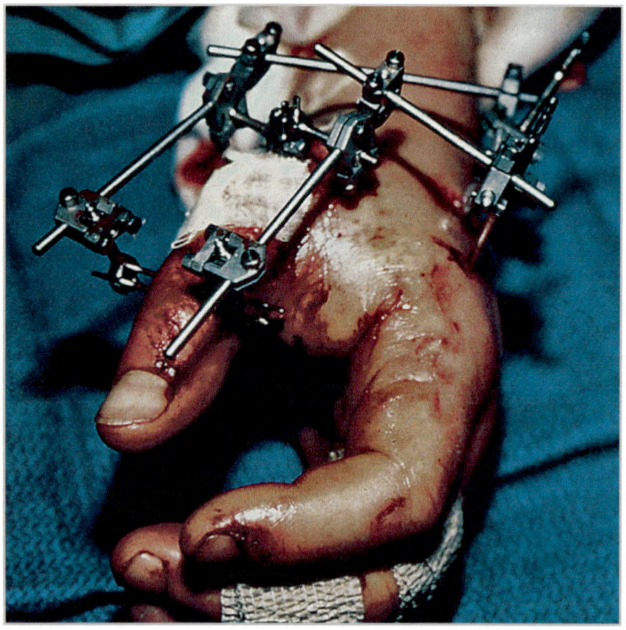

Fig. 10.20
External fixation device.

GENERAL CARE CONSIDERATION WITH FRACTURES OR AMPUTATION

This section examines the general considerations for caring for individuals that have a fracture and require supportive care. It will also examine some of the key issues surrounding amputation and caring for a patient following a significant event such as loss of a limb.

Cast care

Casts are made of plaster of Paris, plastic or fibreglass. Before casting, the part is covered with a stockinette or bandage. This protects the skin. Moistened cast rolls are wrapped around the part (Fig. 10.21).

Plastic and fibreglass casts dry quickly. A plaster of Paris cast dries in 24–48 hours. It is odourless, white and shiny when dry. When wet, it is grey, cool and has a musty smell.

Hip fractures

Fractured hips are common in older people (Fig. 10.22). Healing is slower in older people. Slow healing and other health problems affect the person's condition and care. Postoperative problems present life-threatening risks. They include pneumonia, **atelectasis**, urinary tract infections and thrombi in leg veins. Pressure injuries, constipation and confusion are other risks.

The fracture is fixed in position with a pin, nail, plate, screw or prosthesis (Fig. 10.23). Some people need rehabilitation or subacute care after surgery. Boxes 10.1 and 10.2 describe the care required.

Loss of a limb

An amputation is the removal of all or part of an extremity. Severe injuries, tumours, severe infections, poor wound healing, diabetes and circulatory disorders are common indications that can require the removal of a limb. Vehicle and workplace accidents can cause traumatic amputations. Whatever the situation that causes the loss of a limb, the patient will have significant physical and psychological barriers to overcome.

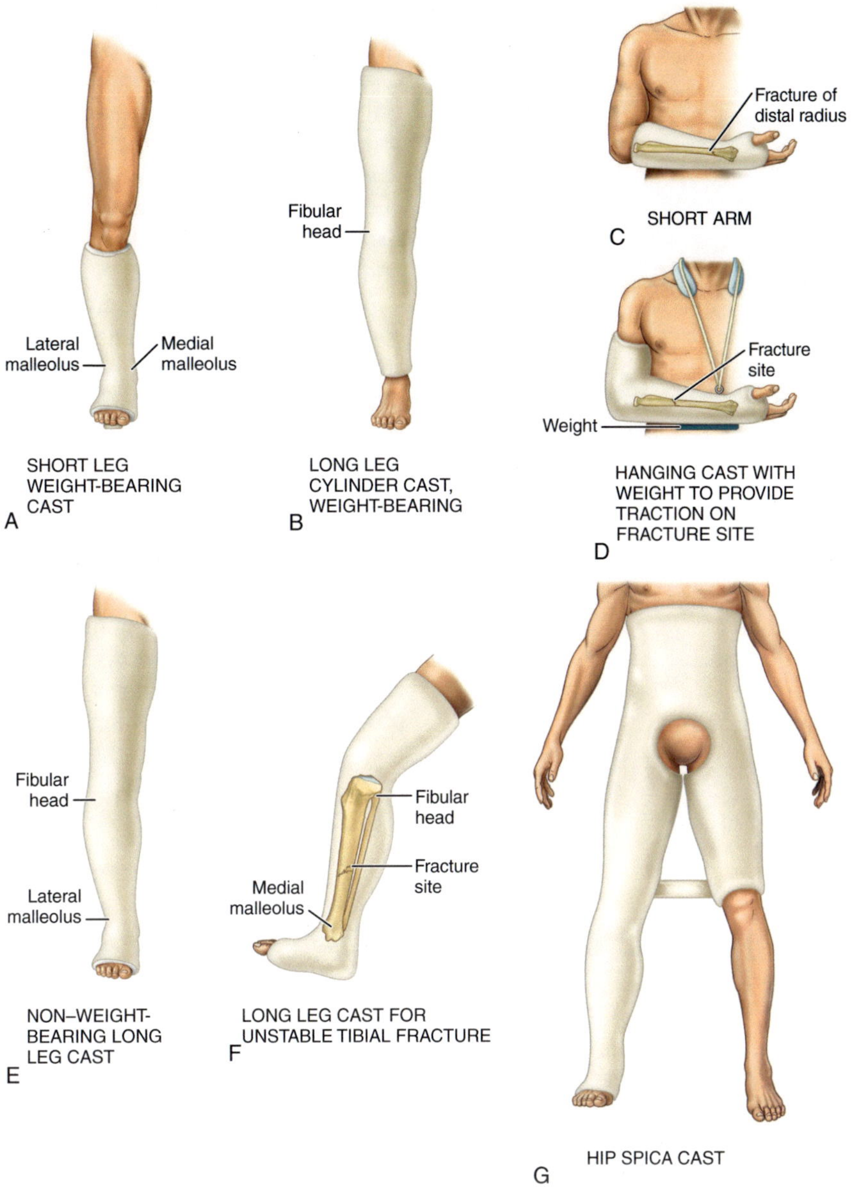

Fig. 10.21
Common casts.

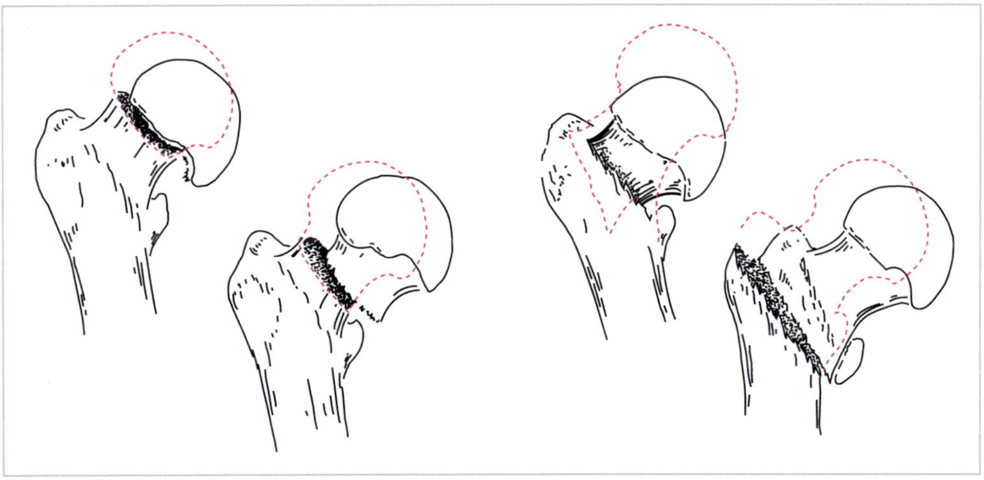

Fig. 10.22
Hip fractures.

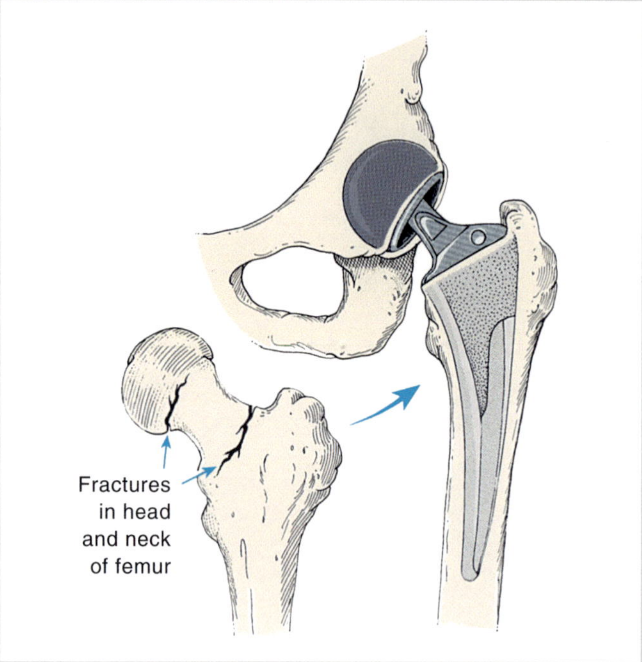

Fig. 10.23
Hip fracture repaired with a prosthesis.

Gangrene is a condition in which there is death of tissue. Causes include infection, injuries and circulatory disorders. These conditions affect blood flow, with tissues not getting enough oxygen and nutrients. Poisonous substances and waste products build up in the tissues. Tissue death results in the tissue becoming black, cold and shrivelled (Fig. 10.24). Surgery is required to remove the dead tissue. If untreated, gangrene spreads through the body and can cause death.

Much support is needed, as amputation affects the person's life. Appearance, daily activities, moving about and work are some areas that are affected.

The person is fitted with a prosthesis (Fig. 10.25). The stump is conditioned so the prosthesis fits. This involves shrinking and shaping the stump into a cone shape (Fig. 10.26). The person is taught exercises to strengthen other limbs. Occupational therapists and physiotherapists help the person to learn to use the prosthesis.

The person may feel that the limb is still there and sometimes may complain of pain in the amputated part. This is called *phantom limb pain.* This is a normal reaction and may occur for a short time after surgery. Some people have phantom limb pain for many years.

BOX 10.1
Caring for a person with a cast

These general rules will assist you in caring for a person with a cast, both immediately after the application of the cast and after a period of time. Casts can take up to 24 hours to dry after application.

- If the cast has been freshly applied and is still damp do not cover it with blankets, plastic or other material. A plaster cast gives off heat as it dries. Covers prevent the heat from escaping. If heat cannot escape, burns can occur.
- Turn the person frequently if the cast has been freshly applied. All cast surfaces need to be exposed to the air at one time or another. Turning promotes even drying.
- Do not place a damp cast on a hard surface. It flattens the cast. The cast must keep its shape. Use pillows to support the entire length of the cast.
- Support a damp cast with your palms when turning and positioning the person. Fingertips can dent the cast. The dents can cause pressure areas that can lead to skin breakdown.
- Protect the person against rough cast edges.
- Keep the cast dry. A wet cast loses its shape.
- Do not let the person insert anything into the cast. Itching under the cast causes an intense desire to scratch. Items used for scratching (pencils, coat hangers, knitting needles, back scratchers) can open the skin. An infection can develop. Scratching items can wrinkle the stockinette or be lost inside the cast. Both can cause pressure and lead to skin breakdown.
- Elevate an arm or leg in a cast on pillows. This reduces swelling.
- Have enough help when turning and repositioning the person. Plaster casts are heavy and awkward. Balance is easily lost.
- Position the person as directed.
- Report these signs and symptoms at once:
  - *pain* – pressure injury, poor circulation or nerve damage
  - *swelling and a tight cast* – reduced blood flow to the part
  - *pale skin* – reduced blood flow to the part
  - *cyanosis* – reduced blood flow to the part
  - *odour* – infection
  - *inability to move the fingers or toes* – pressure on a nerve
  - *numbness* – pressure on a nerve or reduced blood flow to the part
  - *temperature changes* – cool skin means poor circulation; hot skin means inflammation
  - *drainage on or under the cast* – infection
  - *chills, fever, nausea and vomiting* – infection.

BOX 10.2
Care of a person with a hip fracture

- Give good skin care. Skin breakdown can occur rapidly.
- Encourage incentive spirometry and coughing, and deep breathing exercises as directed.
- Turn and reposition the person as directed. Turning and positioning depend on the type of fracture and the surgery performed. Usually the person is not positioned on the operative side.
- Keep the operated leg abducted at all times. The leg is abducted when the person is supine, being turned or in a side-lying position. Use pillows or an abductor splint as directed.
- Prevent external rotation of the hip (turning outwards). Use trochanter rolls, pillows, sandbags or abduction splints as directed.
- Perform range-of-motion exercises as directed. Do not exercise the affected leg.
- Provide a straight-backed chair with armrests. The person needs a high, firm seat. Use pillows or foam cushions as directed. A low, soft chair is not used.
- Place the chair on the unaffected side.
- Follow the nurse's directions for ambulation.
- Do not let the person stand on the leg with a cast applied unless allowed by the doctor.
- Support and elevate the leg as directed when the person is in the chair.
- Apply elastic stockings as directed.
- Remind the person not to cross their legs.

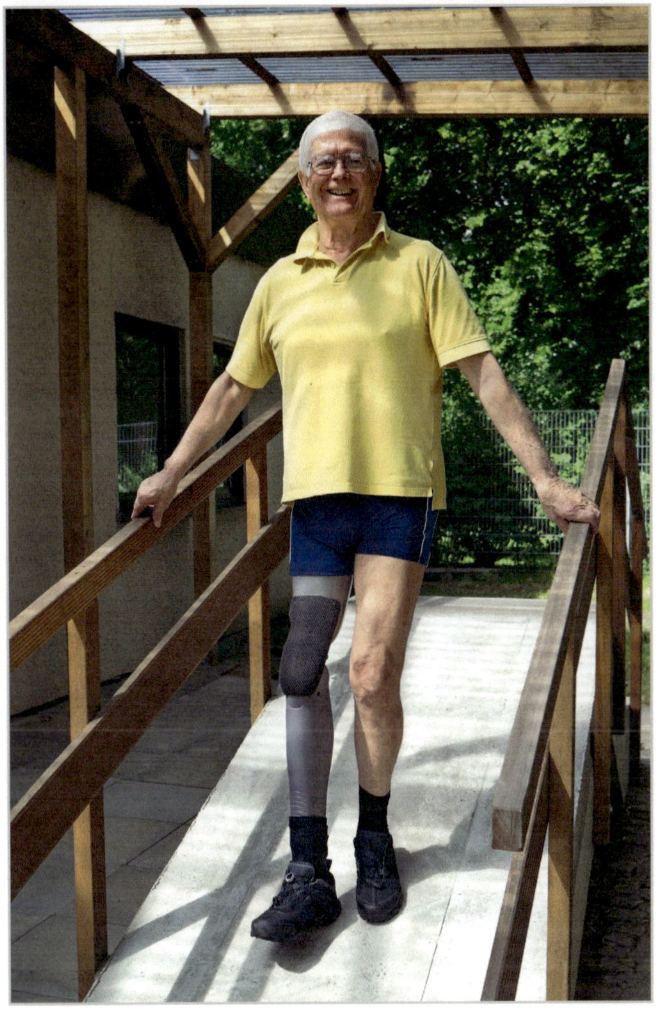

Fig. 10.25
Leg prosthesis.

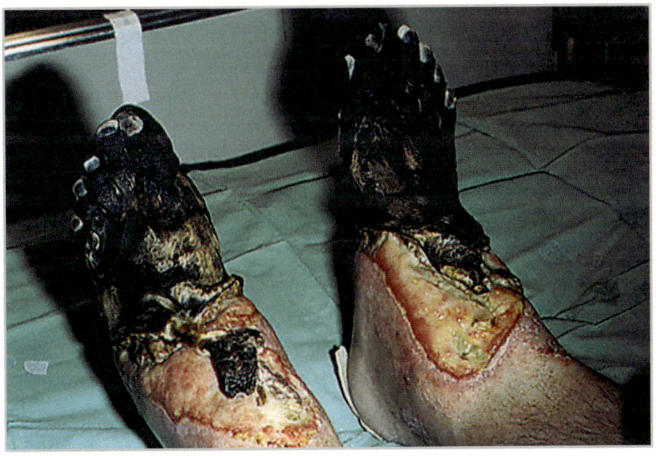

Fig. 10.24
Gangrene.

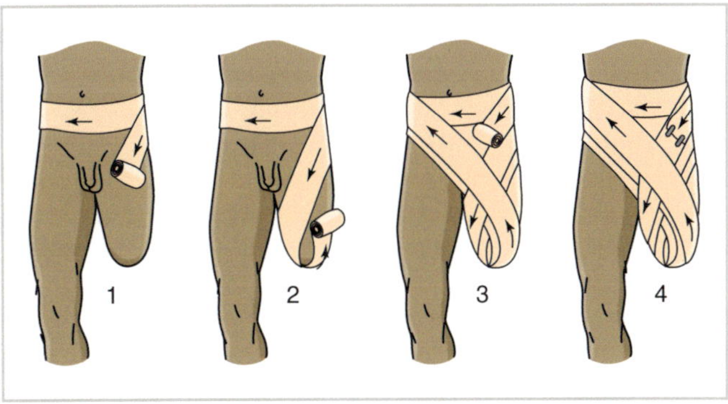

Fig. 10.26
A mid-thigh amputation is bandaged to shrink and shape the stump.

THE NERVOUS SYSTEM

The nervous system controls, directs and coordinates body functions. The two main divisions of the nervous system are:

- **the central nervous system (CNS)** – consists of the brain and spinal cord (Fig. 10.27)
- **the peripheral nervous system** – involves nerves throughout the body (Fig. 10.28).

Nerves carry messages or impulses to and from the brain and are connected to the spinal cord. Nerves are easily damaged and take a long time to heal. Some nerve fibres

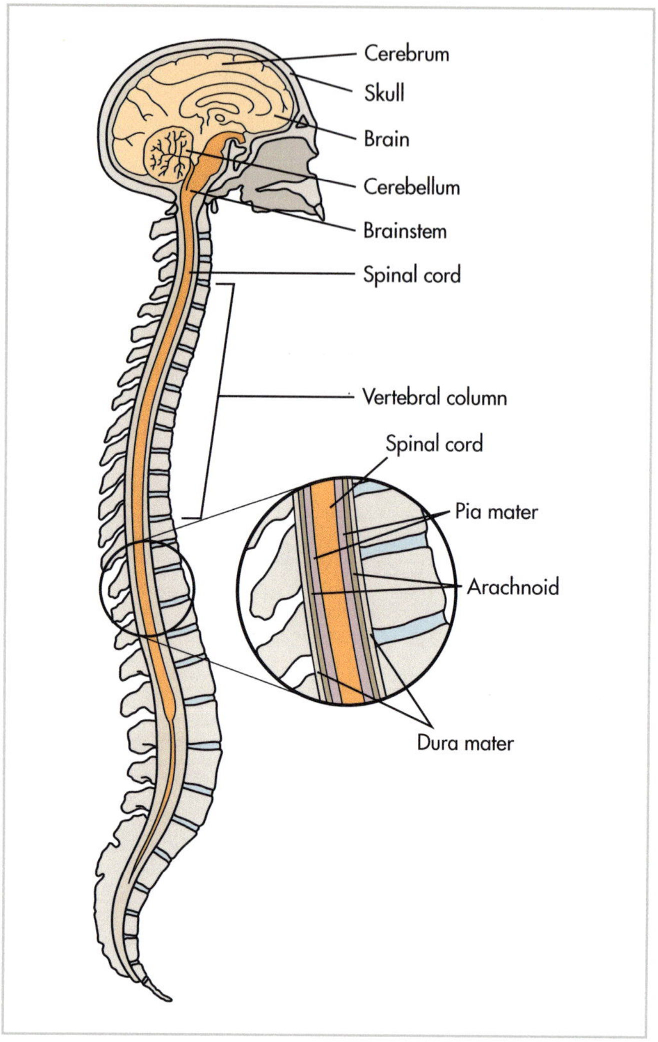

Fig. 10.27
Central nervous system.

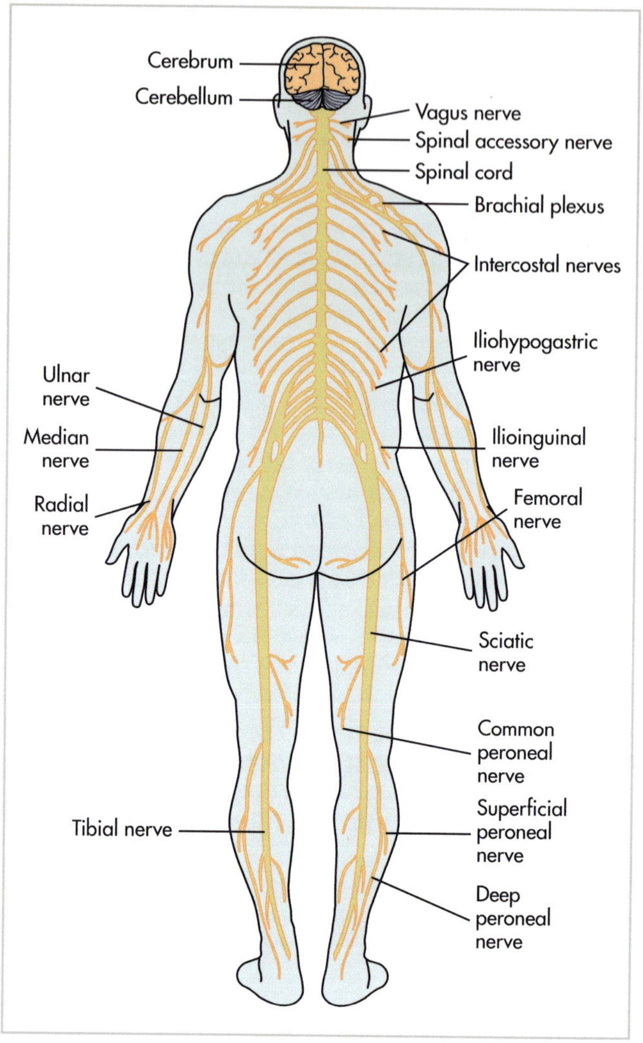

Fig. 10.28
Peripheral nervous system.

have a protective covering called a *myelin sheath*. The myelin sheath also insulates the nerve fibre. Nerve fibres covered with myelin can conduct impulses faster than fibres without the protective covering.

The central nervous system

The central nervous system consists of the brain and spinal cord, which is made up of nervous tissue, such as neuroglia and neurons, which are critical to the functioning of the body. The neuroglial cells support neurons, which help supply them with oxygen and glucose and remove waste products such as carbon dioxide. A neuron cell is composed of three major components: a cell body, an axon and a series of dendrites (Fig. 10.29).

The cell body contains the nucleus of the cell, which directs its activity. When the neuronal cell needs to communicate with a neighbouring cell, its activity increases and produces an electrical signal, which travels down the axon of the neuron and terminates at the dendrites causing the release of neurotransmitters to travel through the synaptic cleft stimulating or inhibiting the neighbouring neuronal cell. This forms the basis of neuronal communication.

The brain is covered by the dura mater, a specialised tissue that functions to support the shape of the brain and maintain a constant pressure within the brain. The dura mater is protected by the skull, which is composed of four main types of bones that are fused together by adulthood, including the frontal, temporal, parietal and occipital bones.

The three main parts of the brain are the cerebrum, the cerebellum and the brainstem (see Fig. 10.30). The *cerebrum* is the largest part of the brain. It is the centre of thought and intelligence. The cerebrum is divided into two halves, called the right and left *hemispheres*. The right hemisphere controls movement and activities on the body's left side. The left hemisphere controls the right side. The outside of the cerebrum is called the *cerebral cortex*. It controls the highest functions of the brain. These include reasoning, memory, consciousness, speech,

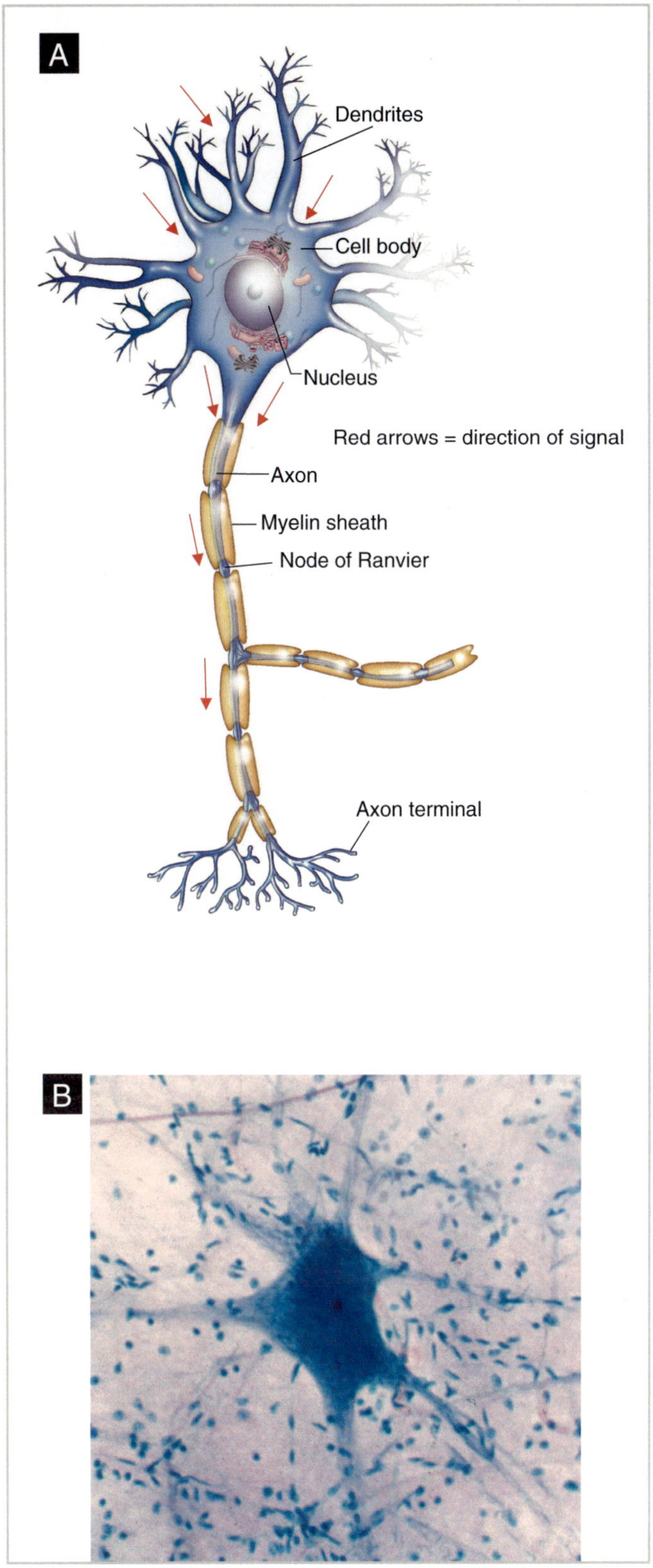

Fig. 10.29
Anatomy of neuron cell.

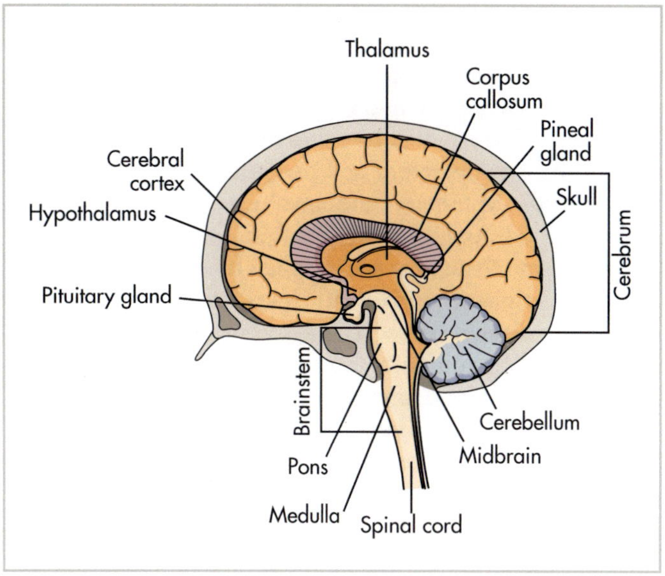

Fig. 10.30
Parts of the brain.

voluntary muscle movement, vision, hearing, sensation and other activities. Fig. 10.30 highlights the anatomy of the cerebral cortex and the associated biological functions governed by the cortex.

The *cerebellum* regulates and coordinates body movements. It controls balance and the smooth movements of voluntary muscles. Injury to the cerebellum results in jerky movements, loss of coordination and muscle weakness.

The *brainstem* connects the cerebrum to the spinal cord. Important structures within the brainstem are the *midbrain*, *pons* and *medulla*. The midbrain and pons relay messages between the medulla and the cerebrum. The medulla is below the pons. The medulla controls heart rate, breathing, blood vessel size, swallowing, coughing and vomiting – each of these complicated biological events takes place with no conscious control, i.e. they are automatic. The brain connects to the spinal cord at the lower end of the medulla.

The spinal cord lies within the vertebral column. The cord is about 43 centimetres long. It contains pathways that conduct messages to and from the brain. The brain and spinal cord are covered and protected by three layers of connective tissue, called the *meninges*:

- The outer layer lies next to the skull. It is a tough covering called the dura mater.
- The middle layer is the arachnoid mater.
- The inner layer is the pia mater.

The space between the middle and inner layers is the *arachnoid space*. The space is filled with fluid called *cerebrospinal fluid*. Cerebrospinal fluid circulates around the brain and spinal cord. It protects the central nervous system by cushioning shocks that could easily injure the structures of the brain and spinal cord.

The peripheral nervous system

The peripheral nervous system has 12 pairs of cranial nerves and 31 pairs of spinal nerves. *Cranial nerves* conduct impulses between the brain and the head, neck, chest and abdomen. They conduct impulses for smell, vision, hearing, pain, touch, temperature and pressure. They also conduct impulses for voluntary and involuntary muscles. *Spinal nerves* carry impulses from the skin, extremities and the internal body structures not supplied by cranial nerves.

Some peripheral nerves with special functions form the *autonomic nervous system*. This system controls involuntary muscles and certain body functions. The functions include the heartbeat, blood pressure, intestinal contractions and glandular secretions. These functions occur automatically.

The autonomic nervous system is divided into the *sympathetic nervous system* and the *parasympathetic nervous system*. These divisions balance one another. The sympathetic nervous system tends to speed up functions. The parasympathetic nervous system slows them down. When you are angry, frightened, excited or exercising, the sympathetic nervous system is stimulated. The parasympathetic system is activated when you relax and when digestion is taking place.

AGEING OF THE NERVOUS SYSTEM

Ageing affects the brain and the nervous system. It is estimated that anatomical and physiological changes in the brain and nervous system start to occur after the age of 30. After age 65 it is common for individuals to start to develop cognitive impairment and changes in mental performance. There are several age-related changes that take place in the nervous system:

- *reduced brain size and weight:* There is a decrease in the volume of the cerebral cortex. This is the outer covering of the brain that is responsible for controlling consciousness, speech, voluntary muscle movement, vision, hearing and sensation. This explains why some of these processes start to decline as the person ages. As there is also a general decline in the number of brain cells over time, this may contribute to the older person having a poorer memory, reduced response times and reduced executive functions.
- *neuron connections change in the brain:* As the individual ages, the connections between neurons change in many areas, including the dendritic branches, spinal branches and interconnections. There may be changes to neurotransmitter function.
- *reduced blood flow to the brain:* The reduction in blood flow is secondary due to atherosclerosis, a condition that leads to the accumulation of fatty lesions in the arterial wall, resulting in reduced blood delivery to the brain. While the reduced blood flow may not directly affect neurons, it can increase the risk of a stroke.
- *internal and external changes in CNS neurons:* As age increases, there can be an accumulation of intracellular deposits called neurofibrillary tangles. These tangles or masses are composed of plaques. The main type is called amyloid beta protein, which is the protein implicated in Alzheimer's disease, although this may be present in older adults who have no cognitive impairment.

NERVOUS SYSTEM DISORDERS

Nervous system disorders affect a person's mental and physical functions. They can affect the ability to speak, understand, feel, see, hear, touch, think, control bowels and bladder and move. Each of these effects is dependent on the specific disorder affecting the person.

Stroke

Stroke is a cardiovascular disease affecting the blood vessels that supply blood to the brain. It is also called a *cerebrovascular accident* (CVA).

The main causes of stroke are:

- *ruptured blood vessel* – bleeding occurs in the brain
- *blood clots* – a blood clot obstructs blood flow to the brain.

Brain cells in the affected area do not get oxygen and nutrients (glucose). Brain cells die and brain damage occurs. Functions controlled by that part of the brain are lost or impaired. Stroke occurs in all age groups, but the risk increases as the individual ages.

SAFETY ALERT

How to recognise the common signs of a stroke – think FAST!

The Australian Stroke Foundation recommends using the FAST test as an easy way to recognise and remember the most common signs of a stroke.

Face – Check their **face**. Has their mouth drooped?
Arms – Can they lift both **arms**?
Speech – Is their **speech** slurred? Do they understand you?
Time – Is critical. If you see any of these signs, call 000 straight away

Source: Stroke Foundation (2021).

Risk factors for a stroke include:

- age – older people are at greater risk than younger people
- gender – men are at higher risk than women
- ethnic group – Indigenous Australians and Māori people are at greater risk
- hypertension (high blood pressure)
- family history of stroke
- cardiovascular disease
- smoking
- diabetes
- high blood cholesterol
- inactivity
- obesity
- excessive alcohol use
- medication abuse.

Stroke can occur suddenly. The person may have nausea, vomiting and memory loss. Unconsciousness, noisy breathing, high blood pressure, slow pulse, redness of the face and seizures may occur. So, can paralysis on one side of the body (**hemiplegia**). The person may lose bowel and bladder control and the ability to speak. **Aphasia** is the inability (*a*) to speak (*phasia*).

Stroke is the third leading cause of death in Australia and New Zealand and is a leading cause of disability in adults. See Box 10.3 for warning signs. The person needs emergency care.

Sometimes warning signs last a few minutes. This is called a *transient ischaemic attack* (*TIA*). (*Transient* means temporary or short term; *ischaemic* means to hold back (*ischein*) blood (*haemic*).) Blood supply to the brain is interrupted for a short time. Medical care is needed.

If the person survives, some brain damage is likely. The functions lost depend on the area of brain damage (Fig. 10.31). The effects of a stroke include:

- loss of face, hand, arm, leg or body control
- hemiplegia
- changing emotions (crying easily or mood swings, sometimes for no reason)
- difficulty swallowing (**dysphagia** means difficulty (dys) swallowing (phagia))
- dimmed vision
- aphasia
- slow or slurred speech
- changes in sight, touch, movement and thought
- impaired memory
- urinary frequency, urgency or incontinence
- depression
- frustration.

Behavioural changes occur and the person may forget or ignore the weaker side. This is called 'neglect'. It stems from loss of vision or movement and feeling on that side. Sometimes thinking is affected. The person may not recognise or know how to use common items. ADLs and other tasks are hard to do. The person may forget what to do and how to do them. If the person does know, the body may not respond.

Rehabilitation starts at once. The person may depend in part or totally on others for care. The health team helps the person regain the highest possible level of function (Box 10.4).

Aphasia

There are two basic types of aphasia. **Expressive aphasia** is difficulty expressing or sending out thoughts. Thinking is clear. There are problems speaking, spelling, counting, gesturing or writing. The person thinks one thing but says another. For example, the person thinks about food but

BOX 10.3
Warning signs of stroke

- Sudden numbness or weakness of the face, arm or leg, especially on one side of the body.
- Sudden confusion, trouble speaking or understanding.
- Sudden trouble walking, dizziness or loss of balance or coordination.
- Sudden trouble seeing in one or both eyes.
- Sudden, severe headaches with no known cause.

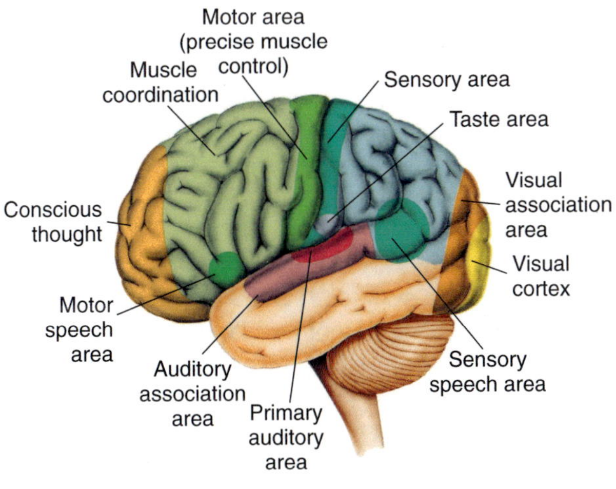

Fig. 10.31
Functions lost from a stroke depend on the area of the brain that has received damage.

BOX 10.4
Care of the person with a stroke

- The lateral position prevents aspiration.
- Coughing and deep breathing are encouraged.
- The bed is kept in **semi-Fowler's position**.
- Turning and repositioning are carried out at least every 2 hours.
- Food and fluid needs are met. Always find out if they need thickened fluids or a modified diet.
- Elastic stockings prevent thrombi (blood clots) in the legs.
- Range-of-motion exercises prevent contractures.
- A catheter is inserted or a bladder training program is started.
- A bowel training program may be needed.
- Safety precautions are practised. Use bed rails according to the care plan.
- The person does as much self-care as possible. Assist as needed.
- Communication methods are established. Magic slates, pencil and paper, a picture board or other methods are used. Limit questions to those that have 'yes' or 'no' answers. Speak slowly. Allow the person time to respond.
- Good skin care prevents pressure injuries.
- Speech therapy, physiotherapy and occupational therapy are ordered.
- Assistive devices are used as needed.
- Support, encouragement and praise are given.

asks for a book. People are called the wrong names, even when names are known. Some people produce sounds and no words. The person may cry or swear for no reason.

Receptive aphasia relates to difficulty receiving information. The person has trouble understanding what is said or read. People and common objects are not recognised. The person may not know how to use a fork, toilet, cup, television, telephone or other items.

With receptive aphasia, messages are not interpreted. With expressive aphasia, messages are not sent. Some people have both types. This is called **expressive–receptive aphasia**.

The person has many emotional needs. Frustration, depression and anger are common. Communication is needed to function and relate to others. The person wants to communicate but cannot. You must be patient and kind.

Parkinson's disease

Parkinson's disease is a slow, progressive disorder and has no cure. Degeneration of a part of the brain occurs. People over 50 years old are at risk. Signs and symptoms become worse over time (Fig. 10.32). They include:

- tremors – these often start in one finger and spread to the whole arm; pill-rolling movements (rubbing of the thumb and index finger) may occur; tremors may occur in the legs, jaw and face
- stiff muscles – in the arms, legs, neck and trunk
- slow movement – the person has a slow, shuffling gait

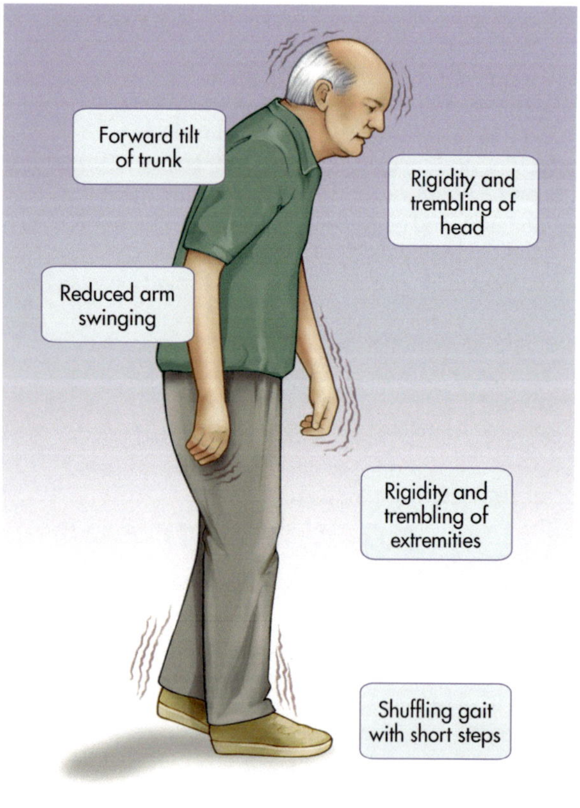

Fig. 10.32
Signs of Parkinson's disease.

- stooped posture and impaired balance – it is hard to walk; falls are a risk
- mask-like expression – the person cannot blink or smile; a fixed stare is common.

Other signs and symptoms can also develop over time. They include swallowing and chewing problems, constipation and bladder problems. Sleep problems and depression can occur. So can memory loss, slow thinking and emotional changes (fear and insecurity). Speech changes occur. They include slurred, monotone and soft speech. Some people talk too fast or repeat what they have said.

The doctor orders medications for Parkinson's disease. Exercise and physiotherapy are ordered to improve strength, posture, balance and mobility. Therapy is needed for speech and swallowing problems. The person may need help with eating and self-care. Normal elimination is a goal. Safety measures prevent injury.

Multiple sclerosis (MS)

Multiple sclerosis (MS) is a chronic disease. *Multiple* means many; *sclerosis* means hardening or scarring. The myelin (which covers nerve fibres) in the brain and spinal cord is destroyed. Nerve impulses are not sent to and from the brain in a normal manner. Functions are impaired or lost. There is no cure.

Symptoms usually start between the ages of 20 and 40. More women are affected than men. Caucasians are at greater risk than are other groups. It is more common in southern Australia and New Zealand.

MS can present as follows:

- *Benign form* – little or no symptom progress after the first attack.
- *Relapsing–remitting* – the person has a series of attacks. Then symptoms lessen or disappear (remission). At some point there are flare-ups (relapses). With each flare-up, more symptoms can occur.
- *Primary progressive* – the person's condition gradually declines. There are no remissions.
- *Secondary progressive* – the person has flare-ups and remissions. After many years, the person's condition declines.
- *Progressive–relapsing* – the person's condition gradually declines. Acute attacks occur. They leave new symptoms and more damage.
- *Malignant* – decline is swift and rapid. Severe disability or death occurs shortly after onset.

Symptoms depend on the damaged areas. Vision problems may occur. Muscle weakness and balance problems affect standing and walking. Paralysis can occur. Tremors, numbness and tingling, loss of feeling, speech problems, dizziness and poor coordination are common. Problems with concentration, attention, memory, judgement and behaviour may occur. Fatigue increases such problems. Bowel, bladder and sexual function problems occur. Respiratory muscle weakness is common. So are anger and depression.

People with MS are kept active for as long as possible. They need to do as much self-care as possible. The care plan reflects the person's changing needs. Skin care, hygiene and range-of-motion exercises are important. So are turning, positioning, coughing and deep breathing. This will help to prevent injuries and complications from bed rest. Bowel and bladder elimination is promoted.

HEAD INJURIES

Head injuries can involve the scalp, skull and brain tissue. Some injuries are minor. They cause only temporary loss of consciousness. Others are more serious. Brain tissue is bruised or torn. Bleeding can occur in the brain or nearby structures. Permanent brain damage or death may result.

Causes include falls, accidents and sports injuries. Often there are other injuries. Spinal cord injuries are likely. If the person survives, some permanent damage is likely. Paralysis, cognitive impairment and personality changes may be permanent. The same is true for speech, breathing, bowel and bladder problems.

Rehabilitation is required and some people need lifelong care. The care plan is based on the person's needs and abilities.

Spinal cord injuries

Spinal cord injuries can permanently damage the nervous system. The most common causes are falls, motor vehicle accidents, sports injuries and violence – blunt and penetrating trauma or bullet wounds.

Problems depend on the level of injury. The higher the level of injury, the more functions are lost (Fig. 10.33). With lumbar injuries, leg function is lost. Injuries at the thoracic level cause loss of function below the chest. Injuries at the lumbar or thoracic levels cause paraplegia. **Paraplegia** is paralysis from the waist down. Cervical injuries cause loss of function to the arms, chest and below the chest. **Tetraplegia** (formerly quadriplegia) is paralysis of both arms and legs.

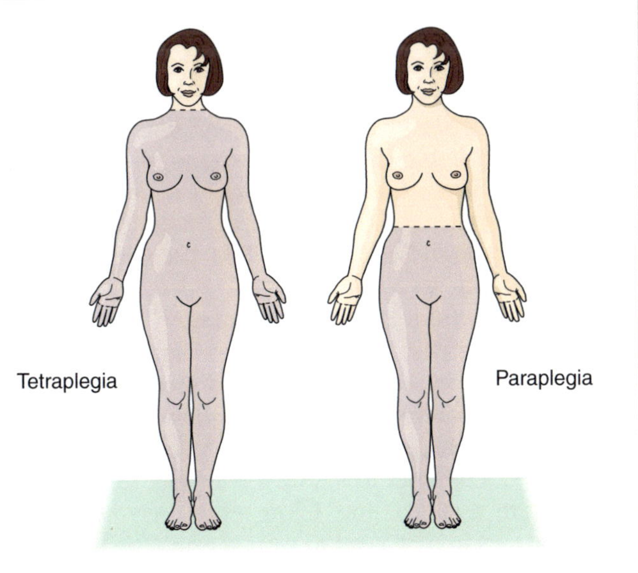

Fig. 10.33
Tetraplegia and paraplegia. The shaded areas show areas of paralysis.

If the person survives, they will need rehabilitation. The person learns to function at his or her highest possible level. Some need to use self-help, assistive and other devices. People who are paralysed often need the care listed in Box 10.5. Pay attention to their emotional needs. Reactions to paralysis and the loss of function are often severe.

Some people return home and live independently. Others need long-term care, home care or assisted-living settings.

THE SENSE ORGANS

The five major senses are sight, hearing, taste, smell and touch. Receptors for taste are in the tongue and are called *taste buds*. Receptors for smell are in the nose. Touch receptors are found in the dermis, especially in the toes and fingertips.

The eye

Receptors for vision are in the eyes (see Fig. 10.34). The eye is easily injured. The skull bones, eyelids, eyelashes and tears protect the eyes from injury.

The eye has three layers:

- The sclera, the white of the eye, is the outer layer. It is made of tough connective tissue.
- The choroid is the second layer. It is made up of blood vessels, the ciliary muscle and the iris. The iris gives the eye its colour. The opening in the middle of the iris is the pupil. Pupil size varies with the amount of light entering the eye. The pupil constricts (narrows) in bright light and dilates (widens) in dim or dark places.
- The retina is the inner layer. It contains receptors for vision and the nerve fibres of the optic nerve.

BOX 10.5
Care of the person with paralysis

- Prevent falls. Follow the care plan for safety measures and bed rail use. (Please note that bed rails are deemed to be a restraint and can only be used if ordered.)
- Keep the bed in low position.
- Keep the call bell within reach. If unable to use the call bell, check the person often.
- Prevent burns. Check bath water, heat applications and food for proper temperature.
- Turn and reposition at least every 2 hours.
- Prevent pressure injuries. Follow the care plan.
- Maintain good alignment at all times. Use supportive devices according to the care plan.
- Follow bowel and bladder training programs.
- Maintain muscle function and prevent contractures. Assist with range-of-motion and other exercises as directed.
- Assist with food and fluids as needed. Provide self-help devices as ordered.
- Give emotional and psychological support.
- Follow the person's rehabilitation plan.

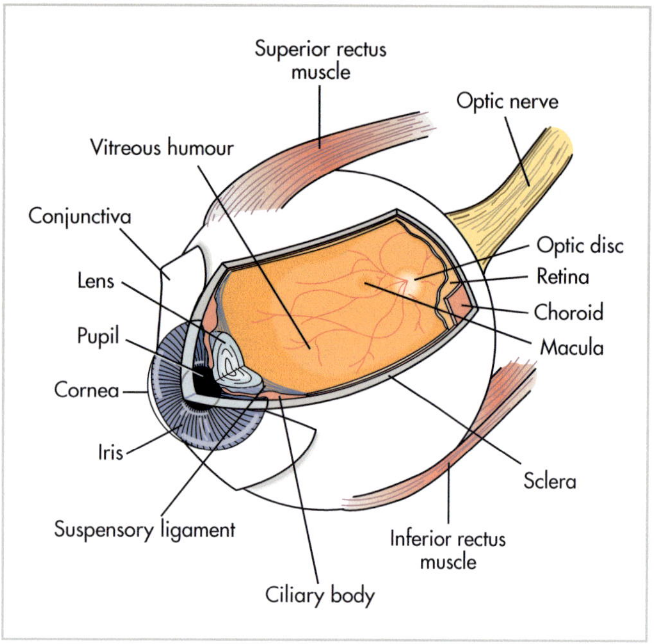

Fig. 10.34
The eye.

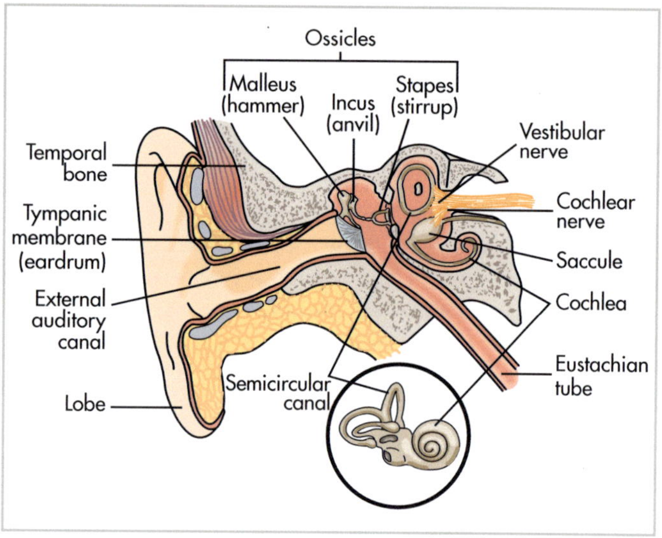

Fig. 10.35
The ear.

Light enters the eye through the *cornea*. This is the transparent part of the outer layer that lies over the eye. Light rays pass through it to the *lens*, which lies behind the pupil. The light is then reflected to the retina, and from there these signals or images are carried to the brain by the optic nerve.

The *aqueous chamber* separates the cornea from the lens. The chamber is filled with a fluid called *aqueous humour*. The fluid helps the cornea keep its shape and position. The *vitreous humour* is found behind the lens. It is a gelatine-like substance that supports the retina and maintains the shape of the eye.

The ear

The ear is a sense organ (Fig. 10.35). It functions in hearing and balance. It is divided into the external ear, middle ear and inner ear.

The *external ear* (outer part) is called the *pinna* or *auricle*. Sound waves are guided through the external ear into the *auditory canal*. Glands in the auditory canal secrete a waxy substance called *cerumen*. The auditory canal extends about 2.5 centimetres to the eardrum. The *eardrum* (tympanic membrane) separates the external ear and the middle ear.

The *middle ear* is a small space. It contains the *Eustachian tube* and three small bones called ossicles. The Eustachian tube connects the middle ear and the throat. Air enters the Eustachian tube so that there is equal pressure on both sides of the eardrum. The ossicles amplify sound received from the eardrum and transmit it to the inner ear. The three ossicles are:

- the malleus – this looks like a hammer
- the incus – looks like an anvil
- the stapes – looks like a stirrup.

The *inner ear* consists of the *semicircular canals* and the *cochlea*. The cochlea looks like a snail shell and contains fluid. The fluid carries sound waves received from the middle ear to the auditory nerve. The auditory nerve then carries the message to the brain.

The three semicircular canals are involved with balance. They sense the position of the head and changes in position and send messages to the brain.

AGEING OF THE SENSORY ORGANS

Ageing affects the senses of touch, smell, taste, sight and hearing. Touch and sensitivity to pain are reduced, as is the ability to feel heat and cold. These changes increase the risk of injury, as the person may not notice painful injuries and diseases.

- *Taste declines:* Taste and smell become dulled and appetite decreases. Taste buds decrease in number. The tongue senses only sweet, salty, bitter and sour tastes. Sweet and salty tastes are lost first. Older people often complain that food has no taste and like more salt or sugar on their food. The visual appeal of food is very important, to encourage residents to maintain healthy eating habits.
- *Eye function declines:* The eyelids become thin and wrinkled. Tear secretion decreases and so eye irritation easily occurs from dust and pollutants. The pupils become smaller and less responsive to light. This causes decreased vision at night or in dark rooms, as the eyes take longer to adjust to changes in the amount of light. Vision problems also occur when going from a dark room into a brighter room, or when going from a bright room into a darker one. Clear vision may be reduced and the person may need to wear glasses. The lens of the eye yellows, which makes it harder to see greens and blues. Older people develop age-related far-sightedness, called **presbyopia** (presby relates to ageing; opia means

'eye'). The lens becomes more rigid with age, which makes it harder for the eye to shift from far vision to near vision and from near to far vision. These changes increase the risk of falls and accidents. The risk increases on stairs and where lighting is poor. Make sure the person wears glasses as needed. Rooms need to be well lit. Night-lights help during the night.

- *Ear and auditory processes decline:* Changes also occur in the ear. The auditory nerve changes and the eardrums atrophy. It becomes hard to hear high-pitched sounds. If these changes progress, severe hearing loss occurs and a hearing aid may be needed. It must be clean and correctly placed in the ear. Wax secretion decreases and the wax becomes harder and thicker. This wax easily becomes impacted (wedged in the ear), which can increase hearing loss. A doctor or nurse can remove the wax if it interferes with hearing.

GENERAL CARE CONSIDERATION FOR SENSORY DEFICIT

It is important to take the following into consideration when caring for an individual who has lost function to the sensory organs:

- Protect older persons from injury.
- Follow safety measures for heat and cold.
- Check for signs of skin breakdown.
- Give good skin care.
- Prevent pressure injuries.

EAR DISORDERS

Otitis media

Otitis media is infection (*itis*) of the middle (*media*) ear (*ot*). It can be acute or chronic. Chronic otitis media can damage the tympanic membrane (eardrum) or the ossicles. These structures are needed for hearing. Permanent hearing loss can occur.

Fluid build-up occurs in the ear, which causes pain and hearing loss. Fever and ringing in the ears (**tinnitus**) also occur. This is treated with antibiotics by the doctor.

Ménière's disease

Ménière's disease is a chronic disease of the inner ear. The increased fluid causes pressure in the inner ear. Tinnitus, hearing loss and vertigo occur. **Vertigo** means dizziness. Whirling and spinning sensations are felt, with the severe dizziness causing nausea and vomiting. Attacks can last a few minutes or many hours. Medications, fluid restriction and a low-salt diet decrease fluid in the ear. Safety is needed during vertigo and the person must lie down. Prevent falls by using bed rails, according to the care plan. (Please note that bed rails are deemed to be a restraint and can only be used if ordered.) The person needs to keep their head still and avoid turning it. To talk to the person, stand directly in front of them. When the person needs to move, they will need to do so slowly, avoiding sudden movements. Avoid bright or glaring lights. Assist with ambulation, as the person should not walk alone in case vertigo occurs.

Hearing problems

Hearing loss occurs in all age groups and is common in older people. Causes include ageing, chronic exposure to loud noises, heredity and some illnesses. Temporary hearing loss can be caused by earwax (*cerumen*) blocking the ear canal. Hearing improves after the earwax is removed. A doctor or a registered nurse can remove this wax.

Hearing problems range from slight hearing loss to complete deafness. Clear speech, responding to others, safety and awareness of one's surroundings all require hearing. Many people deny having a hearing problem as they relate hearing loss to ageing.

Effects on the person

A person may not notice hearing problems that develop gradually. Others may see changes in the person's behaviour. They may not relate hearing problems to the changes. Symptoms of hearing loss include:

- speaking too loudly
- leaning forwards to hear
- turning and cupping the better ear towards the speaker
- answering questions or responding inappropriately
- asking for words to be repeated.

Psychological and social effects are less clear. A person may give wrong answers or responses. They may tend to avoid social events. Often, they feel lonely, bored and left out as only parts of conversations are heard. They may become suspicious and think they are being talked about. Alternatively, they may think that others are talking softly on purpose. Some fear being labelled 'senile' because of their poor responses. Some control the conversation to avoid answering questions. Straining and working to hear can cause fatigue, frustration and irritability.

Hearing is needed for speech. How you pronounce words and project your voice depend on how you hear yourself. Hearing loss may result in slurred speech and incorrect pronunciation of words. Some people have monotone speech or drop word endings. It may be hard to understand the person. Do not assume or pretend that you understand what the person says, or serious problems could result. Follow the guidelines in Boxes 10.6 and 10.7.

Communication

Hearing-impaired people may wear hearing aids (Fig. 10.36) or read lips. They watch facial expressions, gestures and body language. Follow the measures in Box 10.6. They help the person hear or speech read (lip-read). Some people learn sign language (Figs 10.37 and 10.38).

Some people have hearing assistance dogs (hearing guide dogs). The dog alerts the person to sounds. These sounds include telephones, doorbells, smoke detectors, alarm clocks, sirens and oncoming cars.

BOX 10.6
Communicating with the hearing-impaired person

- Gain the person's attention. Alert the person to your presence. Raise an arm or hand or lightly touch the person's arm. Do not startle the person or approach them from behind.
- Face the person when speaking. Do not turn or walk away while you are talking.
- Stand or sit in good light. Shadows and glare affect the ability to see your face clearly.
- Speak clearly, distinctly and slowly.
- Speak in a normal tone of voice. Do not shout.
- Do not cover your mouth, smoke, eat or chew gum while talking. Mouth movements are affected.
- Stand or sit on the side of the better ear.
- State the topic of conversation first.
- Use short sentences and simple words.
- Write out important names and words.
- If the person does not seem to understand you, say things in another way.
- Keep conversations and discussions short. This avoids tiring the person.
- Repeat and rephrase statements as needed.
- Be alert to the messages sent by your facial expressions, gestures and body language.
- Reduce or eliminate background noises.

BOX 10.7
Communicating with the speech-impaired person

- Listen and give the person your full attention.
- Ask questions to which you know the answer. This helps you become familiar with the person's speech.
- Determine the subject being discussed. This helps you to understand the main points.
- Ask the person to repeat or rephrase statements if necessary.
- Repeat what the person has said. Ask the person if your understanding is correct.
- Ask the person to write down key words or the message.
- Watch the person's lip movements.
- Watch facial expressions, gestures and body language for clues to what is being said.

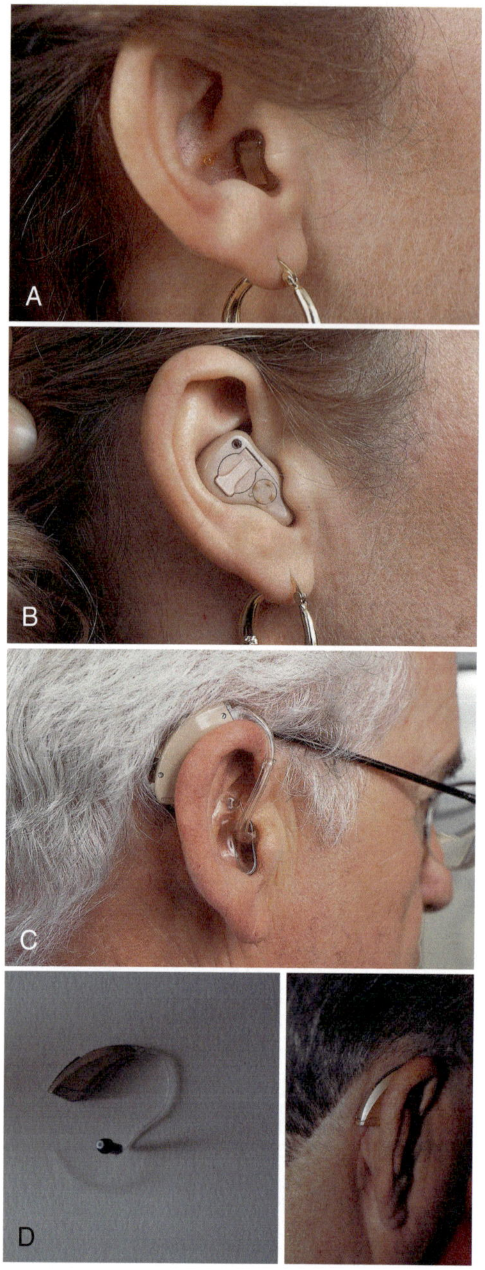

Fig. 10.36
Different types of hearing aids. **A.** Completely-in-canal (CIC). **B.** In the ear (ITE). **C.** Behind the ear (BTE). **D.** Digital hearing aid.

Hearing aids

A hearing aid makes sounds louder; however, it does not correct or cure the hearing problem. The person's ability to hear does not improve. However, the person hears better because the hearing aid makes sounds louder. Background noise and speech are also louder; however, modern hearing aids are able to moderate the amount of background noise by offering a range of adjustable settings. The measures in Box 10.7 apply.

Sometimes hearing aids do not seem to work properly. Try these simple measures:

- Check that the hearing aid is on. It has an on/off switch.
- Check the battery position.
- Insert a new battery, if needed.
- Clean the ear mould if necessary.

As hearing aids are costly, handle and care for them properly. Report lost or damaged hearing aids to the nurse at once. Check with the nurse before cleaning a hearing aid. Also, follow the manufacturer's instructions. Remove the battery at night if it uses standard batteries. If the aids take

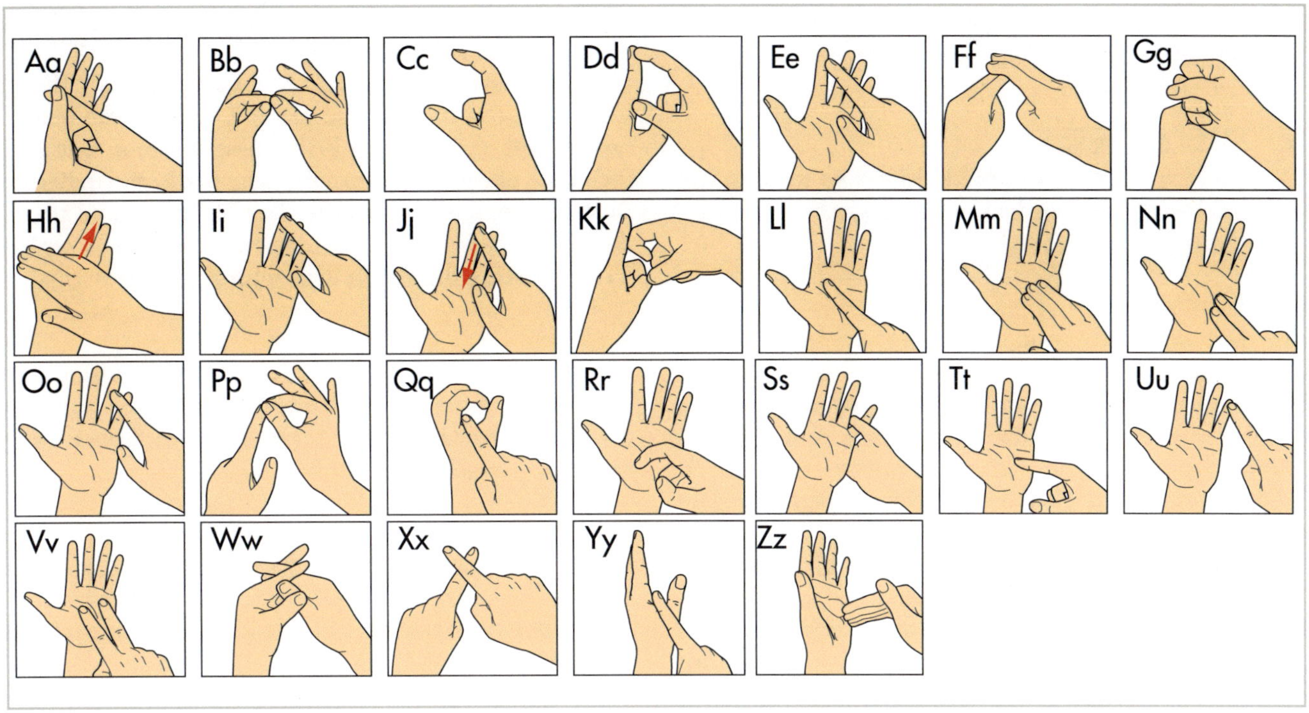

Fig. 10.37
The Auslan alphabet.

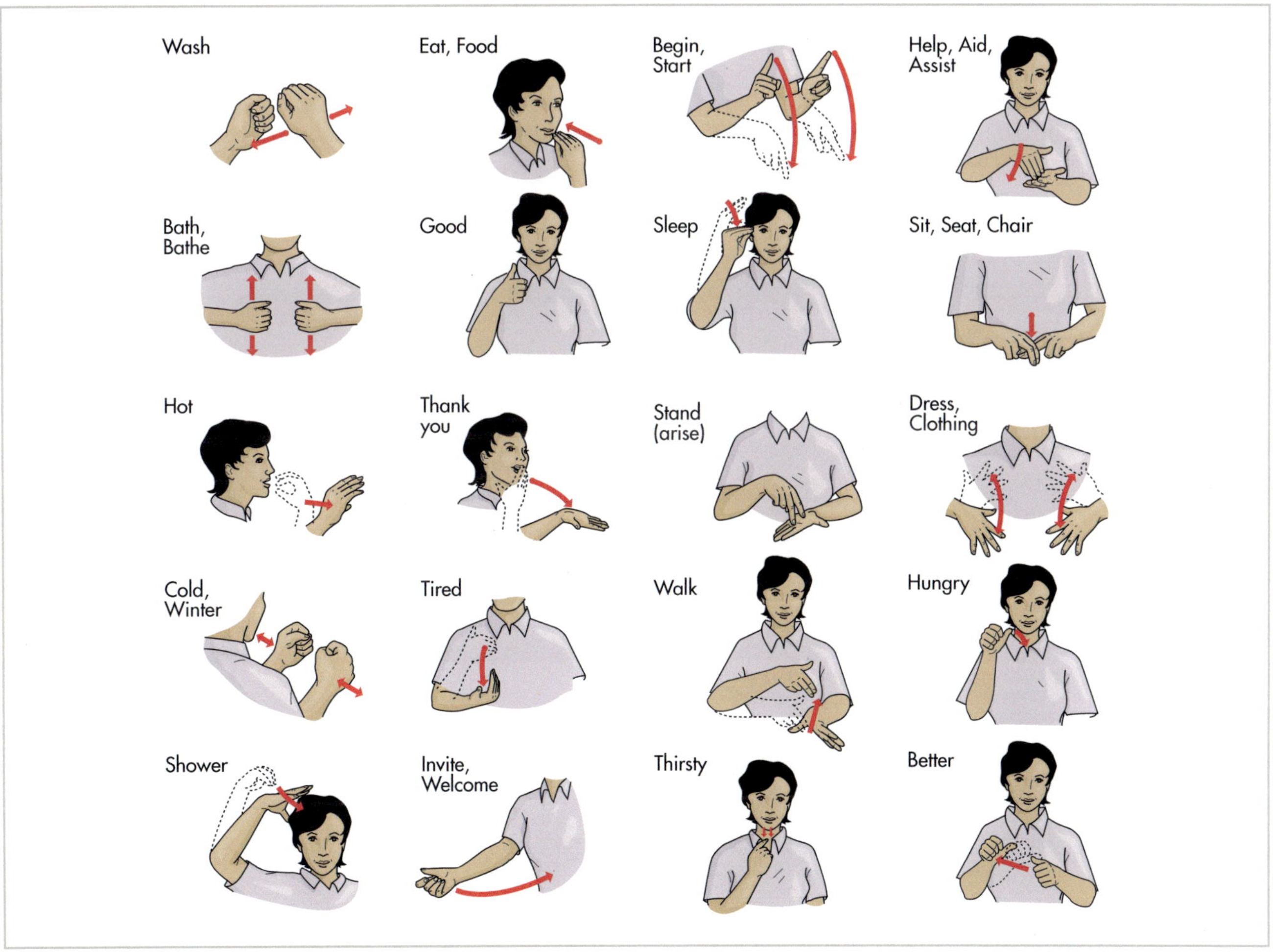

Fig. 10.38
Sign language examples.

rechargeable batteries, make sure they are fully charged each night (in a special charging unit). When not in use, turn the hearing aid off.

EYE DISORDERS

Vision problems range from mild vision loss to complete blindness. Vision loss can be sudden or gradual in onset. One or both eyes are affected.

Glaucoma

With *glaucoma*, fluid pressure within the eye increases and this damages the optic nerve. Vision loss with eventual blindness occurs. Onset can be gradual or sudden. The person loses peripheral vision; that is, they cannot see to the side. The person sees through a tunnel (Fig. 10.39). Blurred vision, haloes around lights and sensitivity to glare also occur.

Glaucoma is the second leading cause of permanent blindness in Australia and New Zealand. People aged over 40 are at risk. Indigenous Australians and Māori people are at greater risk than those of European descent. Other risk factors include a family history of the disease, diabetes and past eye injuries or surgery.

Treatment involves medication therapy and sometimes surgery. The goal is to prevent further damage to the optic nerve. Prior damage cannot be reversed.

Cataracts

A *cataract* is a disorder in which the lens of the eye becomes cloudy (opaque). Light cannot enter the eye (Fig. 10.40). Cataract comes from the Greek word meaning waterfall. Trying to see is like looking through a waterfall. Vision blurs and dims and print and colours look faded. The person is sensitive to light and glare. A cataract can occur in one or both eyes. Ageing is the most common cause. The incidence of cataract formation is higher in the Indigenous Australian population than in the non-Indigenous population. Surgery is the only treatment. The lens is replaced with a plastic lens. Vision then returns to near normal.

Corrective lenses

Glasses and contact lenses can correct many vision problems. Some people wear glasses for reading or seeing at a distance. Others wear them for all activities. Contact lenses are usually worn only while awake.

Glasses

Lenses are made of plastic or hardened glass. Clean them daily and as needed. Wash glass lenses with warm water and dry them with soft tissue. Plastic lenses scratch easily. Use special cleaning solutions, tissues and cloths.

Glasses are expensive, so protect them from breakage or other damage (Fig. 10.41). When not worn, put them in their case.

Contact lenses

Contact lenses fit directly on the eye. A variety of lenses are available, including hard, soft, gas permeable, extended wear, daily wear and disposable, but they are easily lost. To remove and clean contact lenses, follow the manufacturer's

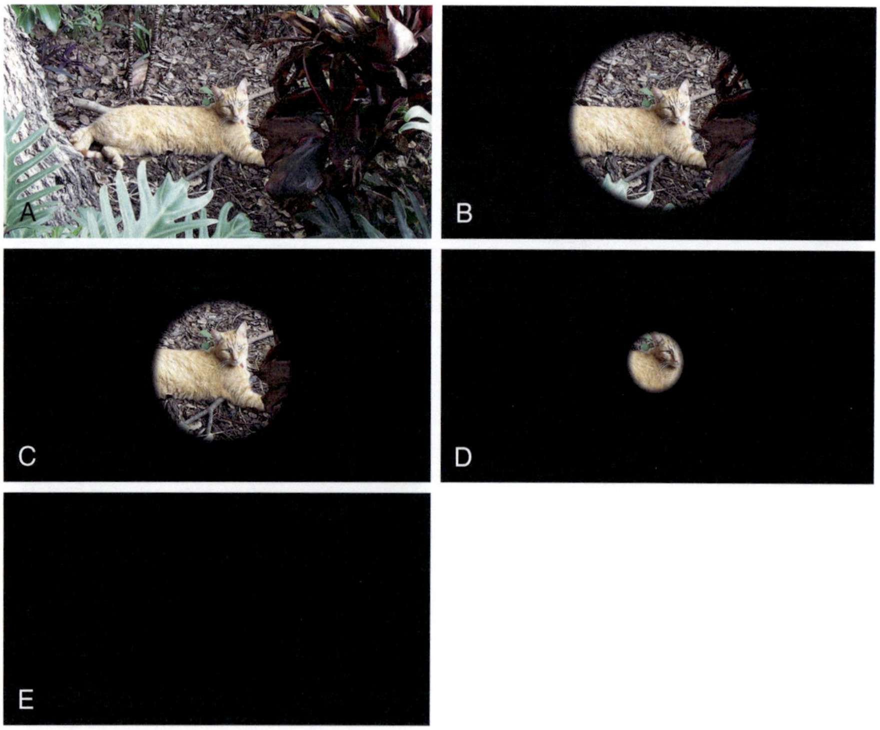

Fig. 10.39
Progression of glaucoma. **A.** Normal vision. **B.** Peripheral vision is lost (tunnel vision). **C. D. E.** Vision loss continues, with eventual blindness.

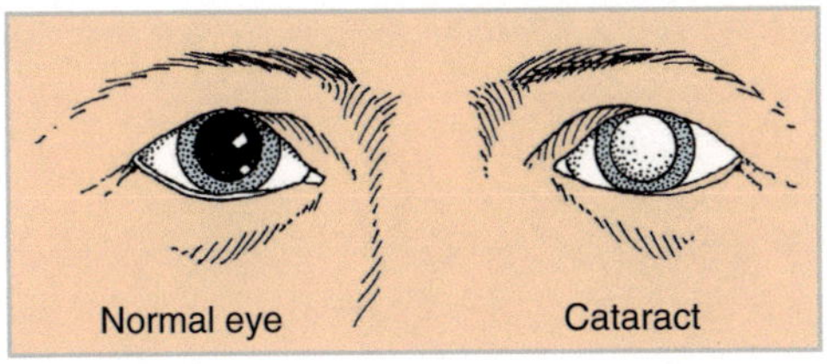

Fig. 10.40
One eye is normal. The other eye has a cataract.

instructions and facility procedures. Only the recommended solutions should be used for cleaning. Report redness, drainage from the eyes, complaints of eye pain or blurred vision at once.

Artificial eyes

Removing an eyeball is sometimes done because of injury or disease. The person is fitted with an ocular (eye) prosthesis (Fig. 10.42). It matches the other eye in colour and shape. The person cannot see through the artificial eye. The other eye may have normal or impaired vision.

Some ocular prostheses are permanent implants, while others are removable. If removable, the person is taught to remove, clean and insert it. The prosthesis is the person's property. Protect it from loss or damage. Follow these measures if the eye is not inserted after removal:

- Wash the eye with a mild soap and warm water. Rinse well.
- Line a container with a soft cloth or gauze. This prevents scratches and damage to the eye.
- Fill the container with water or a 0.9 per cent saline solution.
- Place the eye in the container. Close the container.
- Label the container with the person's name and room number.
- Place the labelled container in the bedside stand.
- Wash the eye socket with warm water or saline. Use a washcloth or gauze square. Remove excess moisture with a gauze square.

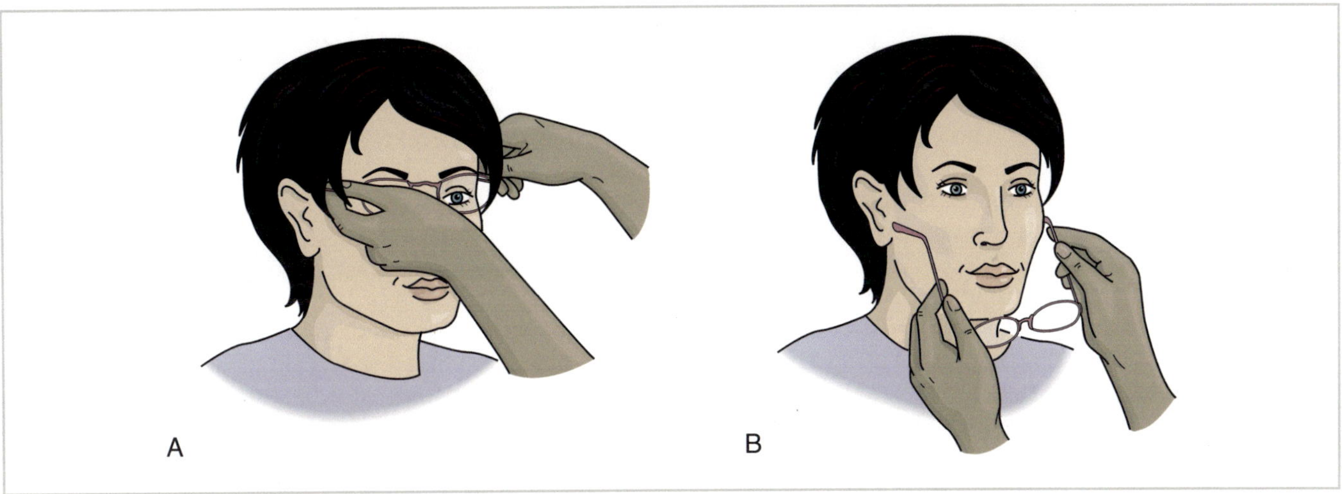

Fig. 10.41
A. To remove glasses, hold the frames in front with both hands. **B.** Lift the frames from the ears and bring the glasses down away from the face.

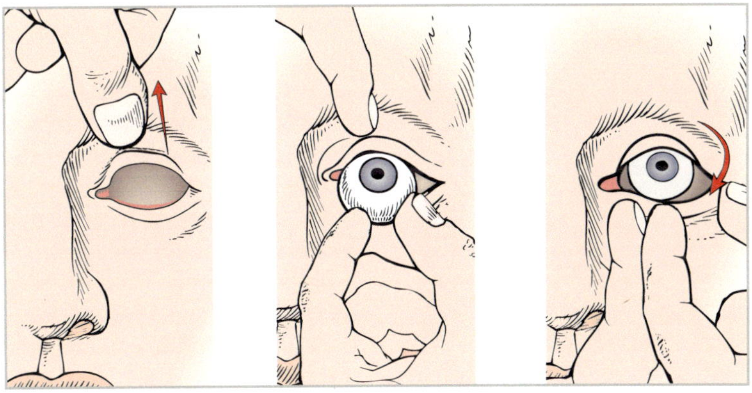

Fig. 10.42
An ocular prosthesis is inserted.

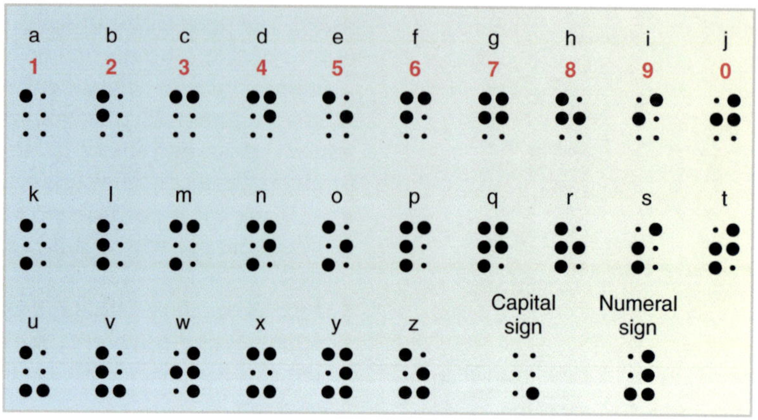

Fig. 10.43
Braille.

- Wash the eyelid with mild soap and warm water. Clean from the inner to the outer aspect of the eyelid. Dry the eyelid.

Visual impairment and blindness

Birth defects, accidents and eye diseases are among the many causes of visual impairment and blindness. It is also a complication of some other diseases. The level of visual impairment varies; some people are totally blind, while others sense some light but have no usable vision. Still others have some usable vision but cannot read newsprint. *Legally blind* is a term used by governments to define conditions for which a person is able to receive some government assistance and benefits.

Loss of sight is serious and adjustments are hard and long. Special education and training are needed. Moving about, daily activities, reading Braille and using a guide dog (seeing eye dog) all require training.

Braille is a tactile writing system that uses raised dots. Dots are arranged for each letter of the alphabet. The first 10 letters also represent the numbers zero to nine (Fig. 10.43). Braille is read with the fingers (Fig. 10.44). Many books, magazines and newspapers are available in Braille.

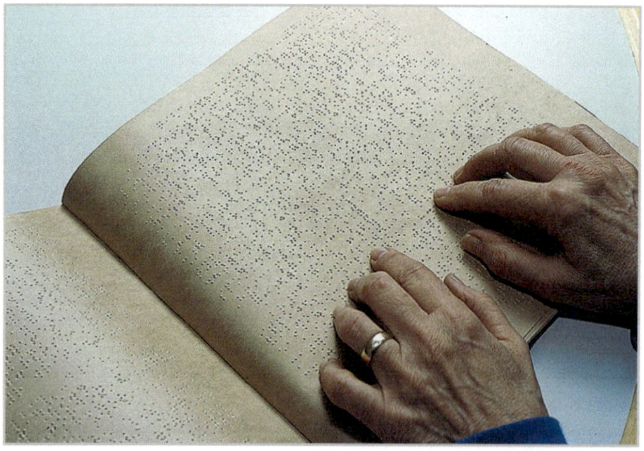

Fig. 10.44
Reading Braille with the fingers.

Some older people may find Braille hard to learn. They may prefer audio books. Blind people learn to move about using a cane. Some use guide dogs, which 'see' for them. These are specially trained dogs that are aware of danger and guide the person around obstacles. Treat the person with a vision impairment with respect and dignity – not pity. Most blind people adjust well and lead independent lives (Box 10.8).

THE CIRCULATORY SYSTEM

The circulatory system is made up of the heart, blood and blood vessels. The heart pumps blood through the blood vessels. The circulatory system has many important functions.

- Blood carries food, oxygen and other substances to the cells.
- Blood also removes waste products from cells.
- The blood and blood vessels aid regulation of body temperature. Heat from muscle activity is carried by the blood to other body parts. Blood vessels in the skin dilate if the body needs cooling and constrict if the body needs to retain heat.
- The circulatory system produces and carries cells that defend the body from disease-causing microorganisms.

Blood

The blood consists of blood cells and a liquid called *plasma*. Plasma is mostly water and carries the blood cells to other body cells. It also carries other substances needed by cells for proper functioning. Food (proteins, fats and carbohydrates), hormones, chemicals and waste products are among the many substances carried in the plasma.

Red blood cells are called erythrocytes. They give the blood its red colour because of a substance in the cell called **haemoglobin**. As red blood cells circulate through the lungs, the haemoglobin picks up oxygen. The haemoglobin then carries the oxygen to the cells around the body. When the blood is bright red, haemoglobin in the red blood cells is saturated (filled) with oxygen. As blood circulates through the body, oxygen is given to the cells. The cells release carbon dioxide (a waste product), which is picked up by the

BOX 10.8
Caring for a visually impaired person

- Ask the person how much he or she can see. Do not assume the person is totally blind or that they have some vision.
- Provide lighting as the person prefers. Tell the person when the lights are on or off.
- Adjust blinds and shades to prevent glare. Sunny days and bright cloudy days cause glare.
- Face the person when speaking. Speak slowly and clearly.
- Use a normal tone of voice. Do not shout or speak loudly. Blindness does not mean the person has a hearing impairment.
- Identify yourself. Give your name, title and reason for being there. Do not touch the person until you have indicated your presence.
- Identify others. Explain where each person is located and what the person is doing.
- Address the person by name. This tells the person that you are directing a comment or question to him or her.
- Do not avoid using the words 'see', 'look' or 'read'.
- Orient the person to the room. Describe the layout. Also describe the location and purpose of furniture and equipment.
- Let the person move about. Let them touch and find furniture and equipment.
- Do not leave the person in the middle of a room. Make sure he or she can reach a wall or furniture.
- Do not rearrange furniture and equipment.
- Keep doors open or shut. Never leave them partially open.
- Give step-by-step explanations of procedures as you perform them. Indicate when the procedure is over.
- Offer assistance. Simply say, 'May I help you?' Respect the person's answer.
- Tell the person when you are leaving the room.
- Assist the person in walking. Offer an arm and walk slightly ahead of him or her. Tell the person which arm is offered. Never push, pull or guide the person in front of you. Walk at a normal pace.
- Tell the person when you are coming to a kerb or steps. State whether you will step up or down.
- Inform the person of doors, turns, furniture and other obstructions when assisting with ambulation.
- Give specific directions. Say 'right behind you', 'on your left' or 'in front of you'. Avoid phrases like 'over here' or 'over there'.
- Keep hallways and walkways free of carts, equipment and other items.
- Assist in food selection. Read the menu to the person.
- Avoid plates, napkins, place mats and tablecloths with patterns and designs. These items should be solid colours and provide contrast. For example, place a white plate on a dark place mat or tablecloth.
- Explain the location of food and beverages. Use the face of a clock. Or guide the person's hand to each item on the tray.
- Cut meat, open containers, butter bread and perform similar activities if needed.
- Keep the call bell within the person's reach.
- Provide a radio, compact disks or audiotapes, television and Braille books.
- Let the person perform self-care if they are able.

haemoglobin. Red blood cells saturated with carbon dioxide make the blood look dark red. Mature red blood cells do not contain a nucleus or other organelles as they need a large amount of space to carry haemoglobin, which supports the oxygen-carrying capacity of the cell.

There are about 25 trillion red blood cells in the body. A cubic millimetre of blood (the size of a tiny drop) contains about 4–5 million cells. These cells live for 3 or 4 months. As they wear out, they are destroyed by the liver and spleen. New red blood cells are produced in the bone marrow, with about 1 million new red blood cells produced every second.

White blood cells are called *leucocytes*. They protect the body against infection. There are 5000–10,000 white blood cells in a cubic millimetre of blood. At the first sign of infection, white blood cells rush to the site of the infection where they begin to multiply rapidly. White blood cells are also produced by the bone marrow. There are several different white blood cells that form part of the immunological system, including antigen-presenting cells (which present the antigen components of the bacteria to the immune cells), effector cells (neutrophils, which initiate phagocytosis, a process that destroys pathogens) and lymphocytes (specialised white cells that form part of the acquired immune system, which produce antibodies and take place in other complex immunological processes).

Platelets (*thrombocytes*) are needed for blood clotting. They are produced by the bone marrow. There are about 200,000–400,000 platelets in a cubic millimetre of blood. A platelet lives for about 4 days.

The heart

The heart is a muscle that pumps blood through the blood vessels to the tissues and cells. The heart lies in the middle to lower part of the chest cavity, towards the left side (see Fig. 10.45). It is hollow and has three layers (Fig. 10.46):

1. The *pericardium* is the outer layer. It is a thin sac covering the heart.
2. The *myocardium* is the second layer. This is the thick muscular portion of the heart.
3. The *endocardium* is the inner layer. It is the membrane lining the inner surface of the heart.

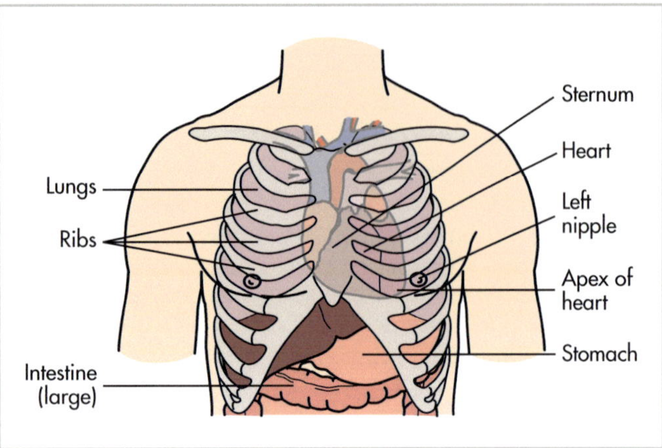

Fig. 10.45
Location of the heart in the chest cavity.

The heart has four chambers (see Fig. 10.46). The two upper chambers receive blood and are called the *atria*. The right atrium receives deoxygenated blood from body tissues and the left atrium receives oxygenated blood from the lungs. The two lower chambers are called *ventricles*. The ventricles pump the blood. The right ventricle pumps blood to the lungs for oxygen. The left ventricle pumps blood to all parts of the body.

Between the atria and the ventricles there are valves that allow blood to flow in one direction only. This prevents blood from flowing back into the atria from the ventricles and from the ventricles to the blood vessels. The *tricuspid valve* is between the right atrium and the right ventricle. The *mitral valve* (*bicuspid valve*) is between the left atrium and the left ventricle. The *aortic valve* is between the left ventricle and the aorta.

There are two main phases of heart action, related to blood filling:

1 *Diastole* – this is the resting phase, when the heart chambers are filling with blood.
2 *Systole* – this is the working phase when the heart is contracting. The contraction pumps blood through the blood vessels.

The heart muscle or myocardium is composed of two different types of muscle cells. The first type are called conductile cells and the second type of cells are called contractile cells. These cells operate to promote cardiovascular function. The heart muscle itself is stimulated by sympathetic and parasympathetic fibres. The sympathetic fibres *increase* the work rate of the cardiovascular system, which increases heart rate, stroke volume, blood pressure and cardiac output. The parasympathetic fibres *decrease* the heart rate, stroke volume, blood pressure and cardiac output.

Blood vessels

Blood flows to body tissues and cells through the blood vessels. There are three groups of blood vessels: arteries, capillaries and veins.

Arteries carry blood away from the heart. Arterial blood is rich in oxygen. The largest artery is the *aorta*. The aorta receives blood directly from the left ventricle. The aorta branches into other arteries that carry blood to all parts of the body (Fig. 10.47). The coronary arteries branch off at the base of the aorta and supply the myocardium with oxygenated blood. These arteries branch into smaller parts within the tissues. The smallest branch of an artery is called an *arteriole*.

Arterioles connect with blood vessels called **capillaries**. Capillaries are very tiny vessels. Food, oxygen and other

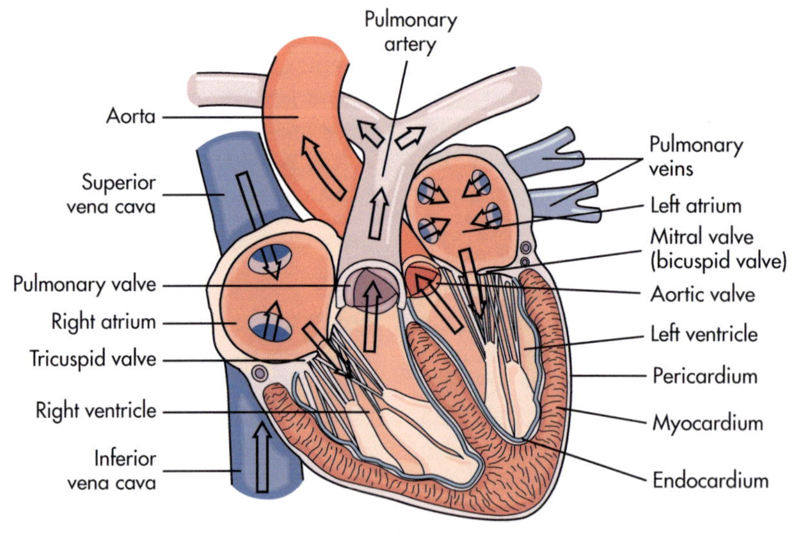

Fig. 10.46
Structures of the heart.

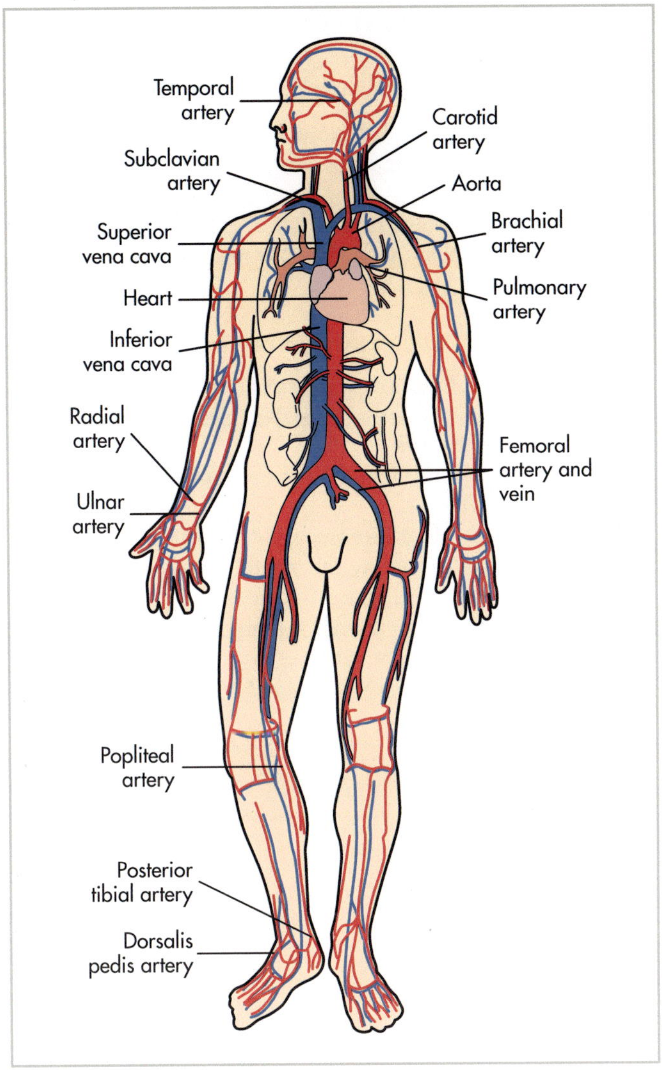

Fig. 10.47
Arterial and venous systems.

substances pass from capillaries into the cells. Waste products, including carbon dioxide and hydrogen ions, are picked up from cells by the capillaries. Waste products are carried back to the heart by the veins.

Veins return blood to the heart. They are connected to the capillaries by venules, or small veins. Venules begin branching together to form veins. The many branches of veins also branch together as they near the heart, to form two main veins (Fig. 10.47). The two main veins are the inferior vena cava and the superior vena cava. Both empty into the right atrium. The *inferior vena cava* carries blood from the legs and trunk. The *superior vena cava* carries blood from the head and arms. Venous blood is dark red because it contains little oxygen and a lot of carbon dioxide.

Blood flow through the heart and circulatory system is shown in Figs 10.46 and 10.47. It is summarised as follows:

1. Venous blood, poor in oxygen, empties into the right atrium.
2. Blood flows through the tricuspid valve into the right ventricle.
3. The right ventricle pumps the blood into the lungs to pick up oxygen.
4. Oxygen-rich blood from the lungs enters the left atrium.
5. Blood from the left atrium passes through the mitral valve into the left ventricle.
6. The left ventricle pumps the blood to the aorta, which branches off to form other arteries.
7. The arterial blood is carried to the tissues by arterioles and to the cells by capillaries.
8. The cells and capillaries exchange oxygen and nutrients for carbon dioxide and waste products.
9. Capillaries connect with venules.
10. Venules carry blood that contains carbon dioxide and waste products.
11. The venules form veins.
12. Veins return blood to the heart.

FUNCTION AND CONTROL OF THE CARDIOVASCULAR SYSTEM

The cardiovascular system is an organ system used by the body to carry blood, oxygen and nutrients to organs and tissues, as well as carry waste and carbon dioxide for removal from the body. The heart is composed of two types of muscle cells: specialised muscle cells of the conducting system, which control and coordinate the heat beat; and contractile cells, which produce powerful contractions that propel blood and are stimulated by the conducting system. Each heart beat is generated at the sinoatrial (SA node – a set of specialised cells), an integral part of the conducting system that kick-starts the electrical activity in the heart. This electrical impulse is then propagated along the length of the conducting system. As these electrical events take place they stimulate the contractile cells – which then push the blood in the right direction through the heart from atria to ventricles to either the pulmonary or the systemic circulations. If the conduction or contractile systems are not working properly the heartbeat and blood flow will not work properly, leaving the person susceptible to arrhythmias. An arrhythmia is a problem with the rate or rhythm of the heartbeat.

AGEING OF THE CARDIOVASCULAR SYSTEM (BLOOD, HEART AND BLOOD VESSELS)

Ageing affects the cardiovascular system in all of the major components, including the blood, the heart and the blood vessels. The changes that take place during the ageing process are:

- *heart changes:* The most obvious change in cardiovascular function as the person ages is the reduction in cardiac output. The conductile cells become less efficient and the heart muscle is less elastic. This affects the heart's ability to contract and relax.

- *blood vessel changes:* Blood vessels have a decreased ability to respond to changes in blood pressure. This is frequently caused by a loss in the elasticity of the blood vessel wall, which can lead to a number of serious medical conditions, including an aneurysm, a stroke, a myocardial infarction or massive blood loss. The weakened blood vessel wall can be due to deposits of calcium salts, which can then increase the risk of stroke or myocardial infarction. As there are more atherosclerotic plaques in the older individual there can be a greater risk of thrombi breaking off and causing a myocardial infarction.
- *blood changes:* One of the biggest changes is the pooling of blood that occurs in the lower half of the body since the valves in the veins and venules are not working properly. The peripheral veins can become blocked by a thrombus, which can detach and become stuck in the smaller blood vessels in the heart (causing a heart attack) and/or in the lungs (causing a pulmonary embolism).

CARDIOVASCULAR DISORDERS

Cardiovascular disorders are the leading cause of death in Australia. Indigenous Australians and Māori people are disproportionately at risk. The pathology of the condition can occur in the heart and the blood vessels.

Hypertension

With hypertension (high blood pressure), the resting blood pressure is too high. The systolic pressure is 140 mmHg or higher. Alternatively, the diastolic pressure is 90 mmHg or higher. This needs to occur on two or more occasions before the person is diagnosed as having hypertension. See Box 10.9 for risk factors.

Narrowed blood vessels are a common cause. When vessels narrow, the heart has to pump with more force to move blood through the vessels. Kidney disorders, head injuries, some pregnancy problems and adrenal gland tumours are other causes.

Hypertension can damage other organs and can lead to stroke, heart attack, heart failure, kidney failure and blindness. Signs and symptoms develop over time and include headache, blurred vision, dizziness and nosebleeds. Medication is often used to lower blood pressure. A healthy diet, a healthy weight and regular exercise are important. Alcohol and caffeine intake should be limited and if the person is a smoker, they must stop smoking. Managing stress and sleeping well will also lower blood pressure.

BOX 10.9
Risk factors for hypertension

Factors that cannot be changed

- Age – 45 years or older for men; 55 years or older for women
- Sex (gender) – younger men are at greater risk than younger women; the risk increases for women after menopause
- Ethnic origin
- Family history – tends to run in families

Factors that can be changed

- Being overweight – related to diet, lack of exercise and atherosclerosis
- Stress – increased sympathetic nervous system activity
- Tobacco use – nicotine narrows blood vessels
- High-salt diet – sodium causes fluid retention; increased fluid raises the blood volume
- Excessive alcohol – increases chemical substances in the body that increase blood pressure
- Lack of exercise – increases risk of being overweight

Coronary artery disease (CAD)

The coronary arteries are in the heart and supply the heart with blood. In coronary artery disease (CAD), the coronary arteries narrow. One or all can be affected. Therefore, the heart muscle gets less blood. The most common cause is atherosclerosis (Fig. 10.48). The narrowed arteries partially or totally block blood flow. Permanent damage occurs in the part of the heart receiving its blood supply from the blocked artery.

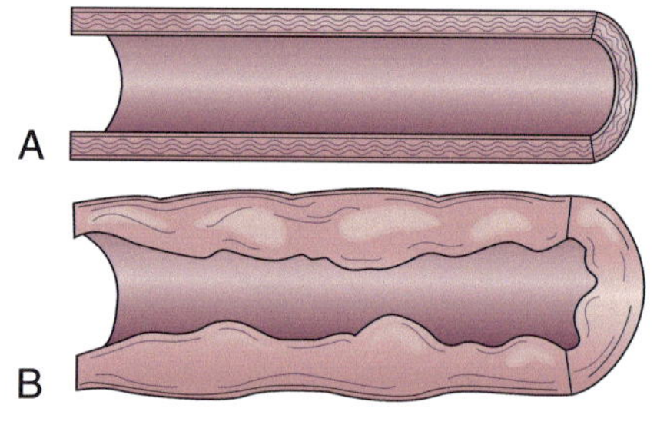

Fig. 10.48
A. Normal artery. **B.** Fatty deposits collect on arterial walls in atherosclerosis.

The major complications of CAD are angina pectoris and myocardial infarction (heart attack). Treatment involves reducing risk factors. Some risk factors cannot be controlled:

- gender – men are at greater risk than women
- age – CAD is more common in older people
- family history
- ethnicity – Indigenous Australians and Māori people are at greater risk.

Other factors can be controlled:

- weight
- smoking
- lack of exercise
- high blood cholesterol level

- hypertension
- diabetes
- stress.

Angina pectoris

Angina (pain) *pectoris* (of the chest) means chest pain. The chest pain is from reduced blood flow to a part of the heart muscle (myocardium). It is commonly called *angina*. It occurs when the heart needs more oxygen. Normally, blood flow to the heart increases when the need for oxygen increases. Exertion, a heavy meal, stress and excitement increase the heart's need for oxygen. In CAD, narrowed vessels prevent increased blood flow.

Chest pain is described as a tightness or pressure. Some complain of discomfort in the chest (Fig. 10.49). Pain in the jaw, neck and down one or both arms is common. The person may be pale, feel faint and perspire. **Dyspnoea** (shortness of breath) is common. The person stops activity to rest, which often relieves symptoms in 3–15 minutes. Rest reduces the heart's need for oxygen; therefore, blood flow returns to normal and heart damage is prevented.

Besides rest, medication is required when an angina attack occurs. The medication is placed under the tongue, where it dissolves and is rapidly absorbed into the bloodstream. Tablets or sprays are kept with the person at all times. The person who is self-medicating takes the medication and then tells the nurse.

Avoid situations that cause angina pectoris. These include overexertion, heavy meals, overeating and emotional stress. The person needs to stay indoors during cold weather or during hot, humid weather. Exercise programs are helpful. However, these must be done under medical supervision.

Surgery can open or bypass the diseased part of the artery (Fig. 10.50) to increase blood flow to the heart. Angina pectoris often leads to heart attack. Chest pain that is not relieved by rest and medication may signal a heart attack.

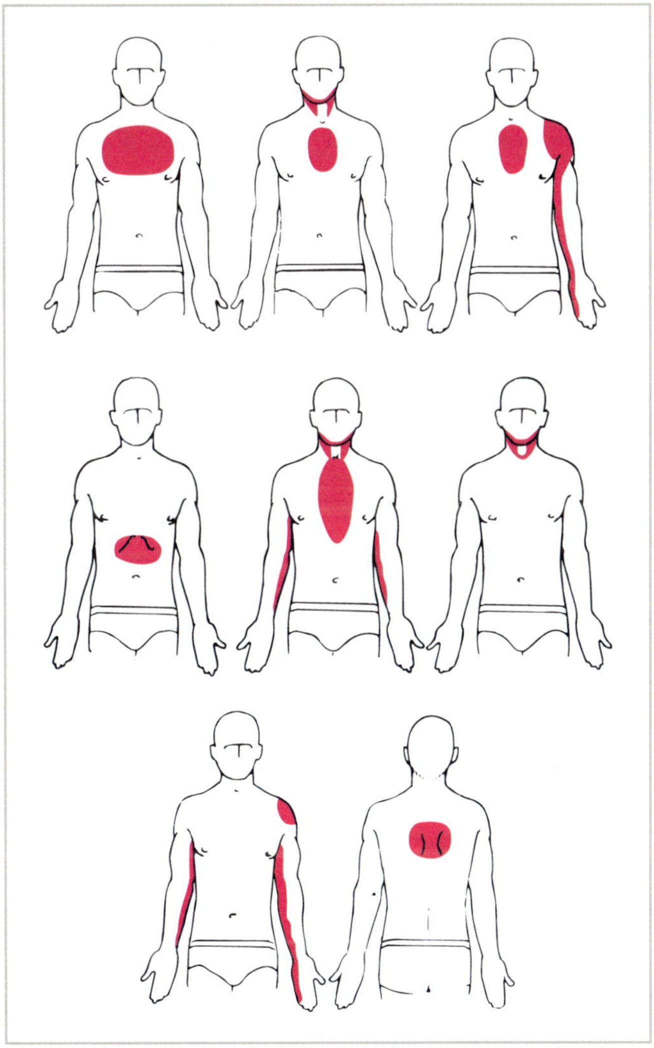

Fig. 10.49
Shaded areas show where the pain of angina pectoris is located.

Myocardial infarction (MI)

Myocardial refers to the heart muscle. *Infarction* means tissue death. With a myocardial infarction (MI), part of the heart muscle dies. This is due to lack of blood flow to the heart muscle.

Common terms for MI are heart attack, coronary, coronary thrombosis and coronary occlusion. Blood flow to the heart muscle is suddenly blocked. A thrombus (blood clot) obstructs blood flow through an artery with atherosclerosis. The area of damage may be small or large (Fig. 10.51). Sudden cardiac death (cardiac arrest) can occur.

Signs and symptoms of MI are listed in Box 10.10. MI is an emergency. Efforts are made to:

- relieve pain
- stabilise vital signs
- give oxygen (only with oxygen levels on 'low')
- calm the person
- prevent life-threatening problems.

The goal is to prevent another heart attack.

Heart failure

Heart failure, or congestive heart failure (CHF) (or congestive cardiac failure, CCF), occurs when the heart is unable to maintain cardiac output of blood to meet sufficient blood and oxygen requirements for the body. This results in the body tissues becoming ischaemic; that is, the tissues start to degenerate and die due to the reduced blood flow and thus oxygen delivery decreases. A damaged or weakened heart usually causes heart failure. MI, hypertension and damaged heart valves are common causes.

Medications are used to strengthen the heart. They also reduce the amount of fluid in the body. A sodium-controlled diet (no added salt) is ordered. **Semi-Fowler's** or **Fowler's position** is preferred for breathing (Fig. 10.52). If acutely ill, the person needs hospital care. You may assist with these aspects of the person's care by:

- maintaining bed rest or a limited activity program
- measuring intake and output

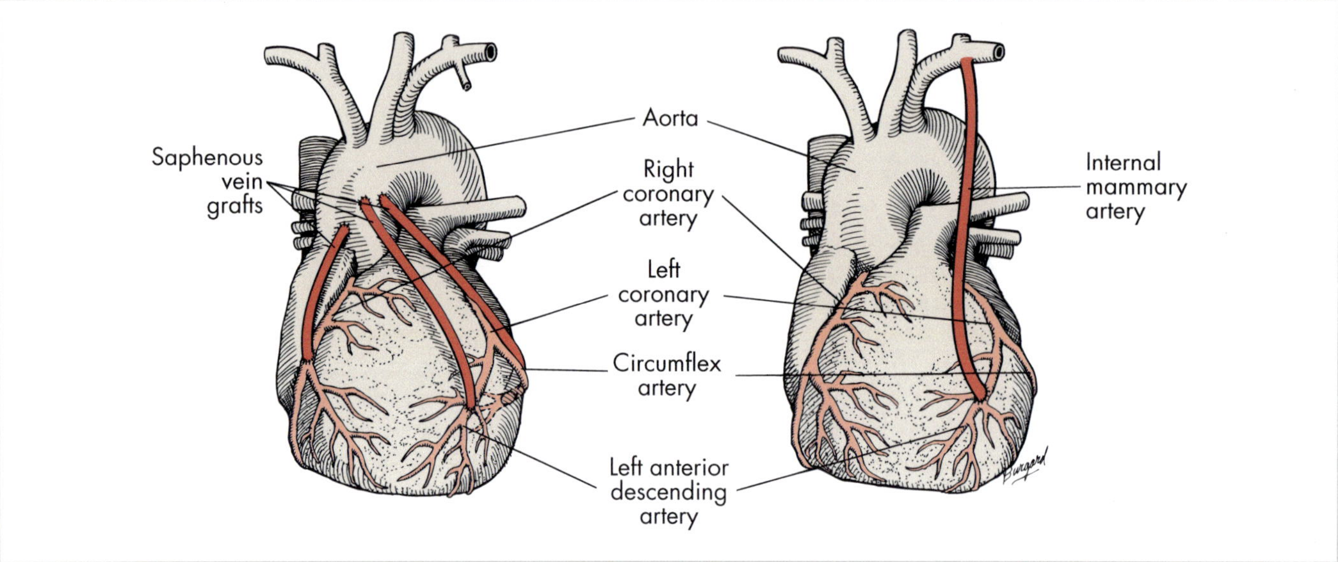

Fig. 10.50
Coronary artery bypass surgery.

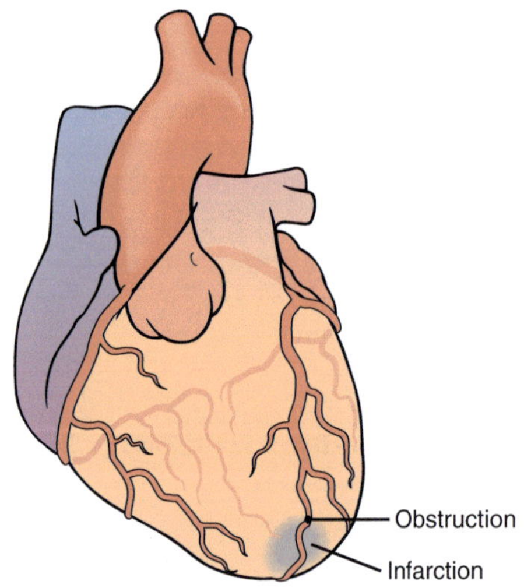

Fig. 10.51
Myocardial infarction.

BOX 10.10
Signs and symptoms of myocardial infarction

- Sudden, severe chest pain
  - Pain is usually on the left side
  - Pain is described as crushing, stabbing or squeezing; some describe it as like someone sitting on your chest
  - Pain may radiate to the neck, jaw and teeth and down the shoulder or to other sites
  - Pain is more severe and lasts longer than angina pectoris
  - Pain is not relieved by rest and nitroglycerine
- Indigestion
- Dyspnoea
- Nausea and vomiting
- Dizziness
- Severe sweating
- Pallor
- Cyanosis
- Cold and clammy skin
- Low blood pressure
- Weak and irregular pulse
- Unsteadiness
- Confusion
- Fear and apprehension
- A feeling of doom

- measuring weight daily
- preventing skin breakdown and pressure injuries
- assisting with transfers or ambulation
- assisting with self-care measures
- maintaining body alignment
- applying elastic stockings.

THE RESPIRATORY SYSTEM

We need oxygen for survival. Every cell in our bodies needs oxygen. Air contains about 21 per cent oxygen, which is enough to meet our body's needs under normal conditions. The respiratory system brings oxygen into the lungs and eliminates carbon dioxide. The process of supplying the cells with oxygen and removing carbon dioxide from them is called **respiration**. Respiration involves *inhalation* (breathing in) and *exhalation* (breathing out). The terms *inspiration* (breathing in) and *expiration* (breathing out) are also used (Fig. 10.53).

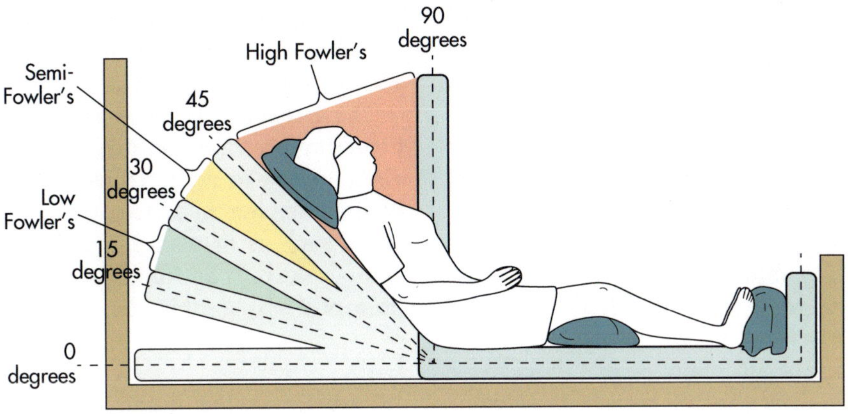

Fig. 10.52
Head of bed positioning for low-Fowler's, semi-Fowler's, and high Fowler's positions.

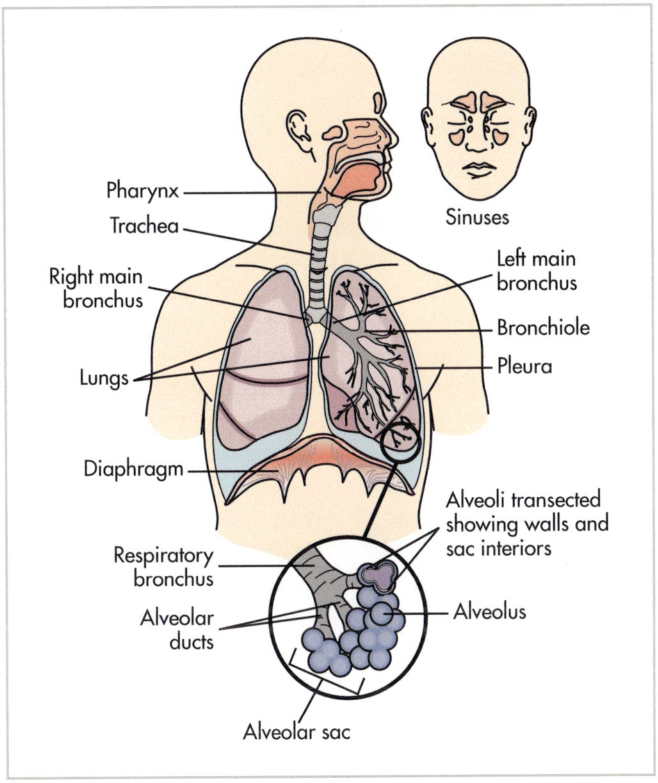

Fig. 10.53
Respiratory system.

Air enters the body through the nose and then passes into the *pharynx* (throat). The pharynx is a tube-shaped passageway for both air and food. Air passes from the pharynx into the *larynx* (the voice box). A piece of cartilage called the *epiglottis* acts like a lid over the larynx. The epiglottis prevents food from entering the airway during swallowing. During inhalation, the epiglottis lifts up to let air pass over the larynx. Air passes from the larynx into the *trachea* (the windpipe).

The trachea divides at its lower end into the *right bronchus* and *left bronchus.* Each bronchus enters a lung. Upon entering the lungs, the bronchi further divide many times into smaller branches. The smaller branches are called *bronchioles.* Eventually the bronchioles subdivide and end in tiny one-celled air sacs called alveoli.

Alveoli look like small clusters of grapes (see Fig. 10.52). They are supplied by capillaries. Oxygen and carbon dioxide are exchanged between the alveoli and capillaries. Alveoli pick up carbon dioxide from the blood in the capillaries for exhalation. Blood in the capillaries picks up oxygen from the alveoli, then returns to the left side of the heart. From there it is pumped to the rest of the body.

The lungs are spongy tissues filled with alveoli, blood vessels and nerves. Each lung is divided into lobes. The right lung has three lobes, the left lung has two. The lungs are separated from the abdominal cavity by a muscle called the *diaphragm.* Each lung is covered by a two-layered sac called the *pleura.* One layer is attached to the lung and the other to the chest wall. The pleura secretes a very thin fluid that fills the space between the layers. The fluid prevents the layers from rubbing together during inhalation and exhalation. The lungs are protected by a bony framework consisting of the ribs, sternum and vertebrae.

AGEING OF THE RESPIRATORY SYSTEM

Ageing affects the respiratory system with many factors interacting to reduce its efficiency. Age-related changes in the respiratory system are:

- *decline in lung movement:* As an individual ages, the elastic tissue deteriorates throughout the body and restricts the compliance (expansion and contraction of the lungs), thus decreasing the capacity of the lungs to uptake oxygen and remove carbon dioxide. Difficult, laboured or painful breathing (dyspnoea) may occur with activity.
- *restriction of chest movement:* Arthritic changes occurring in the cartilage that help protect the lungs, and also help them expand and relax, decrease the flexibility of the lungs. This increase in stiffness prevents the person's ability to cough and clear the airway of secretions. Thus

respiratory infections and diseases are more likely to occur in the elderly. Normal breathing needs to be actively promoted. Heavy bed linen should not cover the chest, as it can prevent normal chest expansion. Turning, repositioning and deep breathing are important, as they help prevent respiratory complications from bed rest. Breathing is usually easier in the semi-Fowler's position. The person should be as active as possible. People who have chronic breathing difficulties should be assessed by a physiotherapist to determine whether regular breathing exercises may be of assistance.

- *emphysema:* By the age of 50, many people show some degree of emphysema, depending on their lifetime exposure to cigarette smoke and other respiratory irritants. The pathological changes to lung tissue that occur during emphysema are discussed below.

RESPIRATORY DISORDERS

The respiratory system brings oxygen (O_2) into the lungs and removes carbon dioxide (CO_2) from the body. Respiratory disorders interfere with this function and threaten life.

Chronic obstructive airway disease (COAD)

The three forms of chronic obstructive airway disease (COAD) are chronic bronchitis, emphysema and asthma. They interfere with oxygen and carbon dioxide exchange in the lungs. They obstruct airflow.

Chronic bronchitis

Chronic bronchitis occurs after repeated episodes of bronchitis. Bronchitis means inflammation (itis) of the bronchi (bronch). Smoking is the major cause. Other causes are infection, air pollution and industrial dusts.

Smoker's cough in the morning is often the first symptom. At first, the cough is dry. Over time the person coughs up mucus, which may contain pus. The cough becomes more frequent and the person has difficulty breathing and tires easily. Mucus and inflamed breathing passages obstruct air flow into the lungs, resulting in the body not getting normal amounts of oxygen.

The person must stop smoking. Oxygen therapy and breathing exercises are often ordered and the person is advised on how to avoid respiratory tract infections. Measures include staying hydrated; practising good hygiene measures, such as handwashing; managing stress and getting enough sleep. If an infection occurs, it needs to be treated promptly with antibiotics.

Emphysema

In *emphysema*, the alveoli enlarge and become less elastic. They do not expand and shrink normally with breathing in and out. As a result, some air is trapped in the alveoli when exhaling. Trapped air is not exhaled. Over time, more alveoli are involved. Therefore, more air is trapped in the alveolar tissue – the air space increases and the efficiency for oxygen and carbon dioxide exchange diminishes. Fig. 10.54 below compares the difference in the structure between normal healthy lung tissue versus lung tissue affected with emphysema. It can be seen in Fig. 10.54A that there are many alveoli that have a very similar structure, whereas Fig. 10.54B shows massive air spaces and reduced surface area that has a very poor ability to exchange oxygen and carbon dioxide.

The most common and preventable cause of emphysema is smoking. The person will experience several symptoms, including shortness of breath and a persistent cough. At first, shortness of breath occurs with exertion. However, over time it can start to occur even at rest as the condition spreads throughout the lungs, reducing its function. Sputum may also contain pus, a sign of infection. One of the most important biological roles of the lungs is to remove trapped bacteria – with emphysema, the ability to clear mucus and bacteria is reduced, thus increasing the risk of serious lung infections. As more air becomes trapped in the lungs, the person develops a barrel-like shaped chest (Fig. 10.55). For those suffering from barrel chest, it is easier to breathe sitting upright and slightly

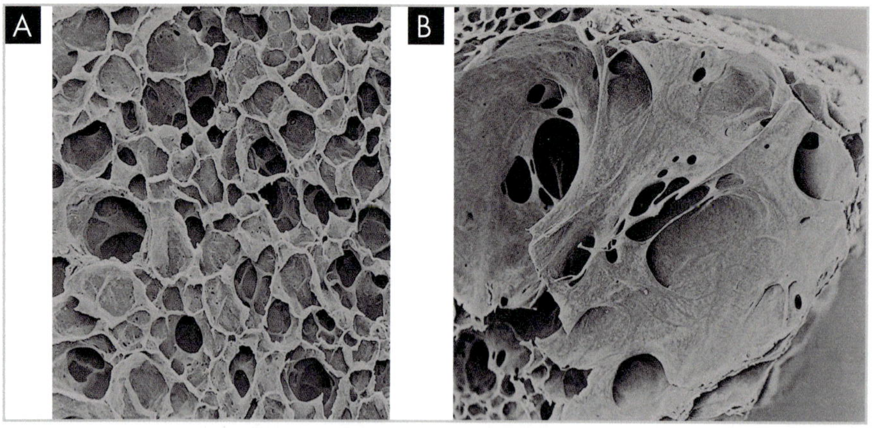

Fig. 10.54
Comparison of: **A.** Normal lung tissue and **B.** Lung tissue affected by emphysema.

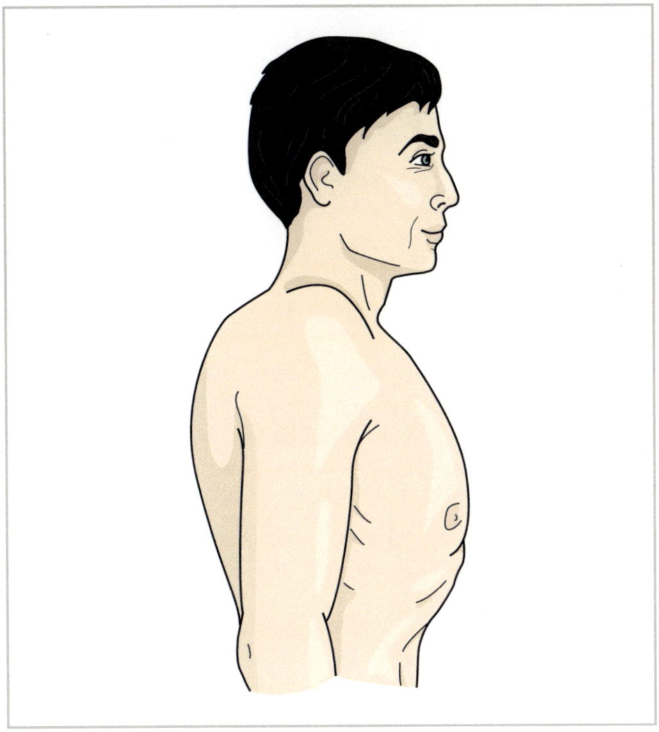

Fig. 10.55
Barrel chest from emphysema.

forward. Respiratory therapy, breathing exercises, oxygen and medication therapy are also generally ordered to help maintain respiration. If smoking is the primary cause of emphysema it is important that the person stops smoking to prevent further worsening of the condition.

Asthma

The airway narrows with *asthma* and dyspnoea results. Allergies and emotional stress are common causes, as well as smoking, respiratory infections and exertion. Symptoms are mild to severe and include wheezing and a cough.

Sudden attacks (asthma attacks) can occur. There is shortness of breath, wheezing, coughing, rapid pulse, sweating and cyanosis. The person gasps for air and can be very frightened. Panicking makes the attack worse.

Asthma is treated with medications. Severe attacks may require emergency department treatment. The person and family are taught how to prevent asthma attacks. Repeated attacks can damage the respiratory system.

Pneumonia

Pneumonia is an inflammation and infection of lung tissue. Affected tissues fill with fluid. Oxygen and carbon dioxide exchange is affected.

Bacteria, viruses and aspiration are some of the causes. Immobility will make the person more vulnerable to pneumonia. The person is very ill. Fever, chills, painful cough, chest pain on breathing and a rapid pulse occur. Cyanosis may be present. Sputum is thick and green, yellowish or rust coloured. The colour depends on the cause.

Medications are ordered for infection and pain. Fluid intake is increased because of fever. Fluids also thin the mucus secretions and they become easier to cough up. Intravenous (IV) fluids and oxygen may be needed. The person needs plenty of rest. The semi-Fowler's position eases breathing. Frequent position changes prevent pooling of secretions in the lung. Standard Precautions are followed. Mouth care is important and frequent linen changes are needed because of fever.

Older people are at risk. Medications and other diseases can mask signs and symptoms of pneumonia. Aspiration pneumonia is common in older people. Dysphagia, decreased cough, gag reflexes and nervous system disorders are risk factors. So are substances that depress the brain – narcotics, sedatives and alcohol. Pneumonia can lead to death.

Tuberculosis (TB)

Tuberculosis (TB) is a bacterial infection. Although it affects the lungs, it can also occur in the kidneys and bones. If untreated, it can lead to death. TB medication therapy was introduced in the 1940s and the number of cases declined after that. Even though the incidence of TB has declined in Australia and New Zealand in past decades, it remains problematic among older Indigenous Australians, Māori people and immigrants from countries where TB is endemic (widespread). TB is a notifiable disease; that is, the health department must be notified of any new or active cases.

TB is spread via airborne droplets associated with coughing, sneezing, speaking and singing. Nearby persons can inhale the bacteria. Those who have close, frequent contact with an infected person are at risk. TB is more likely to occur in close, crowded living areas. Age, poor nutrition and HIV infection are other risk factors.

An active infection may not occur for many years. Chest X-ray and TB skin testing can detect the disease. Signs and symptoms include tiredness, loss of appetite, weight loss, fever, night sweats and coughing. The cough becomes more frequent over time. Sputum production also increases and chest pain occurs.

TB is treated with medication. Cover the mouth and nose with tissues when coughing or sneezing. Flush tissues down the toilet. Alternatively, place them in a paper bag to be burned. In healthcare facilities, tissues are placed in a biohazard bag. It is essential to wash hands after contact with sputum. Practise Standard Precautions and Airborne Precautions. Most aged care facilities do not admit people with active TB.

THE DIGESTIVE SYSTEM

The digestive system breaks down food physically and chemically so it can be absorbed for use by the cells. This process is called **digestion**. The digestive system is also called the *gastrointestinal system* (*GI system*). The system also eliminates solid wastes from the body.

The digestive system consists of the *alimentary canal* (*GI tract*) and the accessory organs of digestion (Fig. 10.56). The alimentary canal is a long tube extending from the

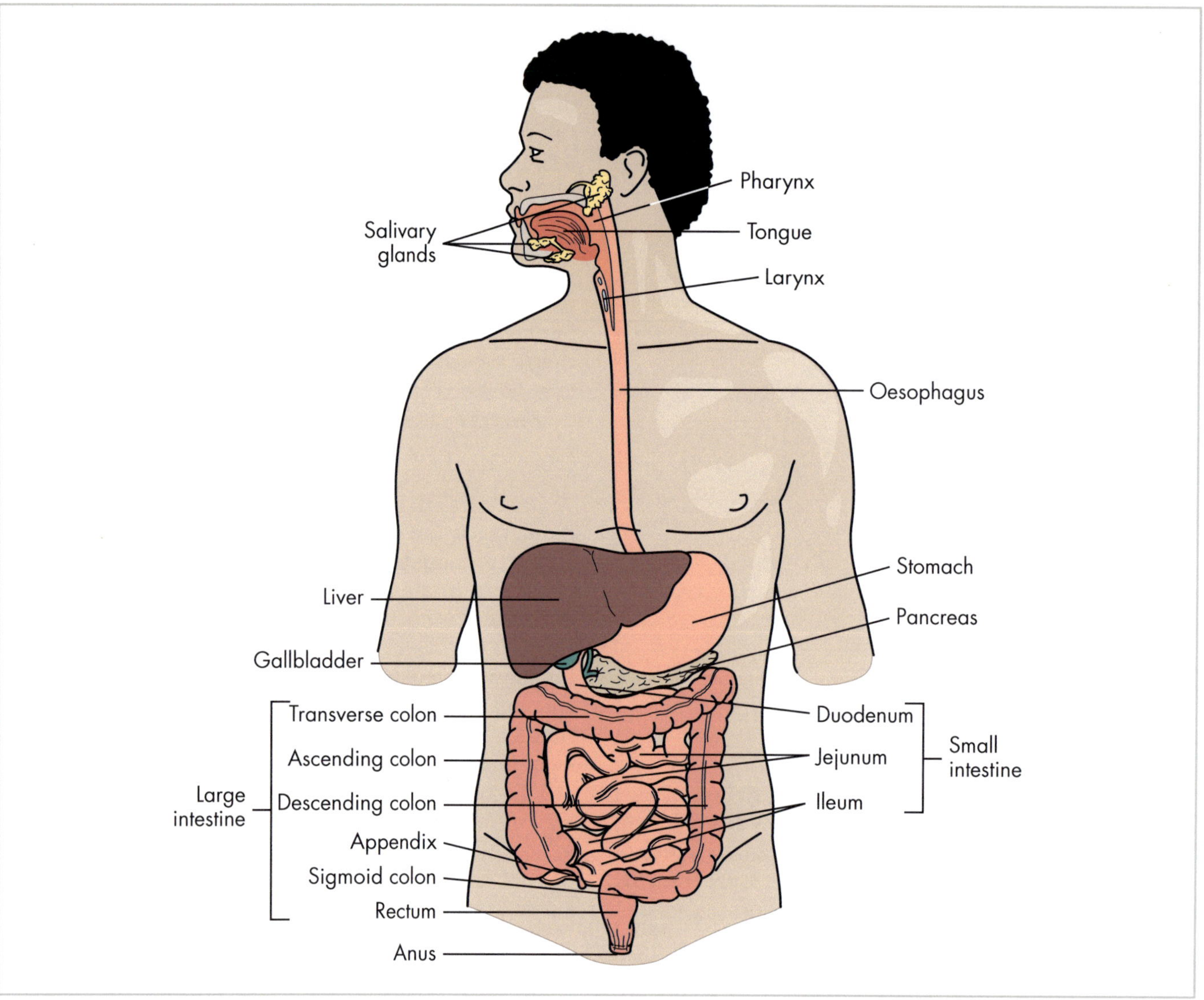

Fig. 10.56
Digestive system.

mouth to the anus. Its major parts are the mouth, pharynx, oesophagus, stomach, small intestine and large intestine. The accessory organs of digestion are the teeth, tongue, salivary glands, liver, gallbladder and pancreas.

Digestion begins in the mouth. The mouth is also called the *oral cavity*. The oral cavity receives food and prepares it for digestion. Using chewing motions, the teeth cut, chop and grind food into smaller particles for digestion and swallowing. The tongue aids in chewing and swallowing. Taste buds on the tongue's surface contain nerve endings, which allow sweet, sour, bitter and salty tastes to be sensed. Salivary glands in the mouth secrete saliva. This moistens food particles for easier swallowing and begins to digest food. During swallowing, the tongue pushes food into the pharynx.

The pharynx (throat) is a muscular tube. The act of swallowing is continued as the pharynx contracts. Contraction of the pharynx pushes food into the *oesophagus*, a muscular tube about 25 centimetres long. It extends from the pharynx to the stomach. Involuntary muscle contractions called **peristalsis** move food down the oesophagus into the stomach.

The *stomach* is a muscular, pouch-like sac in the upper left part of the abdominal cavity. Strong stomach muscles stir and churn food to break it up into even smaller particles. The stomach is lined with a mucous membrane containing glands that secrete gastric juices. Food is mixed and churned with the gastric juices to form a semi-liquid substance called *chyme*. Through peristalsis, the chyme is pushed from the stomach into the small intestine.

The *small intestine* is about 6 metres long and consists of three parts. The first part is the *duodenum*, where more digestive juices are added to the chyme. One of these juices is called *bile*, a greenish liquid produced by the liver and stored in the gallbladder. Juices from the pancreas and small intestine are also added to the chyme. The digestive juices chemically break down food so it can be absorbed.

Peristalsis moves the chyme through the two remaining portions of the small intestine: the *jejunum* and the *ileum*. Tiny projections called *villi* line the small intestine. Villi absorb the digested food into the capillaries. Most of the absorption of food takes place in the jejunum and ileum.

Some chyme is not digested and passes from the small intestine into the *large intestine* (*large bowel* or *colon*). The colon absorbs most of the water from the chyme. The remaining semi-solid material is called *faeces*. Faeces contain a small amount of water, solid wastes and some mucus and germs. These are the waste products of digestion. Faeces pass through the colon into the rectum by peristalsis and out of the body through the anus.

AGEING OF THE DIGESTIVE SYSTEM

Ageing affects all components of the digestive tract. The changes that take place during the ageing process are:

- *decline in the rate of cell production:* The epithelium cells of the digestive tract do not replicate as quickly as required and leave the tract susceptible to damage by acids or enzymes. The most likely condition to occur due to ageing are peptic ulcers (described below). Since the stem cells in the epithelium divide less frequently, tissue repair is less efficient and the stratified epithelium in the mouth, oesophagus and anus become thinner and more fragile.
- *decrease in smooth muscle cell tone:* The digestive tract is composed of smooth muscle cells that are responsible for contraction of the small intestine, an important process in moving food through the digestive tract. Since this tone decreases with age, the motility of the tract decreases together with peristaltic contraction. These changes result in a slow rate of faecal movement through the bowel, resulting in constipation (described below). High-fibre foods help prevent constipation; however, they are hard to chew and can irritate the intestines. These foods include apricots, celery and fruits and vegetables with skins and seeds. Foods that provide soft bulk are often needed for people who have chewing problems or constipation. They include wholegrain cereals and cooked fruits and vegetables. Older people need fewer calories than when younger, as their energy and activity levels are lower. More fluids are needed to aid chewing, swallowing and digestion. Foods are needed that prevent constipation and bone changes. High-protein foods are needed for tissue growth and repair. Weakening of the smooth muscle tone can also contribute to weakening of the lower oesophageal sphincter promoting acid reflux and the development of gastro-oesophageal reflux disease (GORD).
- *cumulative damage:* The cumulative effects as ageing takes place most commonly result in the loss of teeth, increasing the risk of gingivitis. Loss of teeth and ill-fitting dentures cause chewing problems, which cause digestion problems. Avoid hard-to-chew foods; ground or chopped meat is easier to chew and swallow. Ill-fitting dentures need not be tolerated. They can be adjusted so that the person can eat efficiently and enjoy their food. Another cumulative condition that can occur due to alcohol intake is cirrhosis of the liver.
- *increased rates of cancer:* There is an increased risk of cancer in the digestive tract as the individual ages and is more common in stem cells that divide to maintain epithelial cell populations. Thus, rates of cancer are more common in the colon and stomach of the ageing individual, with oral, oesophageal and pharyngeal types of cancers more prevalent in elderly people who smoke.
- *reduced saliva secretion:* As the person ages the amount of saliva produced reduces, making swallowing more difficult – potentially leading to dysphagia.
- *decreased sense of taste and smell:* As the person ages there is a decline in the ability to taste. Oral hygiene and denture care can improve the person's ability to taste. Some clients do not have teeth or dentures and their food is pureed or ground.

DIGESTIVE DISORDERS

The digestive system breaks down food so the body can absorb it. Solid wastes are eliminated.

Vomiting

Vomiting means expelling stomach contents through the mouth. It signals illness or injury and can be life threatening. The vomitus (material vomited) can be aspirated and obstruct the airway. Vomiting large amounts of blood can lead to shock. The following measures are needed:

1. Follow Standard Precautions.
2. Turn the person's head well to one side. This prevents aspiration.
3. Place a kidney basin under the person's chin.
4. Move vomitus away from the person.
5. Provide oral hygiene. This helps remove the bitter taste of vomitus.
6. Eliminate odours.
7. Change linen as necessary.
8. Observe vomitus for colour, odour and undigested food.
9. Measure, report and record the amount of vomitus.
10. Save a specimen for laboratory study.
11. Dispose of vomitus after the nurse observes it.

Gastro-oesophageal reflux disease

Gastro-oesophageal reflux disease (GORD) is the most common chronic condition affecting the oesophagus; it is classified as an inflammatory disease. GORD presents with a frequent reflux of the contents in the stomach (that can include chyme and hydrochloric acid) back up through the gastro-oesophageal sphincter into the oesophagus, causing a burning sensation. Other symptoms include dysphagia, coughing, chest pain and wheezing. GORD is often referred to as reflux or heartburn, which commonly occurs around the intake of food. Fig. 10.57

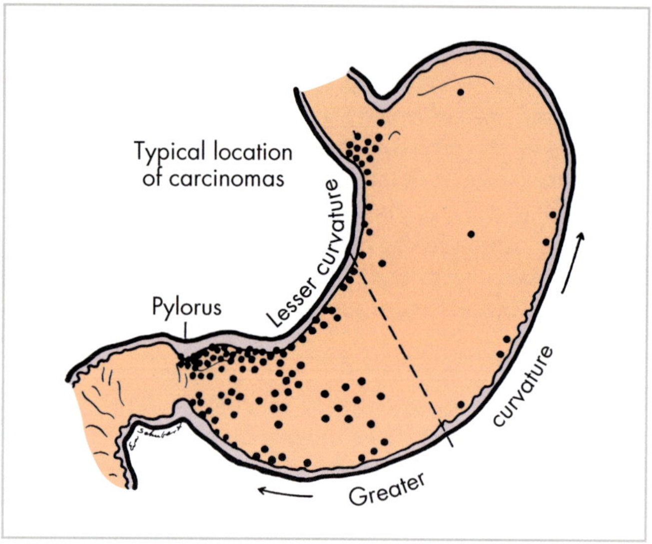

Fig. 10.57

Factors and pathophysiology of GORD.

Weakening of the lower oesophageal sphincter contributes to the symptoms of GORD.

shows the causes of GORD and the weakening of the lower oesophageal sphincter, which contributes to the symptoms experienced by individuals who suffer this condition.

There are numerous factors that increase the likelihood of developing GORD, including: eating a large meal, eating a large meal then performing physical activity, dietary considerations (avoiding coffee, alcohol, chocolate, dietary fats, garlic, onion, tomato, citrus, chilli, peppermint and fizzy drinks), anxiety and stress, smoking, genetics, non-steroidal anti-inflammatory drugs (NSAIDs), irritable bowel syndrome, peptic ulcers and obesity. Ageing also increases the risk of developing GORD, since there is a reduced ability to keep the lower oesophageal sphincter (LOS) closed during digestion because of the decrease in smooth muscle tone. It is important to reduce the factors that increase the likelihood of GORD from developing. The easiest things to modify are the risk factors, in particular the dietary considerations described above.

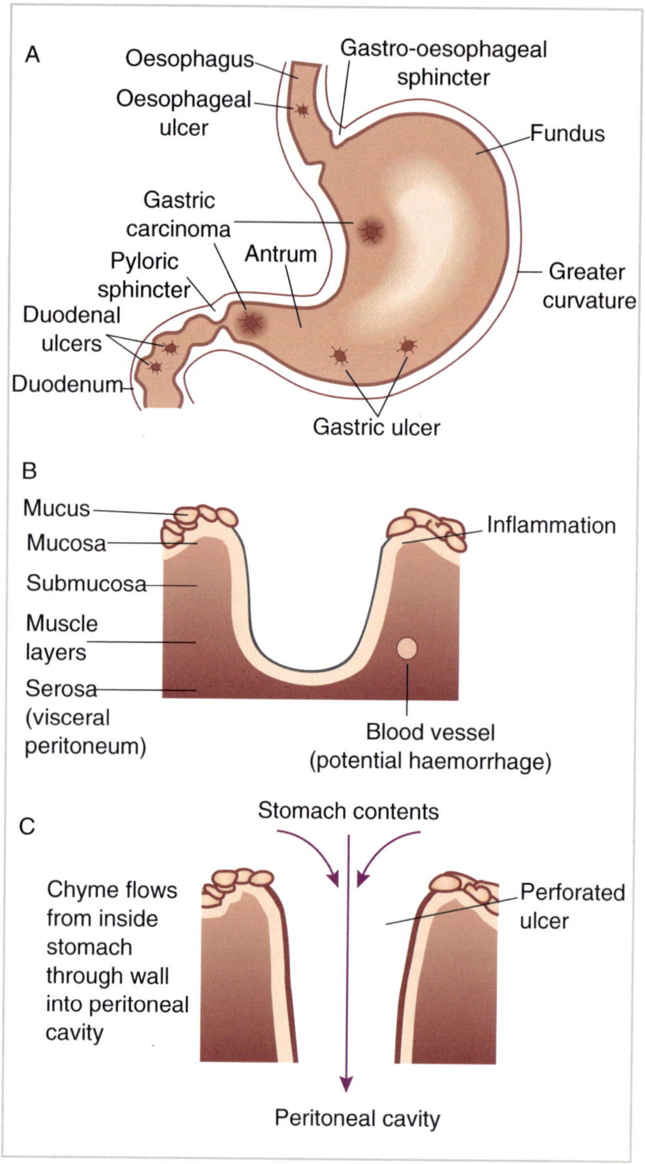

Fig. 10.58

Peptic ulcers.

A. Common sites in which peptic and duodenal ulcers occur.

B. A diagrammatic formation of an ulcer. **C.** The perforation of the ulcers.

Peptic ulcers

Peptic ulcers are breaks in the mucosal membrane lining of the stomach, distal oesophagus or small intestine. Peptic ulcers can be classified as acute, which develop due to gastritis or as a complication to severe stress or a result of extreme hyperacidity. They can also be classified as chronic, usually due to inflammation caused by bacteria *Helicobacter pylori* (*H. pylori*).

H. pylori bacteria are the cause of over 95 per cent of duodenal ulcers and 70 per cent of stomach ulcers; they are considered to be the key factor for the development of these ulcers in the respective parts of the human body. The *H. pylori* secretes urease, an enzyme that acts to protect the bacteria, but at the same time damages the mucosal lining of the stomach or duodenum. The breakdown of the lining in the stomach is the major event that results in the formation of peptic ulcers.

H. pylori and the use of NSAIDs (such as aspirin) appear to increase the risk of peptic ulcer bleeding, a major complication of peptic ulcers. Stress, poor diet (alcohol, caffeine, spicy food) or disturbed sleep can increase the susceptibility to ulcers. Since the rate of epithelial production in the gastrointestinal tract declines with age, this increases the risk of peptic ulcers developing. Reducing dietary factors that can increase the susceptibility of developing peptic ulcers is encouraged. Fig. 10.58 shows the common places where peptic ulcers occur in the digestive tract, together with how the condition leads to perforation of the digestive tract.

THE URINARY SYSTEM

Wastes are removed from the body through the respiratory system, the digestive system and the skin. The digestive system rids the body of solid wastes. The lungs rid the body of carbon dioxide. Water and other substances are contained in sweat. However, there are other waste products in the blood as a result of body cells burning food for energy. The functions of the urinary system (Fig. 10.59) are to:

- remove waste products from the blood
- maintain water balance within the body.

The kidneys are two bean-shaped organs in the upper abdomen. They lie against the muscles of the back, on each side of the spine. They are protected by the lower edge of the rib cage.

Each kidney has over a million tiny nephrons (Fig. 10.60). The nephron is the basic working unit of the kidney. It has a convoluted tubule, which is a tiny coiled tubule. Each convoluted tubule has a *Bowman's capsule* at one end. The capsule partially surrounds a cluster of capillaries called a *glomerulus*. Blood passes through the glomerulus and is filtered by the capillaries. The fluid portion of the blood is squeezed into the Bowman's capsule. The fluid then passes into the tubule. Most of the water and other necessary substances are reabsorbed by the blood and recirculated through the body. The rest of the fluid and the waste products form urine in the tubule – this is also referred to as the glomerular filtration rate (GFR). Urine flows through the tubule to a collecting tubule. All the collecting tubules within the millions of nephrons drain into the renal pelvis within the kidney.

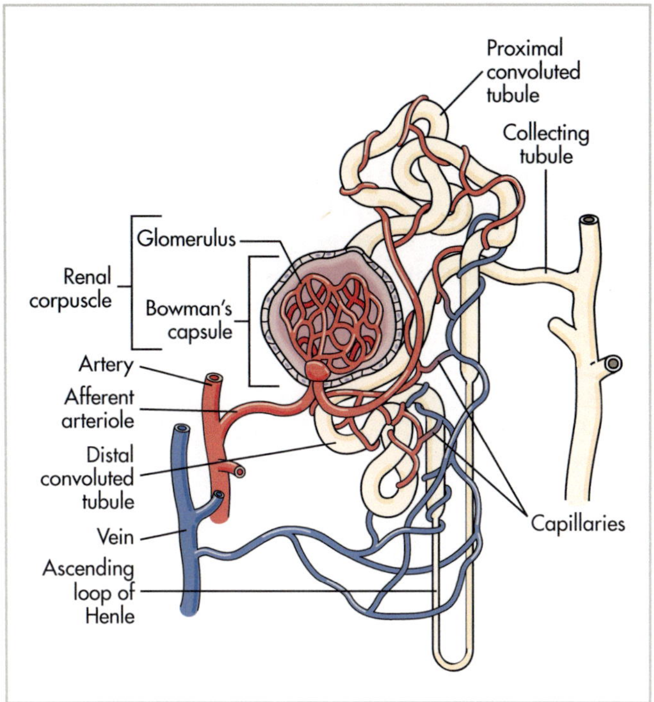

Fig. 10.60
A nephron.

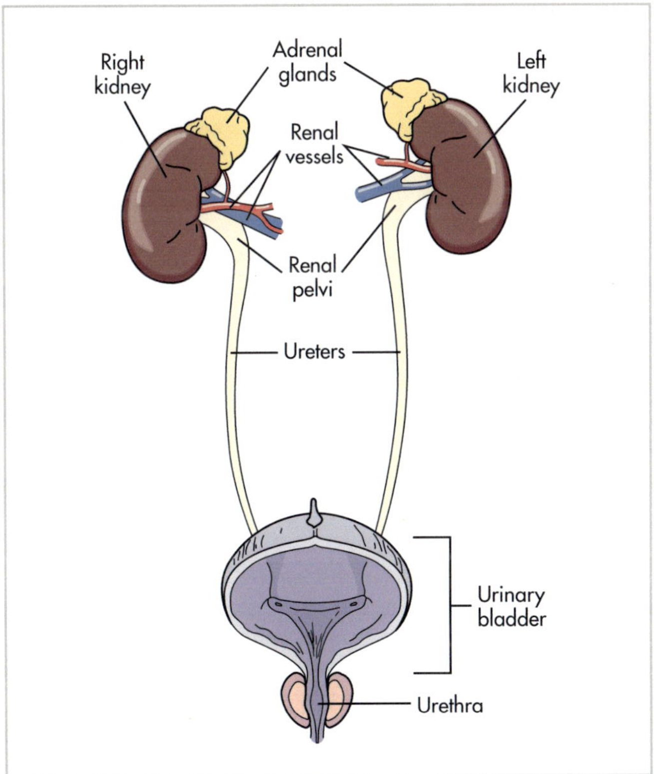

Fig. 10.59
Urinary system.

A tube, called the ureter, is attached to the renal pelvis of the kidney. Each ureter is about 25–30 centimetres long. The ureters carry urine from the kidneys to the bladder. The bladder is a hollow muscular sac situated towards the front in the lower part of the abdominal cavity.

Urine is stored in the bladder until the desire to urinate is felt. The need to urinate usually occurs when there is about 250 mL of urine in the bladder. Urine passes from the bladder through the urethra. The opening at the end of the urethra is the *meatus*. Urine passes from the body through the meatus. Urine is a clear, yellowish fluid.

AGEING OF THE URINARY SYSTEM

Ageing affects several different kidney processes as the individual ages:

- *a decline in number of nephrons:* The total number of nephrons reduces by 30–40 per cent as the individual ages.
- *a decline in the ability of the nephrons to work efficiently:* The kidney is less able to respond to the effects of the anti-diuretic hormone which suppresses excessive urinary secretion.
- *abnormal micturition reflex:* There are a number of factors that lead to abnormal micturition reflex, including: (a) sphincter muscle control loss, (b) loss of control of micturition reflex, which usually happens after a stroke, and (c) in males, urinary retention may take place if there is an enlargement of the prostate gland, which compresses the urethra restricting the flow of urine.

URINARY SYSTEM DISORDERS

The kidneys, ureters, bladder and urethra are the major urinary system structures. Disorders can occur in these structures.

Urinary tract infections

Urinary tract infections (UTIs) are common. Infection in one area can involve the entire system. Microbes can enter the system through the urethra. Catheterisation, urological examinations, intercourse, poor perineal hygiene and poor fluid intake are common causes. UTIs are common nosocomial infections.

Women are at high risk as microbes can easily enter the short female urethra. Prostate gland secretions help protect men from UTIs. In older men, an enlarged prostate increases the risk of a UTI.

Cystitis

Cystitis is a bladder (*cyst*) infection (*itis*) caused by bacteria. Common signs and symptoms are:

- urinary frequency
- oliguria – scant (*olig*) urine (*uria*)
- urgency
- dysuria – difficult or painful (*dys*) urination (*uria*)
- pain or burning on urination
- foul-smelling urine
- haematuria – blood (*haemat*) in the urine (*uria*)
- pyuria – pus (*py*) in the urine (*uria*)
- fever.

Antibiotics are used to treat the infection. Fluids are encouraged – usually 2000 mL per day. If untreated, cystitis can lead to pyelonephritis.

Pyelonephritis

Pyelonephritis is inflammation (*itis*) of the kidney (*nephr*) pelvis (*pyelo*). Infection is the most common cause. Cloudy urine may contain pus, mucus and blood. Chills, fever, back pain and nausea and vomiting can occur. The signs and symptoms of cystitis often also occur. Treatment involves antibiotics and fluids.

Renal calculi

Renal calculi are kidney (*renal*) stones (*calculi*). Caucasian males between the ages of 20 and 40 are at greatest risk. Bed rest, immobility and poor fluid intake are risk factors. Stones vary in size. Signs and symptoms include:

- severe, cramping pain in the back and side, just below the ribs
- pain in the abdomen, thigh and urethra
- nausea and vomiting
- fever and chills
- dysuria – difficult or painful (*dys*) urination (*uria*)
- urinary frequency
- urinary urgency
- oliguria – scant (*olig*) urine (*uria*)
- haematuria – blood (*haemat*) in the urine (*uria*)
- foul-smelling urine.

Medications are given for pain relief. The person needs to drink about 2000–3000 mL of fluid a day, as increased fluids help stones pass through the urine. All urine is strained to detect passed stones. Surgical removal of a stone may be necessary. Sometimes dietary changes can prevent stones.

Renal failure

In renal failure (kidney failure), the kidneys do not function or are severely impaired. Waste products are not removed from the blood and the body retains fluid. Heart failure and hypertension often result. Renal failure may be acute or chronic.

Acute renal failure

Acute renal failure is sudden. There is severe decreased blood flow to the kidneys. Causes include severe bleeding, myocardial infarction (heart attack), heart failure, burns, infection and severe allergic reactions. Hospital care is needed.

At first, *oliguria* (scant amount of urine) occurs. Urine output is less than 400 mL in 24 hours. This phase lasts from a few days to 2 weeks. Then diuresis occurs. *Diuresis* means the process (*esis*) of passing (*di*) urine (*ur*). Large amounts of urine are produced – 1000–5000 mL a day. Kidney function improves and returns to normal during the recovery phase. This can take from 1 month to 1 year. Some people develop chronic renal failure.

Every system is affected by the build-up of waste products in the blood and death can occur. Treatment involves medications, restricted fluids and diet therapy. The diet is high in carbohydrates and low in protein and potassium.

Chronic renal failure

In chronic renal failure, the kidneys cannot meet the body's needs. Nephrons of the kidney are destroyed over many years. Hypertension and diabetes are common causes. Other causes include infections, urinary tract obstructions and tumours.

Signs and symptoms appear when 80–90 per cent of kidney function is lost (Box 10.11). Every body system is affected as waste products build up in the blood.

Treatment includes fluid restriction, diet therapy, medications and dialysis. Dialysis is the process of removing waste products from the blood. It requires specially trained nurses. Some people have kidney transplants.

Care of the person in chronic renal failure is listed in Box 10.12.

THE REPRODUCTIVE SYSTEM

Human reproduction results from the union of a female sex cell and a male sex cell. The structures of the male and female reproductive systems are different. The differences allow for the process of reproduction.

Male reproductive system

The structures of the male reproductive system are shown in Fig. 10.61. The testes (testicles) are the male sex glands.

BOX 10.11
Signs and symptoms of chronic renal failure

- Yellow, tan or dusky skin
- Dry, itchy skin
- Thin, brittle skin
- Bruises
- Bad breath (halitosis)
- Stomatitis (inflammation of the mouth)
- Nausea and vomiting
- Loss of appetite (anorexia)
- Weight loss
- Diarrhoea or constipation
- Decreased urine output
- Bleeding tendencies
- Susceptibility to infection
- Hypertension
- Congestive heart failure
- Gastric ulcers
- Gastrointestinal bleeding
- Irregular pulse
- Abnormal breathing patterns
- Burning sensation in the legs and feet
- Muscle twitching
- Leg cramps at night
- Fatigue
- Sleep disorders
- Headaches
- Convulsions
- Confusion
- Coma

BOX 10.12
Care of the person in chronic renal failure

- A diet low in protein, potassium and sodium
- Fluid restriction
- Measuring blood pressure in the supine, sitting and standing positions
- Measuring weight daily
- Measuring and recording intake and output
- Turning and repositioning
- Measures to prevent pressure injuries
- Range-of-motion exercises
- Measures to prevent itching (bath oils, lotions and creams)
- Measures to prevent injury and bleeding
- Frequent oral hygiene
- Measures to prevent infection
- Measures to prevent diarrhoea or constipation
- Measures to meet emotional needs
- Measures to promote rest

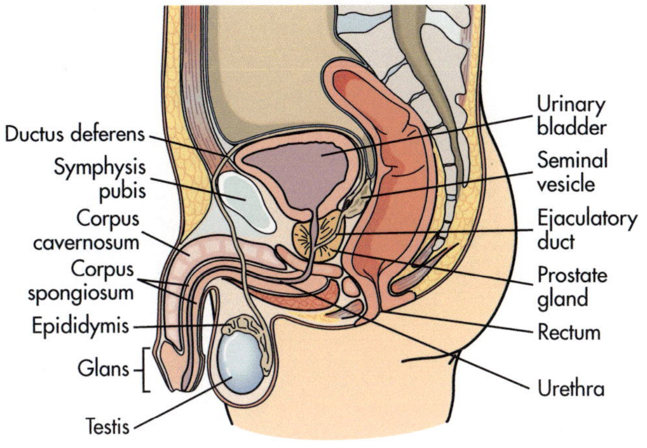

Fig. 10.61
Male reproductive system.

Sex glands are also called *gonads*. The two testes are oval or almond-shaped glands. Male sex cells, called sperm cells, are produced in the testes.

Testosterone, the male **hormone**, is also produced in the testes. This hormone is needed for the functioning of the reproductive organs. It is also needed for the development of the male secondary sex characteristics: facial hair; pubic and axillary hair; hair on the arms, chest and legs; deepening of the voice; and increase in neck and shoulder size.

The testes are suspended between the thighs in a sac called the scrotum. The scrotum is made of skin and muscle. Sperm travel from the testis to the *epididymis*. The epididymis is a coiled tube on top and to the side of the testis. From the epididymis, sperm travel through a tube called the *ductus deferens*. Eventually, each ductus deferens joins a *seminal vesicle*. The two seminal vesicles store sperm and produce semen. Semen is a fluid that carries sperm from the male reproductive tract. The ducts of the seminal vesicles unite to form the ejaculatory duct. The ejaculatory duct passes through the prostate gland and joins the urethra.

The prostate gland lies just below the bladder and is shaped like a doughnut. It secretes fluid into the semen. The urethra runs through the prostate and is the outlet for both urine and semen. The urethra is contained within the penis.

The penis is outside the body and has erectile tissue. When a man becomes sexually excited, blood fills the erectile tissue. This causes the penis to become enlarged, hard and erect. The erect penis can enter the vagina of the female reproductive tract. The semen, which contains sperm, is then released into the vagina.

Female reproductive system

The structures of the female reproductive system are shown in Fig. 10.62. The female gonads are two almond-shaped glands called ovaries. There is an ovary on each side of the uterus in the abdominal cavity.

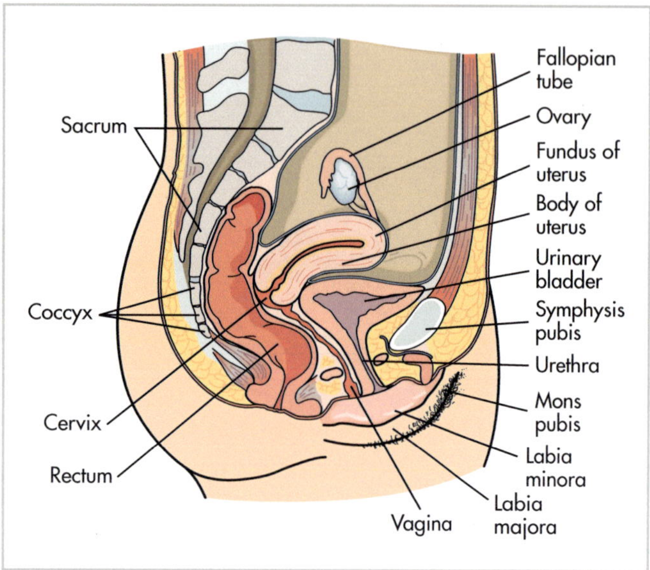

Fig. 10.62
Female reproductive system.

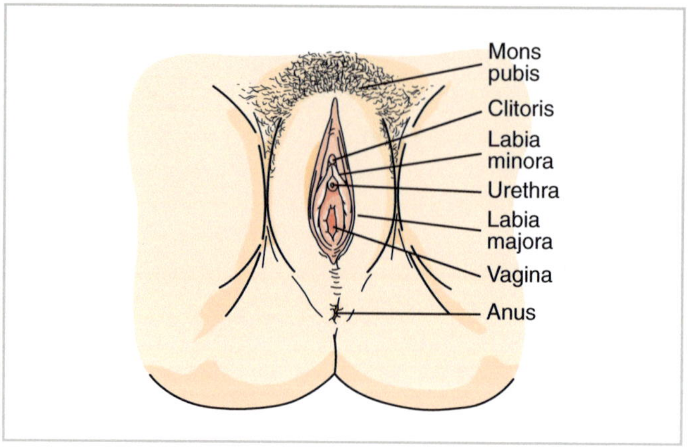

Fig. 10.63
External female genitalia.

The ovaries contain *ova*, or eggs. Ova are the female sex cells. One ovum (egg) is released monthly during the reproductive years. Release of an ovum from an ovary is called ovulation.

The ovaries also secrete the female hormones *oestrogen* and *progesterone*. These hormones are needed for the functioning of the reproductive system. They are also needed for the development of secondary sex characteristics in the female. These include increase in breast size, pubic and axillary hair, slight deepening of the voice and widening and rounding of the hips.

When an ovum is released from an ovary, it travels through a *fallopian tube*. There are two fallopian tubes, one on each side. The tubes are attached at one end to the uterus. The ovum travels through the fallopian tube to the uterus. The uterus is a hollow, muscular organ shaped like a pear. It is in the centre of the pelvic cavity, behind the bladder and in front of the rectum. The main part of the uterus is the fundus. The neck or narrow section of the uterus is the cervix. Tissue lining the uterus is called the endometrium. There are many blood vessels in the endometrium. If sex cells from the male and female unite into one cell, that cell implants into the endometrium, where it grows into a baby. The uterus serves as a place for the unborn baby to grow and receive nourishment.

The cervix of the uterus projects into a muscular canal called the vagina. The vagina opens to the outside of the body. It is located just behind the urethra. The vagina receives the penis during sexual intercourse. It also serves as part of the birth canal. Glands in the vaginal wall keep it moistened with secretions. In young girls, the external vaginal opening is partially closed by a membrane called the hymen. The hymen ruptures when the female has intercourse for the first time.

The external genitalia of the female are referred to as the vulva (Fig. 10.63).

- The mons pubis is a rounded fatty pad over a bone called the symphysis pubis. In the adult female, the mons pubis is covered with hair.
- The labia majora and labia minora are two folds of tissue located on each side of the vaginal opening.
- The clitoris is a small organ composed of erectile tissue. The clitoris becomes hard when the woman is sexually stimulated.

The mammary glands (breasts) secrete milk after childbirth. They are on the outside of the chest. They are made up of glandular tissue and fat (Fig. 10.64). The milk drains into ducts that open onto the nipple.

Menstruation

The endometrium is rich in blood, to nourish the cell that grows into an unborn baby (fetus). If pregnancy does not occur, the endometrium breaks up. It is then discharged through the vagina to the outside of the body. This process is called menstruation. Menstruation occurs about every 28 days. Therefore, it is also called the menstrual cycle.

The first day of the cycle begins with menstruation. Blood flows from the uterus through the vaginal opening. Menstrual flow usually lasts three to seven days. The next phase is ovulation. During ovulation, an ovum that has matured in an ovary is released. Ovulation usually occurs on or about day 14 of the cycle.

Meanwhile, oestrogen and progesterone (the female hormones) are secreted by the ovaries. These hormones cause the endometrium to thicken for possible pregnancy. If pregnancy does not occur, the hormones decrease in amount. Blood supply to the endometrium decreases because of the decrease in hormones. The endometrium breaks up and is discharged through the vagina and another menstrual cycle begins.

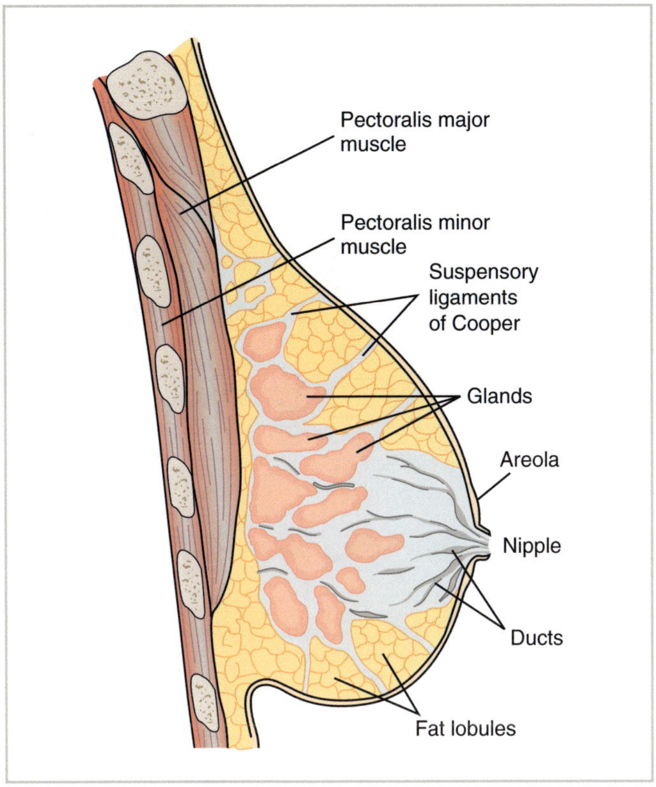

Fig. 10.64
The female breast.

AGEING OF THE REPRODUCTIVE SYSTEM

The main changes that take place in the female reproductive system are the decline in hormones – this is called menopause, which is a normal part of a woman's ageing process. In menopause the ovaries stop producing the hormones oestrogen and progesterone; the ovaries no longer release ova (eggs). The menstrual periods stop and after menopause it is unlikely that pregnancy can occur. As the hormone levels fall there are physical changes, including the walls of the vagina becoming thin, dry, less elastic and possibly more irritated. Because of these physical changes there are higher risks of vaginal yeast infections. There are also changes in the external genitals, including a decrease in the tissue and thinness.

Men also experience changes to their fertility rates as they age. The age-related changes in men occur more gradually in a process called andropause, which primarily occurs in the testes. The size of the testicular mass decreases in size and levels of the male sex hormone testosterone can decrease over time. The tubes that carry sperm may become less elastic and while the testes produce sperm, there is a decrease in semen volume and total sperm count.

It is common for the prostate to enlarge over time in a condition called benign prostatic hypertrophy (as described below), which causes problems with the release of urine and ejaculation. This in part explains why erectile dysfunction (the inability to achieve or maintain an erection) is common in men as they age.

REPRODUCTIVE DISORDERS

There are several reproductive disorders for both men and women that are more likely to occur as they increase with age, including ovarian and breast cancer, benign prostatic disease and prostate cancer.

- **Ovarian cancer:** This is the third most common cancer to occur in the female reproductive system. It is considered the most dangerous type of cancer since it is seldom diagnosed in its early stages, with typical diagnosis taking place in later stages of the disease process. As such, the symptoms of the condition are very subtle, including bloating, pelvic pain, difficulty eating and frequent urination. The prognosis (outcome) of the condition is generally good if the cancer originates in ovarian tissue – which responds well to treatment, including surgery, chemotherapy and radiation. However, in many cases the cancers develop from epithelial cells, which arise from the surface of the ovary and have a poor response to treatment and a poor prognosis.
  There are several causes that contribute to the development of ovarian cancer; however, the exact cause remains to be identified and include:
  - older women who have never given birth
  - genetics
  - infertile women and those with the condition called endometriosis (where endometrial tissue grows outside of the reproductive organs, in the bowel).
- **Breast cancer:** This is a malignant tumour of the mammary glands and has been reported to occur in both men and women. It is more common in women over the age of 50. Mortality from breast cancer has decreased in women from 74 deaths per 100,000 in 1991 to 40 deaths per 100,000 in 2018 (AIHW 2021). However, it remains the most common type of cancer in women. The overall five-year survival rate in 2020 was 91 per cent. If the cancer remains limited to the breast, 96 per cent of patients survived 5 years, while if the cancer spreads to the lymph nodes the number reduces to 80 per cent (Cancer Council Victoria 2021).
  - There are a number of risk factors that are notable for the development of breast cancer, including:
    - family history of breast cancer
    - first pregnancy after the age of 30
    - early menarche (commencement of menstruation) or late menopause.
  - Early detection of breast cancer is essential for a good outcome. Mammography is a technique that uses X-rays to examine the breast tissue; ultrasound can also be used to gather information about the breast tissue, but it lacks the detail of mammography. If breast cancer is suspected, a biopsy will be taken to determine the Stage and Grade, and best course of treatment.

Treatment options depend on the size and grade of the cancer and are rated from Stage 0 to Stage IV, and Grades 1, 2 and 3 (Cancer Council Victoria 2020). In Stage I the tumour is less than 2 cm and has not yet spread to the lymph nodes; it is classed as early breast cancer. Treatment is most successful when the breast cancer is identified as small and has not spread to other regions of the body. Treatment for higher stage breast cancer involves surgical removal of the affected breast tissue with a number of different techniques utilised, depending on the nature of the breast cancer:

  - Lumpectomy: only a part of the breast is removed
  - Total mastectomy: the entire breast is removed
  - Axillary lymph node dissection: the axillary region is checked to identify if there is any cancer present; if cancer is present within the axillary region, the lymph nodes will be removed.
- Usually a combination of chemotherapy, radiation and hormone treatments are used to supplement the surgical approach to treatment.

- **Benign prostatic hyperplasia (BPH):** BPH is an enlargement of the prostate causing obstruction of the flow of urine from the bladder to the urethra, which ultimately prevents the elimination of urine from the body. As the name suggests, the condition is benign, but the number of cells can actually increase. This condition usually involves an abnormal increase in the number of cells taking place in both lobes of the prostate gland. As the urethra runs through the prostate gland, it is very easy to see how the changes in the prostate can impact on the compression of the urethra.
- **Prostate cancer:** Prostate cancer is the most common form of cancer in men and occurs most commonly in those aged 50 years and older. It is usually a very slow-growing cancer and can grow for up to 15–20 years with no symptoms. Typically, men tend to die with prostate cancer because of the secondary cancers (metastasis) that develop from it. Metastasis generally occurs in the vertebrae, ribs or pelvic bones.

THE ENDOCRINE SYSTEM

The endocrine system is made up of glands called the endocrine glands (Fig. 10.65). The glands secrete chemical substances called hormones into the bloodstream. Hormones regulate the activities of other organs and glands in the body.

The pituitary gland is called the master gland. About the size of a cherry, it is at the base of the brain, behind the eyes. The pituitary gland is divided into the anterior pituitary lobe and the posterior pituitary lobe. The anterior pituitary lobe secretes the following hormones:

- *Growth hormone* – needed for the growth of muscles, bones and other organs. It is needed throughout life to maintain normal-sized bones and muscles. Growth is stunted if a baby is born with deficient amounts of the growth hormone. Too much of the hormone causes excessive growth.

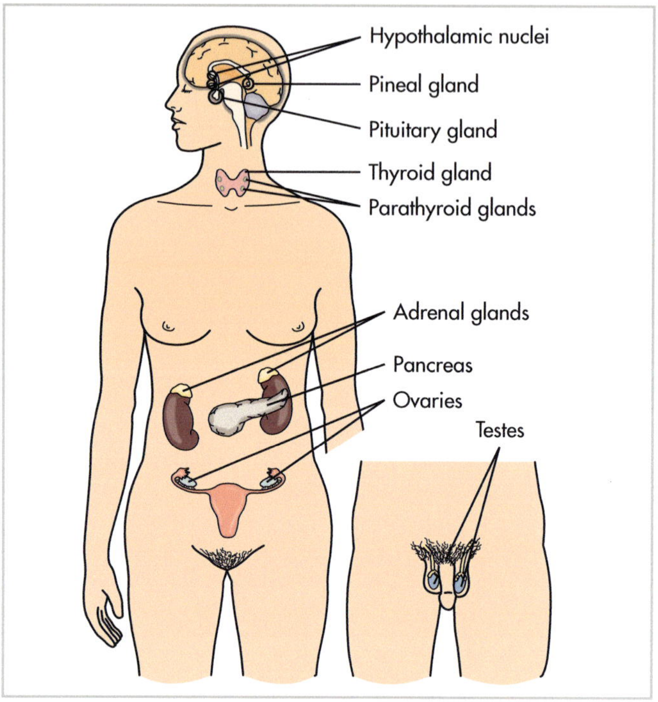

Fig. 10.65
Endocrine system.

- *Thyroid-stimulating hormone* (TSH) – needed for thyroid gland function.
- *Adrenocorticotrophic hormone* (ACTH) – stimulates the adrenal gland.

The anterior lobe also secretes hormones that regulate the growth, development and function of the male and female reproductive systems.

The *posterior pituitary lobe* secretes antidiuretic hormone (ADH) and oxytocin. ADH prevents the kidneys from excreting excessive amounts of water. Oxytocin causes the uterine muscles to contract during childbirth.

The *thyroid gland*, shaped like a butterfly, is in the neck in front of the larynx. Thyroid hormone (thyroxine) is secreted by the thyroid gland. It regulates metabolism. **Metabolism** is the burning of food for heat and energy by the cells. Too little thyroxine results in slowed body processes, slowed movements and weight gain. Too much thyroxine causes increased metabolism, excess energy and weight loss. Some babies are born with deficient amounts of thyroxine and have stunted physical and mental growth as a result.

The four *parathyroid glands* are in pairs on each side of the thyroid gland. They secrete parathormone (parathyroid hormone), which regulates the body's use of calcium. Calcium is needed for nerve and muscle function. Insufficient amounts of calcium cause tetany. Tetany is a state of severe muscle contraction and spasm. If untreated, tetany can cause death.

There are two *adrenal glands*, one on the top of each kidney. The adrenal gland has two parts: the adrenal medulla and the adrenal cortex. The adrenal medulla secretes adrenaline and noradrenaline. These hormones stimulate the body to quickly produce energy during emergencies: heart rate, blood pressure, muscle power and energy all increase.

The *adrenal cortex* secretes three groups of hormones needed for life. The glucocorticoids regulate the metabolism of carbohydrates. They also control the body's response to stress and inflammation and have the ability to decrease the innate immune system cells (including the natural killer cells). The mineralocorticoids regulate the amount of salt and water that is absorbed and lost by the kidneys. The adrenal cortex also secretes small amounts of male and female sex hormones.

The pancreas secretes insulin. Insulin regulates the amount of sugar in the blood available for use by the cells. Insulin is needed for sugar to enter the cells. If there is too little insulin, sugar cannot enter the cells. If sugar cannot enter the cells, excess amounts of sugar build up in the blood. This condition is called diabetes mellitus.

The gonads are the glands of human reproduction. Male sex glands (testes) secrete testosterone. Female sex glands (ovaries) secrete oestrogen and progesterone.

AGEING OF THE ENDOCRINE SYSTEM

The endocrine system undergoes very few changes as the individual ages. The most dramatic change involves the reproductive hormones. Blood and tissue concentrations of many hormones, including TSH, thyroid hormones, ADH, parathyroid hormone, prolactin and glucocorticoids remain unchanged. While these concentrations may be within normal limits, it is also known that some endocrine tissues are less responsive to certain stimulation. For example, it is known that smaller amounts of growth hormone and insulin are secreted after a carbohydrate-rich meal. There have also been noted reductions in tissue sensitivity to glucocorticoids and ADH.

ENDOCRINE SYSTEM DISORDERS

Diabetes mellitus is the most common endocrine disorder.

Diabetes mellitus

In this disorder the body cannot produce or use insulin properly. Insulin is a hormone secreted by the pancreas and is needed for the breakdown of sugar. Sugar builds up in the blood and cells do not have enough sugar for energy. They cannot perform their functions.

There are two major types of diabetes:

- Type 1 – occurs most often in children and young adults. The pancreas produces little or no insulin. Onset is rapid. There is increased thirst and urination, constant hunger, weight loss, blurred vision and extreme fatigue.
- Type 2 – occurs in adults. People over 40 years of age are at risk. Obesity and hypertension are risk factors. The pancreas still secretes some insulin, but the body cannot use it effectively. Onset is slow. Common signs and symptoms include fatigue, nausea, frequent urination, increased thirst, weight loss and blurred vision. Infections are frequent and wounds heal slowly.

Diabetes must be controlled, otherwise complications occur, such as blindness, renal failure, nerve damage, hypertension and circulatory disorders. Circulatory disorders can lead to stroke, heart attack and delayed wound healing. Foot and leg wounds are serious complications. Infection and gangrene can occur and sometimes amputation is required.

Risk factors include a family history of the disease. For type 1, Caucasians are at greater risk than non-Caucasians. Type 2 is more common in older and overweight people.

Type 1 diabetes is treated with daily insulin therapy, healthy eating and exercise. Type 2 diabetes is treated with healthy eating and exercise. Many people take oral medications. Some need insulin. Overweight people need to lose weight.

Both types require blood glucose monitoring. Good foot care is needed as corns, blisters and calluses can lead to an infection and the potential for amputation.

The person's blood sugar level can fall too low or go too high:

- **Hypoglycaemia** means low (*hypo*) sugar (*glyc*) in the blood (*aemia*).
- **Hyperglycaemia** means high (*hyper*) sugar (*glyc*) in the blood (*aemia*).

See Table 10.1 for the causes, signs and symptoms of hypoglycaemia and hyperglycaemia. Both can lead to death if not corrected.

THE IMMUNE SYSTEM

The immune system defends against threats inside and outside the body. It protects the body from diseases and infection. Infection is caused by microorganisms (bacteria, viruses and other germs) in the environment. The immune system provides the body with immunity. **Immunity** means that a person has protection against a disease and will not get it or be affected by it.

- *Specific immunity* is the body's reaction to a specific threat.
- *Non-specific immunity* is the body's reaction to anything it does not recognise as a normal body substance.

Special cells and substances function to produce immunity.

- *Antibodies* are normal body substances that recognise abnormal or unwanted substances. They attack and destroy such substances.
- *Antigens* are abnormal or unwanted substances. An antigen causes the body to produce antibodies. The antibodies then attack and destroy the antigens.
- *Phagocytes* are white blood cells that digest and destroy microorganisms and other unwanted substances.
- *Lymphocytes* are white blood cells that produce antibodies. Lymphocyte production increases as the body responds to an infection.
- *B lymphocytes* (*B cells*) cause the production of antibodies that circulate in the plasma. The antibodies react to specific antigens.

Table 10.1
Hypoglycaemia and hyperglycaemia

	Causes	Signs and symptoms
Hypoglycaemia	• Too much insulin or diabetic medication • Omitting a meal • Delayed meal • Eating too little food • Increased exercise • Vomiting	• Hunger • Weakness • Trembling; shakiness • Sweating • Headache • Dizziness • Faintness • Slurred speech • Drowsiness • Rapid pulse • Low blood pressure • Rapid, shallow respirations • Confusion • Changes in vision • Cold, clammy skin • Emotional changes • Convulsions • Unconsciousness
Hyperglycaemia	• Undiagnosed diabetes • Not enough insulin or diabetic medication • Eating too much food • Too little exercise • Physical or emotional stress	• Weakness • Drowsiness • Thirst • Hunger • Frequent urination • Leg cramps • Flushed face • Sweet breath odour • Slow, deep and laboured respirations • Rapid, weak pulse • Low blood pressure • Dry skin • Blurred vision • Headache • Nausea and vomiting • Convulsions • Coma

- *T lymphocytes* (*T cells*) are cells that destroy invading cells. Killer T cells produce poisonous substances near the invading cells. Some T cells attract other cells and these other cells destroy the invaders.

When the body senses an antigen (an unwanted substance), the immune system is activated. Phagocyte and lymphocyte production increases. Phagocytes destroy the invaders through digestion. The lymphocytes produce antibodies that attack and destroy the unwanted substances.

AGEING OF THE IMMUNE SYSTEM

There are several changes that take place in the immune system as it ages, with the major changes being a less efficient way of combating disease. All of these changes have been listed below:

- The ability of the body to respond to threats within the body declines as the individual ages, with a decline in natural killer cells representing this.
- T cells become less responsive to antigens with fewer cytotoxic T cells being able to respond to infection.
- Number of helper T cells is reduced.
- B cells are less responsive so antibody levels do not rise as quickly after the exposure to antigen exposure.

DISORDERS OF THE IMMUNE SYSTEM

As the older person has a reduced resistance to infectious diseases, vaccination for acute viral diseases, such as the flu, are strongly recommended. The elderly are at increased risk of influenza, pulmonary infection and autoimmune diseases. Several bacterial and autoimmune diseases have already been described above including influenza, rosacea and SLE.

Acquired immunodeficiency syndrome (AIDS)

Acquired immunodeficiency syndrome (AIDS) is caused by the human immunodeficiency virus (HIV). The virus attacks the immune system and the person's ability to fight other diseases is affected. Many new medications have been developed to help reduce complications and prolong life. At present, there is no vaccine or cure for AIDS and it is treated like a chronic disease with medications.

The virus is spread through certain body fluids – blood, semen, vaginal secretions and breast milk. Saliva, tears, sweat, sneezing, coughing, insects or casual contact do not spread HIV. The virus is capable of affecting a number of tissues.

There are several systemic effects that HIV causes in the human body. Fig. 10.66 illustrates the major systems and conditions that occur due to a HIV infection.

The virus is transmitted by:

- unprotected sex with an infected person ('unprotected' means without a new latex or polyurethane condom)
- needle and syringe sharing among IV medication users
- HIV-infected mothers before or during childbirth
- HIV-infected mothers through breastfeeding.

The virus enters the bloodstream through several different orifices of the human body (including the vagina, penis, mouth, anus or skin breaks). The virus can enter the bloodstream through breaks in the mucous membrane (mouth, vagina and rectum). The virus can enter the bloodstream when infected body fluids are exposed to open skin areas. The virus can also be transmitted by contaminated blood left in needles or syringes. When the devices are shared, contaminated blood enters the bloodstream. Needle stick injuries pose a threat to the health team and care needs to be taken when using needles to administer medication or take blood samples when caring for patients who are HIV-positive.

The virus is very fragile and cannot live outside the body. HIV is not spread by casual, everyday contact, such as using public telephones, restrooms, swimming pools or hot tubs. HIV is not spread by food prepared by an infected person.

People with AIDS develop other diseases. Their immune system is damaged and so they cannot fight other diseases. The person is at risk of developing pneumonia, TB, Kaposi's sarcoma (a cancer) and central nervous system damage.

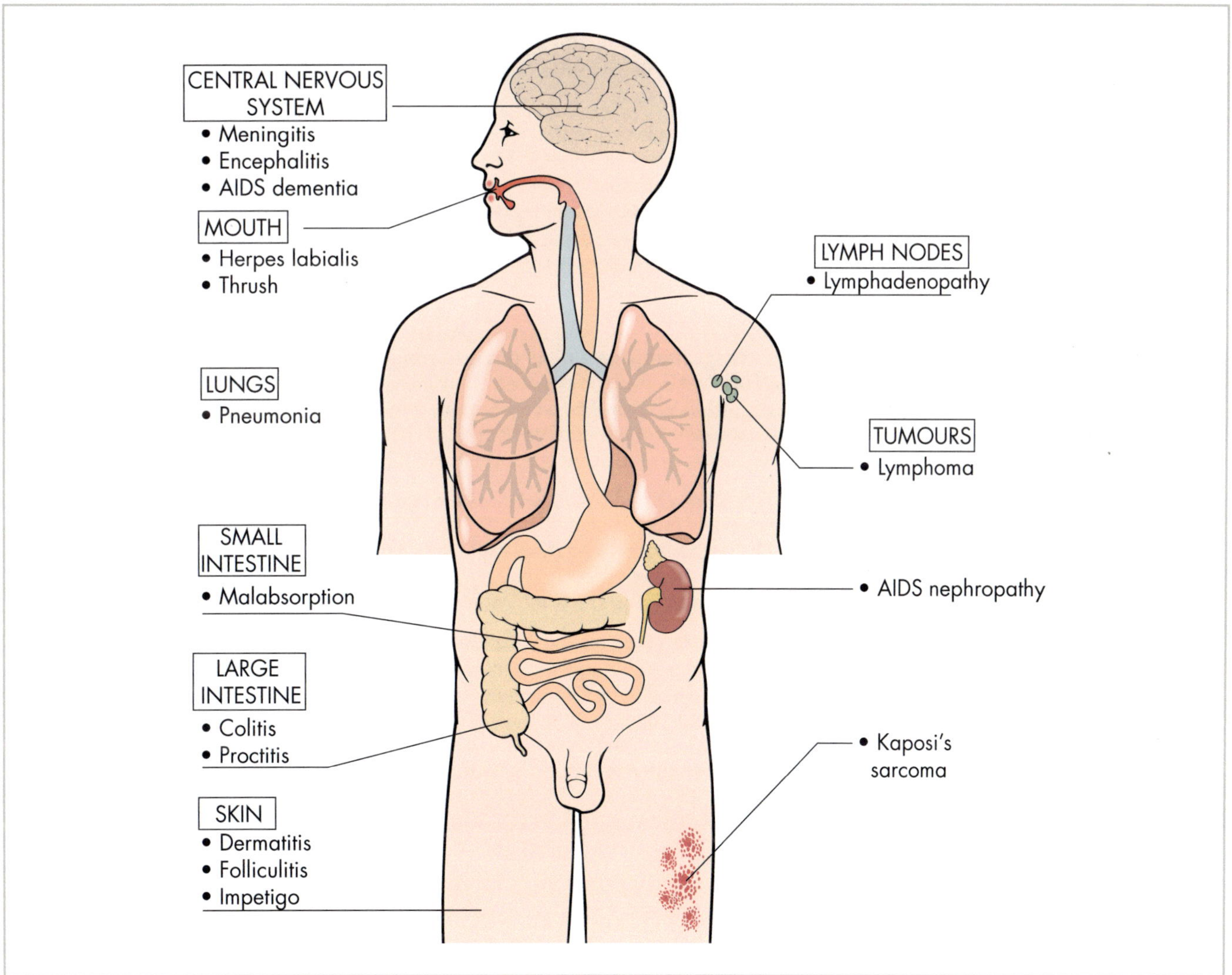

Fig. 10.66
Changes due to acquired immunodeficiency syndrome.

Memory loss, loss of coordination, paralysis, mental health disorders and dementia are also associated with AIDS.

The human body is incredible, and this chapter shows how complex and integrated it is, but also how disease can impact a person's quality of life. As we age, there is the potential for more disease, but also many diseases can be prevented or mitigated through diet, exercise and other lifestyle modifications.

CASE STUDY

Case study 1

You are caring for Miss Sacco, who is close to death. When administering to her hygiene needs, you notice that her urine output has decreased and is very dark, and that her hands and feet are very cold to touch. Her skin is pale and her lips are slightly blue. From your knowledge of anatomy and physiology, you know that her circulatory system is not supplying her skin and tissues with enough oxygen-rich blood. You also know that a decrease in urine output could mean that her urinary system is failing.

You report your observations to your supervisor, who contacts Miss Sacco's family, as it is felt that Miss Sacco has little time left. The family also want their parish priest to be notified. Miss Sacco dies within hours, with her family and priest present.

Case study 2

You visit Mr Stehbens in his home on a regular basis to assist with some wound care. Mr Stehbens is an active 75-year-old who lives by himself and has a history of heart disease. He loves to go for a long walk every morning. During your visit to Mr Stehbens, he tells you that he is getting chest pains and has some shortness of breath. From your understanding of the cardiovascular system, you realise that chest pain is serious and you report this immediately to your supervisor. He is admitted to hospital for further tests and undergoes heart surgery. Following some recuperation, he is able to go home and resumes his long walks each day.

Case study 3

Ms Jasinski is 35 years of age and lives in a high-care residential facility due to multiple sclerosis (MS), which has deteriorated rapidly over the past year. This disease has affected Miss Jasinski's nervous system, requiring full care of many physical functions. You understand that although she needs a lot of assistance physically, her mind is clear and she has full cognitive ability. Working with a multidisciplinary team, a holistic care plan is established to ensure that all of her needs are being met. Ms Jasinski is taking part in a medical trial of a new drug treatment for MS and, although this may not reverse her disease, it may help people newly diagnosed with MS.

Case study 4

Mrs Watson has primary, progressive multiple sclerosis, but has managed to remain in the community as her disease has progressed. She lives in her own ground-level unit with a great deal of assistance from the community team. As part of this team, you have just been assigned to take over Mrs Watson's daily hygiene needs and meal preparation. Due to her deteriorating condition, she has had a catheter inserted and the care plan instructs that you need to empty it on arrival and prior to leaving. She requires the use of the hoist to transfer in and out of bed and likes to be showered three times per week. On the other days, she has a full sponge bath in bed.

During the day, Mrs Watson sits in a specially designed chair that can be wheeled into the courtyard garden, where she enjoys watering her plants when she has the strength. Although she does not like to eat breakfast, she always enjoys a coffee when you visit. Due to her increasing dysphagia, the community-based speech therapist has advised that she needs to commence on level two thickened fluids and a soft diet. The specially prepared, thickened coffee, juice and water arrived last week and she is tolerating them well.

After her morning hygiene care, she likes to listen to some music while you prepare a hot meal for her lunch and usually a sandwich for her dinner. You both enjoy a chat and a coffee while you prepare the food. Her youngest daughter, Melanie, also visits every evening for a short while to ensure that she receives her dinner. Melanie is very close to her mother and is grateful for your support. She stays in frequent contact with you and always ensures that the communication channels are kept open. This helps to make you feel valued and appreciated for the important job that you do. Ultimately, this makes for improved outcomes and ensures that a good quality of life is provided for Mrs Watson.

REVIEW QUESTIONS

Circle the BEST answer:

1 Skeletal muscles:
   a are under involuntary control
   b appear smooth
   c are under voluntary control
   d appear striped and smooth

2 The highest functions of the brain take place in the:
   a cerebral cortex
   b medulla
   c brainstem
   d spinal nerves

3 The liquid part of blood is the:
   a haemoglobin
   b red blood cell
   c plasma
   d alveolus

4 Which of the following carry blood away from the heart?
   a Capillaries
   b Veins
   c Venules
   d Arteries

5 Oxygen and carbon dioxide are exchanged:
   a in the bronchi
   b between the alveoli and the capillaries
   c between the lungs and the pleura
   d in the trachea

6 Most food absorption takes place in the:
   a stomach
   b small intestine
   c colon
   d large intestine

7 The male sex gland is the:
   a semen
   b ovum
   c testis
   d sperm

8 Which of the following are functions of bone?
   a Formation of blood
   b Assist with movement
   c Protect soft tissue
   d All of the above

9 With ageing, changes occur in the nervous system. Which of the following statements is true?
   a More sleep is needed than when younger
   b Recent events are remembered better than past events
   c Sensitivity to pain is reduced
   d Confusion occurs in all older people

10 Older people should avoid very dry foods because of:
   a a decrease in the amount of saliva produced
   b loss of teeth or ill-fitting dentures
   c decreased amounts of digestive juices
   d decreased peristalsis

Answers to these questions are on p. 454.

References

Australian Institute of Health and Welfare (AIHW) (2021). BreastScreen Australia Monitoring Report 2020. Online 20 September 2021. Available: www.aihw.gov.au/reports/cancer-screening/breast-screen-australia-monitoring-report-2020/related-material)

Cancer Council Victoria (2021). Types of cancer: breast cancer. Online 20 September 2021. Available: www.cancer.org.au/cancer-information/types-of-cancer/breast-cancer

Cancer Council Victoria (2020). Diagnosing breast cancer. Online 20 September 2021. Available: www.cancervic.org.au/cancer-information/types-of-cancer/breast_cancer/diagnosing_breast_cancer.html

Healthy Bones Australia (2021). Osteoporosis. Online 7 March 2021. Available Bone Health – Bone Health Website (healthybonesaustralia.org.au)

Stroke Foundation (2021). Stroke symptoms. Online 7 March 2021. Available: strokefoundation.org.au/About-Stroke/Stroke-symptoms

CHAPTER 11
Health assessment

By Karen Scott

AFTER READING THIS CHAPTER, YOU SHOULD BE ABLE TO:

- define the key terms listed in this chapter
- understand why vital signs are measured
- understand the factors affecting vital signs
- know the normal ranges for the temperature sites
- know when to use each temperature site
- know the sites for taking a pulse
- know what to observe about the pulse and respirations
- understand the factors affecting blood pressure
- know how to measure blood pressure
- know how to take a blood glucose measurement
- know what to do before and after a physical examination
- know what equipment is used during a physical examination
- know how to prepare a person for an examination
- know the rules for assisting with a physical examination
- know the procedures described in this chapter
- know how to promote quality of life.

Key terms

blood glucose level: Glucose that the bloodstream carries to all the cells in the body to supply energy

blood pressure: The amount of force exerted against the walls of an artery by the blood

body temperature: The amount of heat in the body, which is a balance between the amount of heat produced and the amount lost by the body

bradycardia: A slow (*brady*) heart rate (*cardia*); the rate is less than 60 beats per minute

diastole: The period of heart muscle relaxation

diastolic pressure: The pressure in the arteries when the heart is at rest

hypertension: Persistent blood pressure measurements above (*hyper*) the normal systolic (140 mmHg) or diastolic (110 mmHg) pressures

hypotension: When the systolic blood pressure is below (*hypo*) 110 mmHg and the diastolic pressure is below 60 mmHg

laryngeal mirror: An instrument used to examine the mouth, teeth and throat

nasal speculum: An instrument used to examine the inside of the nose

ophthalmoscope: A lighted instrument used to examine the internal structures of the eye

otoscope: A lighted instrument used to examine the external ear and the eardrum (tympanic membrane)

percussion hammer: An instrument used to tap body parts to test reflexes; reflex hammer

pulse: The beat of the heart felt at an artery as a wave of blood passes through the artery

pulse rate: The number of heartbeats or pulses felt in 1 minute

respiration: The act of breathing air into (inhalation) and out of (exhalation) the lungs

respiratory rate: The number of respirations undertaken in 1 minute

sphygmomanometer: A cuff and measuring device used to measure blood pressure

stethoscope: An instrument used to listen to the sounds produced by the heart, lungs and other body organs

systole: The period of heart muscle contraction

systolic pressure: The amount of force needed to pump blood out of the heart into the arterial circulation

tachycardia: A rapid (*tachy*) heart rate (*cardia*); the heart rate is over 100 beats per minute

tuning fork: An instrument vibrated to test hearing

vaginal speculum: An instrument used to open the vagina so it and the cervix can be examined

vital signs: The basic signs of life which include: temperature, pulse, respirations, oxygen saturation and blood pressure

Undertaking a physical examination and measuring vital signs are important components of determining the health status of a person. Although the carer does not perform a formal physical assessment of a person, they may be asked to assist in one. Carers in some facilities are expected to measure the vital signs of clients.

PHYSICAL EXAMINATION

Doctors and registered nurses (RNs) perform physical examinations. Routine health examinations are done to promote health, determine a person's fitness for work, assist in diagnosis and treat disease. In aged care facilities, consumers have ongoing examinations to ensure any issues are identified to ensure their optimum health. You may be asked to assist a doctor or nurse with an examination in a residential aged care service or when accompanying a person on a visit to their general practitioner (GP).

What you do depends on centre policies and procedures. It also depends on the examiner's preferences. You may do some or all of the following:

- Collect linen to drape the person and for the procedure.
- Collect examination equipment.
- Prepare the room for the examination.
- Provide lighting.
- Transport the person to and from the examination room.
- Provide psychological support and comfort to the patient during the procedure.
- Measure vital signs, height and weight.
- Position and drape the person.
- Hand equipment and instruments to the examiner.
- Label specimen containers.
- Dispose of soiled linen and discard supplies.
- Clean equipment.
- Help the person dress or assume a comfortable position after the examination.

EQUIPMENT

If you are required to assist, you need to know the instruments shown in Fig. 11.1.

- **ophthalmoscope** – a lighted instrument used to examine the internal structures of the eye
- **otoscope** – a lighted instrument used to examine the external ear and the eardrum (tympanic membrane); some scopes have parts for examining eyes and ears, and are changed into an ophthalmoscope or otoscope
- **percussion hammer** – used to tap body parts to test reflexes; also called a reflex hammer
- **vaginal speculum** – used to open the vagina so it and the cervix can be examined
- **nasal speculum** – used to examine the inside of the nose
- **tuning fork** – vibrated to test hearing
- **laryngeal mirror** – used to examine the mouth, teeth and throat.

Some centres have examination trays in the supply department. If not, collect the items listed.

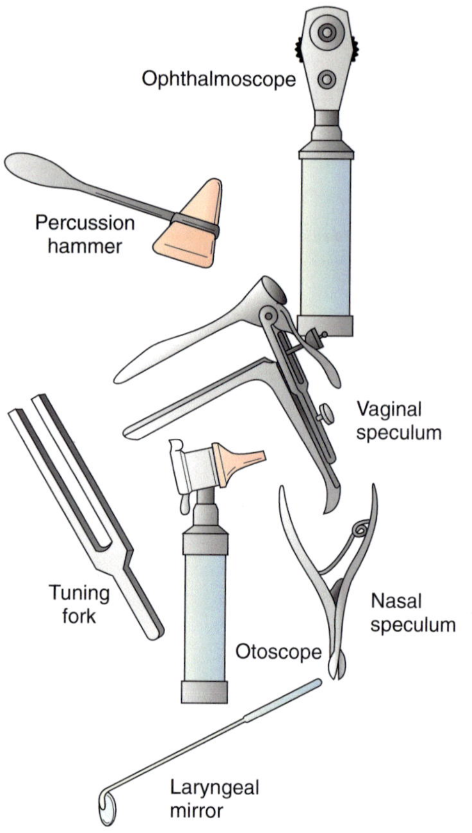

Fig. 11.1
Instruments used for a physical examination.

SAFETY ALERT

Preparing for an examination

- Warmth is a major concern during an examination.
- Protect the person from becoming chilled. Have an extra blanket nearby. Take measures to prevent draughts.
- Protect the person from falls and injury. Do not leave the person unattended.

DELEGATION GUIDELINES

Preparing for an examination

Before preparing a person for an examination, you need the following information from the nurse and the care plan:

- When to prepare the person.
- Where the examination will be done – person's room, consumer's room or doctor's surgery.
- How to position the person.
- What equipment and supplies are needed.
- Whether you need to measure and record height and weight.

PREPARING THE PERSON

People who are to have a physical examination often worry about the possible findings. Some are confused or fearful about what the examiner will do. Discomfort, embarrassment, fear of exposure and not knowing the procedure can all cause anxiety. You must be sensitive to the person's feelings and concerns. The person is prepared physically and psychologically for the examination. The person has the right to know who will do the examination, why it is done and what to expect. The doctor or nurse explains these things to the person. As the carer, you may be required to prepare the examination environment or assist the nurse to prepare the person.

The person has the right to personal choice, and the procedure must be explained before it begins. The examination is done only if the person gives consent. The person may want a different examiner or a family member present. Some people want the examination results explained with a family member present.

The right to privacy is also protected. The person is screened and the room door closed. Clothing is only removed when necessary. If a complete examination is required and all clothes need to be removed, the person is then dressed in a hospital gown. This reduces the naked feeling and the fear of exposure. The person is covered with a paper drape, bath blanket, sheet or drawsheet. Explain that only the body part being examined is exposed.

The person voids before the examination. An empty bladder lets the examiner feel the abdominal organs. A full bladder can change the normal position and shape of organs. It also causes discomfort, especially when the abdominal organs are felt. Confirm with the nurse whether a urine specimen is needed. If it is, the nurse will obtain it at this time.

POSITIONING

Sometimes a special position is needed for the examination. Some examination positions are uncomfortable and embarrassing. It is the responsibility of the nurse to position the person. You may be required to assist with positioning or to help the person maintain the position.

Common examination positions include:

- dorsal recumbent
- lithotomy position
- modified left lateral recumbent position.

The *dorsal recumbent* (horizontal recumbent) or supine position (Fig. 11.2A) is used to examine the abdomen, chest and breasts. The person is supine with the legs straight or knees bent and legs in an outward position. To examine the perineal area, the knees are flexed and hips externally rotated. The person is covered as for perineal care.

The *lithotomy position* (Fig. 11.2B) may be used to examine the vagina. The woman lies on her back. Her hips are brought to the edge of the examination table. The knees are flexed and the hips externally rotated. The feet are supported in stirrups. The person is covered as for the dorsal recumbent position. Some centres provide socks to cover the feet and calves. Some women cannot assume this position. This is not usually undertaken within an aged care facility or the consumer's home, as specialist equipment is required.

The *modified left lateral recumbent position* (Fig. 11.2C) is sometimes used to examine the rectum or vagina.

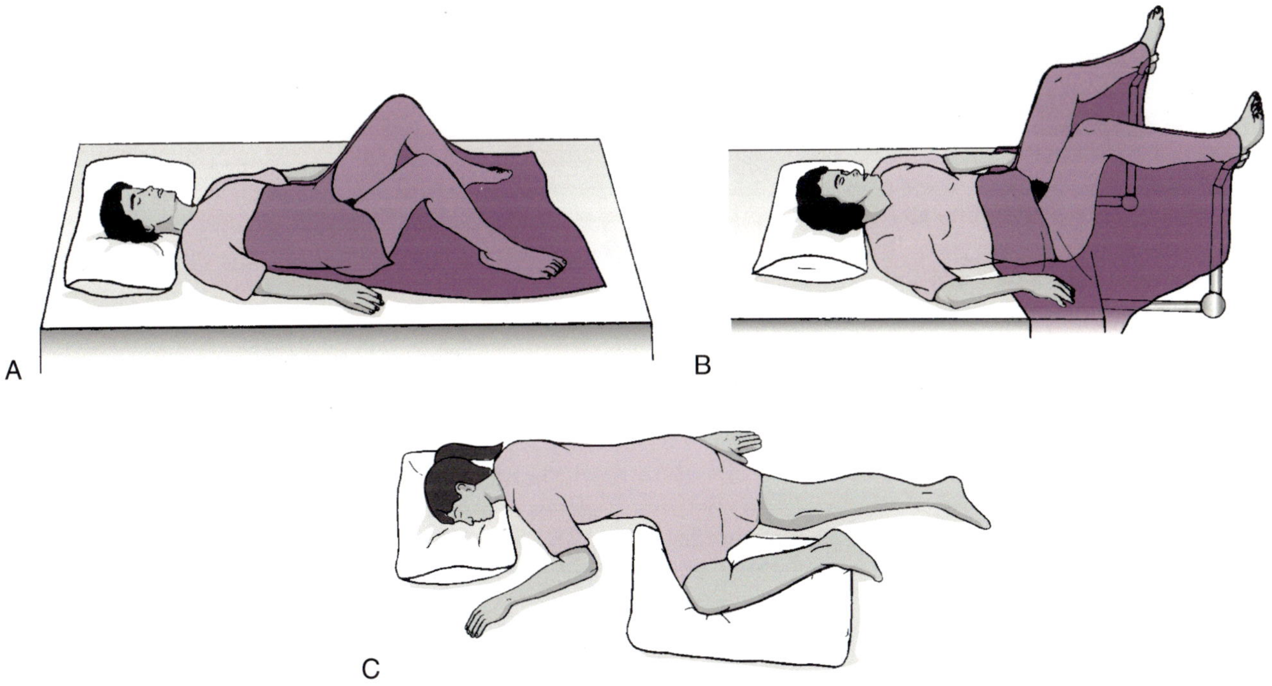

Fig. 11.2
Positioning and draping for the physical examination.
A. Dorsal recumbent position. **B.** Lithotomy position. **C.** Modified left lateral recumbent position.

BOX 11.1
Rules for assisting with the physical examination

- Wash your hands before and after the examination.
- Provide for privacy. This is done by screening, closing doors and draping. Expose only the body part being examined.
- Assist with positioning as directed by the examiner.
- Place instruments and equipment near the examiner.
- Stay in the room when a female is examined (unless you are a male), if a female nurse is not available. When a male examines a female, another female stays in the room. This is for the legal protection of the female and the male examiner. A female attendant also adds to the psychological comfort of the woman. A female examiner may want a male attendant present when she examines a male. This is also for her legal protection. Your role in assisting with an examination will depend on your agency's policies and procedures.
- Protect the person from falling.
- Reassure the person throughout the examination.
- Anticipate the examiner's need for equipment and supplies.
- Follow Standard Precautions.

ASSISTING WITH THE EXAMINATION

You may be asked to assist in preparing and positioning the person (Box 11.1). It is the responsibility of the nurse to assist the doctor with the examination.

AFTER THE EXAMINATION

After the examination, the person dresses or returns to bed. As lubricant is used to examine the vagina and rectum, ensure that the area is wiped or cleaned before the person dresses or returns to bed. You also need to:

- discard disposable items
- replace supplies for the next examination
- clean reusable items according to centre policy. Return them to the tray or storage place. This includes the otoscope and ophthalmoscope tips and stethoscope
- cover the examination table with a clean drawsheet or paper
- take the specimens labelled by the nurse/doctor to the designated area with a requisition slip
- clean and straighten the person's unit or examination room. Follow centre policy for soiled linen.

VITAL SIGNS

Vital signs reflect the function of three processes needed for life: regulation of body temperature, breathing and heart function. The five vital signs of body function are:

- temperature
- pulse
- respiration rate
- blood pressure
- oxygen saturations.

DELEGATION GUIDELINES

Measuring vital signs

The role of carers in taking vital signs varies among states/territories and agencies. Before you perform any of these procedures, make sure that:

- your state or territory allows you to take vital signs
- taking vital signs is within your job description
- you have the necessary training and education
- a nurse is available to answer questions and to supervise you.

Measuring and reporting vital signs

A person's vital signs vary within certain limits. Sleep, activity, eating, weather, noise, exercise, medications, fear, anxiety, pain, environment/surroundings and illness affect them.

Vital signs are measured to detect changes in normal body function and for monitoring and comparison of previous or recent changes in vital signs. They tell about the person's response to treatment. They often signal life-threatening events. Vital signs are part of assessment in the nursing process. Box 11.2 discusses measuring the vital signs of a consumer with dementia.

Vital signs are measured:

- during physical examinations
- when a person is admitted to the aged care facility
- as often as required by the person's condition
- after some care measures, such as ambulation
- after a fall or other injury
- when medications affect the respiratory or circulatory system

BOX 11.2
Consumers living with dementia

- Measuring vital signs on a person with dementia may be difficult. The person may move about, hit at you and grab equipment. This is not safe for the person or for you. Two carers may be needed. One uses touch and a soothing voice to calm and distract the person. The other measures the vital signs.
- You may need to try the procedure when the person is calmer. Or take the pulse and respirations at one time. Then take the temperature and blood pressure later.
- Always approach the person calmly. Use a soothing voice. Tell the person what you are going to do. Do not rush the person. Follow the care plan. If you cannot measure vital signs, tell the nurse immediately.

- when there are complaints of pain, dizziness, light-headedness, shortness of breath, rapid heart rate, not feeling well or other reported abnormalities
- as stated within the observation section of the care plan.

Vital signs show even minor changes in a person's condition. Accuracy is essential when you measure, record and report vital signs. If unsure of your measurements, promptly ask the nurse to take them again. Unless otherwise ordered, take vital signs with the person lying down or sitting.

The person is at rest when vital signs are measured. Report the following to the nurse at once:

- any vital sign that is changed from a previous measurement
- vital signs above the normal range
- vital signs below the normal range
- any other concerns you may have noticed when taking the person's observations, e.g. you may have noticed the person has raspy breathing.

Vital signs are recorded on graph sheets. If measured often, a flow sheet is used. The nurse or doctor compares current and previous measurements.

Body temperature

Body temperature is the amount of heat in the body. It is a balance between the amount of heat produced and the amount lost by the body. Heat is produced as cells use food for energy. It is lost through the skin, breathing, urine and faeces. Body temperature stays within a narrow range. It is usually lower in the morning and higher in the afternoon and evening. Factors affecting body temperature include age, weather, exercise, emotions, stress and illness. Pregnancy and the menstrual cycle are other factors.

Thermometers are used to measure temperature. It is measured using the Celsius (C) scale. Temperature sites are the mouth, axilla (underarm) and ear (tympanic membrane). Normal body temperature depends on the site. Each site has a normal range (Table 11.1).

Older people have lower body temperatures than younger adults. A temperature that is considered to be within the acceptable range in younger adults (e.g. an oral temperature of 37°C) may indicate a fever in the older adult. Always report temperatures that are not within the normal range to the nurse in charge.

Taking temperatures

Temperatures may be taken using oral, tympanic membrane or axillary sites. Special measures are needed for each site.

Table 11.1
Normal body temperatures

Site	Baseline	Normal range
Oral	36.5°C	36–37.5°C
Axillary	36.5°C	36–37.0°C
Tympanic membrane	37°C	35.5–37°C

Oral temperature

The thermometer remains in place according to centre policy or manufacturer's directions. Oral temperatures are not taken if the person:

- is an infant or a child under 6 years of age
- is unconscious
- has had surgery or an injury to the face, neck, nose or mouth
- is receiving oxygen
- breathes through the mouth
- has a nasogastric tube
- is delirious, restless, confused or disoriented
- is paralysed on one side of the body
- has a sore mouth
- has a convulsive disorder.

Axillary temperature

Axillary temperatures are less reliable than the other sites. They are used when the other sites cannot be used. The axilla must be dry. Do not use this site straight after bathing. Hold the thermometer in place for the time required by centre policy or the manufacturer's directions (Fig. 11.3).

DELEGATION GUIDELINES

Taking temperatures

When taking temperatures is delegated to you, you need the following information from the nurse and the care plan:

- Which site to use: oral, axillary or tympanic.
- Which type of thermometer to use.
- How long to leave the thermometer in place.
- When to take temperatures.
- What other vital signs to measure.
- Which people are at risk of elevated temperatures.
- What observations to report and record.

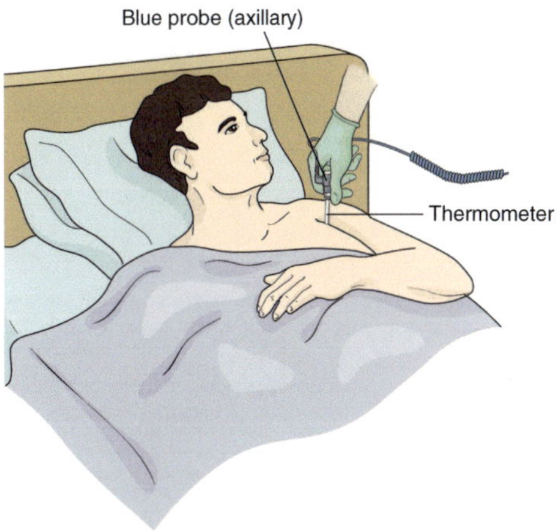

Fig. 11.3
The thermometer is held in place in the axilla by bringing the person's arm over their chest.

SAFETY ALERT

Taking temperatures

Thermometers are never inserted into the mouth of an individual who is confused or unconscious, or who has dementia.

Electronic thermometers

Electronic thermometers are battery-operated. They measure temperature in a few seconds. The temperature is shown on the front of the device. The hand-held unit is kept in a battery charger when not in use.

Electronic thermometers have oral and axillary probes. A disposable cover (sheath) covers the probe. It is discarded after use. This prevents the spread of infection.

Tympanic membrane thermometers

Tympanic membrane thermometers (Fig. 11.4) measure temperature at the tympanic membrane in the ear. The covered probe is gently inserted into the ear (Fig. 11.5). The temperature is measured in 1–3 seconds. The disposable cover is then removed and disposed of as per organisation policy and procedure.

Tympanic membrane thermometers are comfortable. They are useful for confused people because of their speed and comfort (Box 11.3). There are fewer microbes in the ear than in the mouth. Therefore, the risk of spreading infection is reduced. These thermometers are not used if there is any ear discharge.

Other thermometers

Other types of thermometers are used. Follow the manufacturer's instructions.

- *Digital thermometer* (Fig. 11.6) – the temperature is shown on the front of the thermometer. The temperature is measured within 60 seconds. Some have a memory mechanism that recalls the last temperature reading. The device is battery-operated and shuts off after about 10 minutes.
- *Temperature-sensitive tape* – changes colour in response to body heat. The tape is applied to the forehead or abdomen. The measurement takes about 15 seconds.
- *Digital infrared thermometers* may be used for residents and visitors in aged care. It is a non-invasive method whereby an infrared beam is directed to the forehead of the person and a temperature is displayed immediately on the device.

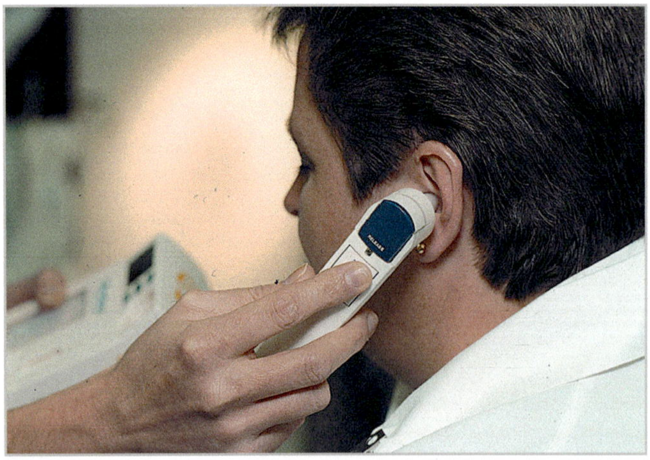

Fig. 11.4
Tympanic membrane thermometer.

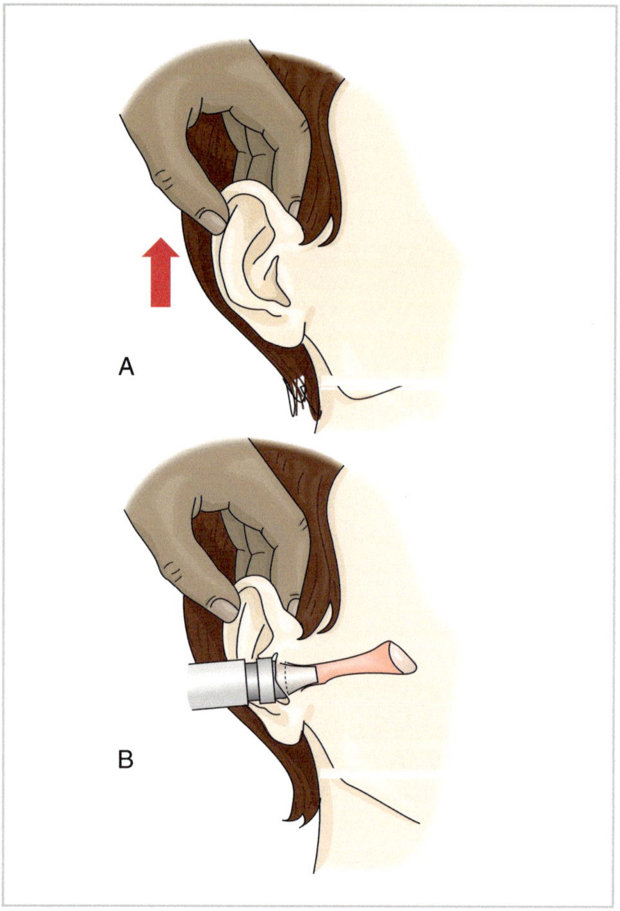

Fig. 11.5
Using a tympanic membrane thermometer.
A. The ear is pulled upwards and back. **B.** The probe is inserted into the ear canal.

BOX 11.3
Consumers living with dementia

A tympanic membrane thermometer is used for people who are confused and resist care. An electronic thermometer can injure the mouth and teeth if the person moves about or bites down on it.

Pulse

The **pulse** is the beat of the heart felt at an artery as a wave of blood passes through the artery. A pulse is felt every time the heart beats.

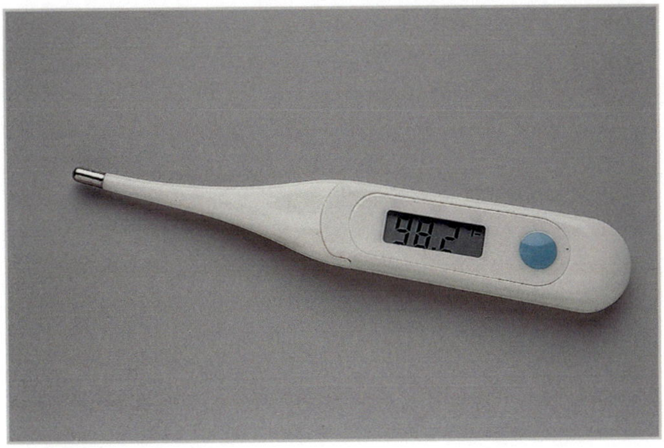

Fig. 11.6
Digital thermometer.

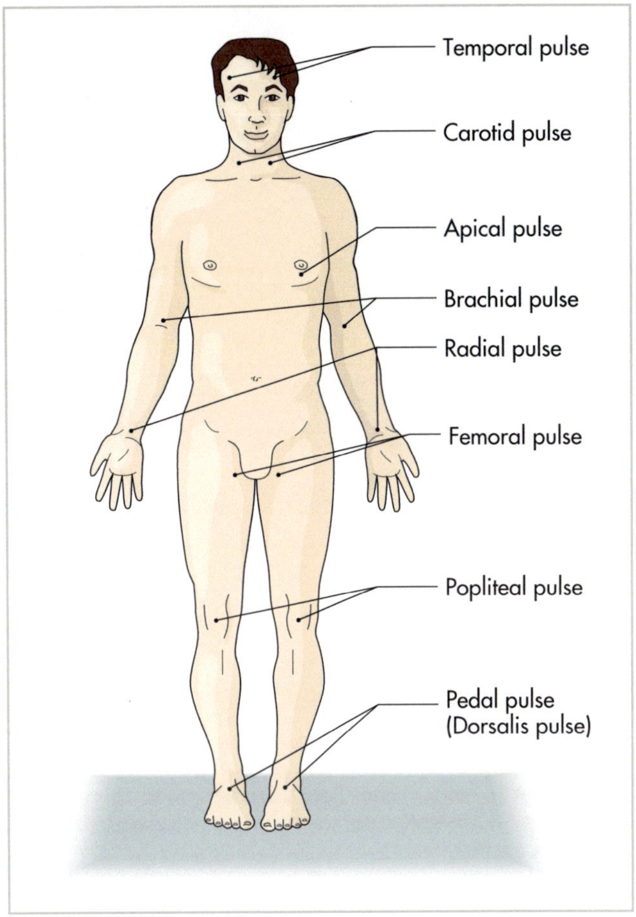

Fig. 11.7
The pulse sites.

Sites for taking a pulse

The temporal, carotid, brachial, radial, femoral, popliteal and dorsalis pedis (pedal) pulses are on both sides of the body (Fig. 11.7). Pulses are easy to feel at these sites, as the arteries are close to the body's surface and lie over a bone.

The radial site is used most often, as it is easy to reach and find. You can take a radial pulse without disturbing or exposing the person. The carotid pulse may be taken in an emergency.

The apical pulse is felt over the apex (apical) of the heart. The apex is at the tip of the heart, just below the left nipple. The apical pulse is taken with a stethoscope.

Using a stethoscope

A **stethoscope** is an instrument used to listen to the sounds produced by the heart, lungs and other body organs. It is used for measuring apical pulse and blood pressure. The device amplifies sounds for easy hearing.

Follow these measures when using a stethoscope:

- Wipe the earpieces (Fig. 11.8) and diaphragm with antiseptic wipes before and after use.
- Warm the diaphragm in your hand (Fig. 11.9).
- Place the earpiece tips in your ears. The bend of the tips points forwards. Earpieces should fit snugly to block out noises. They should not cause pain or ear discomfort.
- Place the diaphragm over the artery. Hold it in place as shown in Fig. 11.10.
- Prevent noise. Do not let anything touch the tubing. Ask the person to be silent.

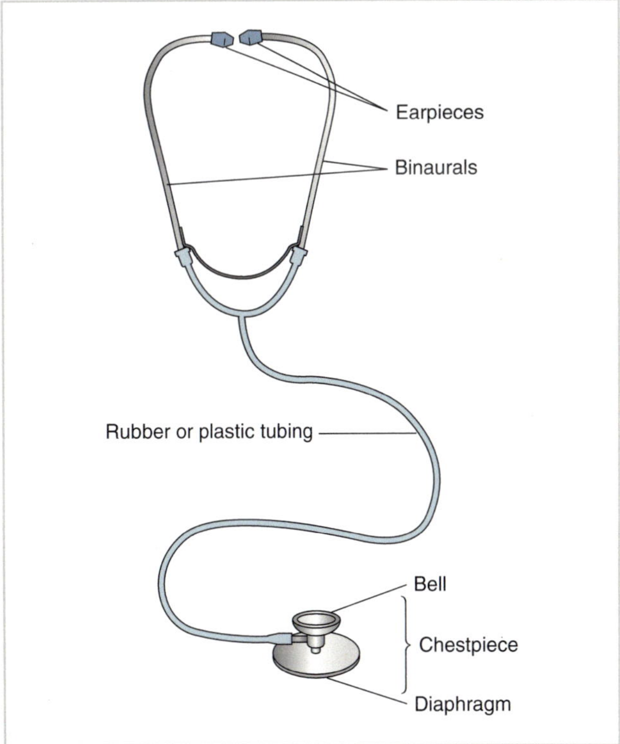

Fig. 11.8
Parts of a stethoscope.

SAFETY ALERT

Stethoscopes

Stethoscopes are in contact with many consumers and staff. Therefore, you must prevent infection. Wipe the earpieces and diaphragm with antiseptic wipes before and after use.

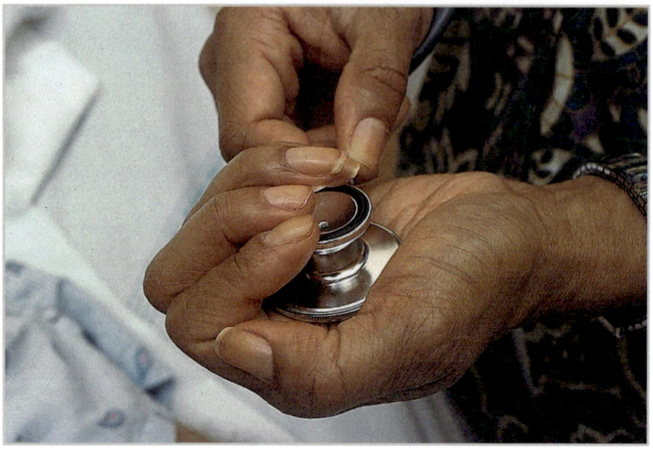

Fig. 11.9
The diaphragm of the stethoscope is warmed in the palm of the hand.

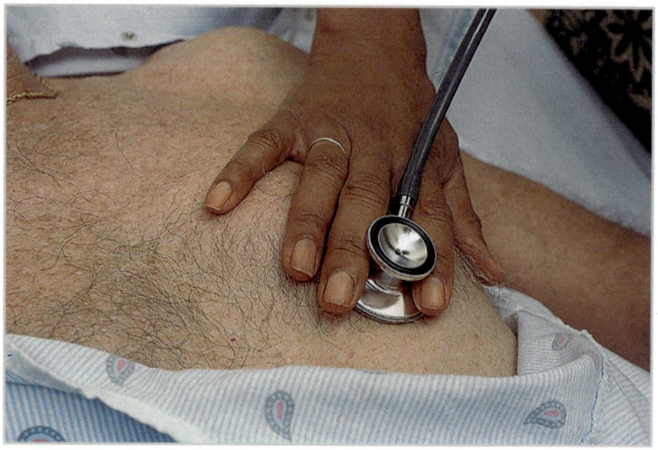

Fig. 11.10
The stethoscope is held in place with the fingertips of the index and middle fingers.

TAKING A TEMPERATURE WITH AN ELECTRONIC THERMOMETER

Quality of life

Remember to respect the client's privacy while doing any procedure. Address the person by name and ensure they know your name.

Pre-procedure

1 Follow the delegation guidelines.
2 Explain the procedure to the person. For an oral temperature, ask the person not to eat, drink, smoke or chew gum for at least 15–20 minutes beforehand.
3 Collect the following:
- thermometer (electronic or tympanic membrane)
- probe
- probe covers
- towel (axillary temperature).

4 Plug the probe into the thermometer. (This is not done for a tympanic membrane thermometer.)
5 Wash your hands.
6 Identify the person. Call the person by name.

Procedure

7 Provide for privacy. Position the person for an oral, axillary or tympanic membrane temperature reading.
8 Put on gloves if contact with blood, body fluids or secretions is likely.
9 Insert the probe into a probe cover.
10 For an oral temperature:
- a ask the person to open their mouth and raise the tongue.
- b place the covered probe at the base of the tongue.
- c ask the person to lower the tongue and close their mouth.

11 For an axillary temperature:
- a help the person remove an arm from the gown. Do not expose the person.
- b dry the axilla with the towel.
- c place the covered probe in the axilla.
- d place the person's arm over their chest.

12 For a tympanic membrane temperature:
- a ask the person to turn their head so the ear is in front of you.
- b insert the covered probe gently. Pull back on the ear to straighten the ear canal.

13 Start the thermometer.
14 Hold the probe in place until you hear a tone or see a flashing or steady light.
15 Read the temperature on the display and record the finding.
16 Remove the probe. Press the eject button to discard the cover.
17 Return the probe to the holder.

Post-procedure

18 Place the signal light within reach (if applicable).
19 Remove any screens from around the person.
20 Return the thermometer to the charging unit.
21 Wash your hands.
22 Record the measurement in the proper place. Note the temperature site. Report an abnormal temperature.

Pulse rate

The **pulse rate** is the number of heartbeats or pulses felt in 1 minute. The rate varies for each age group. The pulse rate is affected by many factors. These include elevated body temperature (fever), exercise, fear, anger, anxiety, excitement, heat, position and pain.

These and other factors cause the heart to beat faster. Some medications also increase the pulse rate. Other medications slow down the pulse.

- The normal adult pulse rate is between 60 and 100 beats per minute. A rate of less than 60 or greater than 100 is not normal. Report abnormal rates to the nurse at once.
- **Tachycardia** is a rapid (*tachy*) heart rate (*cardia*). The heart rate is over 100 beats per minute.
- **Bradycardia** is a slow (*brady*) heart rate (*cardia*). The rate is less than 60 beats per minute.

Rhythm and force of the pulse

The rhythm of the **pulse** should be regular. That is, the pulse is felt in a pattern. The same time interval occurs between beats. An irregular pulse occurs when the beats are unevenly spaced or beats are skipped. Report an irregular pulse to the nurse immediately.

Force relates to pulse strength. A forceful pulse is easy to feel. It is described as strong, full or bounding. Hard-to-feel pulses are described as weak, thready or feeble. Report any abnormalities in relation to pulse strength to the nurse.

Electronic blood pressure equipment can also count pulses. The pulse rate and blood pressure are shown. Information is not given about pulse rhythm and force. You need to feel the pulse to determine rhythm and force.

Taking a radial pulse

The *radial pulse* is used for routine vital signs. Place the first two or three middle fingers of one hand against the radial artery (Fig. 11.11). The radial artery is on the thumb side of the wrist. Count the pulse for 30 seconds. Then multiply the number by two. This gives the number of beats per minute (Table 11.2). If the pulse is irregular, count it for 1 minute.

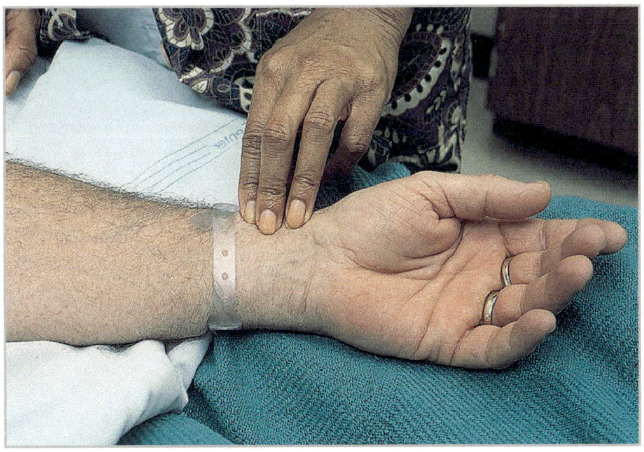

Fig. 11.11
The first two or three middle fingers are used to take the radial pulse.

Table 11.2
Pulse ranges for different ages

Age	Pulse rate (beats per minute)
Birth to 1 year	80–190
1–2 years	80–160
2–5 years	80–120
5–12 years	70–110
12 years and older	60–100

In some centres, all radial pulses are taken for 1 minute. Follow centre policy.

SAFETY ALERT

Radial pulses

Do not use your thumb to take a pulse. The thumb has a pulse. You could mistake the pulse in your thumb for the person's pulse. Reporting the wrong pulse rate can harm the person.

TAKING A RADIAL PULSE

Quality of life

Remember to respect the client's privacy while doing any procedure. Address the person by name and ensure they know your name.

Pre-procedure

1. Follow the delegation guidelines.
2. Wash your hands.
3. Call the person by name.
4. Explain the procedure to the person.
5. Provide for privacy.

Procedure

6. Have the person sit or lie down.
7. Locate the radial pulse. Use your first two or three middle fingers.
8. Note whether the pulse is strong or weak, and regular or irregular.
9. Count the pulse for 30 seconds. Multiply the number of beats by 2. Or count the pulse for 1 minute as directed by the nurse or if required by centre policy.
10. Count the pulse for 1 minute if it is irregular.

Post-procedure

11. Provide for comfort.
12. Place the signal light within reach (if applicable)
13. Remove any screens from around the person.
14. Wash your hands.
15. Report and record the pulse rate and your observations. Report an abnormal pulse.

DELEGATION GUIDELINES

Taking a pulse

Before taking a pulse, you need the following information from the nurse and the care plan:

- What pulse to take – radial or brachial.
- When to take the pulse.
- What other vital signs to measure.
- Whether the nurse has concerns about certain clients.
- What observations to report and record:
  - a pulse rate less than 60 or more than 100 beats per minute (report this at once)
  - if the pulse is regular or irregular
  - the pulse rate
  - pulse force – strong, full, bounding, weak, thready or feeble.

Respiration

Respiration is the act of breathing air into (*inhalation*) and out of (*exhalation*) the lungs. Oxygen enters the lungs during inhalation. Carbon dioxide leaves the lungs during exhalation. Each respiration involves one inhalation and one exhalation. The chest rises during inhalation. It falls during exhalation.

The healthy adult has 12–20 respirations per minute. The **respiratory rate** is affected by the same factors that affect temperature and pulse. Heart and respiratory diseases usually increase the respiratory rate.

Respirations are normally quiet, effortless and regular. Both sides of the chest rise and fall equally.

Count respirations when the person is at rest. Position the person so you can see their chest rise and fall. To a certain extent, a person can control the depth and rate of breathing. As people tend to change breathing patterns when they know their respirations are being counted, they should not know that you are counting them.

Respirations are counted right after taking a pulse. Keep your fingers or stethoscope over the pulse site. (The person assumes you are taking their pulse.) To count respirations, watch the chest rise and fall. Count them for 30 seconds. Multiply the number by two for the number of respirations in 1 minute. If an abnormal pattern is noted, count the respirations for 1 minute.

COUNTING RESPIRATIONS

Quality of life

Remember to respect the client's privacy while doing any procedure. Address the person by name and ensure they know your name.

Pre-procedure

1. Follow the delegation guidelines.
2. Wash your hands.
3. Explain the procedure to the person.
4. Identify the person. Call them by name.

Procedure

5. Continue to hold the person's wrist after taking their radial pulse.
6. Do not tell the person you are counting respirations.
7. Begin counting when the chest rises. Count each rise and fall of the chest as one respiration.
8. Note the following:
   a. if respirations are regular
   b. if the person has pain or difficulty breathing including the use of accessory muscles to breathe, e.g. movement of shoulders
9. Count respirations for 30 seconds. Multiply the number by 2.
10. Count respirations for 1 minute if they are abnormal or irregular.

Post-procedure

11. Provide for comfort.
12. Place the signal light within reach.
13. Wash your hands.
14. Report and record your observations. Report an abnormal respiration rate.

DELEGATION GUIDELINES

Counting respirations

Before counting respirations you will need the following information from the nurse and the care plan:

- When to count respirations.
- What other vital signs to measure.
- What observations to report and record:
  - the respiratory rate
  - whether the respirations were regular or irregular
  - if the person has pain or difficulty breathing.

Blood pressure

Blood pressure is the amount of force exerted against the walls of an artery by the blood. Blood pressure is controlled by:

- the force of heart contractions
- the amount of blood pumped with each heartbeat
- how easily the blood flows through the blood vessels.

The period of heart muscle contraction is called **systole.** The period of heart muscle relaxation is called **diastole.**

Systolic and diastolic pressures are measured. The **systolic pressure** is the higher pressure. It represents the amount of force needed to pump blood out of the heart into the arterial circulation. The **diastolic pressure** is the lower pressure. It reflects the pressure in the arteries when the heart is at rest.

Blood pressure is measured in millimetres (mm) of mercury (Hg). The systolic pressure is recorded over the diastolic pressure. The average adult has a systolic pressure of 120 mmHg and a diastolic pressure of 80 mmHg. This is written as 120/80 mmHg.

Factors affecting blood pressure

Blood pressure can change from minute to minute. Factors affecting blood pressure are listed in Box 11.4.

Because it varies easily, blood pressure has normal ranges:

- systolic pressure – less than 120 mmHg
- diastolic pressure – less than 80 mmHg.

Persistent measurements above the normal systolic and diastolic pressures are abnormal. This condition is called **hypertension**. In young and middle-aged adults, report any systolic pressure above 120 mmHg to the nurse. A diastolic pressure above 80 mmHg is also reported. Likewise, systolic pressures below 110 mmHg and diastolic pressures below 60 mmHg are reported. This is called **hypotension**. Some people normally have low blood pressure. However, hypotension may signal a life-threatening problem.

Systolic and diastolic pressures are normally higher in older people. Arteries narrow and are less elastic. The heart works harder to pump blood through the vessels. A blood pressure of 160/110 mmHg is normal for many older people. Older people are also at risk of orthostatic hypotension. Orthostatic hypotension is a sudden drop in blood pressure when there is a change in posture or position (especially standing up).

Blood pressures are taken and reported before the nurse gives certain medications. The nurse and care plan tell you when this is needed.

BOX 11.4
Factors affecting blood pressure

- *Age* – blood pressure increases with age. It is lowest in infancy and childhood. It is highest in adulthood.
- *Gender* (male or female) – women usually have lower blood pressure than men do. Blood pressure rises in women after menopause.
- *Blood volume* – this is the amount of blood in the system. Severe bleeding lowers the blood volume. Therefore, the blood pressure lowers. Infusing intravenous (IV) fluids rapidly increases the blood volume and thus the blood pressure rises.
- *Stress* – includes anxiety, fear and emotions. Blood pressure increases as the body responds to stress.
- *Pain* – generally increases blood pressure. However, severe pain can cause shock. Blood pressure is seriously low in a state of shock.
- *Exercise* – increases blood pressure. Blood pressure is not measured immediately after exercise.
- *Weight* – blood pressure is higher in overweight people. Blood pressure lowers with weight loss.
- *Ethnicity* – Indigenous Australians have a higher rate of hypertension than European Australians.
- *Diet* – a high-sodium diet increases the amount of water in the body. The extra fluid volume increases blood pressure.
- *Medications* – medications can be given to raise or lower blood pressure. Other medications can cause high or low blood pressure as a side-effect.
- *Position* – blood pressure is lower when lying down. It is higher when standing. Sudden position changes can cause sudden changes in blood pressure (orthostatic hypotension). If a person stands suddenly, their blood pressure can drop suddenly. Dizziness and fainting can occur.
- *Smoking* – increases blood pressure. Nicotine in cigarettes causes blood vessels to narrow. The heart works harder to pump blood through narrowed vessels.
- *Alcohol* – excessive alcohol intake can raise blood pressure.

Equipment

A stethoscope and a sphygmomanometer are used to measure blood pressure. The **sphygmomanometer** has a cuff and a measuring device. There are three types of sphygmomanometer:

- The *aneroid* type has a round dial and a needle that points to the calibrations (Fig. 11.12A).
- The *mercury* type is more accurate than the aneroid type. It has a column of mercury within a calibrated tube (Fig. 11.12B).
- The *electronic* type shows the systolic and diastolic blood pressures on the front of the device (Fig. 11.12C). It also shows the pulse rate. Follow the manufacturer's instructions.

The blood pressure cuff is wrapped around the upper arm. Tubing connects the cuff to the sphygmomanometer. Another tube connects the cuff to a small hand-held bulb. A valve on the bulb is turned so the cuff inflates as the bulb is squeezed. The inflated cuff causes pressure over the brachial artery. The valve is turned the other way for cuff deflation. Blood pressure is measured as the cuff is deflated.

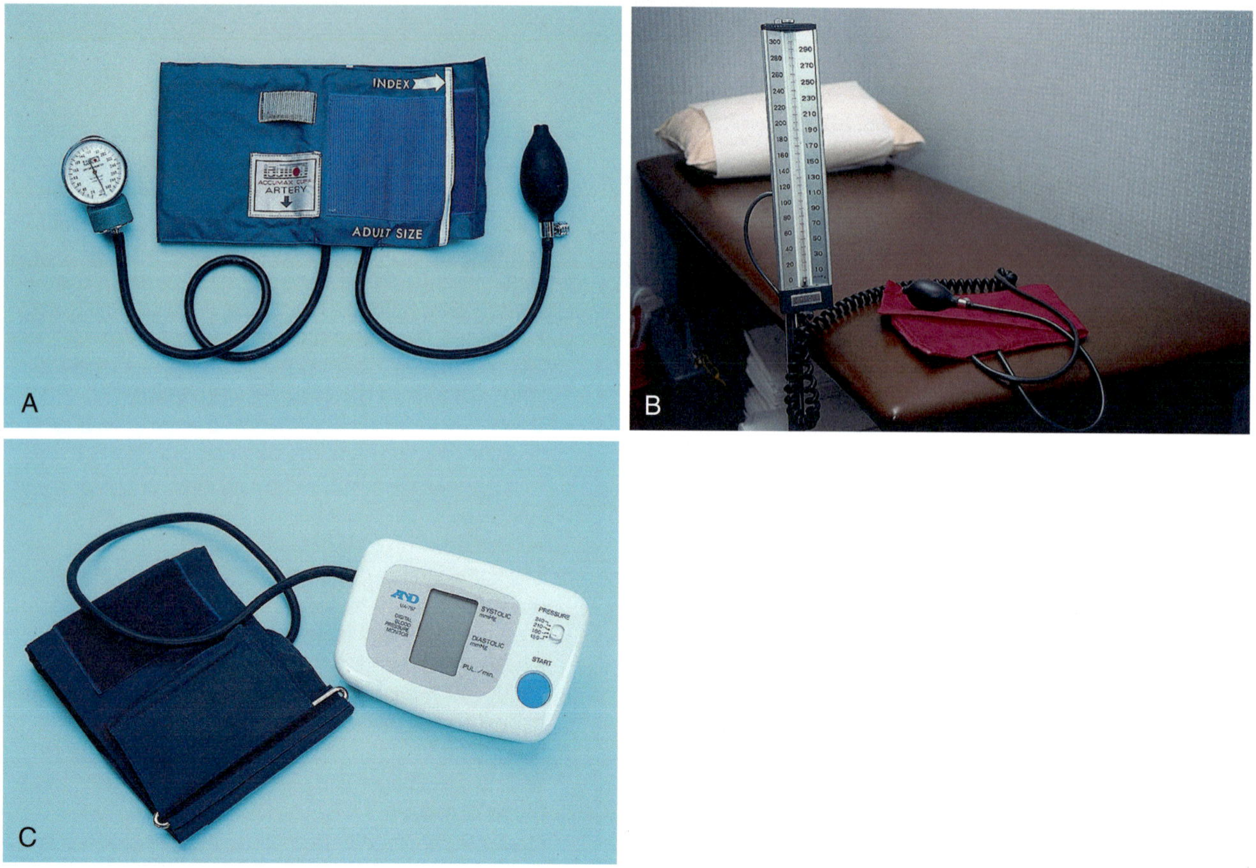

Fig. 11.12
Blood pressure equipment.
A. Aneroid manometer and cuff. **B.** Mercury manometer and cuff. **C.** Electronic sphygmomanometer.

Sounds are produced as blood flows through the arteries. The **stethoscope** is used to listen to the sounds in the brachial artery as the cuff is deflated. A stethoscope is not needed with an electronic device.

A person with very small arms may need paediatric blood pressure cuffs. Those with very large arms may need extra-large cuffs. You need the right size cuff for accuracy. The care plan or the nurse will tell you if a special cuff is needed.

Measuring blood pressure

Blood pressure is normally measured in the brachial artery. Box 11.5 lists the guidelines for measuring blood pressure.

DELEGATION GUIDELINES

Measuring blood pressure

Before measuring blood pressure (BP), you need the following information from the nurse and care plan:

- When to measure blood pressure.
- Whether the person needs to be lying down, sitting or standing.
- Whether a lying and standing BP needs to be recorded to assess if there is a postural drop/orthostatic hypotension.
- What size cuff to use – regular, paediatric or extra-large.
- What observations to report and record.

SAFETY ALERT

Blood pressure

You need to know the normal blood pressure ranges for each person. Report any blood pressure above or below the person's normal range.

BOX 11.5
Guidelines for measuring blood pressure

- Do not take blood pressure on an arm with an IV infusion, a cast, a dressing or a dialysis access site. If a person has had breast surgery, do not take blood pressure on that side. Avoid taking blood pressure on an injured or bruised arm.
- Let the person rest for 10–20 minutes before measuring the blood pressure.
- Measure blood pressure with the person sitting or lying down. Sometimes the doctor orders blood pressure to be measured in the standing position.
- Use the correct size of blood pressure cuff. For example, use a paediatric cuff for a very small arm.
- Apply the cuff to the bare upper arm. Clothing can affect the measurement.
- Make sure the cuff is snug. Loose cuffs can cause inaccurate readings.
- Place the diaphragm of the stethoscope firmly over the artery. The entire diaphragm must have contact with the skin.
- Make sure the room is quiet. Talking, television, radio and sounds from the hallway can affect the accuracy of the measurement.
- Have the sphygmomanometer clearly visible.
- Measure the systolic and diastolic pressures. Expect to hear the first blood pressure sound at the point where you last felt the radial or brachial pulse. The first sound is the systolic pressure. The point where the sound disappears is the diastolic pressure.
- Take the blood pressure again if you are not sure of an accurate measurement. Wait 30–60 seconds before repeating the measurement.
- Notify the nurse at once if you cannot hear the blood pressure.

MEASURING BLOOD PRESSURE

Quality of life

Remember to respect the client's privacy while doing any procedure. Address the person by name and ensure they know your name.

Pre-procedure

1 Follow the delegation guidelines.
2 Collect the following:
   - sphygmomanometer
   - stethoscope
   - antiseptic wipes.
3 Wash your hands.
4 Call the person by name.
5 Explain the procedure to the person.
6 Provide for privacy.

Procedure

7 Wipe the stethoscope earpieces and diaphragm with the wipes.
8 Have the person sit, stand or lie down as per instructions from the care plan or nurse.
9 Position the person's arm level with the heart. The palm is up.
10 Stand no more than 50 cm away from the sphygmomanometer. A mercury model is vertical, on a flat surface and at eye level. The aneroid type is directly in front of you.
11 Expose the upper arm. Remove any constrictive clothing.
12 Squeeze the cuff to expel any remaining air. Close the valve on the bulb.
13 Find the brachial artery at the inner aspect of the elbow.
14 Place the arrow on the cuff over the brachial artery. Wrap the cuff around the upper arm at least 2.5 cm above the elbow. It should be even and snug (Fig. 11.13).
15 Place the stethoscope earpieces in your ears.
16 Locate the radial or brachial pulse.
17 Inflate the cuff until you can no longer feel the pulse. Note this point.
18 Inflate the cuff 30 mmHg beyond the point where you last felt the pulse.
19 Place the diaphragm over the brachial artery. Do not place it under the cuff.
20 Deflate the cuff at an even rate of 2–4 millimetres per second. Turn the valve counter-clockwise to deflate the cuff.
21 Note the point where you heard the first sound. This is the systolic reading. It is near the point where the radial pulse disappeared.
22 Continue to deflate the cuff. Note the point where the sound disappears. This is the diastolic reading.
23 Deflate the cuff completely. Remove it from the person's arm. Remove the stethoscope.
24 Return the cuff to the case or wall holder.

Post-procedure

25 Provide for comfort.
26 Place the signal light within reach (if applicable).
27 Remove the screens from around the person.
28 Clean the earpieces and diaphragm with wipes.
29 Return the equipment to its proper place.
30 Wash your hands.
31 Report and record the blood pressure.

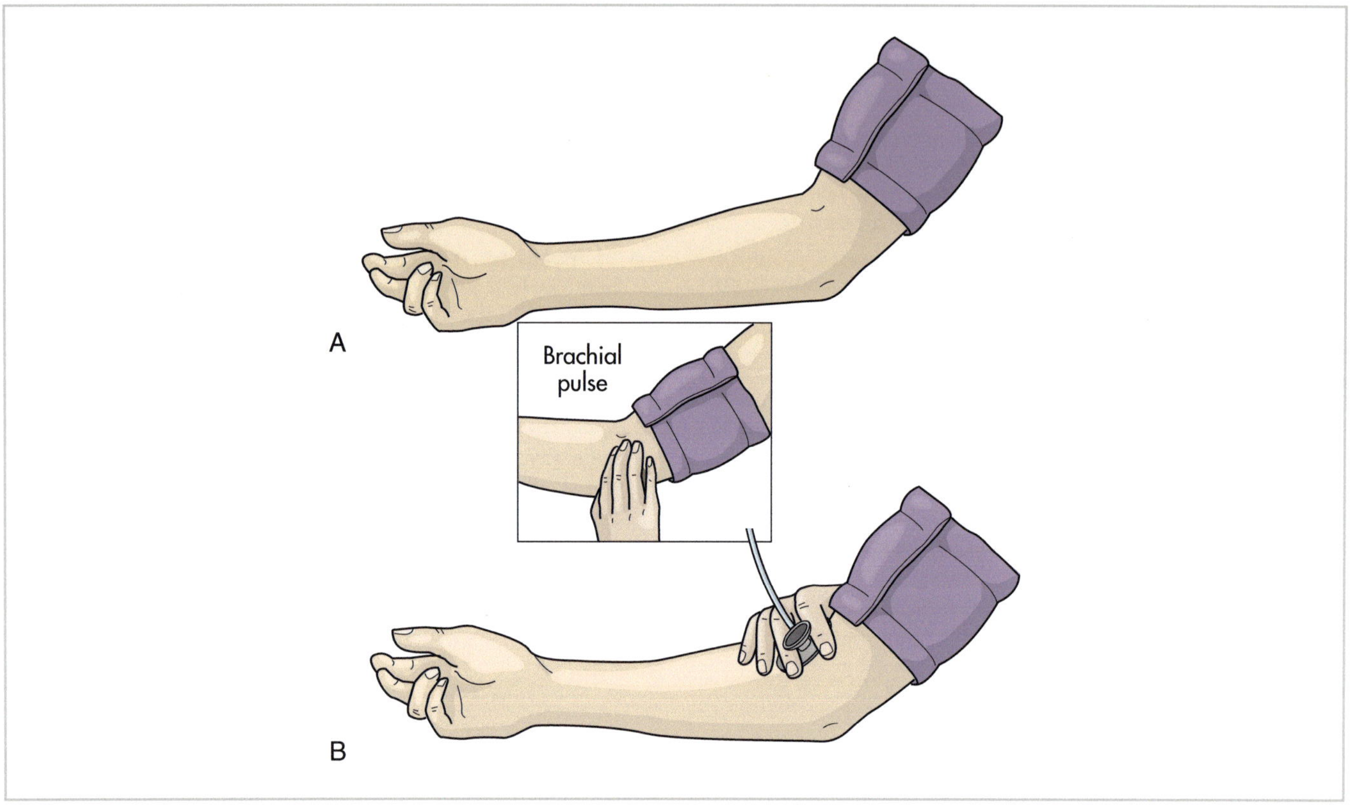

Fig. 11.13
Measuring blood pressure.
A. The cuff is over the brachial artery. **B.** The diaphragm of the stethoscope is over the brachial artery.

CASE STUDY

A new client has arrived at the aged care service where you work. You are asked to prepare the room for an admission examination. In the examination room you ensure that you have collected and set up all the necessary equipment in accordance with the organisation's policies and procedures. You check that you have closed windows and doors and that the curtains are drawn to promote privacy for the client, that a supply of blankets or draw sheets/sheets is available and that the lighting is appropriate for the examination. Prior to starting the examination, you place an 'Examination in progress' sign on the door. You are then required to assist the client to the examination room and explain the procedures to him or her. You introduce yourself to the client and show them the way to the procedure room. You must measure and weigh the client first. You are then required to assist them to disrobe and put on a gown. You measure the client's vital signs. By measuring respiration, blood pressure, temperature and pulse you are providing a baseline for further care in the facility. It is your responsibility to reassure the client at all times. You assist the client on to the bed and remain with them at all times. After the examination is complete, you assist the client to change back into his or her clothes and return to their room. You return to the examination room, discard disposable items, restock trolleys or cupboards and clean all equipment as per organisation policy. Follow Standard Precautions at all times when handling equipment and soiled linen.

BLOOD GLUCOSE MEASUREMENTS

People with diabetes need to constantly monitor the level of glucose in their blood. Blood glucose monitoring allows both the healthcare professionals and the person to identify patterns of blood glucose changes. This helps in the planning of meals and activities and to ensure that medications and/or diet taken by the person are working effectively. It also helps to ensure that any complications of diabetes are minimised by early detection of abnormal blood glucose measurements.

Carers are often trained to undertake this testing, especially if they are supporting people in their homes or in the community in supported living units.

Blood glucose is measured in mmol/L. Normal **blood glucose levels** are between 4.0 and 6.0 mmol/L when fasting and can rise to 7.8 mmol/L 2 hours after eating.

ASSESSING BLOOD GLUCOSE MEASUREMENTS

Quality of life

Remember to respect the client's privacy while doing any procedure. Address the person by name and ensure they know your name.

Pre-procedure

1 Follow the delegation guidelines.
2 Wash your hands.
3 Collect the following:
   - blood glucose monitor
   - test strips
   - lancet
   - gauze
   - gloves.
4 Explain the procedure to the person.
5 Identify the person. Call them by name.
6 Ensure that the person's hands are cleaned prior to testing.

Procedure

7 Insert the test strip into the monitor and turn the monitor on.
8 Put on the gloves.
9 Remove safety cap from the lancet.
10 Prick the side of the tip of the person's finger.
11 Squeeze the person's finger gently to produce a droplet of blood.
12 Touch the tip of the test strip against the blood droplet.
13 Place gauze over the pricked site.
14 Note the reading from the blood glucose meter.
15 Dispose of the lancet.

Post-procedure

16 Wash your hands.
17 Report and record your observations.

QUALITY OF LIFE

Client care is given in a way that promotes dignity, self-esteem and physical, mental and social wellbeing. You must protect the person's right to privacy when assisting with an examination or measuring vital signs. Do not expose the person unnecessarily. Always keep their body covered.

Fears about who will perform an examination and how it will be done are common. So are fears about the need for the examination. Is the person dying? Will cancer be found? Will surgery be needed? Will more medications be needed? Will an illness be found? All these factors affect the person's dignity, self-esteem and wellbeing.

Remember, the person has the right to personal choice. The person also has the right to privacy and confidentiality. Always keep client information confidential. Vital signs and the results from a physical examination are just as private as other information. Share this information only with the nurse. Refer questions from family and visitors to the nurse.

The person needs to feel safe and secure. Protect the person from falls and other injuries. Also, keep the person covered. This provides warmth and protects the person from chills and draughts. The person must also feel covered and protected from exposure.

Safety and security affect mental wellbeing. Knowing the reasons for any examination or measuring of vital signs will help the person feel safe and secure.

Unless ordered otherwise, vital signs are measured with the person sitting or lying down. Let the person choose the position. The person may also prefer that you use the right or left arm for pulse and blood pressure. If safe to do so, use the arm the person prefers.

REVIEW QUESTIONS

Circle the BEST answer:

1 Which statement is false?
   a The vital signs are temperature, pulse, respirations and blood pressure
   b Vital signs detect changes in body function
   c Vital signs change only during illness
   d Sleep, exercise, medications, emotions and noise affect vital signs

2 Which gives the least accurate measurement of body temperature?
   a Oral site
   b Axillary site
   c Tympanic membrane site
   d Rectal site

3 Which of the following does not describe normal respirations?
   a There are 12–20 per minute
   b They are quiet and effortless
   c They are regular, with both sides of the chest rising and falling equally
   d Noises occur on inhalation

4 Which blood pressure is normal for an adult?
   a 88/54 mmHg
   b 210/100 mmHg
   c 120/78 mmHg
   d 152/116 mmHg

5 When taking blood pressure, what should you not do?
   a Take the blood pressure in the arm with an intravenous infusion
   b Apply the cuff to a bare upper arm
   c Turn off the television and radio
   d Locate the brachial artery

6 Which is the systolic blood pressure?
   a The point where the pulse is no longer felt
   b The point where the first sound is heard
   c The point where the last sound is heard
   d The point 30 mmHg above where the pulse was felt

7 The otoscope is used to examine:
   a The internal structures of the eye
   b The external ear and the eardrum
   c Reflexes
   d The vagina

8 Mrs Porter is having a physical examination. Which part of Mrs Porter's examination can you do?
   a Test her reflexes
   b Inspect her mouth, teeth and throat
   c Measure her height, weight and vital signs
   d Observe her perineum and rectum

Circle T if the statement is true or F is the statement is false:

9 T / F A pulse should not be taken using the thumb

10 T / F A sphygmomanometer is a device designed to measure blood pressure

11 T / F The nurse has asked carer A to take the observations of a person, yet the person has refused to allow the carer to perform the task. The observations must be done even without the consent of the client as it is a delegated task.

Answers to these questions are on p. 454.

Further reading

Chester JG (2011). Vital signs in older patients: Age-related changes, Journal of the American Medical Directors Association, 12(5):337–43.

Goldberg C (2021). A practical guide to clinical medicine. University of California, San Diego. Online 21 September 2021. Available: meded.ucsd.edu/clinicalmed/vital.htm

Medline Plus (2021). Blood pressure measurement. Online 8 March 2021. Available: www.nlm.nih.gov/medlineplus/ency/article/007490.htm

CHAPTER 12
Caring for the person

By Dianne Cheeseman

THIS CHAPTER HAS ESSENTIAL INFORMATION ON CARING FOR AN AGED CARE CLIENT. AS IT IS A FAIRLY LENGTHY CHAPTER, IT HAS BEEN DIVIDED INTO SECTIONS THAT EASILY IDENTIFY DIFFERING ASPECTS OF CARE. THESE INCLUDE ASSISTING WITH:

- hygiene needs
- grooming skin and nail care
- bowel evacuation and management
- urinary elimination and management
- wound care
- identifying and managing pain
- feeding and drinking
- exercise.

Key terms

abrasion: A partial-thickness wound caused by the scraping away or rubbing of the skin

acetone: Ketone body that appears in the urine from the rapid breakdown of fat for energy

acute pain: Pain that is felt suddenly from injury, disease, trauma or surgery; it lasts for less than 6 months

afternoon care: Care given after lunch or after the evening meal

alopecia: Hair loss

ambulation: The act of walking

anal incontinence: Faecal incontinence

anorexia: Loss of appetite

anticoagulant: A medication that prevents or slows (*anti*) blood clotting time (*coagulate*)

arterial ulcer: An open wound on the lower legs and feet caused by poor arterial blood flow

aspiration: Breathing fluid or an object into the lungs

atrophy: A decrease in size or a wasting away of tissue

bruise: A contusion

catheter: A tube used to drain or inject fluid through a body opening

catheterisation: Inserting a catheter

chronic pain: Pain lasting longer than 6 months; it may be constant or occur off and on

chronic wound: A wound that does not heal easily

circulatory ulcer: An open wound on the lower legs and feet caused by decreased blood flow through arteries or veins; vascular ulcer

clean wound: A wound that is not infected; microbes have not entered the wound

clean-contaminated wound: An infection following surgical entry of the urinary, reproductive, respiratory or gastrointestinal systems, which are not sterile

closed wound: A wound in which tissues are injured but the skin is not broken

colostomy: A surgically created opening (*stomy*) between the colon (*colo*) and the abdominal wall

comfort: A state of wellbeing; the person has no physical or emotional pain and is calm and at peace

constipation: The passage of a hard, dry stool

contaminated wound: A wound that has been contaminated by infection

contracture: The lack of joint mobility caused by abnormal shortening of a muscle

contusion: A closed wound caused by a blow to the body; bruise

dandruff: An excessive amount of dry, white flakes from the scalp

defecation: The process of excreting faeces from the rectum through the anus; a bowel movement

dehiscence: The separation of wound layers

dehydration: A decrease in the amount of water in body tissues

diarrhoea: The frequent passage of liquid stools

dirty wound: An infected wound

discomfort: A feeling of aching, hurting or soreness; pain

distraction: Something that changes a person's centre of attention

dysphagia: Difficulty (*dys*) swallowing (*phagia*)

dysuria: Painful or difficult (*dys*) urination (*uria*)

embolus: A blood clot that travels through the vascular system until it lodges in a distant vessel

enema: The introduction of fluid into the rectum and lower colon

enteral nutrition: Giving nutrients through the gastrointestinal tract (*enteral*)

enuresis: Urinary incontinence in bed at night

evening care: Care given in the evening at bedtime

evisceration: The separation of a wound along with the protrusion of abdominal organs

external rotation: When the legs and hips turn outwards

faecal impaction: The prolonged retention and build-up of faeces in the rectum

footdrop: The foot falls down at the ankle (permanent plantar flexion)

full-thickness wound: The dermis, epidermis and subcutaneous tissue are penetrated; muscle and bone may be involved

gangrene: A condition in which there is death of tissue

gastrostomy: A surgically created opening (*stomy*) in the stomach (*gastro*)

gavage: Tube feeding

glucosuria: Sugar (*glucose*) in the urine (*uria*); also called glycosuria

graduated jug/measuring container: A container used to measure fluids

guided imagery: Creating and focusing on an image

haematuria: Blood (*haem*) in the urine (*uria*)

hirsutism: Excessive body hair in women and children

incision: An open wound with clean, straight edges; usually intentionally produced with a sharp instrument

infected wound: A wound containing large amounts of bacteria and showing signs of infection; a dirty wound

infection: When a microorganism, such as a bacterium or a virus, invades a part of the body where it is not usually present; it may be localised in a wound or spread throughout the body in the blood

intentional wound: A wound created for therapy

jejunostomy: An opening (*stomy*) into the middle part of the small intestine (*jejunum*)

ketone bodies: Acetone

kilojoule: A measure of the amount of energy produced when the body burns food

laceration: An open wound with torn tissues and jagged edges

micturition: The process of emptying urine from the bladder; urination or voiding

morning care: Care given before or after breakfast

muscle atrophy: Loss of muscle strength from inactivity

nasogastric (NG) tube: A tube inserted through the nose (*naso*) into the stomach (*gastro*)

nocturia: Frequent urination (*uria*) at night (*noct*)

nutrient: A substance that is ingested, digested, absorbed and used by the body

nutrition: The many processes involved in the ingestion, digestion, absorption and use of foods and fluids by the body

oedema: Swelling caused by fluid collecting in tissues

oliguria: Scant amount (*olig*) of urine (*uria*); usually less than 500 mL in 24 hours

open wound: The skin or mucous membrane is broken

oral hygiene: Mouth care

orthostatic hypotension: A drop in (*hypo*) blood pressure when the person stands (*ortho* and *static*); postural hypotension

pain: A feeling of aching, hurting or being sore

partial-thickness wound: A wound in which the dermis and epidermis of the skin are broken

pediculosis: Lice infestation

penetrating wound: An open wound in which the skin and underlying tissues are pierced

percutaneous endoscopic gastrostomy (PEG) tube: A tube inserted into the stomach (*gastro*) through a stab or puncture wound (*stomy*) made through (*per*) the skin (*cutaneous*); a lighted instrument (*scope*) allows the doctor to see inside a body cavity or organ (*endo*)

perineal care: Cleaning the genital and anal areas

phantom pain: Pain felt in a body part that is no longer there

phlebitis: Inflammation (*itis*) of a vein (*phleb*)
plantar flexion: Bending the foot
plaque: A thin film that sticks to the teeth; it contains saliva, microbes and other substances
polyuria: Abnormally large amounts (*poly*) of urine (*uria*)
postural hypotension: Orthostatic hypotension
pressure injury: Any injury caused by unrelieved pressure; may also be called a decubitus ulcer, bedsore or pressure sore
pressure ulcer: A wound that occurs because of poor skin care and immobility
puncture wound: An open wound made by a sharp object; entry of the skin and underlying tissues may be intentional or unintentional
purulent drainage: Thick green, yellow or brown drainage
radiating pain: Pain felt at the site of tissue damage and in nearby areas
range of motion (ROM): The movement of a joint to the extent possible without causing pain
regurgitation: The backward flow of food from the stomach into the mouth
relaxation: To be free from mental or physical stress
rest: A state of calmness, ease and relaxation, free from anxiety and stress
sanguineous drainage: Bloody (*sanguis*) drainage
serous drainage: Clear, watery fluid (serum)
serosanguineous drainage: Thin, watery drainage (*sero*) that is blood-tinged (*sanguineous*)
skin tear: A break or rip in the skin; the epidermis separates from the underlying tissue
sleep: A state of unconsciousness, reduced voluntary muscle activity and lowered metabolism
stasis ulcer: An open wound on the lower legs and feet caused by poor blood return through the veins; venous ulcer
syncope: A brief loss of consciousness; fainting
tartar: Hardened plaque
thrombus: A blood clot
trauma: An accident or violent act that injures the skin, mucous membranes, bones and internal organs
unintentional wound: A wound resulting from trauma
urinary frequency: Voiding at frequent intervals
urinary incontinence: The inability to control the loss of urine from the bladder; loss of bladder control
urinary urgency: The need to void immediately
urination: The process of emptying urine from the bladder; micturition or voiding
vascular ulcer: A circulatory ulcer
venous ulcer: A stasis ulcer
voiding: Urination or micturition
wound: A break in the skin or mucous membrane

Prior to commencing this chapter it is advisable to read and understand Chapter 2 of this book. It is also advisable to access and read current work, health and safety (WHS) information sheets on COVID-19 (swa.gov.au/coronavirus (Australia) and www.health.govt.nz/our-work/diseases-and-conditions/covid-19-novel-coronavirus (NZ)).

ASSISTING WITH HYGIENE

After reading this section, you should be able to:

- explain the importance of cleanliness and skin care
- describe the routine care given in the morning, afternoon and evening
- describe the importance of oral hygiene and the observations to report
- describe the rules for bathing and the observations to make
- identify the safety precautions for a person taking a bath or a shower
- explain the purposes of a back massage
- identify the purposes of perineal care
- perform the procedures described in this section.

Personal hygiene promotes comfort, safety and health. The skin is the body's first line of defence against disease. Intact skin prevents microbes from entering the body and causing an infection. Likewise, mucous membranes of the mouth, genital area and anus must be kept clean and intact. Besides cleansing, good hygiene prevents body and breath odours. It also promotes relaxation and increases circulation.

Culture and personal choice affect people's hygiene practices. Some people take showers while others prefer to have baths. Some bathe at bedtime; others bathe in the morning. Bathing frequency also varies from person to person, with some people bathing once or twice a week and others once or twice a day. Some people cannot afford soap, deodorant, shampoo, toothpaste or other hygiene products.

Many factors affect personal hygiene needs: perspiration, urinary and bowel continence, vomiting, drainage from wounds or body openings, bed rest and activity. Illness and ageing can affect self-care abilities. Some people need help with hygiene. The direct care worker, in conjunction with the nurse, uses the nursing process (assess; plan; implement; evaluate) to decide how to meet the person's hygiene needs. The care plan describes the person's individual hygiene needs and how this care should be provided.

Some people may resist your efforts to assist with hygiene. Common reasons include illness, disability, dementia or personal choice. The care plan explains how to work with each person to maximise their independence and choice. Always seek support and guidance from consumer or community care agency supervisors when a person displays unusual or altered behaviours.

CARING ABOUT CULTURE

Hygiene needs may vary from one culture to another. Personal hygiene is very important to East Indian Hindus. Their religion requires at least one bath a day. Some Hindus believe that bathing after a meal causes injury. It is also believed that eye injuries can occur from a bath that is too hot. When preparing a bath, hot water can be added to cold water. Cold water is not added to hot water. After bathing, carefully rub or pat the body dry with a towel. Consider the religious and cultural requirements of your clients and modify their care in consultation with the client, their family and the care team.

Adapted from: JN Giger & RE Davidhizar (2016). Transcultural nursing: assessment and intervention, 7th edn, Mosby, St Louis.

DAILY CARE

Most people have hygiene routines and habits. For example, teeth are brushed and the face and hands are washed on awakening. These and other hygiene measures are often done before and after meals and at bedtime.

A person with a disability or an illness, or a person who is frail, may need help with hygiene. Holistic care recognises the person's hygiene preferences and maximises their independence. Although routine care is given during the day and evening, you are required to provide assistance with personal hygiene whenever it is needed. You must protect the person's right to privacy, dignity and personal choice.

Morning care

Routine **morning care** focuses on assisting the person to get ready for breakfast and to attend to their personal hygiene, grooming and dressing needs. Morning care can occur before or after breakfast, depending on the person's preferences and care setting.

Morning care includes:

- assisting the person to the toilet or offering a commode, bedpan or urinal
- assisting the incontinent person and changing any damp or soiled pads or bed linen
- assisting with hygiene – face and handwashing, oral hygiene, bathing, back massage and perineal care

- assisting with grooming – hair care, shaving and dressing
- positioning the person for breakfast, morning tea and lunch in the dining room, bedside chair or in bed
- straightening the person's room or unit.

Afternoon care

Routine hygiene is done after lunch and after the evening meal. Many people like to attend to their hygiene needs before taking a nap, having visitors or attending activity programs or social gatherings.

Afternoon care involves:

- assisting the person to the toilet or offering a commode, bedpan or urinal
- assisting with hygiene – face and handwashing, oral hygiene, brushing or combing hair and perineal care
- helping the person into pyjamas, dressing gown or clothes
- assisting the person with lying down and getting up from a nap
- changing any damp or soiled bed linen/pads
- assisting with activity – range-of-motion (ROM) exercises and ambulation
- straightening the person's room or unit
- positioning the person for dinner in the dining room, bedside chair or in bed.

Evening care

Evening care is care given in the evening at bedtime. It is designed to be relaxing and to promote rest and sleep.

Measures performed just before the person is ready for sleep include:

- assisting the person to the toilet or offering a commode, bedpan or urinal
- attending to the incontinent person, changing any damp or soiled bed linen/pads and turning down the bed
- assisting with hygiene – face and handwashing, oral hygiene, brushing or combing hair, bathing, back massage and perineal care
- helping the person to undress and change into night attire
- assisting the person into bed if required
- giving a back and/or hand massage
- straightening the person's room or unit.

ORAL HYGIENE

Oral hygiene (mouth care) keeps the mouth and teeth clean, and reduces mouth odours and the risk of oral infections, cavities (dental caries) and periodontal disease (gum disease, pyorrhoea). It also increases comfort and makes food taste better. For mouth care use a soft toothbrush with a small pea-sized amount of high fluoride toothpaste (SA Dental Association 2009). These toothbrushes should be changed every 4 months, with some services using different coloured toothbrushes to indicate the season and to make it obvious when the toothbrush needs changing.

Periodontal disease is an inflammation of the tissues around the teeth. Poor oral hygiene allows the build-up of plaque and tartar. **Plaque** is a thin film that sticks to teeth. It contains saliva, microbes and other substances. Plaque leads to tooth decay (cavities). When plaque hardens it is called tartar. **Tartar** builds up at the gum line near the neck of the tooth. Tartar build-up leads to periodontal disease. The gums become red and swollen, and bleed easily. As the disease progresses, bone is destroyed and the teeth loosen. Tooth loss is common.

Illness, disease and some medications often cause a bad taste in the mouth. Sometimes they cause a whitish coating on the mouth and tongue. Others cause redness and swelling of the mouth and tongue. A dry mouth is common from oxygen, some medications, smoking, decreased fluid intake and anxiety.

The nurse, speech pathologist and/or dietitian may assess the need for mouth care. Oral hygiene is given on awakening, after meals, after administering certain medications and at bedtime. Many people also practise oral hygiene before meals. Some people need mouth care at least every 2 hours. Always follow the person's care plan.

SAFETY ALERT

Oral hygiene

Follow Standard Precautions when giving oral hygiene. You have contact with the person's mucous membranes. Gums may bleed during oral care. In addition, the mouth contains many microbes. Pathogens spread through sexual contact may be in the mouths of some people.

Equipment

A toothbrush, toothpaste, dental floss and mouthwash are needed. The toothbrush should have soft, flat bristles. People with dentures need a denture cleaner, denture cup and denture brush or toothbrush. Use only those products recommended for cleaning dentures. Otherwise you could damage the dentures. Some people prefer to use an electric or battery-operated toothbrush. Pressure-sensitive models and handle adaptations are available to assist people with disabilities.

Sponge or cotton swabs are used for people with sore, tender mouths. They are also used for unconscious people. Use swabs with care. Always check the foam or cotton pad to make sure it is tight on the stick. The person could choke on the pad if it comes off the stick.

You also need a kidney basin or receiving bowl, a glass of water, straw, tissues, towels and gloves.

When assisting with oral hygiene, you need to observe, report and record if a person has:

- dry, cracked, swollen or blistered lips
- mouth or breath odour
- loose teeth
- redness, swelling, irritation, sores or white patches in the mouth or on the tongue

- bleeding, swelling or redness of the gums
- rough, sharp or chipped areas on dentures.

Brushing teeth

Many people perform oral hygiene themselves. Others need help gathering and setting up equipment. You may have to brush the teeth of someone who is very frail or who cannot use or move their arms. Some people are too weak or confused to brush their teeth. Promote independence by prompting and providing encouragement to people as needed.

Flossing

Flossing assists in the removal of plaque and tartar from the teeth. These substances cause serious gum disease that leads to tooth loss. Flossing also removes food from between the teeth. It is usually done after brushing but can be done at other times. Some people floss after meals. If done once a day, bedtime is the best time to floss.

You need to floss for people who cannot tend to oral hygiene. Some older people do not floss their teeth. Follow the person's care plan.

ASSISTING A PERSON TO BRUSH THEIR TEETH

Quality of life

Remember to respect the person's privacy while doing any procedure. Address the person by name and ensure they know your name.

Pre-procedure

1 Explain the procedure to the person before starting and ensure that you verbalise each step as it is carried out during the procedure.
2 Wash your hands.
3 Collect the following:
   - toothbrush
   - toothpaste
   - mouthwash (or solution noted on the care plan) and lip lubricant (if used)
   - dental floss
   - water glass filled with cool water
   - straw
   - kidney basin or receiving bowl
   - face towel
   - paper towels.
4 Place the paper towels on the over-bed table. Arrange items on top of them.
5 Call the person by name and introduce yourself.
6 Provide for privacy.
7 Position the person so they can brush with ease.

Procedure

8 Place the towel over the person's chest. This protects garments and linens from spills.
9 Position the over-bed table in front of the person. Adjust table height.
10 Assist the person to perform oral hygiene. This includes brushing the teeth, rinsing the mouth, flossing, using mouthwash or other solution and applying lip lubricant. (Gloves will be needed.)
11 Remove the towel when the person has finished.
12 Reposition and adjust the height of the over-bed table.

Post-procedure

13 Provide for comfort.
14 Place the call bell within reach.
15 Clean and return items to their proper place. Wear gloves for this step.
16 Wipe off the over-bed table with the paper towels and discard them.
17 Remove any screens from around the person.
18 Follow agency policy for dirty linen or place in client's laundry basket.
19 Wash your hands.
20 Report and record your observations.

BRUSHING THE PERSON'S TEETH

Quality of life

Remember to respect the person's privacy while doing any procedure. Address the person by name and ensure they know your name.

Pre-procedure

1 Explain the procedure to the person before starting and ensure that you verbalise each step as it is carried out during the procedure.
2 Wash your hands.
3 Collect gloves and items listed in 'Assisting a person to brush their teeth'.
4 Place the paper towels on the over-bed table. Arrange items on top of them.
5 Identify the person. Call the person by name and introduce yourself.
6 Provide for privacy.
7 Raise the bed to a height that facilitates good body mechanics or assist the person into a chair.

Procedure

8 Lower the bed rail nearest you (if applicable).
9 Raise the head of the bed so the person can sit comfortably. Position the person on their side, facing you, if they cannot sit up.
10 Place the towel over the person's chest. This protects garments and linens from spills.

11 Position and adjust the height of the over-bed table so you can reach it with ease.
12 Put on the gloves.
13 Apply a pea-sized amount of toothpaste to the toothbrush.
14 Hold the toothbrush over the kidney basin. Pour some water over the brush.
15 Brush the person's teeth gently.
16 Let the person rinse their mouth with water. Hold the kidney basin under the person's chin. Repeat this step as needed.
17 Brush the person's tongue gently (Fig. 12.1), if needed, then rinse.
18 Floss the person's teeth.
19 Assist the person to use mouthwash or other solution. Hold the kidney basin under their chin (Fig. 12.2). Apply lip balm, if used.
20 Remove the towel when done.
21 Remove and discard the gloves and wash your hands.

Post-procedure

22 Provide for comfort.
23 Place the call bell within reach (if applicable)
24 Lower the bed to its lowest position (if applicable).
25 Clean and return equipment to its proper place. Wear gloves for this step.
26 Wipe off the over-bed table with the paper towels and discard them.
27 Reposition and adjust the height of the over-bed table.
28 Remove the screens from around the person.
29 Follow agency policy for dirty linen or place in client's laundry basket.
30 Wash your hands.
31 Report any observations of concern to the nurse on duty.

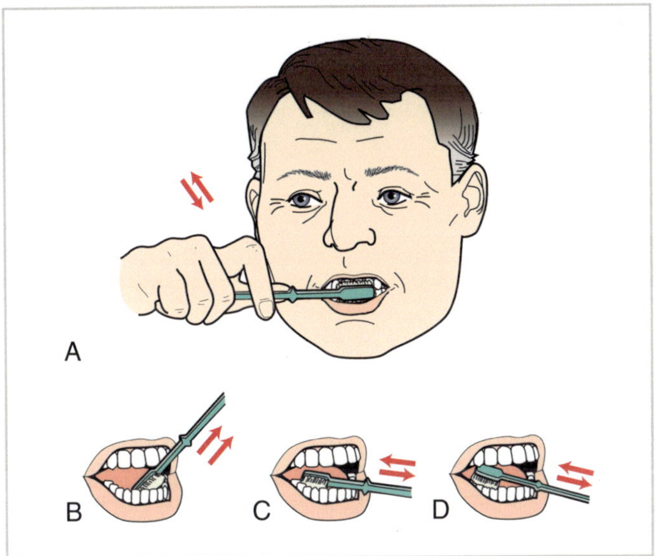

Fig. 12.1
Brushing teeth.
A. Position the brush at a 45-degree angle to the gums. Brush with short strokes. **B.** Position the brush at a 45-degree angle against the inside of the front teeth. Brush from the gum to the crown of the tooth with short strokes. **C.** Hold the brush horizontally against the inner surfaces of the teeth. Brush back and forth. **D.** Position the brush on the biting surfaces of the teeth. Brush back and forth.

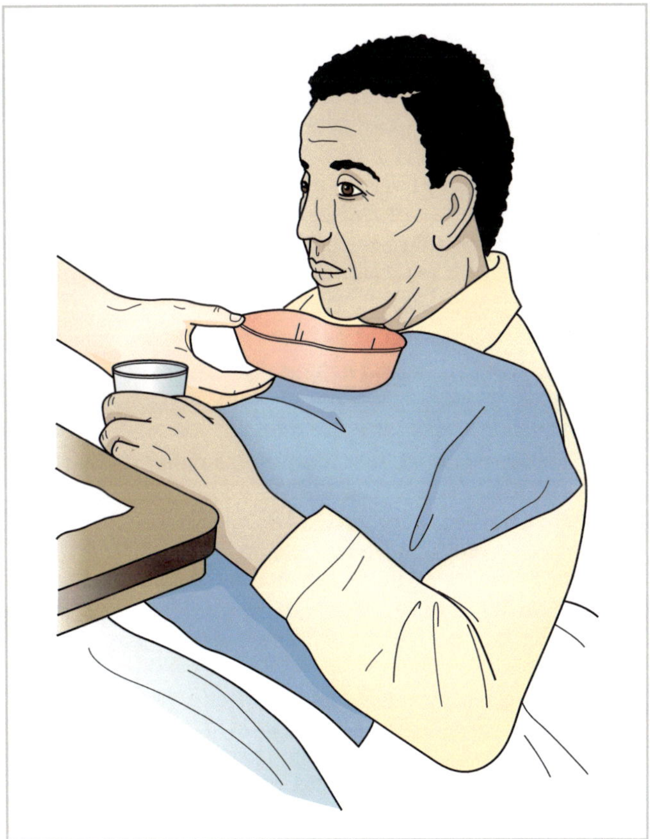

Fig. 12.2
The kidney basin is held under the person's chin.

FLOSSING A PERSON'S TEETH

Quality of life

Remember to respect the person's privacy while doing any procedure. Address the person by name and ensure they know your name.

Pre-procedure

1. Explain to the person what you are going to do.
2. Wash your hands.
3. Collect the following:
   - kidney basin or receiving bowl
   - water glass with cool water
   - dental floss
   - face towel
   - paper towels
   - gloves.
4. Place the paper towels on the over-bed table. Arrange items on top of them.
5. Call the person by name and introduce yourself.
6. Provide for privacy.
7. Raise the bed to a height that facilitates good body mechanics, or assist the person into a chair.

Procedure

8. Lower the bed rail nearest you (if applicable).
9. Raise the head of the bed so the person can sit comfortably (if applicable). Position the person on their side, facing you, if they cannot sit up.
10. Place the towel over the person's chest. This protects garments and linen from spills.
11. Position and adjust the height of the over-bed table so you can reach it with ease.
12. Put on the gloves.
13. Break off a 50-cm piece of floss from the dispenser.
14. Hold the floss between the middle fingers of each hand (Fig. 12.3).
15. Stretch the floss with your thumbs.
16. Start at the upper back tooth on the right side. Work around to the left side.
17. Move the floss gently up and down between the person's teeth. Move the floss up and down from the top of the crown to the gum line and back along the other side.
18. Move to a new section of floss after every second tooth.
19. Floss the lower teeth. Hold the floss with your index fingers. Gently floss up and down from the top of the crown to the gum line and back along the other side. Start on the right side. Work around to the left side.
20. Let the person rinse out their mouth. Hold the kidney basin under their chin. Repeat rinsing as necessary.
21. Remove the towel when done.
22. Remove and discard the gloves and wash your hands.

Post-procedure

23. Follow steps 22 through 31 for 'Brushing the person's teeth'.

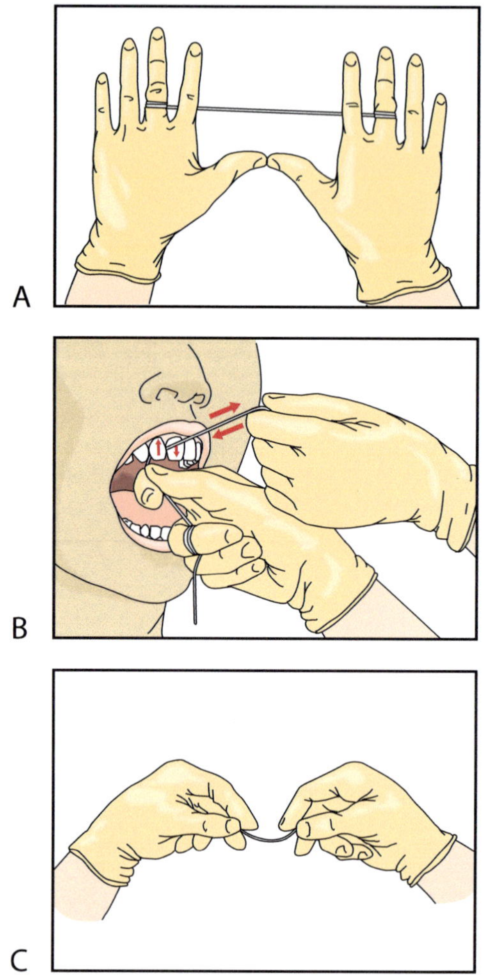

Fig. 12.3
Flossing.
A. Floss is held between the middle fingers to floss the upper teeth. **B.** Floss is moved in up-and-down motions between the teeth. Floss is moved up and down from the crown to the gum line. **C.** Floss is held with the index fingers to floss the lower teeth.

Mouth care for the unconscious person

Unconscious people need special mouth care. They cannot eat or drink and they often breathe with their mouth open. Many receive oxygen, which causes mouth dryness and crusting on the tongue and mucous membranes. Oral hygiene helps keep the mouth clean and moist and helps to prevent infection.

The care plan tells you what cleaning agent to use. Use a sponge or cotton swabs to apply the cleaning agent. Apply a lubricant (check the care plan) to the lips to prevent cracking.

Unconscious people usually cannot swallow and rely on others to protect them from choking and aspiration. **Aspiration** means breathing fluid or an object into the lungs. It can cause pneumonia and death. To prevent aspiration, position the person on one side with the head turned well

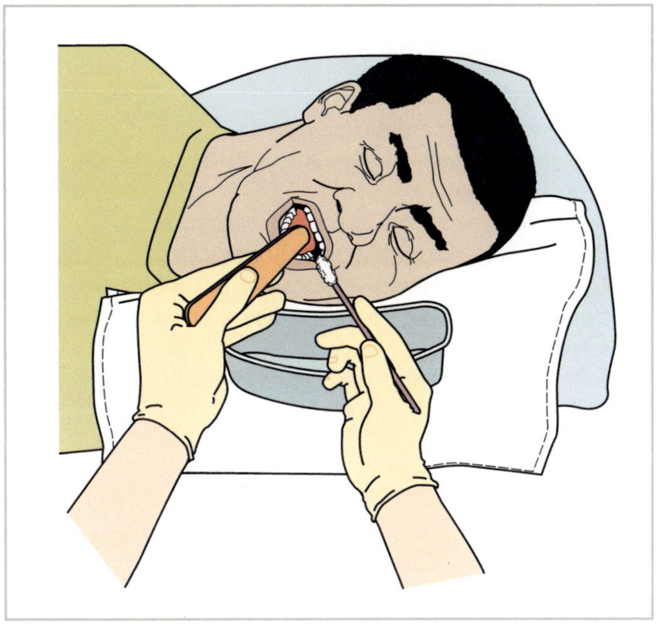

Fig. 12.4
The head of the unconscious person is turned well to the side to prevent aspiration. A padded tongue blade is used to keep the mouth open while cleaning the mouth with swabs.

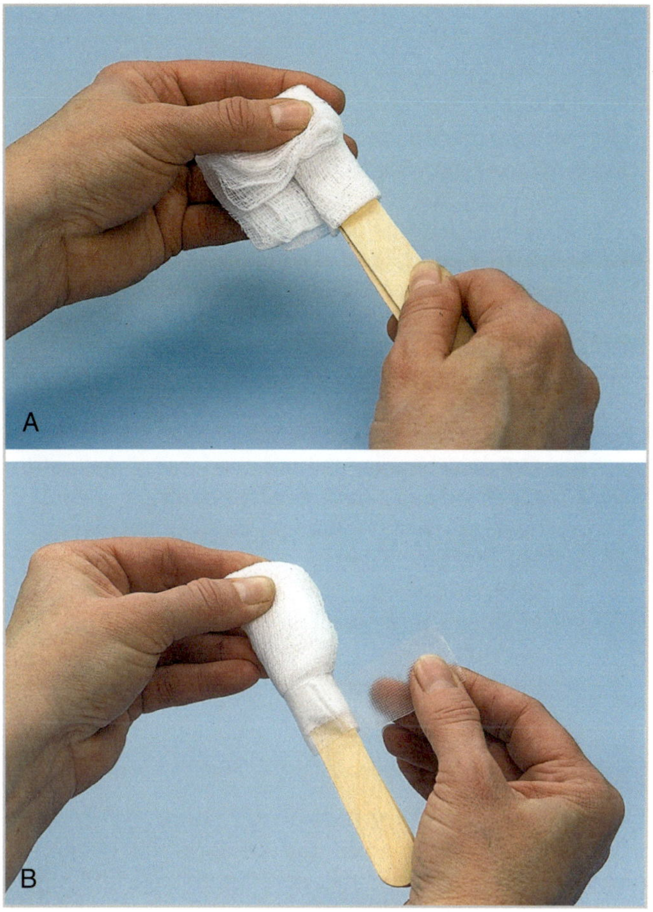

Fig. 12.5
Padded tongue blade.
A. Place two wooden tongue blades together and wrap gauze around the top half. **B.** Tape the gauze in place.

to the side (Fig. 12.4). In this position, excess fluid runs out of the mouth.

When attending to oral hygiene:

- use only a small amount of fluid; sometimes oral suctioning is needed
- keep the person's mouth open with a padded tongue blade (Fig. 12.5). Do not use your fingers to hold the mouth open, as the person may bite down on them. A bite could break your skin and create a portal of entry for microbes. All bites pose a risk of infection. Report and record any bite and seek medical advice promptly.

Unconscious people cannot speak or respond to what is happening. However, some can hear. Always assume that the unconscious person can hear. Explain what you are doing at each step. Also, tell the person when you have finished and when you are leaving the room.

Mouth care is given at least every 2 hours. Follow the care plan. Unconscious people are also repositioned at least every 2 hours. Combining mouth care, skin care and other comfort measures promotes comfort and safety.

PROVIDING MOUTH CARE FOR AN UNCONSCIOUS PERSON

Quality of life

Remember to respect the person's privacy while doing any procedure. Address the person by name and ensure you introduce yourself.

Pre-procedure

1 Wash your hands.
2 Collect the following:
   - cleaning agent (check the care plan)
   - sponge or cotton swabs
   - padded tongue blade (see Fig. 12.5)
   - water glass filled with cool water
   - face towel
   - kidney basin
   - lip lubricant
   - paper towels
   - gloves.
3 Place the paper towels on a stable surface near the client. Arrange items on top of them.
4 Call the person by name and introduce yourself.
5 Explain the procedure to the person before starting and ensure that you verbalise each step as it is carried out during the procedure.
6 Provide for privacy.
7 Raise the bed to a height that facilitates good body mechanics, or assist the person into a chair.

Procedure

8 Put on the gloves.
9 Position the person on their side, facing you.
10 Place the towel under the person's face.
11 Place the kidney basin under their chin.
12 Position and adjust the height of the over-bed table so you can reach it with ease.
13 Separate the upper and lower teeth. Use the padded tongue blade. Be gentle. Never use force. If you have problems, ask the nurse or your supervisor for help.
14 Clean the mouth with swabs moistened with the cleaning agent. Use as many swabs as necessary. Using the swab with a gentle, rotating motion will facilitate full use of the whole swab surface.
   a Clean the chewing and inner surfaces of the teeth.
   b Clean the outer surfaces of the teeth.
   c Swab the roof of the mouth, inside of the cheeks and the lips.
   d Swab the tongue.
   e Moisten a clean swab with water. Swab the mouth to rinse.
15 Place used swabs in the kidney basin.
16 Apply lubricant to the lips.
17 Remove the towel.
18 Remove and discard the gloves.
19 Explain that the procedure is done and that you will reposition them.
20 Reposition the person and provide for comfort.
21 Place the call bell within reach (if applicable).
22 Lower the bed to its lowest position (if applicable).
23 Clean and return equipment to its proper place. Discard disposable items.
24 Remove any screens from around the person.
25 Tell the person that you are leaving.
26 Follow agency policy for dirty linen or place in the client's laundry basket.
27 Wash your hands.
28 Report any observations of concern to the nurse on duty.

Denture care

Dentures are cleaned for people who cannot do so themselves. Mouth care is given and dentures are cleaned as often as for natural teeth. Remember to take care when handling dentures, as they are costly and can easily break or chip if dropped onto a hard surface (e.g. floor, sink). Dentures are very slippery when wet, so hold them firmly. During cleaning, hold them over a basin of water lined with a small hand or face towel. This should prevent the dentures from breaking if accidentally dropped.

Most denture-makers recommend the use of specific denture-cleaning agents and do not recommend the use of normal toothpaste. All denture-specific cleaning agents have manufacturer's instructions. These explain how to use the cleaning agent and what water temperature to use. Do not use hot water to clean or store dentures, as hot water will cause them to warp. If they are not to be worn, store dentures in a container of cool water. Dentures left to dry out will warp and crack.

Dentures are usually removed at bedtime. Some people do not wear their dentures. Others wear them to eat and remove them after meals. Remind these people not to wrap dentures in tissues or napkins, as they may be accidentally discarded.

Many people clean their own dentures. They may need help getting to the bathroom or collecting any cleaning items. Many people do not like being seen without their dentures. Privacy is very important when cleaning dentures. For people who clean their own dentures, allow them privacy. If you clean dentures, return them to the person as quickly as possible.

SAFETY ALERT

Caring for dentures

Dentures are the person's property. They are costly. Handle them very carefully. Also, make sure that the denture cup is labelled with the person's name and, if in a care facility, their room number. Report lost or damaged dentures to the nurse or agency supervisor at once.

PROVIDING DENTURE CARE

Quality of life

Remember to respect the person's privacy while doing any procedure. Address the person by name and ensure they know your name.

Pre-procedure

1 Explain the procedure to the person before starting, and ensure that you verbalise each step as it is carried out during the procedure.
2 Wash your hands.
3 Collect the following:
   - denture brush or toothbrush (hard bristles)
   - denture cup labelled with the person's name
   - denture-cleaning agent
   - water glass with cool water
   - straw
   - mouthwash (or other specified solution: follow the care plan)

- basin
- two face towels
- gauze squares
- gloves.

4 Call the person by name and introduce yourself.
5 Provide for privacy.

Procedure

6 Place a towel over the person's chest. This protects garments and linens from spills.
7 Put on the gloves.
8 Ask the person to remove their dentures. Carefully place them in a basin.
9 Remove the dentures if the person cannot do so. Use gauze squares to get a good grip on the slippery dentures.
 a Grasp the upper denture with your thumb and index finger (Fig. 12.6). Move it up and down slightly to break the seal. Gently remove the denture. Place it in the kidney basin.
 b Grasp and remove the lower denture with your thumb and index finger. Turn it slightly and lift it out of the mouth. Place it in the kidney basin.
10 Take the basin, denture cup, brush and cleaning agent to the sink.
11 Line the sink with a towel. Half-fill the sink with cool water.
12 Rinse each denture under warm running water. Return them to the denture cup.
13 Apply the cleaning agent to brush.
14 Brush the dentures (Fig. 12.7).
15 Rinse dentures under cool running water.
16 Place them in the denture cup. Cover the dentures with cool water.
17 Clean the basin.
18 Take the denture cup and kidney basin to the bedside table.
19 Position the person for oral hygiene.
20 Have the person use mouthwash (or noted solution). Hold the basin under the chin.
21 Ask the person to insert the dentures. Insert them if the person cannot.
 a Hold the upper denture firmly with your thumb and index finger. Raise the upper lip with the other hand. Insert the denture. Gently press on the denture with your index fingers to make sure it is in place.
 b Hold the lower denture securely with your thumb and index finger. Pull the lower lip down slightly. Insert the denture. Gently press down on it to make sure it is in place.

Post-procedure

22 Place the denture cup in the top drawer of the bedside stand if the dentures are not worn.
23 Remove the towel.
24 Remove the gloves. Wash your hands.
25 Provide for comfort.
26 Place the call bell within reach (if applicable).
27 Remove the screens from around the person.
28 Clean and return equipment to its proper place. Discard disposable items.
29 Follow agency policy for dirty linen or place in client's laundry basket.
30 Wash your hands.
31 Report any observations of concern to the nurse on duty.
32 Some people like to soak their dentures overnight. (Please follow manufacturer's instructions if using denture-cleaning products.)

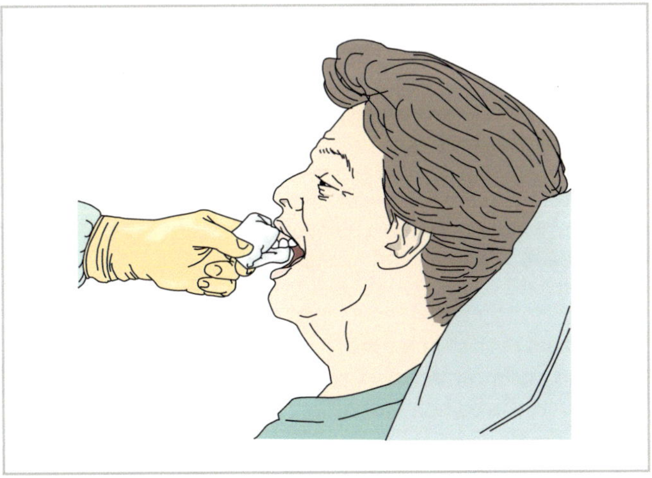

Fig. 12.6
Remove the upper denture. Grasp it with the thumb and index finger of one hand. Use a piece of gauze to grasp the slippery denture. Use upward strokes.

BATHING

Bathing cleans the skin and the mucous membranes of the genital and anal areas. Microbes, dead skin, perspiration and excess oils are removed. A bath is refreshing and relaxing. Circulation is stimulated and body parts are exercised. Observations and assessments are made, and you have time to talk to the person.

Bathing may involve a complete or partial bed bath, a bath or a shower, with or without the use of a shower chair. The method depends on the person's condition, self-care abilities and personal choice. In aged care services, bathing usually takes place in the morning, before or after breakfast. The person's choice of bath time is respected whenever possible. See Box 12.1 for the rules of bathing and Box 12.2 on bathing clients with dementia.

Bathing frequency is a personal matter. Some people bathe daily, while others take a complete bath only once or twice a week. Personal choice, weather, physical activity and illness affect bathing frequency. Illness usually increases the need for bathing because of fever and increased perspiration.

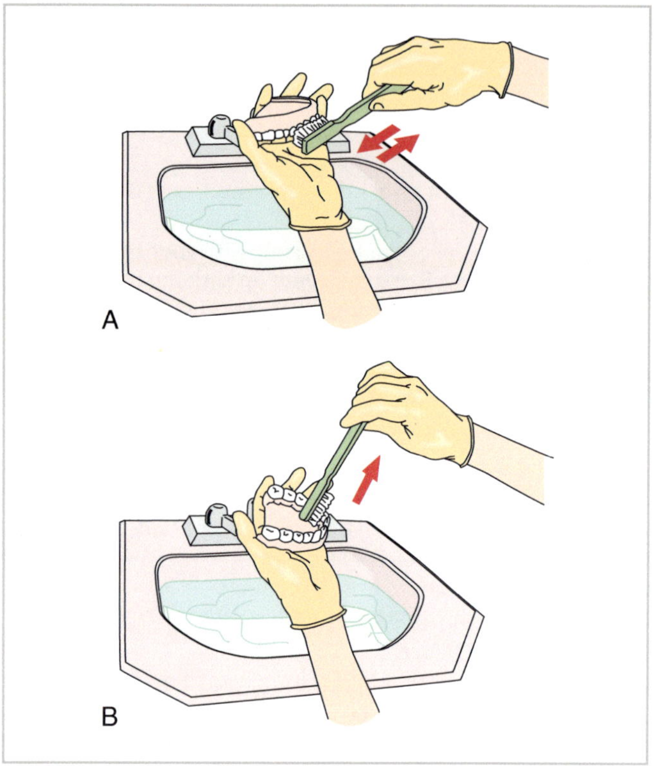

Fig. 12.7
Cleaning dentures. **A.** Brush the outer surface of the upper denture with back-and-forth motions. Note that the denture is held over the sink, which is filled halfway with water and lined with a towel. **B.** Position the brush vertically to clean the inner surfaces of the denture.

Dry skin is easily damaged. Dry skin occurs with ageing and the use of some soap products, so liquid soap-free products are used. Therefore, older people usually need a complete bath or shower twice a week. Partial baths are taken on the other days. Others use products that contain additional moisturisers or are marketed as being hypoallergenic. Thorough rinsing is needed when using all soap or soap-like products. Additional lotions and oils help keep the skin soft and are often used during and after bathing. Follow the care plan.

SAFETY ALERT

Bathing

Hot water can burn delicate and fragile skin. To protect the person from burns, measure the water temperature according to agency policy. If you are unsure whether the water is too hot, ask the nurse or supervisor to check it.

When giving bed baths, protect the person from falls. Also protect the person and yourself from the spread of infection. When giving baths, contact with blood, body fluids, secretions and excretions is likely. Follow Standard Precautions and additional precautions.

BOX 12.1
Rules for bathing

- Follow the care plan for bathing method and skin care products. Allow personal choice whenever possible.
- Follow Standard Precautions. Wear gloves whenever contact with blood, body fluids, secretions or excretions is likely.
- Collect necessary items before starting the procedure.
- Provide for privacy. Screen the person. Close doors, shades or drapes.
- Cover the person for warmth and privacy.
- Reduce draughts by closing doors and windows.
- Protect the person from falling.
- Use good body mechanics at all times.
- Make sure the water temperature is not too hot, particularly for older people.
- Use liquid soap-free cleanser or a sorbolene-based product that has a balanced pH.
- Wash from the cleanest to the dirtiest areas.
- Encourage the person to help as much as is safely possible.
- Rinse the skin thoroughly to remove all cleanser.
- Pat the skin dry to avoid irritating or breaking the skin.
- Remember to dry thoroughly under the breasts, between skin folds, in the perineal area and between the toes.
- Bathe the skin whenever faecal material or urine is on the skin. This helps to prevent skin breakdown and odours.

BOX 12.2
Bathing clients with dementia

Bathing procedures can be threatening to people with dementia. They may not understand what is happening or why and may become fearful and resist care or become agitated and combative.

The care plan also includes measures to help the person through the bathing procedure. Such measures may include the following:

- Involve the person in pre-procedure activities by offering appropriate clothing and product choices. Make environmental changes that enhance the person's comfort and relaxation, such as warming the bath area, playing a favourite song, minimising interruptions and reducing loud noises.
- Do not rush the person.
- Use a calm, pleasant voice.
- Divert the person's attention.
- Be gentle.
- Calm the person by prompting and encouraging their participation.
- If the person continues to resist care, try the bath later.

Skin-care products

Some skin-care products clean the skin. Others protect the skin from drying or friction. The products used depend on personal choice, skin care needs and cost.

Soap-like products cleanse the skin. They remove dirt, dead skin, skin oil, some microbes and perspiration. However, they tend to dry and irritate skin. Dry skin is itchy, uncomfortable and easily injured. Skin needs to be rinsed well to remove all cleansers.

Bath oils keep the skin soft and prevent drying. Bath oils can be added directly to bath water, while some soaps contain bath oils. However, bath oils make showers and bathtubs slippery. Only add the manufacturer's recommended amount of bath oil to the water. Use safety measures to prevent falls. You will need to check the consumer aged care policies in relation to using oils in baths.

Creams and lotions protect the skin from the drying effect of air and evaporation. They do not feel greasy but leave an oily film on the skin. Scented lotions are often used for hand and back massage. Applying lotion to bony points helps prevent skin breakdown. Unless indicated otherwise, you can apply lotion to the hands, back, elbows, knees, buttocks and heels after the person has bathed.

Although powders absorb moisture and can minimise friction when two skin surfaces rub together, they are not used in most aged care services as they cause caking and crusts that irritate the skin.

Deodorants and antiperspirants are applied to the axillae (underarms). Deodorants mask and control body odours. Antiperspirants reduce perspiration. These products do not take the place of bathing. Do not apply them to irritated or broken skin.

SAFETY ALERT

Applying talcum powder

- Most services do not use talcum powder. Check agency guidelines.
- Do not apply talcum powder in designated bath areas, as it can make surfaces slippery and increase the risk of falls. Follow agency guidelines for the safe application of powder.
- Talcum powder is not used near people with respiratory diseases, as inhaling powder can irritate the air passages and lungs. Before applying talcum powder, check the person's care plan. To safely apply talcum powder:
  - do not shake or sprinkle it directly onto the person
  - sprinkle a small amount of powder onto your hands or a cloth
  - apply the powder in a thin, even layer
  - turn your face away from the person so you do not inhale the powder.

DELEGATION GUIDELINES

Bathing

When assisting a person to bathe, you need the following information from the care plan:

- what kind of bath to give: complete bed bath, partial bath, bath, shower, hot towel bath or bag bath
- how much help the person needs (one- or two-person assist), and whether a shower chair, a bathmat or other assistive device is required
- the person's activity or position limits
- what water temperature to use. Bath water cools rapidly, therefore water temperature for a complete bed bath is usually 43–46°C for adults. However, older people have fragile skin and may need lower water temperatures
- what skin care products to use
- what bathing and skin care products the person prefers
- what observations to report:
  - the colour of the skin, lips, nail beds and sclera (whites of the eyes)
  - the location and description of rashes
  - dry skin
  - bruises or torn skin areas
  - pale or reddened areas, particularly over bony parts
  - drainage or bleeding from wounds or body openings
  - swelling of the feet and legs
  - corns or calluses on the feet
  - skin temperature
  - complaints of pain or discomfort.

The complete bed bath

The complete bed bath involves washing the person's entire body in bed. Bed baths are usually needed by people who are unconscious, paralysed or weak from illness. You give complete bed baths to people who cannot bathe themselves. This procedure usually requires two personal carers, especially if the bed sheets need changing after the procedure, unless, of course, the consumer is able to turn themselves in bed on their own.

A bed bath is a new experience for some people. Some are embarrassed to have another person see their bodies and others fear exposure. Check the care plan to identify the person's ability to assist with the bath and any activity or position limits they may have. Explain to the person how a bed bath is given and how you will cover their body for privacy and warmth.

GIVING A COMPLETE BED BATH

Quality of life

Remember to respect the person's privacy while doing any procedure. Address the person by name and ensure they know your name.

Pre-procedure

1 Call the person by name and introduce yourself.
2 Explain the procedure to the person before starting and ensure that you verbalise each step as it is carried out during the procedure.
3 Offer the bedpan or urinal. Provide for privacy.
4 Wash your hands.
5 Collect clean linen for a closed bed. Place linen on a clean surface.
6 Collect the following:
   - washbasin
   - liquid soap-free cleanser
   - bath thermometer
   - orange stick or nail file
   - washcloth
   - two bath towels and two face towels
   - bath blanket
   - gown or pyjamas
   - items for oral hygiene
   - lotion or cream (check the care plan)
   - talcum powder (check care plan as not used for most clients)
   - deodorant or antiperspirant
   - brush and comb
   - other grooming items if requested
   - paper towels
   - gloves
   - clean pad if required
   - plastic bag for disposal of used pads.
7 Position and adjust the height of the over-bed table or side table, so that you can reach it with ease. Arrange items on the over-bed table.
8 Close doors and windows to prevent draughts.
9 Provide for privacy.
10 Raise the bed to a height that facilitates good body mechanics.

Procedure

11 Remove the call bell. Put on gloves.
12 Provide oral hygiene.
13 Cover the person with a bath blanket. Remove top linen.
14 Lower the head of the bed to a level appropriate for the person. Keep it as flat as possible. Let the person have at least one pillow.
15 Cover the over-bed table with paper towels.
16 Fill the washbasin two-thirds full of water. Water temperature is usually 43–46°C for adults. These higher temperatures are needed because the water cools rapidly. Measure the water temperature with a bath thermometer or test the bath water by dipping your elbow or inner wrist into the basin. It should feel comfortably warm, not hot.
17 Place the basin on the over-bed table or side table, on top of the paper towels.
18 Place a bath towel over the person's chest.
19 Make a mitt with the washcloth (Fig. 12.8). Use a mitt throughout the procedure.
20 Wash around the person's eyes with water (Fig. 12.9). Do not use soap or cleansers. Gently wipe from the inner aspect with a corner of the mitt. Clean the far eye first. Repeat this step for the near eye. Use a clean part of the washcloth.
21 Ask the person if you should use cleanser on the face.
22 Wash the person's face, ears and neck. Rinse and pat dry with the towel on the chest.
23 Help the person move to the side of the bed near you. If they are unable to assist, with the help of another personal carer gently roll the person to you with their assistance.
24 Remove the gown. Do not expose the person. (Not removing the gown until this time helps the person feel less exposed and more comfortable with the bath.)
25 Place a bath towel lengthwise under the person's far arm.
26 Support the arm with your palm under the person's elbow. Their forearm rests on your forearm.
27 Use one face cloth for washing and one for rinsing.
28 Wash the arm, shoulder and underarm (axilla) with long, firm strokes, then rinse and pat dry (Fig. 12.10).
29 Place the basin on the towel. Place the person's hand into the water (Fig. 12.11). Wash it well. Clean under the fingernails with an orange stick or nail file.
30 Have the person exercise the hand and fingers.
31 Remove the basin and dry the hand well. Cover the arm with the bath blanket.
32 Repeat steps 25 to 31 for the person's near arm.
33 Place a bath towel over the chest crosswise (Fig. 12.12). Hold the towel in place and pull the bath blanket from under the towel to the waist.
34 Lift the towel slightly and wash the chest. Do not expose the person. Rinse and pat dry, especially under breasts and other skin folds.
35 Move the towel lengthwise over the chest and abdomen (Fig. 12.13). Do not expose the person. Pull the bath blanket down to the pubic area.
36 Lift the towel slightly and wash the abdomen. Rinse and pat dry.
37 Pull the bath blanket up to the shoulders. Both arms are covered. Remove the towel.
38 Change the water if it is soapy or cool.
39 Uncover the far leg. Do not expose the genital area. Place a towel lengthwise under the foot and leg.
40 Bend the knee and support the leg with your arm. Wash it with long, firm strokes. Rinse and pat dry.
41 Place the basin on the towel near the foot.
42 Lift the leg slightly. Slide the basin under the foot.
43 Place the foot in the basin (Fig. 12.14).
   a Wash the foot. Carefully separate the toes. Rinse and pat dry.
   b Clean under toenails with an orange stick or nail file if necessary.

44 Remove the basin. Dry the leg and foot. Cover the leg with the bath blanket. Remove the towel.
45 Repeat steps 39–44 for the person's near leg.
46 Change the water. Do not leave the person unattended at any time.
47 Turn the person onto the side away from you. Keep them covered with the bath blanket.
48 Uncover the back and buttocks. Do not expose the person. Place a towel lengthwise on the bed along the back.
49 Wash the person's back. Work from the back of the neck to the lower end of the buttocks. Use long, firm, continuous strokes (Fig. 12.15). Wash the buttocks and anal area. Rinse and dry well. Place face towel into dirty linen container. Discard gloves.
50 Give a back massage. The person may want the back massage after the bath.
51 Turn the person onto their back.
52 Change the water for perineal care.
53 Let the person wash the genital area. Adjust the over-bed table or side table so they can reach the washbasin, cleanser and towels with ease. Place the call bell within reach. Ask the person to use the call bell when finished. Make sure the person understands what to do. Answer the call bell promptly. Put on gloves and provide perineal care if the person cannot do so and change the pad if the person is wearing one.
54 Give a back massage if you have not already done so.
55 Apply deodorant or antiperspirant as the person requests. Apply lotion or powder as the care plan or person requests.
56 Put a clean gown or pyjamas on the person.
57 Comb and brush the hair.
58 Attend to oral hygiene needs.
59 Make the bed, reposition the over-bed table or side table and place the call bell within the person's reach.

Post-procedure

60 Provide for comfort.
61 Lower the bed to its lowest position (if applicable).
62 Empty and clean the washbasin. Return it and other supplies to their proper place.
63 Wipe off the over-bed table with the paper towels and discard them, also discarding used pads appropriately.
64 Remove the screens from around the person.
65 Follow agency policy for dirty linen or place in the client's laundry basket.
65 Wash your hands.
67 Report any observations of concern to the nurse on duty.

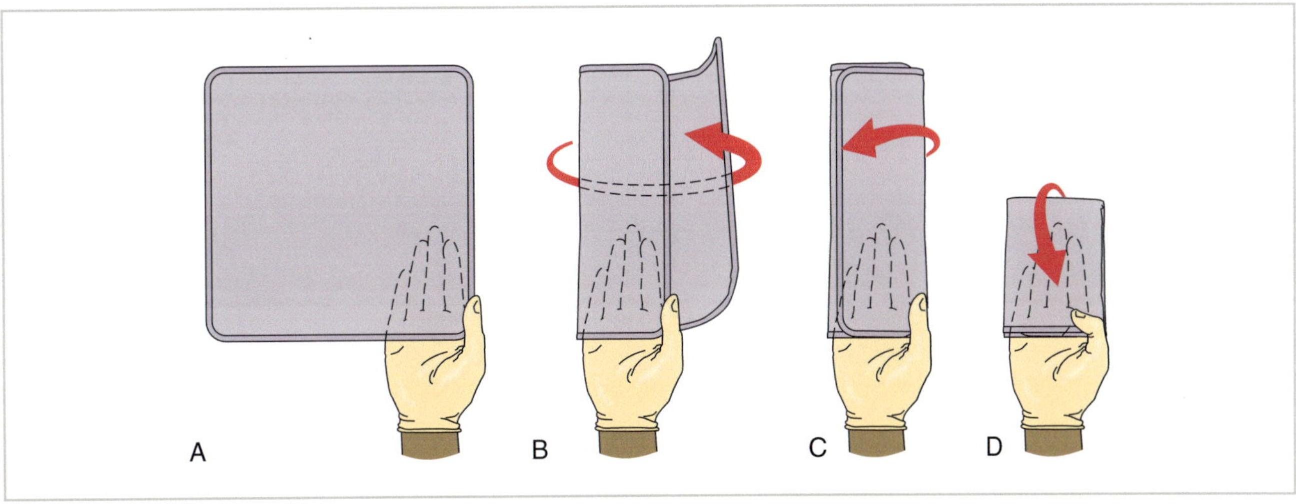

Fig. 12.8
Making a mitted washcloth.
A. Make a mitt with a washcloth by grasping the near side of the washcloth with your thumb. **B.** Bring the washcloth around and behind your hand. **C.** Fold the side of the washcloth over your palm as you grasp it with your thumb. **D.** Fold the top of the washcloth down. Tuck it under next to your palm.

Hot towel baths

Like bed baths, hot towel baths are given to people who cannot bathe themselves. Hot towel baths are well tolerated by people who are immobile, in pain, frail or weak or have limited movement. Hot towel baths are relaxing and soothing. They are often used for people who are on bed rest and for those who are receiving palliative care. People with dementia often respond well to this type of bath.

There are a number of ways to prepare a hot towel bath. The linen pack may contain up to three bath towels and

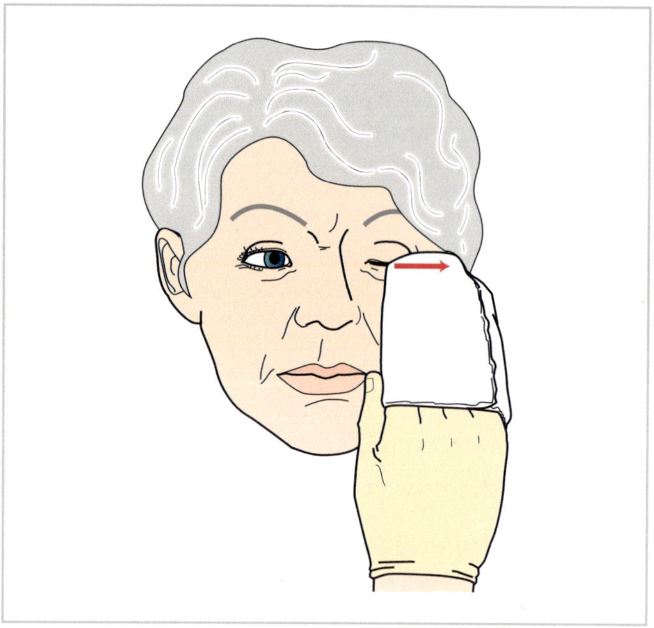

Fig. 12.9
Wash around the person's eyes with a mitted washcloth. Wipe from the inner to the outer aspect of the eye.

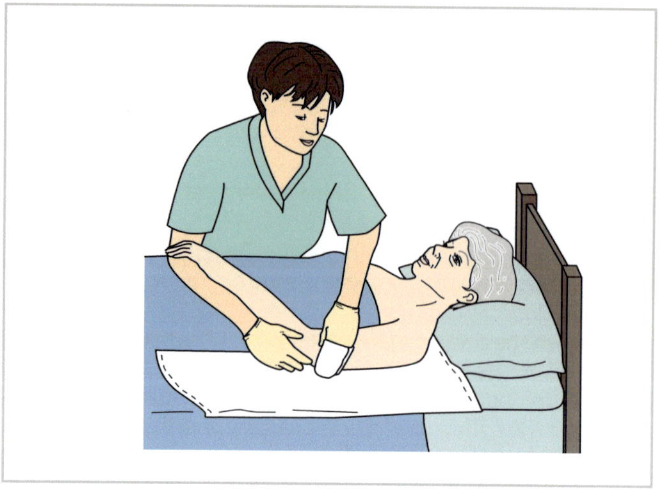

Fig. 12.10
Wash the person's arms with firm, long strokes using a mitted washcloth.

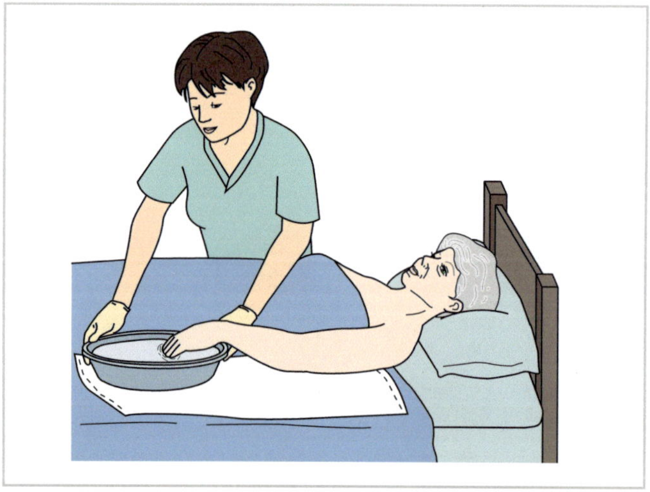

Fig. 12.11
The person's hand is washed by placing the washbasin on the bed.

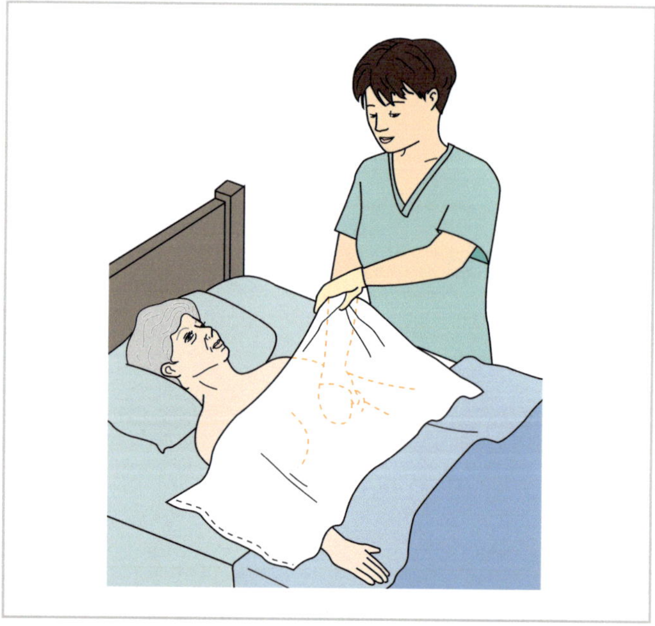

Fig. 12.12
The person's breasts are not exposed during the bath. A bath towel is placed horizontally over the chest area. The towel is lifted slightly to reach under to wash the breasts and chest.

two face towels, or just one large bath towel. The linen pack is placed within a bucket or basin, which is lined with a waterproof plastic bag. Following the manufacturer's directions, a measure of cleansing solution is mixed with a quantity of moderately hot water and poured over the linen pack. Some manufacturers recommend that the saturated linen pack be left for 20 minutes so all the towel(s) are moistened and evenly heated through. The solution contains water, a cleaning agent and a skin-softening agent. It also has a drying agent so the person's body dries quickly.

To give a hot towel bath, carefully follow the manufacturer's directions and the agency policies and procedures.

Bag baths

Bag baths are commercially prepared or prepared at the centre. Eight to 12 washcloths are in a plastic bag. The

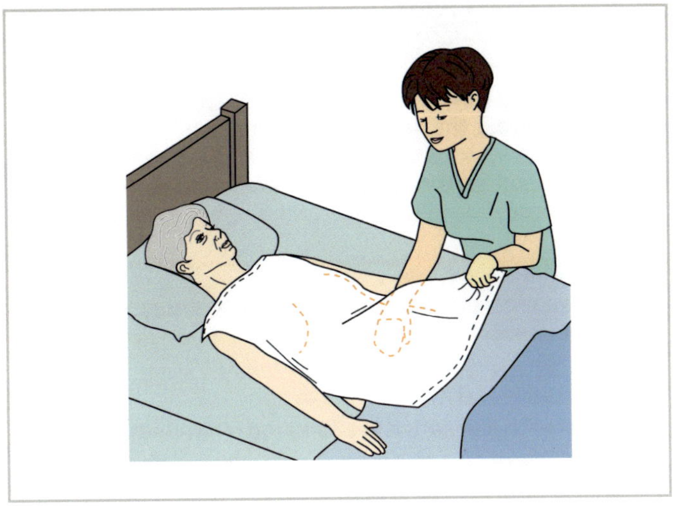

Fig. 12.13
The bath towel is turned vertically so that it covers the breasts and abdomen. The towel is lifted slightly to bathe the abdomen. The bath blanket covers the pubic area.

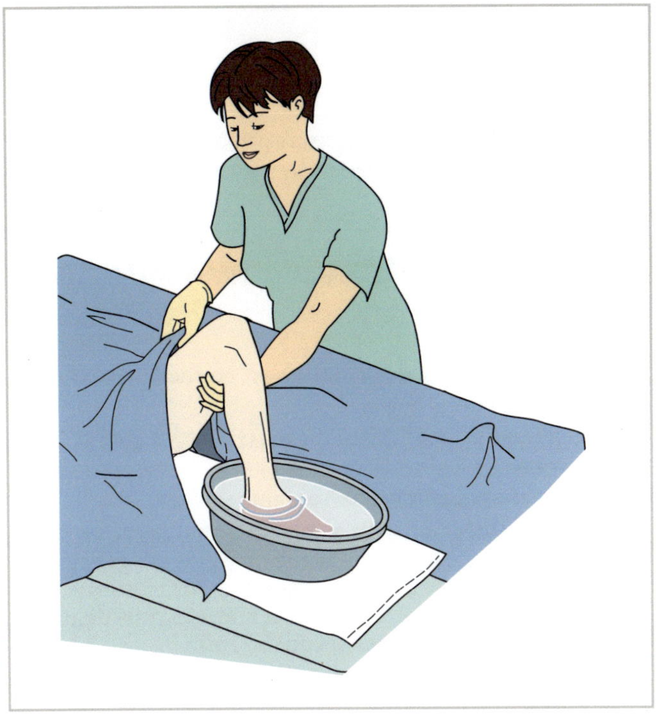

Fig. 12.14
The foot is washed by placing it in the washbasin on the bed.

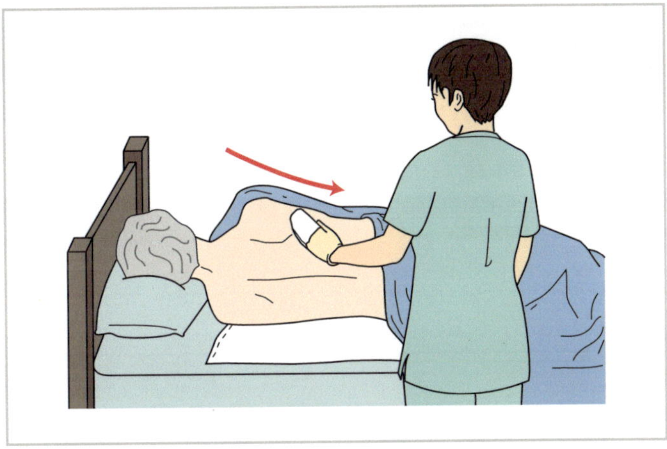

Fig. 12.15
The back is washed with long, firm, continuous strokes. Note that the person is in a side-lying position. A towel is placed lengthwise on the bed to protect the linen from water.

washcloths are moistened with a cleaning agent that does not require rinsing. The washcloths are warmed in a microwave oven. (The manufacturer's and agency instructions list what microwave settings to use.) A new washcloth is used for each body part. The skin air-dries. Towels are not needed.

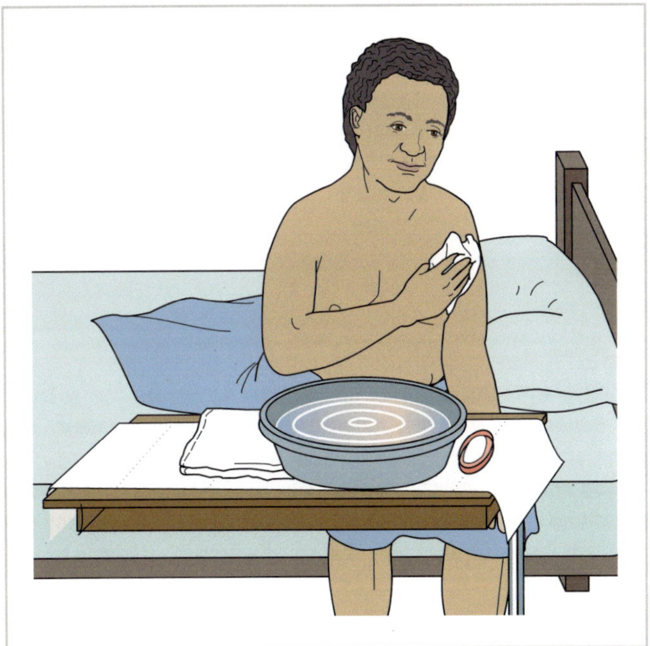

Fig. 12.16
The person is bathing himself in bed. Necessary equipment is within his reach.

The partial bath

The partial bath involves bathing the person's face, hands, axillae (underarms), back, buttocks and perineal area (Fig. 12.16). These areas may develop unpleasant odours or cause discomfort if not clean. Assist people who are able to bathe themselves in bed or at the sink by gathering hygiene items and washing the back. Give partial bed baths to people who cannot bathe themselves.

GIVING A PARTIAL BATH

Quality of life

Remember to respect the person's privacy while doing any procedure. Address the person by name and ensure they know your name.

Pre-procedure

1 Follow steps 1–10 in 'Giving a complete bed bath'. Put on gloves.

Procedure

2 Make sure the bed is in the lowest position (if applicable).
3 Assist with oral hygiene.
4 Remove top linen. Cover the person with a bath blanket.
5 Place the paper towels on a stable surface.
6 Fill the washbasin with water. Water temperature is 43–46°C, or as directed by the care plan or agency supervisor. (Use a bath thermometer to measure water temperature. Alternatively, test bath water by dipping your elbow or inner wrist into the basin.)
7 Place the basin on a stable surface on top of the paper towels.
8 Raise the head of the bed so the person can bathe comfortably (if applicable). Assist them to sit at the bedside if indicated by the care plan.
9 Help the person to undress.
10 Ask the person to wash easy-to-reach body parts. Explain that you will wash the back and areas the person cannot reach.
11 Ask the person to use the call bell if they need help, or when bathing is complete.
12 Leave the room after washing your hands.
13 Return when necessary.
14 Change the bath water.
15 Ask the person what areas they have washed? Wash and dry areas the person could not reach. The face, hands, underarms, back, buttocks and perineal area are washed for the partial bath. Wear gloves if contact with blood, body fluids, secretions or body waste is likely.
16 Give a back massage.
17 Apply lotion, powder and deodorant or antiperspirant as required.
18 Help the person put on clean garments.
19 Assist with oral hygiene needs.
20 Assist with hair care and other grooming needs.
21 Assist the person to a chair. (Lower the bed if the person transfers to a chair.) Otherwise, turn the person onto the side away from you, or as directed by the turning schedule in the care plan, if used.
22 Make the bed. Make sure you raise the bed to a height that facilitates good body mechanics. Adjust the height of the over-bed table to an appropriate level.
23 Lower the bed to its lowest position (if applicable). Assist the person to return to bed, if desired.

Post-procedure

24 Provide for comfort.
25 Empty and clean the basin. Return the basin and supplies to their proper place.
26 Wipe off the over-bed table with the paper towels and discard them.
27 Remove the screens from around the person.
28 Follow agency policy for dirty linen or place in client's laundry basket.
29 Wash your hands.
30 Report any observations of concern to the nurse on duty.

Baths and showers

Many people prefer baths or showers. However, burns from hot water and falls are constant risks. Safety is important. You must prevent slipping, falls, chills and burns. The care plan will provide any special instructions for helping a person with a bath or shower. Always seek support from your agency supervisor if unsure about any aspect of a person's hygiene needs.

DELEGATION GUIDELINES

Baths and showers

Before helping a person with a bath or shower, you need the following information from the care plan:

- whether the person takes a bath or shower
- what water temperature to use (usually 40°C)
- if any special equipment is needed
- how much help the person needs
- what observations to report.

Baths

Baths are relaxing for many people, but because a bath can cause a person to feel faint, weak or tired, it is recommended that they last no longer than 20 minutes. There is a greater risk for people who are immobile.

Some consumer aged care services have portable baths or spas, and many private homes have spa baths. Some baths have sides that can be lowered to transfer the person from the bed to the bath (Fig. 12.17). After the transfer, the sides are raised and the person is transported to the bathroom. The bath is filled and bathing proceeds in the usual manner. Remember to keep the person covered with a bath blanket for privacy and warmth.

Some baths and spas have hydraulic lifts (Fig. 12.18). The person is transferred to a special shower chair or stretcher in their room and then transported to the bathroom, where the chair or stretcher is lifted into the bath (Fig. 12.19). The spa has a whirlpool action that cleans the person's lower body. You wash the upper part of the person's body. Carefully wash under breasts, between skin

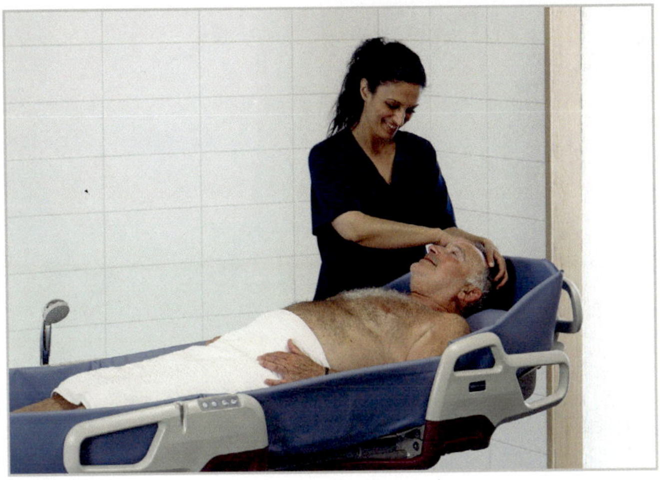

Fig. 12.17
Portable bath. The sides are lowered for transfers into and out of the bath.

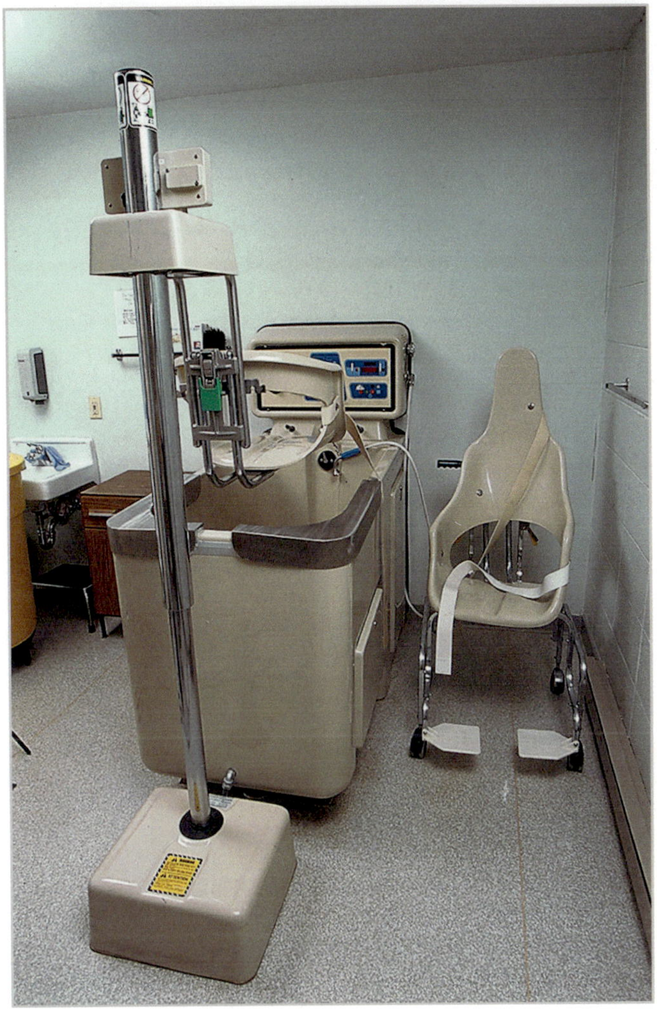

Fig. 12.18
Whirlpool bath with hydraulic lift.

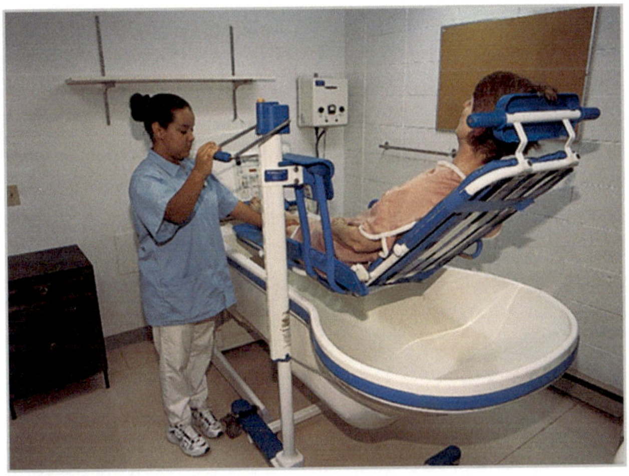

Fig. 12.19
The person and stretcher are lowered into the bath.

folds and in the perineal area. Carefully dry these areas after the bath.

Showers

Most aged care services have purpose-built shower rooms with shower stalls or shower cabinets (Fig. 12.20). The person walks into the stall or cabinet or is wheeled in on a shower chair. An open area on the plastic seat lets water drain off the chair (see Fig. 12.20). The chair is used to transport the person to and from the shower room. The wheels are locked during the shower as this prevents the chair from moving. If fitted, a lap belt should be fastened.

The shower room may have more than one stall or cabinet. Protect the person's right to privacy by screening, covering the person and closing the door. See Box 12.3 for safety measures for baths and showers.

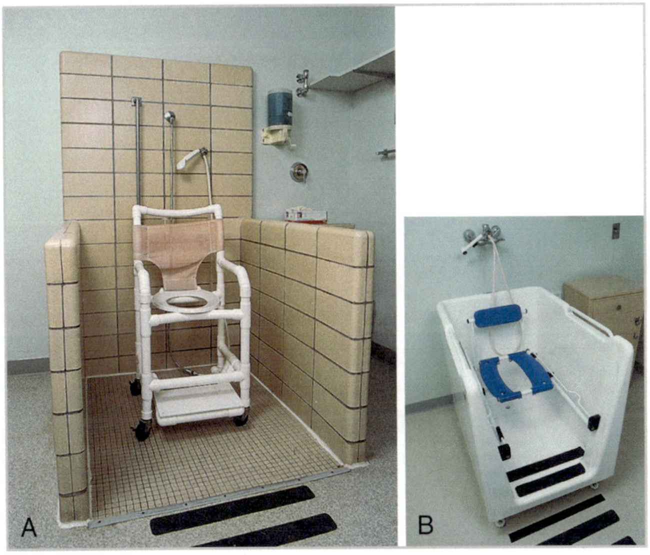

Fig. 12.20
A. Shower chair in a shower stall. **B.** Shower cabinet.

BOX 12.3
Safety measures for baths and showers

- Know what water temperature to use.
- Clean the bath or shower before and after use. This prevents the spread of microbes and infection.
- Make sure the floor of the bath or shower room is dry.
- Check to see that handrails, grab bars, hydraulic lifts and other safety aids are in working order.
- Place a bathmat in the bathtub or on the shower floor unless there are non-skid strips or a non-skid surface (Fig. 12.21).
- Cover the person for warmth and privacy. This includes during transport to and from the bath or shower room.
- Place needed items within the person's reach.
- Place the call bell within the person's reach and show them how to use it.
- Drain the bath before the person gets out, keeping the person covered to protect from exposure and chilling.
- Have the person use safety bars when getting into and out of the bath or shower. Do not let the person use towel rails for support.
- Turn cold water on first, then the hot water. Turn hot water off first, then the cold water.
- Adjust water temperature and pressure to prevent chilling or burns. Do this before the person gets into the shower. If a shower chair is used, position the shower chair before adjusting the water. Use the hand-held nozzle to direct the water away from the person until the desired temperature is reached.
- Fill the bath before the person gets into the bath.
- Measure the water temperature. For showers and baths, use the digital display. Alternatively, you can use a bath thermometer for a bath.
- Keep the water spray directed towards the person during the shower. This helps keep them warm.
- Avoid using bath oils as they make bath and shower surfaces slippery.
- Do not leave weak or unsteady persons unattended in the bath tub or shower.
- Stay within hearing distance if the person can be left alone. You will be nearby if the person calls for you or has an accident.

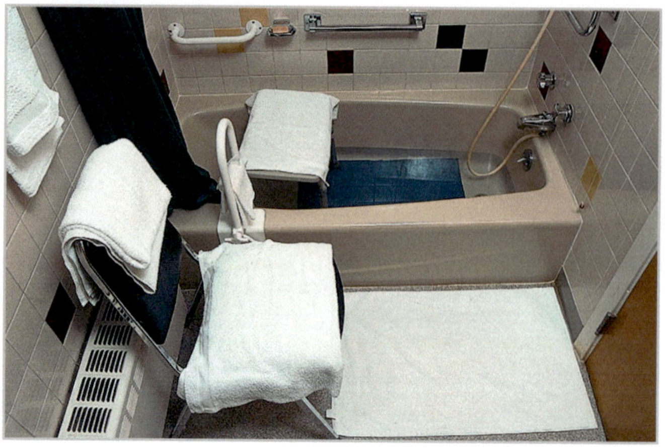

Fig. 12.21
A bathmat is in the bath. The bath is filled halfway with water. A floor mat is in front of the bath.

Showers in private homes can be separate units or positioned over the bath. Useful modifications include hand-held shower hoses, fixed or mobile shower seats and rails. Bath boards that are placed over the bath allow the person to sit while taking or being assisted to take a shower. If the person has to step into the bath to take a shower, make sure there are safety rails for the person to hold on to. People can buy or rent a shower chair for home use. Alternatively, a sturdy plastic chair (e.g. a lawn chair) can be used.

Some people can stand safely in the shower. Encourage them to use handrails for support during the shower.

Most bathtubs, shower stalls and cabinets have non-skid surfaces. If not, a bathmat is used. Ideally, use a shower chair for any person who is very frail or weak, or who may be prone to falls because of a medical condition or the use of some medications. Always follow the care plan.

SAFETY ALERT

Baths and showers

Some people are very weak or very large. Two staff members are needed to safely assist them with baths and showers.

When using portable baths, spa equipment and shower chairs, always follow the manufacturer's instructions. Also protect the person from falls and burns. Follow the safety measures discussed elsewhere within this text. Remember to measure water temperature.

ASSISTING WITH A BATH OR SHOWER

Quality of life

Remember to respect the person's privacy while performing care procedures. Address the person by name and ensure they know your name.

Pre-procedure

1 Reserve the bathtub or shower if necessary.
2 Call the person by name and introduce yourself.
3 Explain the procedure to the person before starting and ensure that you verbalise each step as it is carried out during the procedure.
4 Wash your hands.
5 Collect the following:
   - two face towels and two bath towels
   - liquid soap-free cleanser
   - bath thermometer (for a bath)
   - clean gown, pyjamas or day clothes
   - deodorant and other toilet articles as requested
   - bath robe and non-skid footwear
   - rubber bathmat if needed
   - towelling or disposable bathmat
   - gloves
   - a clean shower chair, if used.

Procedure

6 Place items in the bath or shower room in the space provided, or on a chair. Warm the room as required.
7 Clean the bath or shower if needed.
8 Place a rubber bathmat in the bath or on the shower floor. Do not block the drain.
9 Place the disposable or towelling bathmat on the floor in front of the bath or shower.
10 Put the 'Occupied' sign on the door.
11 Return to the person's room. Provide for privacy.
12 Help the person sit on the side of the bed.
13 Help the person put on a robe and non-skid footwear.
14 Assist or transport the person to the bath or shower room.
15 For a bath:
   a Have the person sit on a chair by the bath.
   b Fill the bath halfway with warm water (40°C). Measure water temperature with the bath thermometer or check the digital display.
16 For a shower:
   a Turn on the shower.
   b Adjust water temperature and pressure.
17 Assist the person to remove their robe, gown or pyjamas and footwear.
18 Help the person into the bath or shower. If using a shower chair, place it in position and lock the wheels. Ask the person to use the call bell when finished or when help is necessary. Remind the person not to stay in the bath longer than 20 minutes.
19 Leave the room only if the person can be left unattended. Otherwise stay in the room or remain nearby. Wash your hands if you leave the room. Check the person every 5 minutes. Return when they activate the call bell and knock before entering.
20 Assist with washing if necessary. Wear gloves if directed by the care plan or if the person is heavily soiled.
21 Place a towel across the chair.
22 Turn off the shower or drain the bath. Place a towel across the person's shoulders to prevent chilling. Help the person out of the bath or shower and onto the chair.
23 Help the person dry off. Pat gently. Remember to dry under breasts, between skin folds, in the perineal area and between toes.
24 Assist with lotion, deodorant or antiperspirant and other grooming items as needed.
25 Help the person to dress and put on footwear.
26 Assist with oral hygiene needs
27 Help the person return to the room. Assist them into a re-made bed or to a chair.
28 Give a back massage if the person returns to bed.
29 Assist with hair care and other grooming needs.

Post-procedure

30 Provide for comfort.
31 Place the call bell within reach.
32 Clean the bath or shower. Remove soiled linen and discard disposable items. Wear gloves for this step.
33 Put the 'Unoccupied' sign on the door. Return supplies to their proper place.
34 Follow agency policy for dirty linen or place in client's laundry basket.
35 Wash your hands.
36 Report any observations of concern to the nurse on duty.

THE BACK MASSAGE

The back massage (back rub) relaxes muscles and stimulates circulation. Massages are given after the bath and with evening care. They should last 3–5 minutes. Observe the skin before starting the massage. Look for breaks in the skin, bruises, reddened areas and other signs of skin breakdown.

Lotion reduces friction during the massage. It is warmed before being applied. Warm the lotion by placing the bottle in warm water or holding it under warm running water for a short time. Alternatively, rub some lotion between your hands.

The prone position is best for a massage. However, the side-lying position may be more comfortable for some people. Use firm strokes and always keep your hands in contact with the person's skin. After the massage, apply some lotion to the elbows, knees and heels to keep the skin soft. These bony areas are at risk of skin breakdown.

SAFETY ALERT

Back massage

Back massages can be dangerous for people with certain heart diseases, back injuries, back surgery, skin diseases and some lung disorders. Check with the agency supervisor, nurse and care plan before giving back massages to any person.

Also, do not massage bony areas that are reddened. Reddened areas signal skin breakdown and pressure ulcers. Massage can lead to further tissue damage.

If the person's skin is not intact, you need to wear gloves. Follow Standard Precautions.

DELEGATION GUIDELINES

Back massage

Before giving a back massage, you need the following information from the care plan:

- Can the person have a back massage?
- How should you position the person?
- Does the person have position limits?
- When should the person receive a back massage?
- Does the person need frequent back massages for comfort, relaxation and/or skin management?
- What observations to report:
  - bruising
  - reddened areas
  - signs of skin breakdown.

GIVING A BACK MASSAGE

Quality of life

Remember to respect the person's privacy while doing any procedure. Address the person by name and ensure they know your name.

Pre-procedure

1. Call the person by name and introduce yourself.
2. Explain the procedure to the person before starting and ensure that you verbalise each step as it is carried out during the procedure.
3. Wash your hands.
4. Collect the following:
   - bath blanket
   - bath towel
   - lotion.
5. Provide for privacy and maintain warmth.
6. Raise the bed to a height that facilitates good body mechanics.

Procedure

7. Position the person in the prone or side-lying position. The back is towards you.
8. Expose the back, shoulders, upper arms and buttocks. Cover the rest of the body with the bath blanket.
9. Lay the towel on the bed along the back.
10. Apply the pre-warmed lotion to your hands or rub some between your hands.
11. Explain that the lotion may feel cool and wet.
12. Apply lotion to the lower back area.
13. Stroke up from the buttocks to the shoulders (Fig. 12.22). Then stroke down over the upper arms. Stroke up the upper arms, across the shoulders and down the back to the buttocks. Use firm strokes. Keep your hands in contact with the person's skin.
14. Repeat step 13 for at least 3 minutes.
15. Knead by grasping skin between your thumb and fingers (Fig. 12.23). Knead half of the back, starting at the buttocks, and move up to the shoulder. Then knead down from the shoulder to the buttocks. Repeat on the other half of the back.
16. Apply lotion to bony areas. Use circular motions with the tips of your index and middle fingers. (Do not massage bony areas that are reddened.)
17. Use fast movements to stimulate and slow movements to relax the person.
18. Stroke with long, firm movements to end the massage. Tell the person you are finishing.
19. Cover the person. Remove the towel and bath blanket.

Post-procedure

20. Provide for comfort.
21. Lower the bed to its lowest position.
22. Place the call bell within reach.
23. Return lotion to its proper place.
24. Remove the screens from around the person.
25. Follow agency policy for dirty linen.
26. Wash your hands.
27. Report any observations of concern to the nurse on duty.

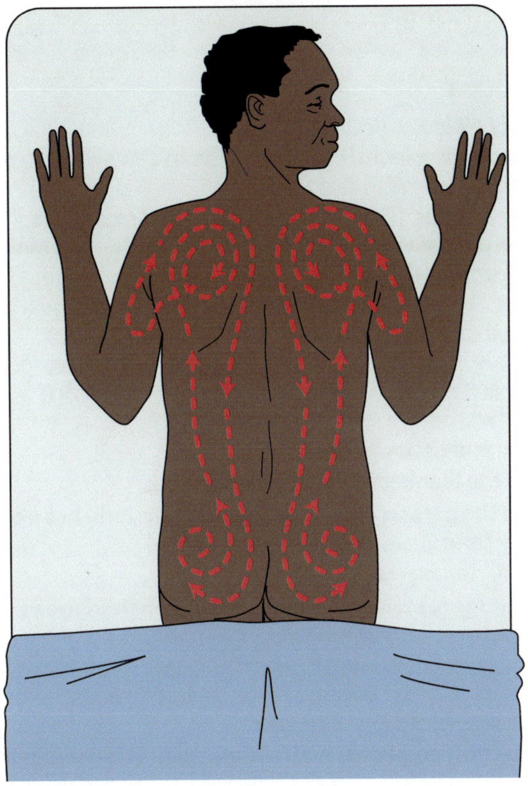

Fig. 12.22
The person lies in the prone position for a back massage. Stroke upwards from the buttocks to the shoulders, down over the upper arms, back up the upper arms, across the shoulders and down the back to the buttocks.

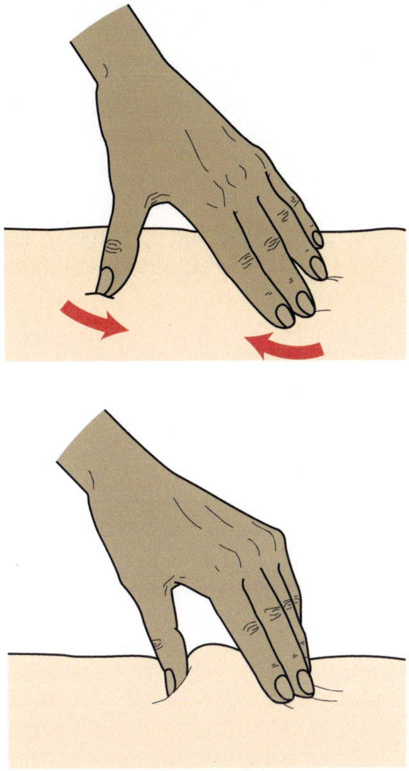

Fig. 12.23
Kneading the back is done by picking up tissue between the thumb and fingers.

PERINEAL CARE

Perineal care (peri-care) involves cleaning the genital and anal areas. These areas provide a warm, moist and dark place for microbes to grow. Cleaning prevents infection, minimises unpleasant odours and promotes comfort.

Perineal care is done daily during the bath. It is also done whenever the area is soiled with urine or faeces. People with certain medical conditions may need perineal care more frequently. The care plan will tell you when the person needs perineal care.

Assistance with perineal care is provided to people who are unable to attend to their own perineal care. Perineal care can be embarrassing for the person and care staff. Sensitivity and a professional approach are required to overcome embarrassment, especially when providing perineal care to a person of the opposite sex.

'Perineum' and 'perineal' are not common terms. Most people understand terms such as 'privates', 'private parts', 'crotch', 'genitals' or 'the area between your legs'. Use terms the person understands. The term must also be in good taste professionally.

Standard Precautions are followed. Work from the cleanest area to the dirtiest. The urethral area (the front) is the cleanest and the anal area (the back) is the dirtiest. Therefore, clean from the urethra to the anal area front to back.

The perineal area is very delicate and easily injured. Use warm water, not hot. Use washcloths, moistened towelettes, cotton balls or swabs according to agency policy and the care plan. Rinse thoroughly. Gently pat dry after rinsing to reduce moisture and to promote comfort.

SAFETY ALERT

Perineal care

Hot water can burn delicate perineal tissues. To prevent burns, measure water temperature according to agency policy. If you are unsure whether the water is too hot, ask the person or other staff member to check it.

Also, protect the person and yourself from the spread of infection. When giving perineal care, contact with blood, body fluids, secretions and excretions are likely. Follow Standard Precautions.

GIVING FEMALE PERINEAL CARE

Quality of life

Remember to respect the person's privacy while doing any procedure. Address the person by name and ensure they know your name.

Pre-procedure

1 Explain the procedure to the person before starting and ensure that you verbalise each step as it is carried out during the procedure.
2 Wash your hands.
3 Collect the following:
- washbasin
- liquid soap-free cleanser
- at least four washcloths
- bath towel
- bath blanket
- bath thermometer
- waterproof pad
- creams or lotions if used (check the care plan)
- gloves
- paper towels.

4 Position and adjust the height of the over-bed table so you can reach it with ease. Cover the over-bed table with paper towels and arrange items on top of them.
5 Identify the person. Call her by name and introduce yourself.
6 Provide for privacy.
7 Raise the bed to a height that ensures good body mechanics (if applicable).
8 Cover the person with a bath blanket (Fig. 12.24). Move top linen to the foot of the bed or place on a chair.
9 Position the person on her back.
10 Place a waterproof pad under her buttocks.
11 Raise the bed rail, if used.
12 Fill the washbasin. Water temperature should be about 40–42°C. Measure water temperature according to agency policy.
13 Place the basin on the over-bed table on top of the paper towels.
14 Help the person flex her knees and spread her legs. Alternatively, if she cannot flex her knees, help her spread her legs as much as possible with her knees straight.
15 Put on the gloves.
16 Fold the corner of the bath blanket between her legs onto her abdomen.
17 Wet the washcloths. Squeeze out excess water from washcloths before using them.

Procedure

18 Apply cleanser to the washcloth.
19 Separate the labia (Fig. 12.25). Clean downwards from front to back with one stroke.
20 Repeat steps 18 and 19 until the area is clean. Use a clean part of the washcloth for each stroke. Use more than one washcloth if needed.
21 Rinse the perineum with a clean washcloth. Separate the labia. Stroke downwards from front to back. Repeat as necessary. Use a clean part of the washcloth for each stroke. Use more than one washcloth if needed.
22 Pat the area dry with the towel.
23 Fold the blanket back between her legs.
24 Help the person lower her legs and turn onto her side away from you.
25 Apply cleanser to a washcloth.
26 Clean the rectal area (Fig. 12.26). Clean from the vagina to the anus with one stroke.
27 Repeat steps 25 and 26 until the area is clean. Use a clean part of the washcloth for each stroke. Use more than one washcloth if needed.
28 Rinse the rectal area with a washcloth. Stroke from the vagina to the anus. Repeat the step as needed using a clean part of the washcloth for each stroke. Use more than one washcloth if needed.
29 Pat the area dry with the towel. Apply any creams or lotions.
30 Remove the waterproof pad.
31 Remove and discard the gloves and wash your hands.

Post-procedure

32 Provide for comfort.
33 Return bed linen to its proper position and remove the bath blanket.
34 Lower the bed to its lowest position.
35 Place the call bell within reach (if applicable).
36 Empty and clean the washbasin.
37 Return the basin and supplies to their proper place.
38 Wipe off the over-bed table with the paper towels and discard them.
39 Remove the screen from around the person.
40 Follow agency policy for dirty linen.
41 Wash your hands.
42 Report any observations of concern to the nurse on duty.

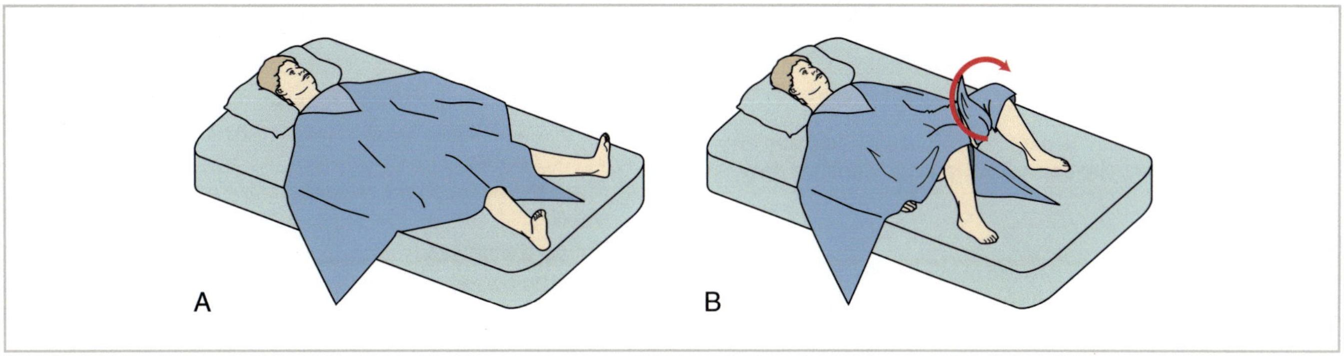

Fig. 12.24
Draping for perineal care.
A. Position the blanket like a diamond: one corner is at the neck, there is a corner at each side and one corner is between the person's legs. **B.** Wrap the blanket around the leg by bringing the corner around under the leg and over the top. Tuck the corner under the hip.

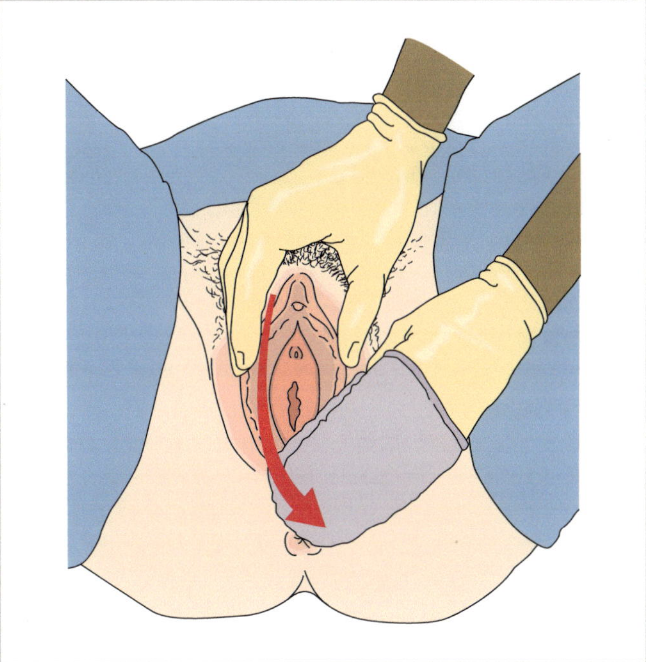

Fig. 12.25
Female perineal care. Separate the labia with one hand. Use a mitted washcloth to clean between the labia with downward strokes.

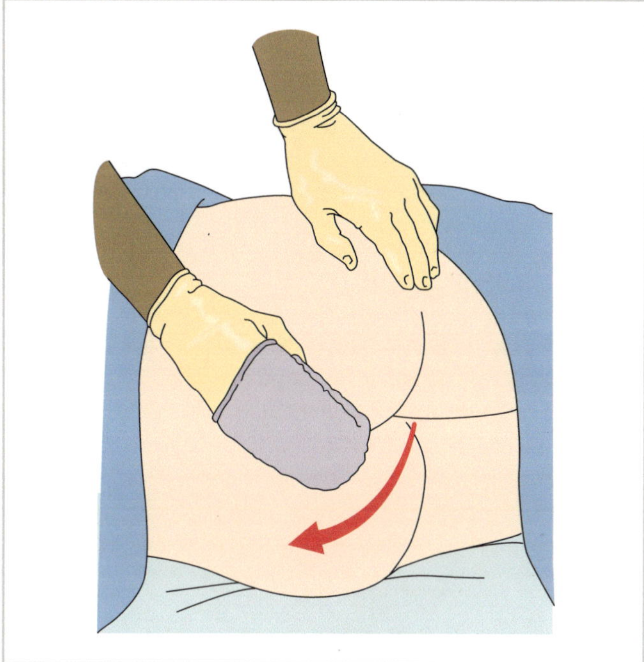

Fig. 12.26
Cleaning the rectal area. Wipe from the vagina to the anus. The side-lying position allows thorough cleaning of the anal area.

DELEGATION GUIDELINES

Perineal care

Before giving perineal care, you need the following information from the care plan:

- when perineal care needs to be done
- what terms the person understands (perineum, privates, private parts, crotch, genitals or area between the legs)
- how much help the person needs
- what water temperature to use (40–42°C)
- any position restrictions or limits
- what observations to report:
  - odours
  - redness, swelling, discharge or irritation
  - complaints of pain, burning or other discomfort
  - signs of urinary or faecal incontinence.

GIVING MALE PERINEAL CARE

Quality of life

Remember to respect the person's privacy while doing any procedure. Address the person by name and ensure they know your name.

Pre-procedure

1. Explain the procedure to the person before starting and ensure that you verbalise each step as it is carried out during the procedure.
2. Wash your hands.
3. Collect the following:
   - washbasin
   - liquid soap-free cleanser
   - at least four washcloths
   - bath towel
   - bath blanket
   - bath thermometer
   - waterproof pad
   - creams or lotions if used (check the care plan)
   - gloves
   - paper towels.
4. Position and adjust the height of the over-bed table so you can reach it with ease. Cover the over-bed table with paper towels and arrange items on top of them.
5. Identify the person. Call him by name and introduce yourself.
6. Provide for privacy.
7. Raise the bed to a height that facilitates good body mechanics (if applicable).
8. Cover the person with a bath blanket (see Fig. 12.24). Move top linen to the foot of the bed or place on a chair.
9. Position the person on his back.
10. Place a waterproof pad under his buttocks.
11. Raise the bed rail, if used.
12. Fill the washbasin. Water temperature should be about 40–42°C. Measure water temperature according to agency policy.
13. Place the basin on the over-bed table on top of the paper towels.
14. Put on the gloves.
15. Fold the corner of the bath blanket onto his abdomen to allow access to his genital area.
16. Wet the washcloths. Squeeze out excess water from washcloths before using them.

Procedure

17. Retract the foreskin if the person is uncircumcised (Fig. 12.27).
18. Grasp the penis.
19. Clean the tip. Use a circular motion (Fig. 12.28). Start at the urethra and work outwards. Repeat this step as necessary. Use a clean part of the washcloth each time.
20. Rinse the area with another washcloth.
21. Return the foreskin to its natural position.
22. Clean the shaft of the penis with firm downward strokes. Rinse the area.
23. Clean the scrotum. Rinse well. Observe for redness and irritation in the skin folds.
24. Gently pat dry the penis and scrotum.
25. Fold the bath blanket back between his legs.
26. Help him lower his legs and turn onto his side away from you.
27. Clean the rectal area. Rinse and dry well.
28. Remove the waterproof pad.
29. Remove and discard the gloves and wash your hands.

Post-procedure

30. Follow steps 32 to 42 in 'Giving female perineal care'.

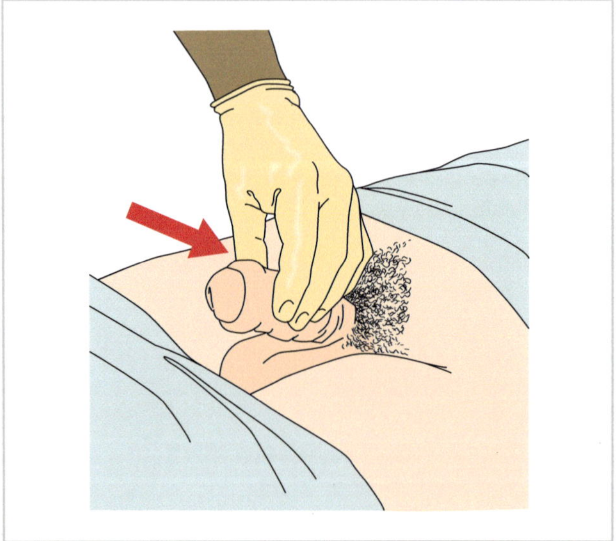

Fig. 12.27
Male perineal care. The foreskin of the uncircumcised male is pulled back. It is returned to its normal position immediately after cleaning.

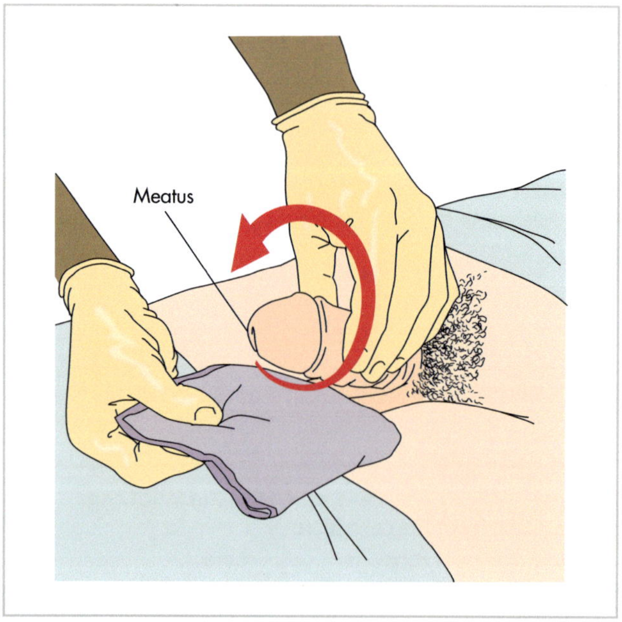

Fig. 12.28
The penis is cleaned with circular motions starting at the urethra.

QUALITY OF LIFE

Client rights are protected and enshrined in legislation. They are intended to improve the person's quality of life, health and safety. You must provide hygiene in a way that maintains or improves the person's quality of life, health and safety. You must protect the person's rights when giving such care.

Protect the right to privacy by:

- not exposing the person
- asking visitors to leave the room before you give care; a family member or friend may want to help – the person must consent to this
- closing doors, privacy curtains and drapes before giving care
- exposing only the body part involved in the procedure
- covering a person when taking them to and from the bath or shower room
- if there is more than one shower stall, protecting the person from being exposed to others who are present.

Everyone has the right to personal choice; they have the right to be involved in the planning of their care and treatment. Hygiene is a very personal matter. People have a voice about when and how hygiene is done. Personal choice is respected in matters such as bath time, products used, what to wear and hair styling.

Everyone has the right to keep and use personal items. You will handle the person's property in hygiene procedures. Protect dentures and glasses from loss or breakage. If jewellery or religious items are removed for care, protect them from loss, damage or theft.

Freedom from restraint (restrictive practices) is another client right. Bed rails are classed as restraints under current aged care legislation. You can only use bedrails if they are identified as permitted within the person's care plan. Always follow the person's care plan for the use of bed rails and ensure that you use them only if permitted when undertaking any care activities. If bed rails are permitted for use, you must ensure that they are up at all times when giving care and only lowered as required so that you can maintain good body mechanics. Do not stretch over the bed rails to give care. If you need to leave the person for any reason at all, you must return the bedrails to the raised position before leaving the bedside. Only lower the bedrail on the side that you are attending to the person. The opposite bedrail must stay up.

FOCUS ON COMMUNITY CARE

Within the community setting, before attending to a client's hygiene needs, always complete a safety audit. Many homes do not have the same level of equipment or modified areas as in consumer care. Many older-style Australian and New Zealand homes do not have showers or have showers that have been placed over the bath. Do not attempt to assist a client into a bath unless you have been shown an appropriate technique to do so. The use of bath boards or seats makes the act of bathing much easier but do not address the issues of getting into and out of the bath. Many people with long-term disabilities are aware of appropriate techniques and will direct you in how to attend to their hygiene needs safely and appropriately. If you are unsure of your ability to get a client into or out of a bath or home shower, it is far safer to assist with their hygiene needs seated by the bath or a basin until you have been taught the appropriate techniques or the environment has been adapted to suit the person's needs.

Reporting

You will make many important observations while assisting people to meet their hygiene needs. Always follow the agency policy for reporting your observations. Report events of concern immediately to your agency supervisor or nurse. Events of concern can include bleeding, dizziness, complaints of feeling ill and unexpected pain or discomfort.

ASSISTING WITH GROOMING, SKIN AND NAIL CARE

After reading this section, you should be able to:

- understand the importance of hair care and shaving
- understand the factors that affect hair care
- know the ways to shampoo hair
- know the measures required when shaving a person
- understand why nail and foot care are important
- know how to dress and undress a person
- perform the procedures described in this section
- know how to promote quality of life.

Hair care, shaving and nail and foot care are important to many clients. Like hygiene, these grooming measures prevent infection and promote comfort. They also affect love, belonging and self-esteem needs.

People vary in their grooming measures. Some only want clean hair, while others want a certain hairstyle. Some only want clean hands, while others want their nails cleaned, manicured and polished. Many men shave and groom their beards. Likewise, many women shave their legs and underarms. Some women have facial hair. They may shave, wax or use creams to remove such hair. Also, be aware of organisation policies and procedures as they vary from one organisation to another in relation to job responsibility, such as who does nail care.

HAIR CARE

A person's appearance and mental wellbeing are affected by how their hair looks and feels. Some cannot care for their own hair and need help with hair care. Many services have a barber or a hairdresser to cut and shampoo hair. It is the carer's role to assist with daily hair care.

The care plan reflects the person's culture, personal choice, skin and scalp condition, health history and self-care ability. The following terms are common in care plans:

- **Alopecia** means hair loss. Hair loss may be complete or partial. Male-pattern baldness occurs with ageing and is hereditary. Hair also thins in some women with ageing. Cancer treatments (radiation therapy to the head and chemotherapy) often cause alopecia in males and females. Skin disease is another cause. Stress, poor nutrition, pregnancy, some medications and hormone changes are other causes. The hair often grows back, except for hair loss from ageing.
- **Hirsutism** is excessive body hair in women and children. It may be hereditary because of abnormal amounts of male hormones.
- **Dandruff** is an excessive amount of dry, white flakes from the scalp. Itching often occurs. Sometimes the eyebrows and ear canals are involved. Medicated shampoos correct the problem.
- **Pediculosis** (lice) is an infestation of lice. *Infestation* means being in or on a host. Lice bites cause severe itching in the affected body area. Pediculosis capitis is the infestation of the scalp (*capitis*) with lice. Pediculosis pubis is the infestation of the pubic (*pubis*) hair with lice. Both head and pubic lice attach their eggs to hair shafts. Pediculosis corporis is the infestation of the body (corporis) with lice. Lice eggs attach to clothing and furniture. Lice spread easily to other people through clothing, furniture, bed linen and sexual contact. They are also spread by sharing combs and brushes. Medicated shampoos, lotions and creams are used to treat lice. All medicated shampoos and hair treatments should be listed on the person's care plan. Thorough bathing is needed, as is washing clothing and linen in hot water. Report any signs of lice to your supervisor or the nurse at once.

Brushing and combing hair

Brushing and combing hair are part of morning, afternoon and evening care. They are also attended to whenever needed. Encourage clients to do their own hair care, but assist as needed. You perform hair care for those who cannot do so. The person chooses how to brush, comb and style their hair. Encouraging them to perform own hair care assists in maintaining independence.

Brushing increases blood flow to the scalp. It also brings scalp oils along the hair shaft. Scalp oils help keep the hair soft and shiny. Brushing and combing prevent tangled and matted hair. When brushing and combing hair that is quite tangled, start at the ends, gently teasing out the knots, and work your way up towards the scalp.

Long hair mats and tangles easily. Daily brushing and combing prevent this problem. Braiding does too. Do not braid hair without the person's consent. Never cut matted or tangled hair. Tell your supervisor or the nurse if the person has matted or tangled hair. You may have to comb or brush through the matting and tangling. Do this as follows:

- Take a small section of hair near the ends.
- Comb or brush through to the hair ends.
- Working up to the scalp, add small sections of hair.
- Comb or brush through each longer section to the hair ends.
- Brush or comb from the scalp to the hair ends.

Special measures are needed for curly, coarse and dry hair. Use a wide-toothed comb for curly hair. Start at the neckline. Working upwards, lift and fluff the hair outwards. Continue until you reach the forehead. Wet the hair or apply a conditioner as directed. This makes combing easier.

The person may have certain practices or hair care products. These become part of the person's care plan. In addition, the person can guide you when giving hair care.

When giving hair care, place a towel across the person's shoulders to protect their garments. If the person is in bed, give hair care before changing the pillowcase. If done after a linen change, place a towel across the pillow to collect falling hair.

CARING ABOUT CULTURE

Care of a person's hair may be a culturally sensitive issue as some cultures do not allow people of the opposite sex to see or care for their hair. Always check with the client, their families or your supervisor if you are unsure.

SAFETY ALERT

Brushing and combing hair

Sharp bristles on a brush can injure the scalp; so can a comb with sharp or broken teeth. Tell your supervisor if you have concerns about the person's brush or comb.

DELEGATION GUIDELINES

Brushing and combing hair

You need the following information from the care plan before brushing and combing hair:

- how much help the person needs
- what to do if hair is matted or tangled
- what measures are needed for curly, coarse or dry hair
- what hair care products to use
- the person's preferences and routine hair care measures
- what observations to report and record:
  - scalp sores
  - flaking
  - the presence of lice
  - patches of hair loss
  - very dry or very oily hair.

BRUSHING AND COMBING HAIR

Quality of life

Remember to respect the person's privacy while doing any procedure. Address the person by name and ensure they know your name. Remember that looking one's best helps people to feel better about themselves.

Pre-procedure

1. Follow the delegation guidelines.
2. Call the person by name.
3. Explain the procedure to the person. Ask the person how to style their hair.
4. Collect the following:
   - comb and brush
   - bath towel
   - other grooming items as requested.
5. Arrange items.
6. Wash your hands.
7. Provide for privacy.

Procedure

8. Help the person to the chair. (If the person is in bed, raise the bed for body mechanics. Assist the person into a semi-Fowler's position if allowed.)
9. Place the towel across the person's shoulders or the pillow.
10. Ask the person to remove their glasses. Put these in the glasses case. Put the case in the bedside stand.
11. Part the hair into two sections (Fig. 12.29). Divide one side into two sections.
12. Brush the hair. Start at the scalp and brush towards the hair ends (Fig. 12.30).
13. Style the hair as the person prefers.
14. Remove the towel.
15. Help the person put on their glasses.

Post-procedure

16. Provide for comfort.
17. Lower the bed to its lowest position if raised for body mechanics (if applicable).
18. Place the call bell within reach.
19. Remove the screens from around the person (if applicable).
20. Clean and return equipment to its proper place.
21. Follow centre policy for dirty linen.
22. Wash your hands.

Shampooing

Clients may need help shampooing. The frequency of shampooing depends on the person's needs and preferences. Usually shampooing is done weekly, on the person's bath or shower day.

Some people use special shampoos and/or conditioners. Others use medicated shampoo ordered by the doctor. If a woman's hair is looked after by the hairdresser, do not shampoo her hair. She will wear a shower cap during the bath or shower.

The shampoo method depends on the person's condition, safety factors and personal choice. The health team decides which method to use. Hair is dried and styled as quickly as possible after the shampoo.

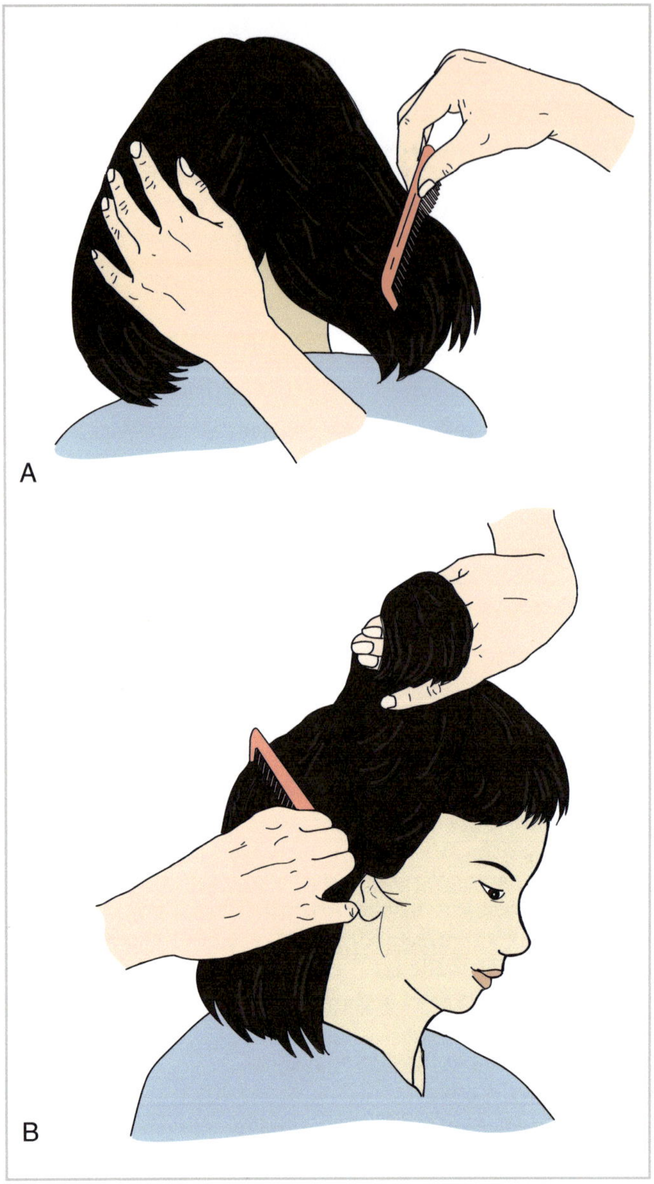

Fig. 12.29
Parting the hair.
A. Part hair down the middle. Divide it into two sections.
B. Then part each section into two smaller sections.

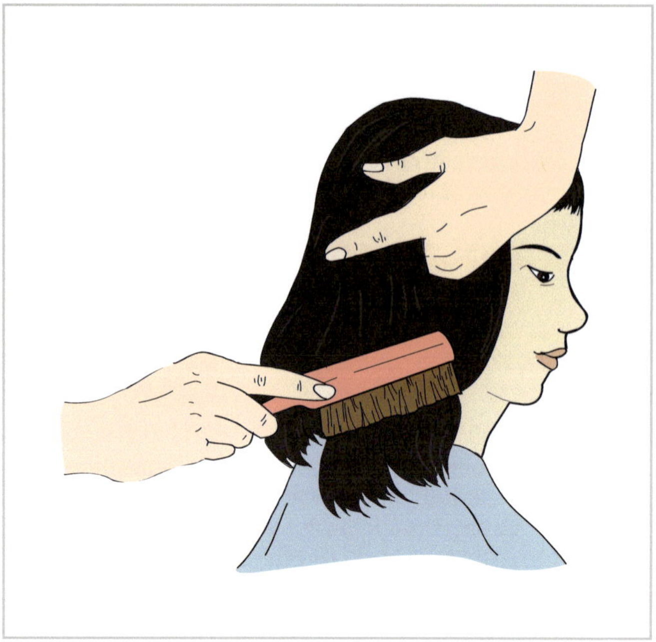

Fig. 12.30
Brush the hair by starting at the scalp. Then brush down to the hair ends.

Women may want their hair curled or rolled up before drying. Check with the nurse before doing so.

- *Shampoo during the shower or bath* – A handheld shower nozzle is used. The person tips their head back to keep shampoo and water out of their eyes. Support the back of the person's head with one hand. Shampoo with your other hand. Some people cannot tip their head back. They lean forwards and hold a folded washcloth over their eyes. Support the forehead with one hand as you shampoo with the other. Be sure that the person can breathe easily.
- *Shampoo at the sink* – The person sits facing away from the sink. A folded towel is placed over the edge of the sink. It protects the person's neck. The person's head is tilted back over the edge of the sink. A water jug or hand-held nozzle is used to wet and rinse the hair. (Many older or disabled persons have limited range of motion in their neck and upper back. This method is not used for them.)
- *Shampoo on a stretcher* – The stretcher is in front of the sink (Fig. 12.31). A towel is placed under the person's neck. The head is tilted over the edge of the sink. The water jug or hand-held nozzle is used to wet and rinse

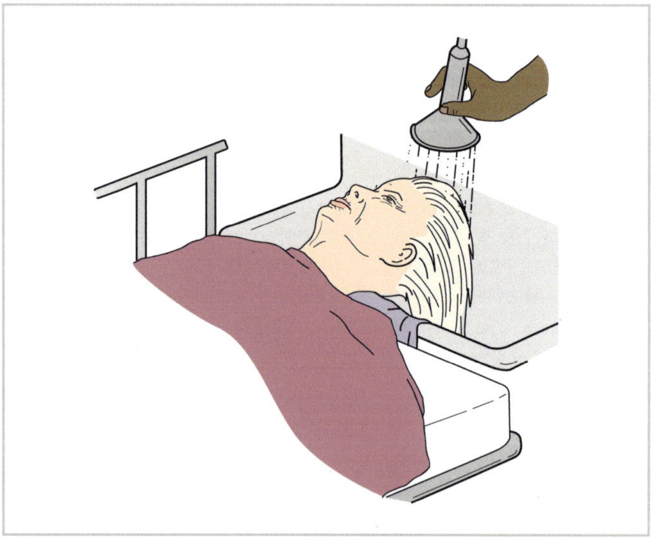

Fig. 12.31
Shampooing while the person is on a stretcher. The stretcher is in front of the sink.

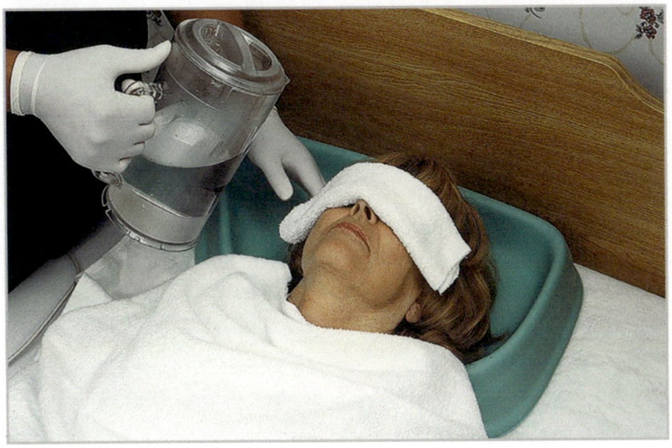

Fig. 12.32
A shampoo tray is used to shampoo a person in bed. The tray is directed to the side of the bed so the water drains into a collecting basin.

the hair. Remember to lock the stretcher wheels and use the safety straps. (This method is not used for persons with limited range of motion in the neck or upper back.)

- *Shampoo in bed* – The person's head and shoulders are moved to the edge of the bed if possible. A shampoo tray placed under the person's head protects the linen and mattress from water (Fig. 12.32). The tray also drains water into a basin placed on a chair next to the bed. Use a water jug to wet and rinse the hair. (This method is used for people who need complete bed baths. It is also used for those who cannot use a chair, wheelchair or stretcher.) A number of products are also available, so that a client can have a 'dry' shampoo in bed.

SAFETY ALERT

Shampooing

It is very important to keep shampoo out of the eyes. The person holds a face towel or washcloth over their eyes. Do not let shampoo get near the eyes. When rinsing, cup your hand at the person's forehead. This keeps soapy water from running down the person's forehead and into their eyes.

If a medicated shampoo or conditioner is used, return it to the nurse. Never leave it at the bedside unless instructed to do so.

If the person has scalp lesions, wear gloves and follow Standard Precautions.

DELEGATION GUIDELINES

Shampooing

Before shampooing a person's hair, you need the following information from the care plan:

- when to shampoo the person's hair
- what method to use (during the shower or bath, at the sink, on a stretcher or in bed)
- what shampoo and conditioner to use
- the person's position restrictions or limits
- what water temperature to use (usually about 40.5°C)
- whether the hair should be curled or rolled up before drying
- what observations to report and record:
  - scalp sores
  - hair falling out in patches
  - how the person tolerated the procedure
  - the presence of lice.

SHAMPOOING A PERSON'S HAIR

Quality of life

Remember to respect the person's privacy while doing any procedure. Address the person by name and ensure they know your name.

Pre-procedure

1. Follow the delegation guidelines.
2. Explain the procedure to the person.
3. Wash your hands.
4. Collect the following:
   - two bath towels
   - face towel or washcloth
   - shampoo
   - hair conditioner (if requested)
   - bath thermometer
   - water jug or nozzle (if needed)
   - shampoo tray (if needed)
   - basin or pail (if needed)
   - waterproof pad (if needed)
   - gloves (if needed)
   - comb and brush
   - hair dryer. (Do not plug in until required.)
5. Arrange items nearby.
6. Call the person by name. Provide for privacy.

Procedure

7. Position the person for the method you will use. Place the waterproof pad and shampoo tray under the head and shoulders if needed.
8. Place a bath towel across the shoulders or across the pillow.

9 Brush and comb the hair to remove snarls and tangles.
10 Raise the bed rail, if used.
11 Obtain water. Water temperature should be about 40.5°C. Test the temperature according to centre policy.
12 Lower the bed rail (if used).
13 Put on gloves (if needed).
14 Ask the person to hold a dampened face towel or washcloth over their eyes. It should not cover the person's nose or mouth. (A damp towel or washcloth is easier to hold. It will not slip.)
15 Use the water jug or nozzle to wet the hair.
16 Use a small amount of shampoo.
17 Work up a lather with both hands. Start at the hairline. Work towards the back of the head.
18 Massage the scalp with your fingertips. Do not scratch the scalp with your fingernails.
19 Rinse the hair.
20 Repeat steps 16 to 19.
21 Rinse the hair completely.
22 Apply conditioner. Follow the directions on the container, and ensure hair is rinsed completely.
23 Squeeze water from the person's hair.
24 Cover the hair with a bath towel.
25 Dry the person's face with the towel.
26 Help the person raise their head if appropriate.
27 Rub the hair and scalp with the towel. Use the second towel if the first is wet.
28 Comb hair to remove snarls and tangles.
29 Dry and style the hair as quickly as possible.

Post-procedure

30 Remove and discard the gloves. Wash your hands.
31 Provide for comfort.
32 Place the call bell within reach (if applicable).
33 Clean and return equipment to its proper place. Discard disposable items.
34 Follow centre policy for dirty linen or place in client's laundry basket.
35 Wash your hands.

SHAVING

Many men shave for comfort and mental wellbeing. Some older women with coarse facial hair want it shaved off, but you must ask first if they want any excess hair removed. Younger women usually shave their legs and underarms. Shaving rules are listed in Box 12.4.

Blade or electric shavers are used. Clients are usually required to have their own electric shavers. Most services will require that any electrical devices brought in by clients are to be checked for safety hazards. If the centre's shaver is used, clean it between each use. Follow facility policy.

Safety razors (blade razors) involve razor blades. Razor blades can cause nicks or cuts. Follow Standard Precautions to prevent contact with blood. Clients should have their own safety razors. If not, use disposable razors and make sure that they are disposed of in the sharps containers.

Safety razors are not used on persons who take anticoagulant medications. An **anticoagulant** is a medication that prevents or slows down (*anti*) blood-clotting time (*coagulate*). Bleeding occurs easily and a nick or cut can cause serious bleeding. Electric shavers are used for people taking such medications. They are also safer for clients with dementia (Box 12.5).

Soften the beard and skin before using a safety razor. Apply a warm washcloth or towel to the face for a few minutes. Then lather the face with soap and water or shaving cream.

BOX 12.4
Rules for shaving

- Follow Standard Precautions.
- Use electric shavers for people taking anticoagulant medications. Never use safety razors.
- Protect bed linen. Place a towel under the part being shaved. Or place a towel across the shoulders to protect clothing.
- Soften the skin before shaving.
- Encourage the person to do as much as safely possible.
- Hold the skin taut as needed.
- Shave in the direction of hair growth when shaving the face and underarms.
- Shave up from the ankles when shaving legs. This is against hair growth.
- Do not cut, nick or irritate the skin.
- Rinse the body part completely.
- Apply direct pressure to nicks or cuts.
- Report nicks, cuts or irritation to the nurse at once.

SAFETY ALERT

Shaving

Safety razors are very sharp. Protect the person and yourself from nicks or cuts. Follow Standard Precautions. Discard used razor blades and disposable shavers in a sharps container. Follow centre policy for disposing of sharps. When using electric shavers, follow safety precautions for electrical equipment.

BOX 12.5
Clients with dementia

Safety razors are not used to shave people with dementia. They may not understand what you are doing. They may resist care and move suddenly. This increases the risk of serious nicks and cuts. Electric shavers are safer for these people.

DELEGATION GUIDELINES

Shaving

You need the following information from the care plan when delegated shaving tasks:

- what shaver to use – electric or safety (blade)
- whether the person takes anticoagulant medications
- when to shave the person.

SHAVING A PERSON WITH A SAFETY RAZOR

Many consumer aged care services no longer use safety razors. Check with your supervisor before using a safety razor.

Quality of life

Remember to respect the person's privacy while doing any procedure. Address the person by name and ensure they know your name.

Pre-procedure

1 Follow the delegation guidelines.
2 Explain the procedure to the person.
3 Wash your hands.
4 Collect the following:
   - washbasin
   - bath towel
   - face towel
   - washcloth
   - safety razor
   - mirror
   - shaving cream, soap or lotion
   - shaving brush
   - aftershave lotion (men only)
   - tissues
   - paper towels
   - gloves.
5 Arrange towels and supplies.
6 Call the person by name.
7 Provide for privacy.
8 Raise the bed for body mechanics (if applicable).

Procedure

9 Fill the basin with warm water.
10 Place the basin on the over-bed table.
11 Lower the bed rail near you if up (if applicable).
12 Assist the person into a semi-Fowler's position if allowed or assist the person into the supine position.
13 Adjust lighting to clearly see the person's face.
14 Place the bath towel over the chest.
15 Ensure items are in easy reach.
16 Tighten the razor blade to the razor.
17 Wash the person's face. Do not dry.
18 Wet a washcloth or face towel. Wring it out.
19 Apply the washcloth or towel to the face for a few minutes.
20 Put on gloves.
21 Apply shaving cream with your hands. Or use a shaving brush to apply lather.
22 Hold the skin taut with one hand.
23 Shave in the direction of hair growth (Fig. 12.33). Use shorter strokes around the chin and lips.
24 Rinse the razor often.
25 Apply direct pressure to any bleeding area.
26 Wash off remaining shaving cream or soap. Dry with a towel.
27 Apply aftershave lotion if requested.
28 Remove the towel and gloves. Wash your hands.
29 Move the over-bed table to the side of the bed.

Post-procedure

30 Provide for comfort.
31 Place the call bell within reach (if applicable).
32 Lower the bed to its lowest position (if applicable).
33 Clean and return equipment and supplies to their proper place. Discard disposable items. Wear gloves for this step.
34 Wipe off the over-bed table with the paper towels. Discard paper towels.
35 Position the table for the person.
36 Remove the screens from around the person (if applicable).
37 Follow centre policy for dirty linen or place in person's laundry basket.
38 Wash your hands.
39 Report nicks or bleeding.

Caring for moustaches and beards

Beards and moustaches need daily care. Food can collect in hair, as can mouth and nose drainage. Daily washing and combing are needed. Ask the person how to groom his beard or moustache. Never trim or shave a beard or moustache without the person's consent.

Shaving female legs and underarms

Many women shave their legs and underarms. This practice varies among cultures. Some women shave only the lower legs. Others shave to mid-thigh or the entire leg.

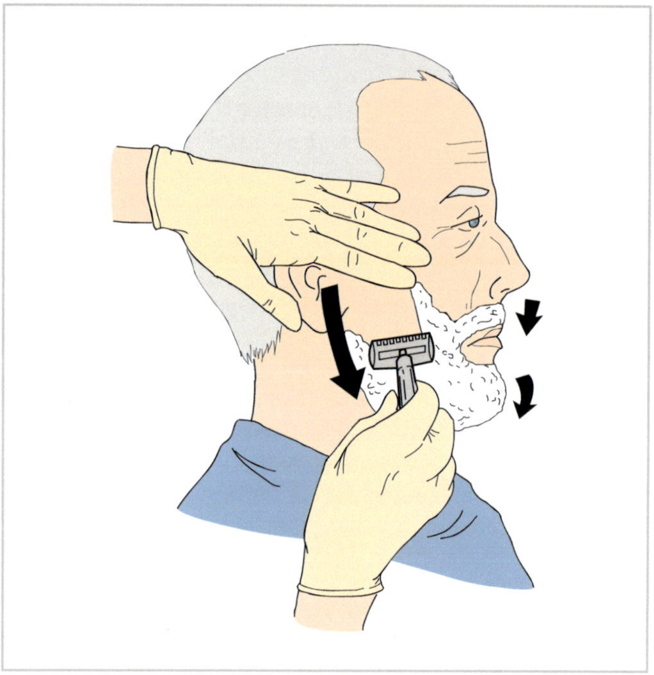

Fig. 12.33
Shave in the direction of hair growth. Use longer strokes on the larger areas of the face. Use short strokes around the chin and lips.

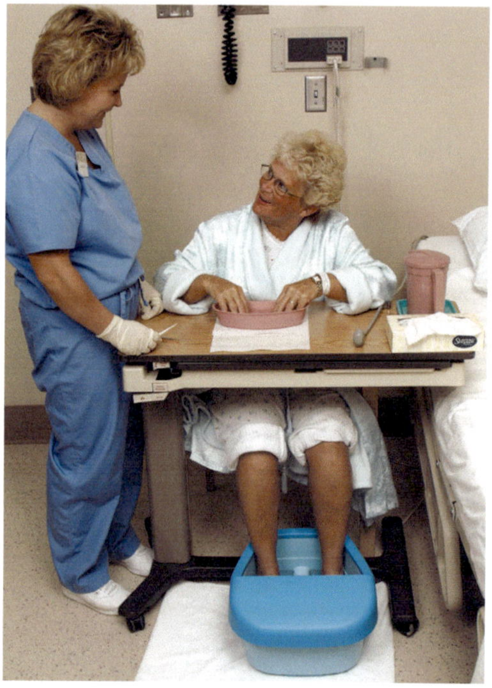

Fig. 12.34
Nail and foot care. The feet soak in a washbasin. The fingers soak in a kidney basin.

Legs and underarms are shaved after bathing because the skin is soft at this time. Soap and water, shaving cream or lotion is used for lather. Collect shaving items with bath items. Use the kidney basin to rinse the razor. Do not use the bath water. The rules in Box 12.4 apply when shaving underarms and legs.

CARE OF NAILS AND FEET

Nail and foot care prevents infection, injury and odours. Hangnails, ingrown nails (nails that grow in at the side) and nails torn away from the skin cause breaks in the skin. Such breaks let microbes enter the body. Long or broken nails can scratch skin or snag clothing.

The feet are easily injured and infected. Dirty feet, socks or stockings can harbour microbes and can also cause foot odours. Shoes and socks provide a warm, moist environment for microbes to grow in. Injuries occur from stubbing toes, stepping on sharp objects or being stepped on. Shoes that fit poorly cause blisters. Shoes that fit properly and have a non-slip sole can help prevent falls and injuries.

Poor circulation prolongs healing. Infections or foot injuries are very serious for older people and those with circulatory disorders. Gangrene and amputation are serious complications. Trimming and clipping toenails can easily cause injuries and cannot be done by care staff, but by trained nursing staff or a podiatrist.

Nails are easier to trim and clean after soaking or bathing (Fig. 12.34). Nail clippers are used to cut fingernails. Never use scissors. Use extreme caution to prevent damage to nearby tissues.

SAFETY ALERT

Nail and foot care

Carers are not to cut or trim toenails, and a patient with any of the following conditions is at risk if toenails are not managed by suitably qualified staff:

- has diabetes
- has poor circulation in the legs and feet
- takes medications that affect blood clotting
- has very thick nails or ingrown toenails.

The registered nurse or a podiatrist cuts toenails and provides foot care for these people.

Remember to check between the toes for cracks and sores. These areas are often overlooked. If left untreated, a serious infection could occur. Breaks in the skin and bleeding can occur. Follow Standard Precautions.

DELEGATION GUIDELINES

Nail and foot care

Before giving nail and foot care, you need the following information from the care plan:

- what water temperature to use.
- how long to soak fingernails and feet (usually 15–20 minutes. However, some people may need to soak for less time as soaking can lead to softening of skin and possible breakdown).
- what observations to report and record:
  - reddened, irritated or calloused areas
  - breaks in the skin
  - corns on top of and between toes
  - very thick nails
  - loose nails.

It is important that that each consumer should have their own nail files and clippers, to prevent cross infection, which are cleaned and stored between use.

GIVING NAIL AND FOOT CARE

Quality of life

Remember to respect the person's privacy while doing any procedure. Address the person by name and ensure they know your name.

Pre-procedure

1. Follow the delegation guidelines.
2. Explain the procedure to the person.
3. Wash your hands.
4. Collect the following:
   - washbasin
   - soap
   - bath towel
   - face towel
   - washcloth
   - bowel or basin
   - nail clippers
   - emery board or nail file
   - lotion or petroleum jelly
   - paper towels
   - disposable bathmat
   - gloves.
5. Arrange paper towels and other items.
6. Call the person by name.
7. Provide for privacy.
8. Assist the person to a chair. Place the call bell within reach (if applicable).

Procedure

9. For foot care, place the bathmat under the person's feet.
10. Fill the wash basin with warm water.
11. Place the basin on the bathmat.
12. Help the person remove shoes and socks.
13. Help the person put their feet into the basin.
14. For hand care adjust the over-bed table in front of the person. Fill the basin.
15. Place the bowl on a stable surface.
16. Put the person's fingers into the basin. Position the arms for comfort.
17. Let the feet and fingernails soak for 15–20 minutes (see Fig. 12.34). Rewarm water as needed.
18. For hand care remove the basin. Dry the hands and between the fingers thoroughly.
19. Put on the gloves.
20. Clean under fingernails.
21. Clip fingernails straight across with nail clippers (Fig. 12.35).
22. Shape nails with an emery board or nail file.
23. Push cuticles back with a washcloth or orange stick (Fig. 12.36).
24. Move the over-bed table to the side.
25. For foot care wash the feet with soap and a washcloth. Wash between the toes.
26. Rinse the feet and between the toes.
27. Remove the feet from the basin. Dry thoroughly, especially between the toes.
28. Apply lotion or petroleum jelly to the tops and soles of the feet. Do not apply between the toes. Warm lotion before applying it.
29. Remove and discard the gloves. Wash your hands.
30. Help the person put on socks and shoes.

Post-procedure

31. Provide for comfort.
32. Place the call bell within reach (if applicable).
33. Clean and return equipment and supplies to their proper places. Discard disposable items. Wear gloves for this step.
34. Remove the screens from around the person.
35. Follow centre policy for soiled linen or place in the client's laundry basket.
36. Wash your hands.
37. Report and record your observations.

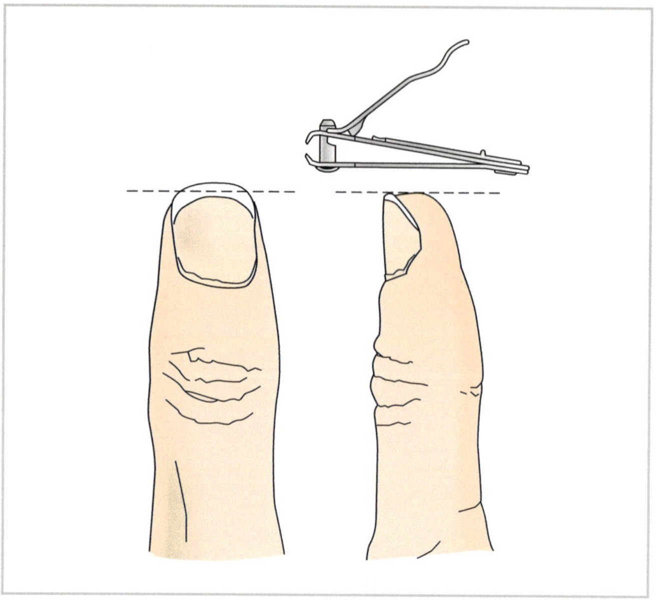

Fig. 12.35
Clip fingernails straight across. Use a nail clipper.

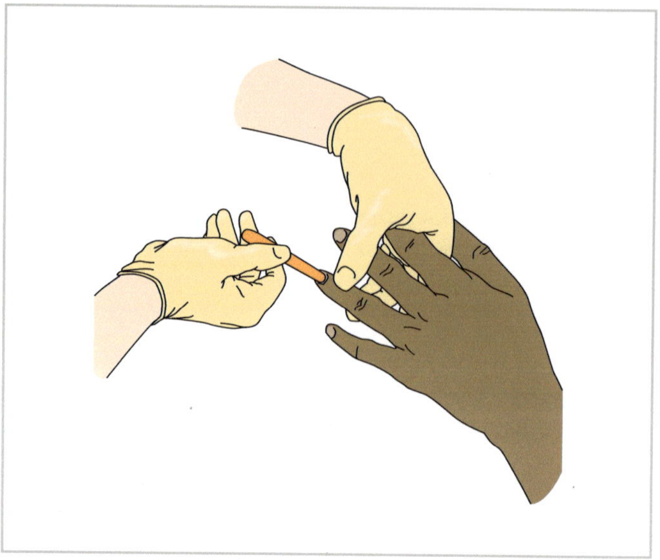

Fig. 12.36
Push the cuticle back with an orange stick.

CHANGING CLOTHING

Dressing and undressing occur at least daily. Clients change from sleepwear into clothing after morning care. They undress and put on sleepwear at bedtime. Incontinent persons may change garments more often. Some people need help dressing and undressing. Changing is easier for those who can move their arms and legs. Arm or leg injuries or paralysis require special measures. Changing clothing has to been done gently, as it is possible to dislocate a shoulder joint when dressing or undressing a client.

Follow these rules when changing clothing:

- Provide for privacy. Do not expose the person.
- Encourage the person to do as much as possible.
- Let the person choose what to wear. Make sure the right undergarments are chosen.
- Remove clothing from the strong side first.
- Put clothing on the weak side first.
- Support the arm or leg when removing or putting on a garment.

UNDRESSING THE PERSON

Quality of life

Remember to respect the person's privacy while doing any procedure. Address the person by name and ensure they know your name.

Pre-procedure

1. Follow the delegation guidelines.
2. Explain the procedure to the person.
3. Practise hand hygiene.
4. Get a bath blanket.
5. Speak to the person by name.
6. Provide for privacy.
7. Lower the bed rail on the person's weak side (if applicable).
8. Position the person supine.
9. Cover the person with the bath blanket. Fan-fold linen to the foot of the bed.

Procedure

10. Remove garments that open at the back.
    - a Raise the head and shoulders or turn the person onto the side away from you.
    - b Undo buttons, zippers, ties or snaps.
    - c Bring the sides of the garment to the person's sides (Fig. 12.37). If they are in a side-lying position, tuck the far side under them (Fig. 12.38). Fold the near side onto their chest.
    - d Position the person supine.
    - e Slide the garment off the shoulder on the strong side (Fig. 12.39). Remove the garment from the arm.
    - f Repeat step 10e for the weak side.
11. Remove garments that open in the front.
    - a Undo buttons, zippers, snaps or ties.
    - b Slide the garment off the shoulder and arm on the strong side.
    - c Raise the person's head and shoulders. Bring the garment over to the weak side (Fig. 12.40). Lower the person's head and shoulders.
    - d Remove the garment from the weak side.
    - e If you cannot raise the person's head and shoulders:
        - i Turn the person towards you. Tuck the removed part under them.
        - ii Turn the person onto the side away from you.

iii Pull the side of the garment out from under the person. Make sure they will not lie on it when supine.

iv Return the person to the supine position.

v Remove the garment from the weak side.

12 Remove pullover garments.

a Undo any buttons, zippers, ties or snaps.

b Remove the garment from the strong side (Fig. 12.41).

c Raise the person's head and shoulders. Or turn them onto the side away from you. Bring the garment up to the neck.

d Remove the garment from the weak side.

e Bring the garment over the person's head.

f Position the person in the supine position.

13 Remove pants or slacks.

a Remove footwear.

b Position the person supine.

c Undo buttons, zippers, ties, snaps or buckles.

d Remove the belt.

e Ask the person to lift their buttocks off the bed. Slide the pants down over their hips and buttocks (Fig. 12.42). Have the person lower their hips and buttocks.

f If the person cannot raise their hips off the bed:

i Turn the person towards you.

ii Slide the pants off their hip and buttock on the strong side (Fig. 12.43).

iii Turn the person away from you.

iv Slide the pants off the hip and buttock on the weak side (Fig. 12.44).

g Slide the pants down the legs and over the feet.

14 Dress the person.

15 Help the person get out of bed if they are to be up. If the person is to stay in bed:

a Cover the person and remove the bath blanket.

b Provide for comfort.

c Lower the bed to its lowest position.

Post-procedure

16 Place the call bell within reach.

17 Remove the screens from around the person.

18 Follow centre policy for dirty linen or place in the client's laundry basket.

19 Wash your hands.

20 Report and record your observations.

DELEGATION GUIDELINES

Dressing and undressing

Before assisting a person with dressing and undressing, you need the following information from the care plan:

- how much help the person needs
- whether the person needs to wear certain garments
- what observations to report and record:
  - how much help was given
  - how the person tolerated the procedure
  - any client complaints.

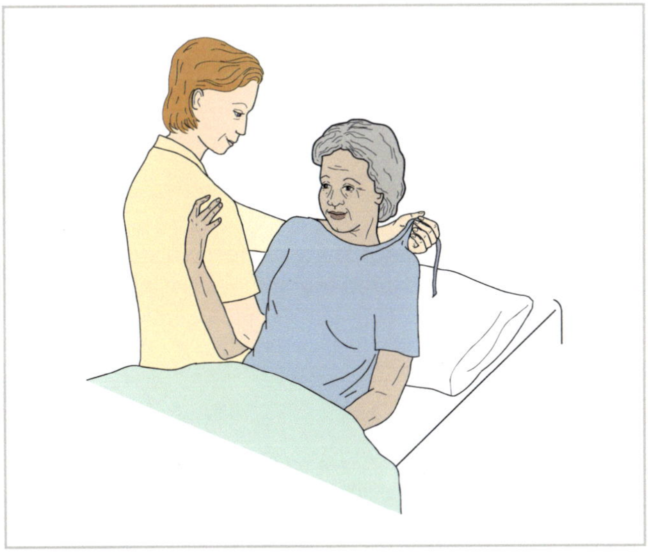

Fig. 12.37

The sides of the garments are brought from the back to the sides of the person.

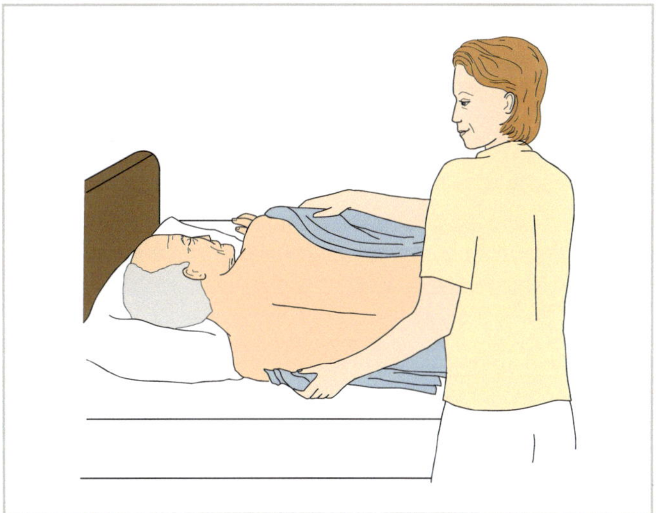

Fig. 12.38

A garment that opens at the back is removed from the person in the side-lying position. The far side of the garment is tucked under the person. The near side is folded onto their chest.

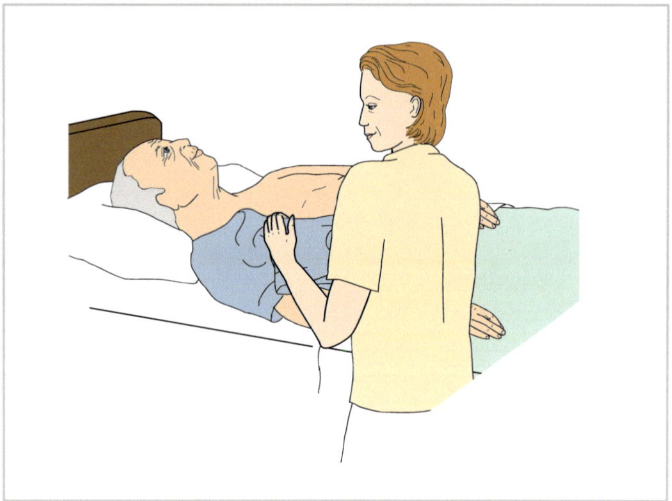

Fig. 12.39
The garment is slid off the shoulder on the person's strong side.

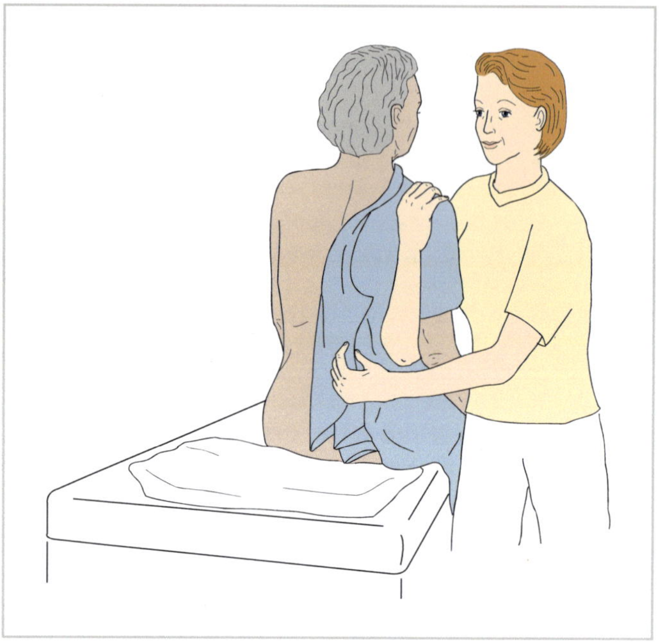

Fig. 12.40
A front-opening garment is removed with the person's head and shoulders raised. The garment is removed from the strong side first. Then it is brought around the back to the weak side.

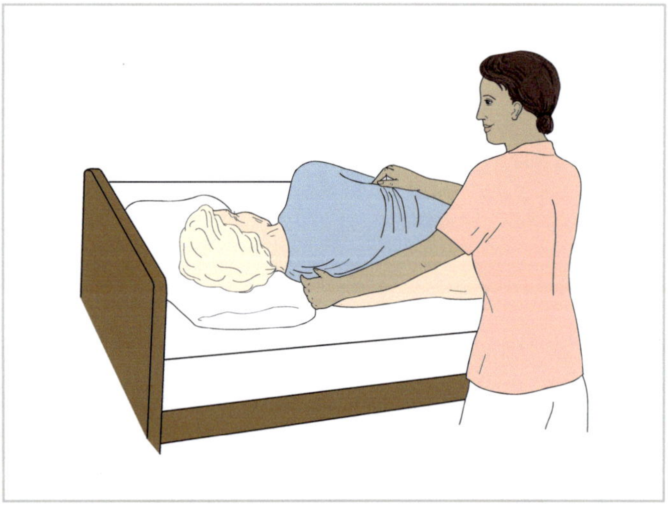

Fig. 12.41
A pullover garment is removed from the strong side first. Then the garment is brought up the person's neck so it can be removed from the weak side.

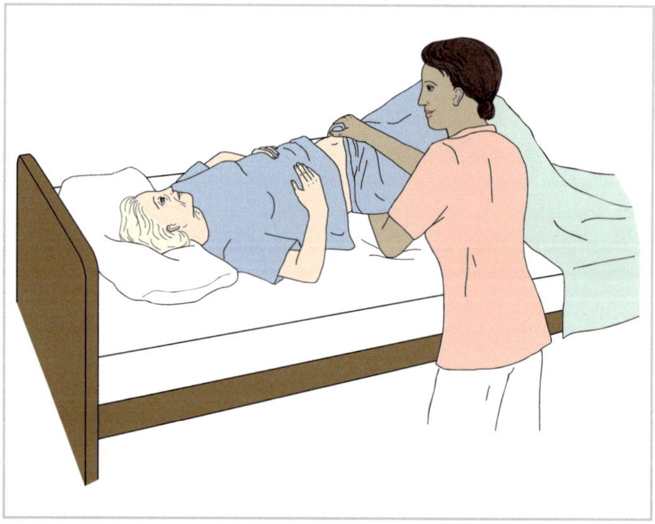

Fig. 12.42
The person lifts their hips and buttocks for removing the pants. The pants are slid down over the hips and buttocks.

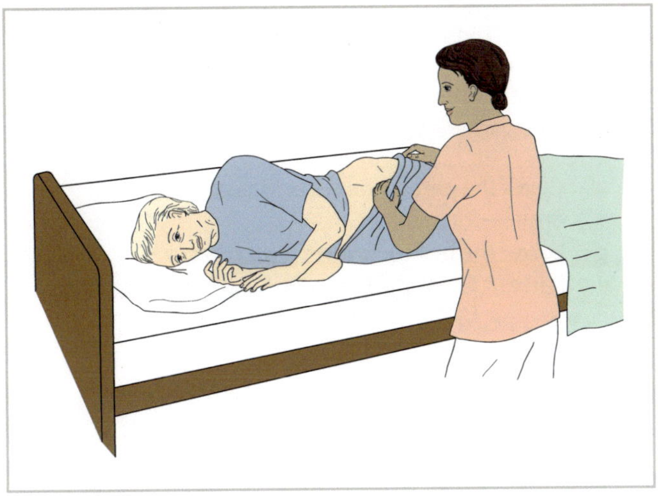

Fig. 12.43
Pants are removed in the side-lying position. They are removed from the strong side first. They are slid over the hips and buttocks.

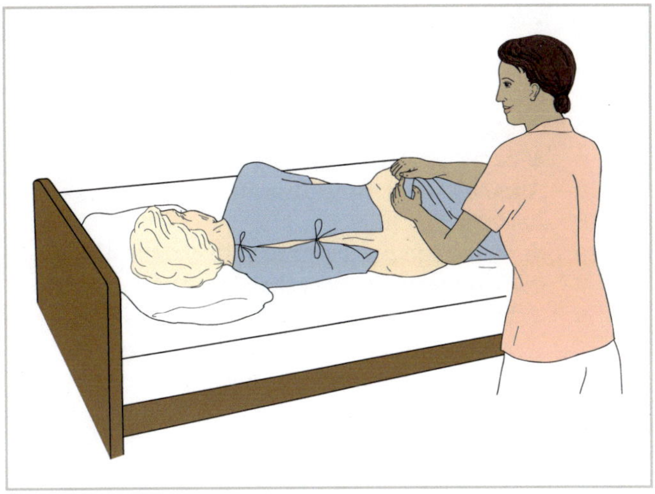

Fig. 12.44
The person is turned onto the other side. The pants are removed from the weak side.

DRESSING THE PERSON

Quality of life

Remember to respect the person's privacy while doing any procedure. Address the person by name and ensure they know your name.

Pre-procedure

1 Follow the delegation guidelines.
2 Explain the procedure to the person.
3 Practise hand hygiene.
4 Get a bath blanket and the clothing requested by the person.
5 Speak to the person by name.
6 Provide for privacy.
7 Undress the person.
8 Position the person supine.

Procedure

9 Cover the person with the bath blanket. Fan-fold linen to the foot of the bed.
10 Put on garments that open at the back (Fig. 12.45):
- a Slide the garment onto the arm and shoulder of the weak side.
- b Slide the garment onto the arm and shoulder of the strong side.
- c Raise the person's head and shoulders.
- d Bring the sides of the garment to the back.
- e If the person is in a side-lying position:
  - i Turn the person towards you.
  - ii Bring the side of the garment to the person's back.
  - iii Turn the person away from you.
  - iv Bring the other side of the garment to the person's back.
- f Fasten buttons, snaps, ties or zippers.
- g Position the person supine.

11 Put on garments that open at the front:
- a Slide the garment onto the arm and shoulder on the weak side.
- b Raise the head and shoulders. Bring the side of the garment around to the back. Lie the person down. Slide the garment onto the arm and shoulder of the strong arm.
- c If the person cannot raise their head and shoulders:
  - i Turn the person towards you.
  - ii Tuck the garment under the person.
  - iii Turn the person away from you.
  - iv Pull the garment out from under the person.
  - v Turn the person back to the supine position.
  - vi Slide the garment over the arm and shoulder of the strong arm.
- d Fasten buttons, snaps, ties or zippers.

12 Put on pullover garments:
- a Position the person supine.
- b Bring the neck of the garment over the head.
- c Slide the arm and shoulder of the garment onto the weak side.
- d Raise the person's head and shoulders.
- e Bring the garment down.
- f Slide the arm and shoulder of the garment onto the strong side.
- g If the person cannot assume a semi-sitting position:
  - i Turn the person towards you.
  - ii Tuck the garment under the person.
  - iii Turn the person away from you.
  - iv Pull the garment out from under the person.
  - v Position the person supine.

  vi Slide the arm and shoulder of the garment onto the strong side.

 h Fasten buttons, snaps, ties or zippers.

13 Put on pants or slacks:

 a Slide the pants over the feet and up the legs.
 b Ask the person to raise their hips and buttocks off the bed.
 c Bring the pants up over the buttocks and hips.
 d Ask the person to lower their hips and buttocks.
 e If the person cannot raise their hips and buttocks:
  i Turn the person onto the strong side.
  ii Pull the pants over the buttock and hip on the weak side.
  iii Turn the person onto their weak side.
  iv Pull the pants over the buttock and hip on the strong side.
  v Position the person supine.
 f Fasten buttons, ties, snaps, the zipper and belt buckle.

14 Put socks and footwear on the person.

15 Help the person get out of bed. If the person is to stay in bed:

 a Cover the person. Remove the bath blanket.
 b Provide for comfort.
 c Lower the bed to its lowest position.
 d Raise or lower the bed rails. Follow the care plan.

Post-procedure

16 Place the call bell within reach.

17 Remove the screens from around the person.

18 Follow centre policy for dirty linen or place in the client's laundry basket.

19 Wash your hands.

20 Report and record your observations.

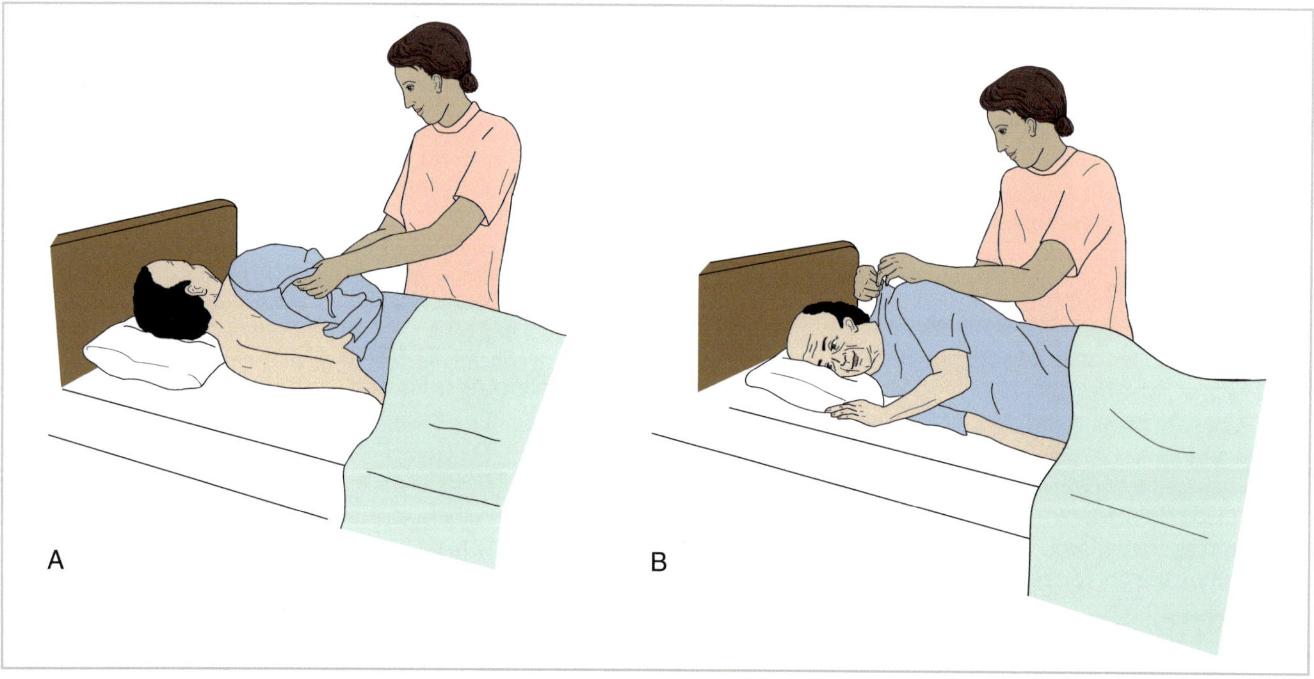

Fig. 12.45

Putting on garments that open at the back.

A. The side-lying position can be used. Turn the person towards you after the garment is put on the arms. The side of the garment is brought to the person's back. **B.** Then turn the person away from you. The other side of the garment is brought to the back and fastened.

ASSISTING WITH BOWEL EVACUATION AND MANAGEMENT

After reading this section, you should be able to:

- understand the normal pattern and frequency of bowel movements
- know what to observe about bowel movements
- understand factors affecting bowel evacuation
- understand the care required for faecal incontinence
- understand common bowel evacuation problems

- know how to promote comfort and safety during defecation
- understand the purpose of bowel training
- know why enemas are given
- know the common enema solutions
- know the rules for administering enemas
- understand how to care for a person with an ostomy
- understand why stool specimens are collected.

Bowel evacuation is a basic physical need. It is the excretion of wastes from the gastrointestinal system. Many factors affect bowel evacuation. They include privacy, personal habits, age, diet, exercise and activity, fluids and medications. Problems occur easily. Promoting normal bowel evacuation is important. You will assist people in meeting their evacuation needs.

NORMAL BOWEL MOVEMENTS

Foods and fluids are partially digested in the stomach. The partially digested foods and fluids are called *chyme*. Chyme passes from the stomach into the small intestine. Then it enters the large intestine (large bowel or colon), where fluid is absorbed. Chyme becomes less fluid and more solid in consistency. Faeces are the semisolid mass of waste products in the colon.

Faeces move through the intestines by *peristalsis*, the alternating contraction and relaxation of intestinal muscles. Faeces move through the large bowel to the rectum. Faeces are stored in the rectum until excreted from the body. **Defecation** (bowel movement) is the process of excreting faeces from the rectum through the anus. *Stool* is the term for excreted faeces.

Some people have a bowel movement every day or once a week, while others have one every two to three days. Some people have two or three bowel movements a day. Many people defecate after breakfast. Others do so in the evening. Many older people expect a bowel movement every day and the slightest irregularity concerns them.

Stools are normally brown. Bleeding in the stomach and small intestine causes black or tarry stools, called melaena. Bleeding in the lower colon and rectum causes red-coloured stools, as does beetroot. A diet high in green vegetables can cause green stools. Diseases and infection can cause clay-coloured or white, pale, orange or green-coloured stools.

Stools are normally soft, formed, moist and shaped like the rectum. They have a normal odour, which is from bacterial action in the intestines. Certain foods and medications also cause odours.

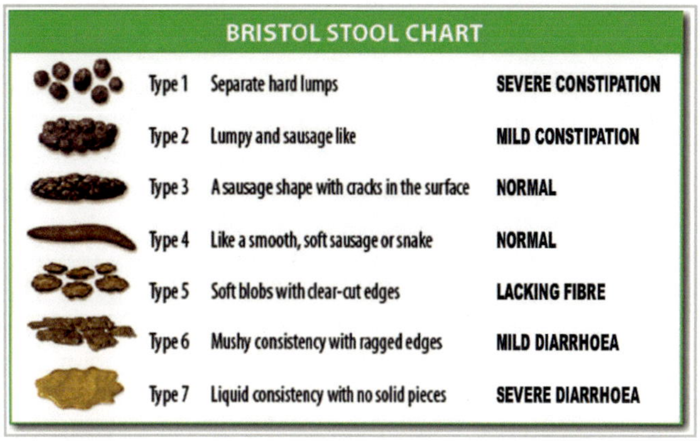

Fig. 12.46
The Bristol Stool Chart is a common method used to describe bowel movements.

Observations

Carefully observe stools before disposing of them. Ask your supervisor or the nurse to inspect any stools that concern you. Observe and report the following:

- colour
- amount
- consistency
- odour
- shape
- size
- frequency of defecation
- complaints of pain or discomfort.

A monthly bowel chart such as the Bristol Stool chart is commonly used to chart bowel movements (Fig. 12.46).

Factors affecting bowel evacuation

The following factors affect the frequency, consistency, colour and odour of stools. The nurse considers these factors when using the nursing process to meet the person's evacuation needs. Normal, regular evacuation is the goal.

- *Privacy* – bowel evacuation is a private act. Odours and sounds are embarrassing. Lack of privacy can prevent defecation, despite having the urge. Imagine using a bedpan or commode in a semi-private room. Some people ignore the urge to defecate when others are present.
- *Personal habits* – many people have a bowel movement after breakfast. Some drink a hot beverage, read or take a walk. These activities are relaxing. Defecation is easier when a person is relaxed, not tense.
- *Diet* – a well-balanced diet and bulk are needed. High-fibre foods leave a residue for needed bulk. Fruits, vegetables and wholegrain cereals and breads are high in fibre. Many older people do not eat enough fruits and vegetables. Some do not have teeth, or have dentures that fit poorly. Therefore, they cannot chew these foods. Some people think that they cannot digest fruits and vegetables, so they refuse to eat them. Often bran is added to cereal, or prunes or prune juice are given in aged care services. These foods provide fibre and help

prevent constipation. Milk causes constipation in some people and diarrhoea in others. Chocolate and other foods cause similar reactions. Wind-forming foods stimulate peristalsis, which aids defecation. Wind-forming foods include onions, beans, cabbage, cauliflower, radishes and cucumbers. Older people often avoid wind-forming foods. Wind may cause 'stomach aches' or 'bloating'.

- *Fluids* – faeces contain water. Stool consistency depends on the amount of water absorbed in the colon. The amount of fluid ingested, urine output and vomiting are factors. Faeces harden and dry when large amounts of water are absorbed or when fluid intake is poor. Hard, dry faeces move slowly through the colon and constipation can occur. Drinking six to eight glasses of water daily promotes normal bowel evacuation. Warm fluids, coffee, tea, cider and warm water increase peristalsis.
- *Activity* – exercise and activity maintain muscle tone and stimulate peristalsis. Irregular evacuation and constipation often occur after inactivity and bed rest. Inactivity may result from disease, surgery, injury and ageing.
- *Medications* – medications can prevent constipation or control diarrhoea. Other medications have diarrhoea or constipation as side-effects. Medications for pain relief often cause constipation. Antibiotics (used to fight or prevent infection) often cause diarrhoea. Diarrhoea occurs when the antibiotics kill normal flora in the colon. Normal flora is needed to form stools.
- *Ageing* – with ageing, faeces pass through the intestines at a slower rate, and constipation results. Some people lose bowel control. Older people may not completely empty the rectum. They often need to defecate again about 30–45 minutes after the first bowel movement.
- *Disability* – some people cannot control bowel movements and they defecate whenever faeces enter the rectum. In this case, a bowel training program is needed. The goal is to have a bowel movement at the same time each day. This keeps the rectum empty and prevents faecal incontinence.

Comfort and safety

The care plan will outline how to meet the person's evacuation needs. The care plan may involve diet, fluids and exercise. The actions in Box 12.6 are practised routinely. They promote comfort and safety during bowel evacuation.

CARING ABOUT CULTURE

Be aware that specific routines must be followed within some cultures in relation to elimination. Always check with your client how they manage their normal elimination functions.

BOX 12.6
Comfort and safety during bowel evacuation

- Assist the person to the toilet or commode or provide the bedpan as soon as requested.
- Wheel the person into the bathroom on the commode if possible. Place the commode over the toilet. This provides privacy.
- Provide for privacy. Ask visitors to leave the room.
- Close doors; pull privacy curtains and close window curtains, blinds or shades.
- If used, make sure the bedpan is warm.
- Position the person in a normal sitting or squatting position.
- Cover the person for warmth and privacy. Allow enough time for defecation. Place the call bell and toilet paper within the person's reach.
- Stay nearby if the person is weak or unsteady. Leave the room if the person can be alone. Provide perineal care if required.
- Dispose of faeces promptly. This reduces odours and prevents the spread of microbes.
- Assist the person with handwashing after evacuation.
- Follow the person's care plan if they have faecal incontinence. The care plan tells you when to assist with evacuation.
- Follow Standard Precautions and blood-borne pathogen standards.

COMMON PROBLEMS

Common problems include constipation, faecal impaction, diarrhoea, faecal incontinence and flatulence.

Constipation

Constipation is the passage of a hard, dry stool. The person usually strains to have a bowel movement. Stools are large or marble sized. Large stools cause pain as they pass through the anus. Constipation occurs when faeces move slowly through the bowel. This allows more time for water absorption. Common causes include a low-fibre diet, ignoring the urge to defecate, decreased fluid intake, inactivity, medications, ageing and certain diseases. Dietary changes, fluids and activity prevent or relieve constipation, along with medications and enemas.

Faecal impaction

Faecal impaction is the prolonged retention and build-up of faeces in the rectum. Faeces are hard or like putty. Faecal impaction results if constipation is not relieved. The person cannot defecate. More water is absorbed from already hard faeces. Liquid faeces pass around the hardened faecal mass in the rectum and seep from the anus.

The person tries many times to have a bowel movement. Abdominal discomfort, nausea and rectal pain are common. Older people may also have poor appetite or mental confusion. Report these signs and symptoms to your supervisor or the nurse.

A nurse or doctor may do a digital (finger) examination to check for an impaction. A lubricated, gloved finger is inserted into the rectum and feels for a hard mass (Fig. 12.47).

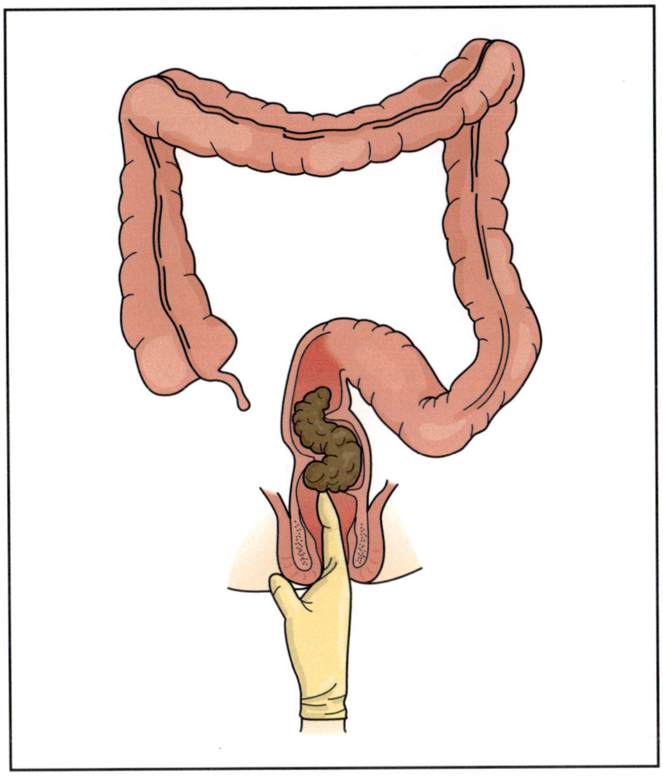

Fig. 12.47
An index finger is used to check for a faecal impaction.

The mass is felt in the lower rectum. Sometimes it is higher in the colon and out of reach. The digital examination often causes the urge to defecate. The doctor may order medications and enemas to remove the impaction. Sometimes the faecal mass is removed with a gloved finger. This is called digital removal of an impaction and must never be performed by the untrained person, as damage can easily occur to the rectal walls. Only a registered nurse or doctor does this procedure, as there are risks to the client.

Diarrhoea

Diarrhoea is the frequent passage of liquid stools. Faeces move through the intestines rapidly. This reduces the time for fluid absorption. The need to defecate is urgent and some people cannot get to a toilet in time. Abdominal cramping, nausea and vomiting may occur.

Causes include infections, some medications, irritating foods and microbes in food and water. Diet or medications reduce peristalsis. You need to do the following:

- Assist with evacuation needs promptly.
- Dispose of stools promptly. This prevents odours and the spread of microbes.
- Give good skin care. Liquid faeces irritate the skin. So does frequent wiping with toilet paper. Skin breakdown and pressure ulcers are risks.
- Replace lost fluids. Otherwise, dehydration occurs. Dehydration is the excessive loss of water from tissues. The person has pale or flushed skin, dry skin, coated tongue and **oliguria** (scant amount of urine). Thirst, weakness, dizziness and confusion also occur. Falling blood pressure and increased pulse and respirations are serious signs. Death can occur. The doctor orders intravenous or subcutaneous fluids in severe cases.

Microbes often cause diarrhoea. Preventing the spread of infection is important. Always practise Standard Precautions when in contact with stools.

Death is a risk from unrecognised and untreated dehydration. The amount of water in the body decreases with ageing. Therefore, diarrhoea is very serious in older people. Report any signs of diarrhoea to the nurse or your supervisor at once. Ask the nurse to observe the stool.

Faecal incontinence

Faecal incontinence (**anal incontinence**) is the inability to control the passage of faeces and wind through the anus. Causes include:

- intestinal diseases
- nervous system diseases and injuries
- faecal impaction
- diarrhoea
- some medications
- chronic illness
- ageing
- mental health problems or dementia – the person may not recognise the need or act of defecating (Box 12.7)
- unanswered call bells when help is needed with evacuation
- not being able to find the toilet when in a new setting.

Faecal incontinence affects the person emotionally. Frustration, embarrassment, anger and humiliation are common emotions. The person may need:

- bowel training
- assistance to establish a routine evacuation using enemas or suppositories
- good skin care
- incontinence products to keep garments and linen clean.

BOX 12.7
Clients with dementia

People with dementia may smear faeces on themselves, or on furniture and walls. A detailed history is required from family so this type of behaviour is known, and a regular toileting program can be planned to minimise problems. They may also resist caregivers' efforts to keep them clean. This can be a very distressing part of care for the family of those with dementia, whether in a consumer or home setting. Family need help to manage faecal incontinence. Use the same approach for people with dementia as for those who are incontinent of urine. Be patient and follow the care plan. Ask for help from co-workers. If you have questions, ask your supervisor or the nurse.

Incontinence products

Incontinence products are primarily aimed to manage urinary incontinence. They are, therefore, not seen as wholly dependable for people with faecal incontinence. However, the products designed for heavy urinary incontinence are most commonly used.

A number of faecal collectors are available on the market. These can be applied to the skin around the anus to collect faecal seepage. However, they are not commonly used and can be difficult for the older person to apply correctly.

Flatulence

Gas and air are normally found in the stomach and intestines. They are expelled through the mouth (belching, eructating) and anus. Gas and air passed through the anus is called flatus. Flatulence is the excessive formation of gas or air in the stomach and intestines. Common causes are:

- swallowing air while eating and drinking – this includes chewing gum, eating fast, drinking through a straw and drinking carbonated beverages; tense or anxious people may swallow large amounts of air when drinking
- bacterial action in the intestines
- gas-forming foods (onions, beans, cabbage, cauliflower, radishes and cucumbers)
- constipation
- bowel and abdominal surgery
- medications that decrease peristalsis.

If flatus is not expelled, the intestines distend. That is, they swell or enlarge from the pressure of the gases. Abdominal cramping or pain, shortness of breath and a swollen abdomen occur. 'Bloating' is a common complaint. Exercise, walking, moving in bed and the left side-lying position often produce flatus. Doctors may order enemas, medications or rectal tubes to relieve flatulence.

BOWEL TRAINING

Bowel training has two goals:

- to gain control of bowel movements
- to develop a regular pattern of evacuation. Faecal impaction, constipation and faecal incontinence are prevented.

Meals, particularly breakfast, stimulate the urge to defecate. The person's usual time of day for a bowel movement is noted on the care plan. Toilet, commode or bedpan use is offered at this time. Factors that promote evacuation are part of the care plan and bowel training program. These include a high-fibre diet, increased fluids, warm fluids, activity and privacy. The nurse tells you about a person's bowel training program.

The doctor or nurse may order a suppository to stimulate defecation. This is only used if oral aperients have not worked. A suppository is a cone-shaped, solid medication that is inserted into a body opening. It melts at body temperature. The rectal suppository is inserted into the rectum (Fig. 12.48) (wrapper from suppository must be removed prior to insertion of suppository). You must never give a suppository unless you have been trained to do so and have checked the relevant policies of your facility. A bowel movement will occur about 30 minutes later.

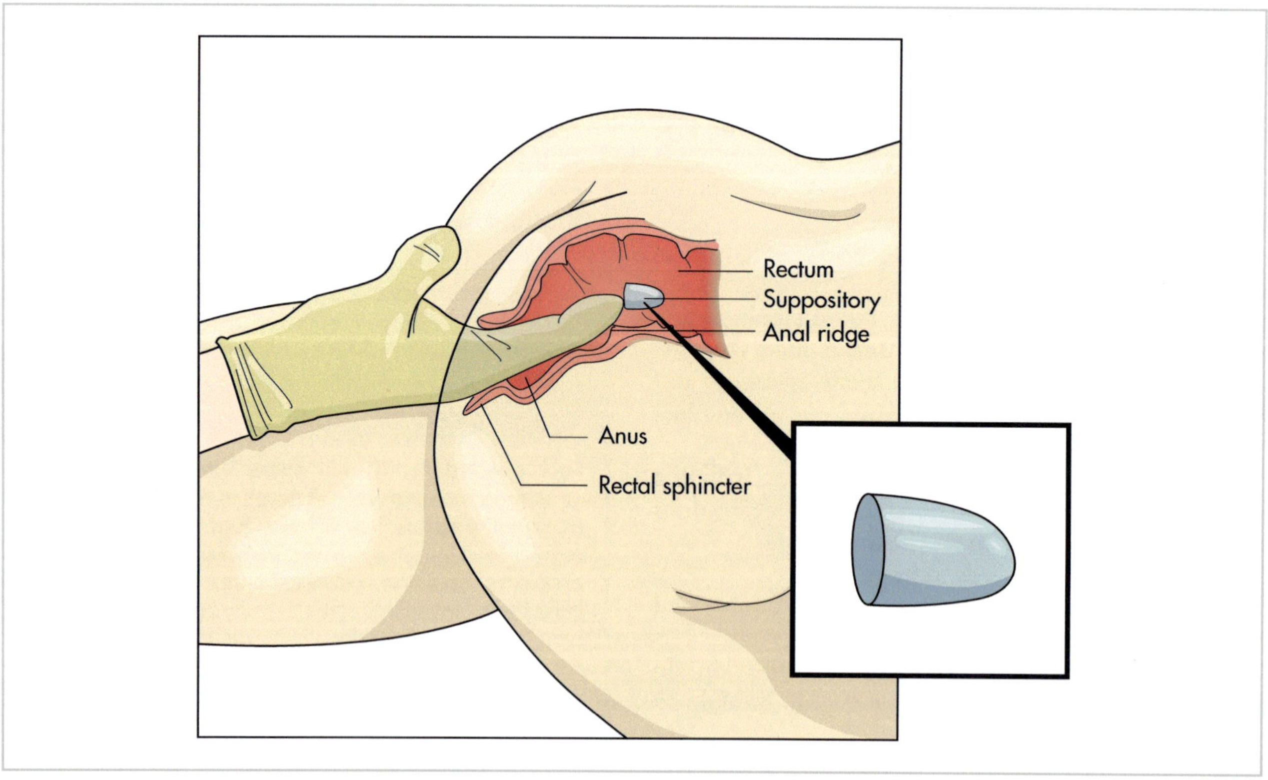

Fig. 12.48
The suppository (inset) is inserted into the rectum.

Enemas

An **enema** is the introduction of fluid into the rectum and lower colon. Doctors and nurses order enemas to:

- remove faeces
- relieve constipation, faecal impaction and flatulence
- clean the bowel of faeces before certain types of surgery and diagnostic procedures.

Comfort and safety measures are practised when giving an enema. Most enemas are commercially prepared. It is rare for any other type to be ordered.

The commercial enema

Commercial enemas are also called small volume or disposable enemas. They irritate and distend the rectum. This causes defecation. They are often ordered for constipation or when the bowel does not need complete cleansing.

The commercial enema is ready to give. The solution is usually given at room temperature. To give the enema, squeeze and roll up the plastic bottle from the bottom. Do not release pressure on the bottle. Otherwise, solution is drawn from the rectum back into the bottle.

Encourage the person to retain the solution until there is an urge to defecate. It usually takes 5–12 minutes for the enema to take effect. Remaining in the modified left lateral recumbent position or left side-lying position helps retain the enema longer.

DELEGATION GUIDELINES

Enemas and suppositories

Some services will allow carers to give enemas. Others do not. When giving a suppository, or an enema is delegated to you, make sure that:

- your facility allows you to perform the procedure
- the procedure is in your job description
- you have the necessary education and training
- you review the procedure with the nurse
- a nurse is available to answer questions and to supervise you.

If the above conditions are met, you need the following information from the nurse before giving a suppository or an enema:

- what type of suppository/enema to give
- what time to give it
- how many times to give it
- how to position the person – in modified left lateral recumbent position or the left side-lying position
- how far to insert the suppository or enema nozzle – usually the length of an average index finger
- how long the person should try to retain the enema
- what to report and record (Fig. 12.49).

Date	Time	
8/7/22	1700	750 mL tap water enema given with the resident in the (L) side-lying position.
		The resident was asked to retain the enema for at least 15 minutes. Bed in low
		position. Call bell within reach. No resident complaints at this time. Resident
		informed that I would return in 15 minutes or when the call bell was used.
		Angie Martinez, EN
	1715	Assisted resident to the bedside commode. Privacy curtain pulled. Call bell and
		toilet tissue within reach. Resident reminded to call when finished expelling the
		enema or if she needs assistance. Angie Martinez, EN
	1722	Resident assisted from the commode to bed. Assisted with perineal care and hand-
		washing. States she feels tired. Denies pain or discomfort. Positioned in semi-
		Fowler's position. Bed in low position. Call bell within reach. Large amt. soft,
		brown stool emptied from the commode. No unusual odour noted. Mary Smith, RN
		asked to observe results. Angie Martinez, EN

Fig. 12.49
Charting sample.

SAFETY ALERT

Enemas and suppositories

Giving a suppository or an enema is usually a safe procedure. Many people give them to themselves at home. However, enemas present dangers for older people and those with certain heart and kidney diseases.

Contact with stools is likely when giving enemas. They may contain microbes and blood. Follow Standard Precautions.

GIVING A COMMERCIAL ENEMA

Quality of life

Remember to respect the person's privacy while doing any procedure. Address the person by name and ensure they know your name.

Pre-procedure

1. Follow the delegation guidelines.
2. Explain the procedure to the person.
3. Wash your hands.
4. Collect the following:
   - commercial enema
   - bedpan or commode
   - waterproof pad
   - toilet paper
   - gloves
   - robe and non-skid footwear
   - bath blanket.
5. Call the person by name.
6. Provide for privacy.

Procedure

7. Cover the person with a bath blanket. Fan-fold top linen to the foot of the bed.
8. Position the person in the modified left lateral recumbent position or left side-lying position.
9. Put on the gloves.
10. Place the waterproof pad under the person's buttocks.
11. Expose the anal area.
12. Position the bedpan near the person.
13. Remove the cap from the enema tip.
14. Separate the buttocks to see the anus.
15. Ask the person to take a deep breath through the mouth.
16. Insert the enema tip the length of an average index finger into the rectum. Do this when the person is exhaling. Insert the tip gently (Fig. 12.50). Stop if the person complains of pain, if you feel resistance or if bleeding occurs.
17. Squeeze and roll the bottle gently. Release pressure on the bottle after removing the tip from the rectum.
18. Put the bottle into the box (tip first).
19. Help the person onto the bedpan; raise the head of the bed. Or assist the person to the toilet or commode. The person wears a robe and non-skid footwear when up. The bed is in the lowest position.
20. Place the call bell and toilet paper within reach. Remind the person not to flush the toilet.
21. Discard disposable items.
22. Remove the gloves and wash your hands.
23. Leave the room if the person can be alone.
24. Return when the person signals. Knock before entering. Wash your hands and lower bed rail, if up.
25. Put on gloves.
26. Observe enema results for amount, colour, consistency and odour.
27. Help the person clean the perineal area.
28. Remove the bed protector.
29. Empty, clean and disinfect the bedpan or commode. Flush the toilet after you have observed the results.
30. Return equipment to its proper place.
31. Remove the gloves and wash your hands.
32. Assist the person with handwashing. Wear gloves if necessary.
33. Return top linen. Remove the bath blanket.

Post-procedure

34. Provide for comfort.
35. Place the call bell within reach.
36. Lower the bed to its lowest position.
37. Remove the screens from around the person.
38. Follow organisational policy for soiled linen and used supplies. Wear gloves for this step.
39. Decontaminate your hands.
40. Report and record your observations.

THE PERSON WITH AN OSTOMY

Sometimes part of the intestines is surgically removed. Common causes include cancer, bowel diseases and trauma (stab or bullet wounds). An ostomy is sometimes necessary. An ostomy is the surgical creation of an artificial opening. The opening is called a *stoma*. The person wears a bag over the stoma to collect faeces and flatus. Stomas do not have nerve endings. Therefore, they are not painful. You will not hurt the person when touching the stoma.

Colostomy

A **colostomy** is a surgically created opening (*stomy*) between the colon (*colo*) and the abdominal wall. Part of the

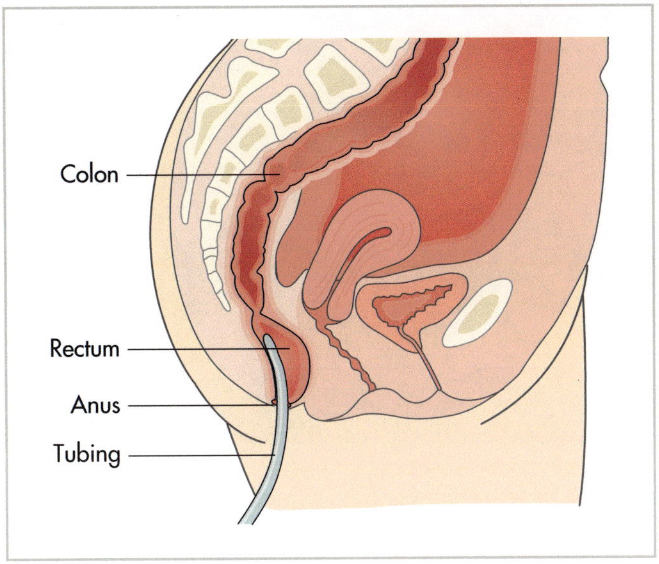

Fig. 12.50
The commercial enema tip is inserted 5 cm into the rectum.

colon is brought out onto the abdominal wall and a stoma made. Faeces and flatus pass through the stoma, not the anus. With a permanent colostomy, the diseased part of the colon is removed. A temporary colostomy gives the diseased or injured bowel time to heal. After healing, the bowel is reconnected by surgery.

The colostomy site (Fig. 12.51) depends on the site of disease or injury. Stool consistency depends on the colostomy site. Stools are liquid to formed. The more colon remaining to absorb water, the more solid and formed the stool. If the colostomy is near the start of the colon, stools are liquid. A colostomy near the end of the colon results in formed stools.

Faeces irritate the skin. Skin care prevents skin breakdown around the stoma. First, the skin is washed and dried. Then a skin barrier is applied around the stoma. It prevents faeces from having contact with the skin. The skin barrier is part of the bag or a separate device.

Ileostomy

An ileostomy is a surgically created opening (*stomy*) between the ileum (small intestine, *ileo*) and the abdominal

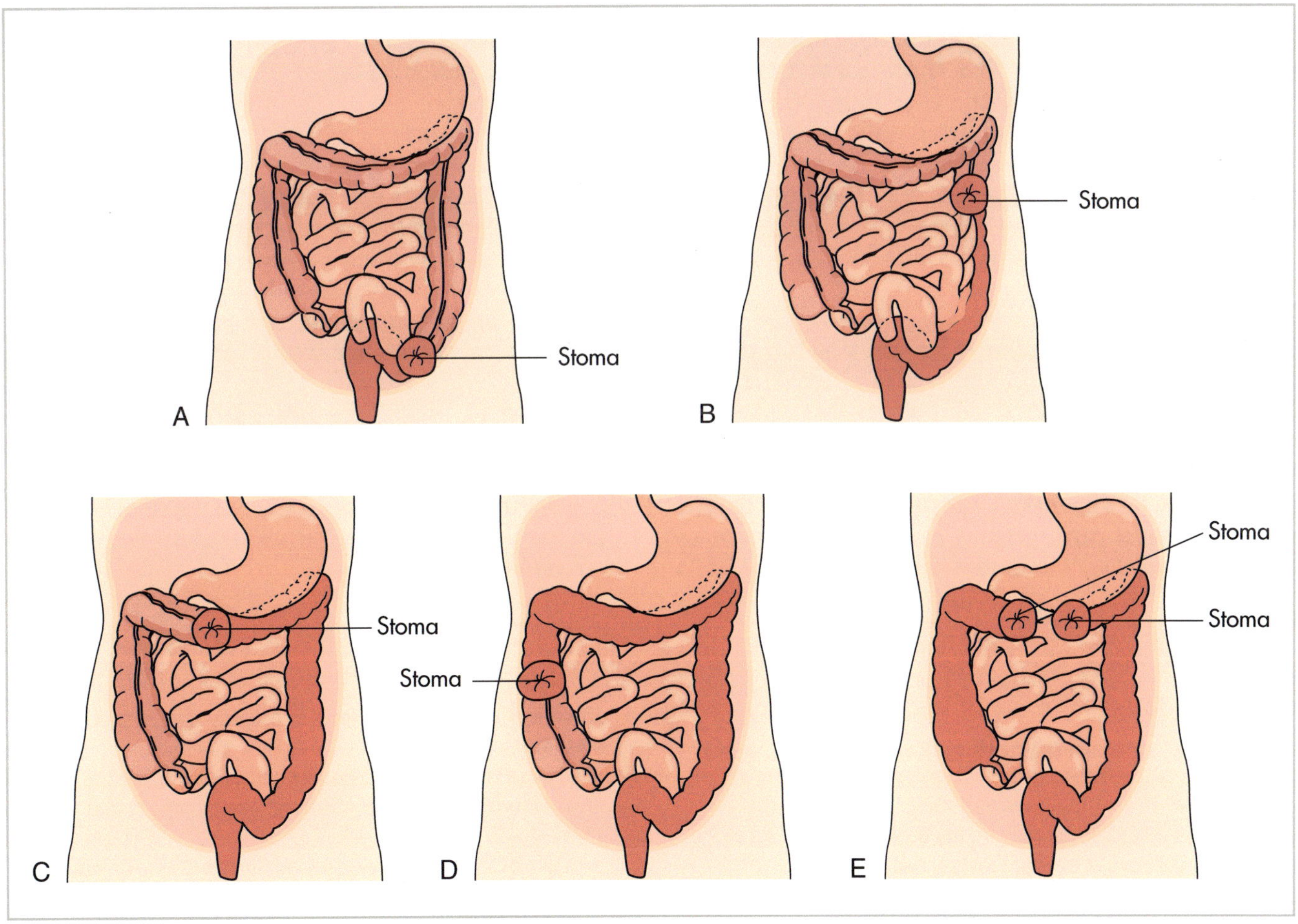

Fig. 12.51
Colostomy sites. Shading shows the part of the bowel that was surgically removed. **A.** Sigmoid colostomy. **B.** Descending colostomy. **C.** Transverse colostomy. **D.** Ascending colostomy. **E.** Double-barrel colostomy. Two stomas are created: one allows for the excretion of faeces. The other is for the introduction of medicine for bowel healing. This type is usually temporary.

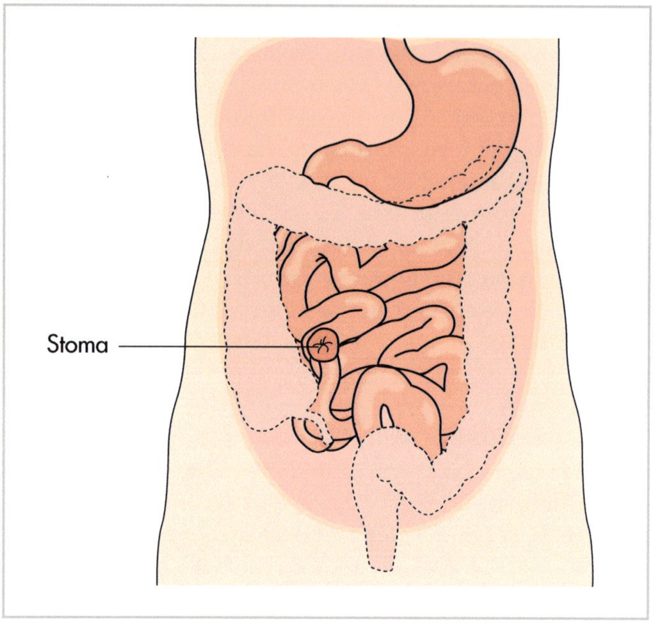

Fig. 12.52
An ileostomy. The entire large intestine is surgically removed.

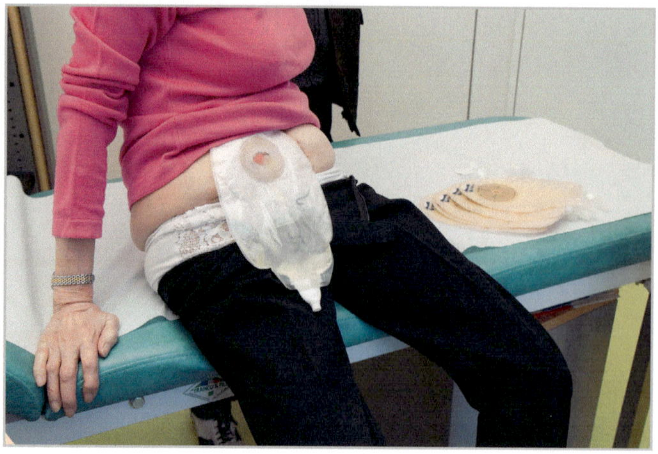

Fig. 12.53
Many types of ostomy bags are available.

wall. Part of the ileum is brought out onto the abdominal wall and a stoma made. The entire colon is removed (Fig. 12.52). Liquid faeces drain constantly from an ileostomy. Water is not absorbed because the colon has been removed. Faeces in the small intestine contain digestive juices that are very irritating to the skin. The ileostomy bag must fit well.

Faeces must not touch the skin. Good skin care is required.

Ostomy bags

The ostomy bag has an adhesive backing that is applied to the skin. Sometimes bags are secured to ostomy belts. Many bags have a drain at the bottom that closes with clips, clamps or wire closures. The drain is opened to empty the bag. The bag is emptied when faeces are present. It is opened when it balloons or bulges with flatus. The drain is wiped with toilet paper before it is closed. There are many types of ostomy bags on the market nowadays (Fig. 12.53). Some are very discreet and can even be worn under bathers when swimming.

The bag is changed every 3 to 7 days, and when it leaks. Some people prefer to have the bag changed daily or whenever soiling occurs. However, frequent bag changes can damage the skin.

Odours are prevented by:

- good hygiene
- emptying the bag
- avoiding gas-forming foods
- putting deodorants into the bag.

The care plan will itemise what to use.

The person can wear regular clothes. However, tight garments can prevent faeces from entering the bag. Also, bulging from faeces or flatus can be seen with tight clothes.

Peristalsis increases after eating. Therefore, stomas are usually quiet before breakfast. That is, expelling faeces is less likely at this time. If the person showers or bathes with the bag off, it is best done before breakfast. Showers and baths are delayed 1 or 2 hours after applying a new bag. This gives the adhesive time to stick to the skin.

Do not flush bags down the toilet. Follow facility policy for disposing of them.

DELEGATION GUIDELINES

Ostomy bags

Many people manage their ostomies without help. Others need assistance. When the nurse delegates changing an ostomy bag to you, make sure that:

- your facility allows carers to perform the procedure
- the procedure is in your job description
- you have the necessary education and training
- you review the procedure with your supervisor or the nurse
- the nurse is available to answer questions and to supervise you
- the nurse tells you what kind of ostomy the person has – colostomy or ileostomy
- the nurse tells you what equipment and supplies to use
- the nurse tells you what observations to report and record:
  - signs of skin breakdown (normally the stoma is red, like mucous membranes)
  - colour, amount, consistency and odour of faeces
  - complaints of pain or discomfort.

SAFETY ALERT

Ostomy bags

When changing an ostomy bag, contact with faeces is likely. They may contain microbes or blood. You must follow Standard Precautions.

CHANGING AN OSTOMY BAG

Quality of life

Remember to respect the person's privacy while doing any procedure. Address the person by name and ensure they know your name.

Pre-procedure

1 Follow the delegation guidelines.
2 Explain the procedure to the person.
3 Wash your hands.
4 Collect the following:
- clean bag with skin barrier
- skin barrier (if not part of the bag)
- bag clamp, clip or wire closure
- clean ostomy belt (if used)
- skin barrier as ordered
- gauze squares or washcloths
- adhesive remover
- cotton balls
- bedpan with cover
- waterproof pad
- bath blanket
- toilet paper
- washbasin
- prescribed soap or cleansing agent
- bag deodorant
- paper towels
- gloves
- disposable bag.

5 Arrange your work area.
6 Identify the person. Call them by their name.
7 Provide for privacy.

Procedure

8 Lower the bed rail near you, if up.
9 Cover the person with a bath blanket. Fan-fold linen to the foot of the bed.
10 Put on the gloves.
11 Place the waterproof pad under the ostomy.
12 Disconnect the bag from the belt if one is worn. Remove the belt.
13 Remove the bag gently. Gently push the skin down and away from the skin barrier. Place the bag in the bedpan.
14 Wipe around the stoma with toilet paper or a gauze square. This removes mucus and faeces. Place soiled tissue in the bedpan. Discard gauze squares into the disposable bag.
15 Moisten a cotton ball with adhesive remover. Clean around the stoma to remove any remaining skin barrier. Clean from the stoma outwards.
16 Cover the bedpan. Take it to the bathroom.
17 Measure faeces as directed by the nurse.
18 Ask the nurse to observe abnormal faeces. Then empty the bag and bedpan into the toilet. Note the colour, amount, consistency and odour of faeces. Put the bag in the disposable bag.
19 Remove the gloves and wash your hands. Put on clean gloves.
20 Fill the washbasin with warm water. Place the basin on the over-bed table on top of the paper towels. Lower the bed rail near you if up.
21 Wash the skin around the stoma. Rinse and pat dry. Use soap or other cleansing agent as directed by the nurse.
22 Apply the skin barrier if it is a separate device.
23 Put a clean ostomy belt on the person (if a belt is worn).
24 Add deodorant to the new bag.
25 Remove adhesive backing on the bag.
26 Centre the bag over the stoma. The drain points downwards.
27 Press around the skin barrier so the bag seals to the skin. Apply gentle pressure from the stoma outwards.
28 Maintain pressure for 1–2 minutes.
29 Connect the belt to the bag (if a belt is worn).
30 Remove the waterproof pad.
31 Remove the gloves. Wash your hands.
32 Cover the person. Remove the bath blanket.

Post-procedure

33 Provide for comfort.
34 Lower the bed to its lowest position.
35 Place the call bell within reach (if applicable).
36 Remove the screens from around the person.
37 Clean the bedpan, washbasin and other equipment. Wear gloves for this step.
38 Return equipment to its proper place.
39 Discard the disposable bag according to centre policy. Follow centre policy for soiled linen.
40 Remove the gloves and wash your hands.
41 Report and record your observations.

STOOL SPECIMENS

When internal bleeding is suspected, faeces are checked for blood. Stools are also studied for fat, microbes, worms and other abnormal contents. The rules for collecting urine specimens apply when collecting stool specimens.

The stool specimen must not be contaminated with urine. Fig. 12.54 shows how to collect a specimen of stool. Some tests require a warm stool. The specimen is taken to the laboratory at once if a warm stool is needed.

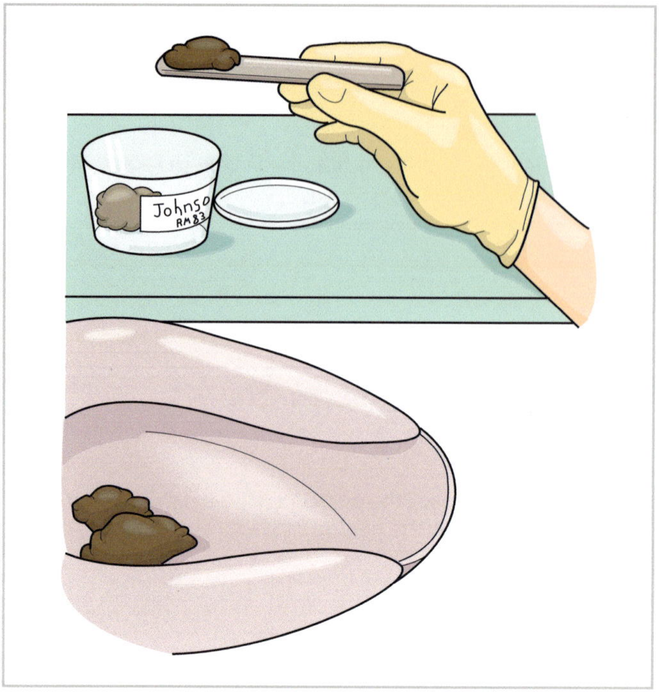

Fig. 12.54
A tongue blade is used to transfer a small amount of stool from the bedpan to the specimen container.

DELEGATION GUIDELINES

Before collecting a stool specimen, you need the following information from your supervisor or the nurse:

- what time to collect the specimen
- what special measures are needed
- what observations to report and record:
  - difficulty in obtaining the specimen
  - colour, amount, consistency and odour of faeces
  - complaints of pain or discomfort.

SAFETY ALERT

Stool specimens

When collecting a stool specimen, contact with faeces is likely. They may contain blood. They may contain microbes. You must follow Standard Precautions.

COLLECTING A STOOL SPECIMEN

Quality of life

Remember to respect the person's privacy while doing any procedure. Address the person by name and ensure they know your name.

Pre-procedure

1. Follow the delegation guidelines.
2. Explain the procedure to the person.
3. Wash your hands.
4. Collect the following:
   - bedpan and cover or commode
   - urinal (or bedpan with cover) for voiding
   - specimen pan or bedpan for the toilet or commode
   - specimen container and lid
   - tongue blade
   - disposable bag
   - gloves
   - toilet paper
   - laboratory requisition slip
   - plastic bag.

Procedure

5. Label the container.
6. Call the person by name.
7. Provide for privacy.
8. Ask the person to void. Provide the bedpan, commode or urinal if the person does not use the toilet. Empty and clean the device.
9. Place the specimen pan or bedpan under the toilet seat if the person uses the toilet (Fig. 12.55).
10. Assist the person onto the bedpan or to the toilet or commode. The person wears a robe and non-skid footwear when up.
11. Ask the person not to put toilet paper in the bedpan, commode or specimen pan. Provide a bag for toilet paper.
12. Place the call bell and toilet paper within reach. Raise or lower bed rails. Follow the care plan.
13. Wash your hands and leave the room.

14 Return when the person signals. Knock before entering. Wash your hands.
15 Lower the bed rail near you if up.
16 Put on the gloves. Remove pan from under the person and provide perineal care if needed.
17 Use a tongue blade to take about two tablespoons of faeces to the specimen container (see Fig. 12.54). Take the sample from the middle of a formed stool. If required by centre policy, take stool from two different places on the specimen.
18 Put the lid on the specimen container. Do not touch the inside of the lid or container. Place the container in the plastic bag.
19 Wrap the tongue blade in toilet paper.
20 Discard the tongue blade.
21 Empty, clean and disinfect equipment.
22 Remove the gloves and wash your hands.
23 Return equipment to its proper place.
24 Help the person with handwashing. Wear gloves if necessary.

Post-procedure

25 Provide for comfort.
26 Place the call bell within reach (if applicable).
27 Lower the bed to its lowest position (if applicable).
28 Remove the screens from around the person.
29 Take the specimen and requisition slip to the nurse.
30 Wash your hands.
31 Report and record your observations.

FOCUS ON COMMUNITY CARE

When managing evacuation needs within a client's home, you will need to always use Standard Precautions. Faecal material on clothing or bed linen should be flushed down the toilet and then the item placed in an appropriate soaking solution (e.g. Napisan or other antibacterial agent). If you are employed to do the washing for your client, wash these items separately from other non-soiled items.

QUALITY OF LIFE

The quality-of-life considerations described for urinary elimination apply for bowel evacuation. As always, you must protect the person's rights. Assist with bowel elimination as directed by the nurse and the care plan.

Bowel evacuation is a very private act. Odours and sounds occur with defecation. Therefore, people want and need privacy. Do all you can to protect the person's right to privacy. Otherwise, normal bowel evacuation can be affected. Constipation and faecal impaction could result.

Bowel control is important to people. Physical and mental wellbeing are related to normal bowel function. Personal routines related to defecation also affect wellbeing. Good hygiene is needed after bowel movements.

Normal bowel evacuation is not always possible. Constipation, faecal impaction, diarrhoea, faecal incontinence and flatulence are common problems. The doctor may order enemas, rectal tubes, medications or diet changes to relieve the problem. You must completely understand the nurse's instructions and the procedure.

Clients have the right to personal choice. People with ostomies manage their care if they are able. Some have had ostomies for a long time. They may have special routines or care measures. Their choices in ostomy care are followed.

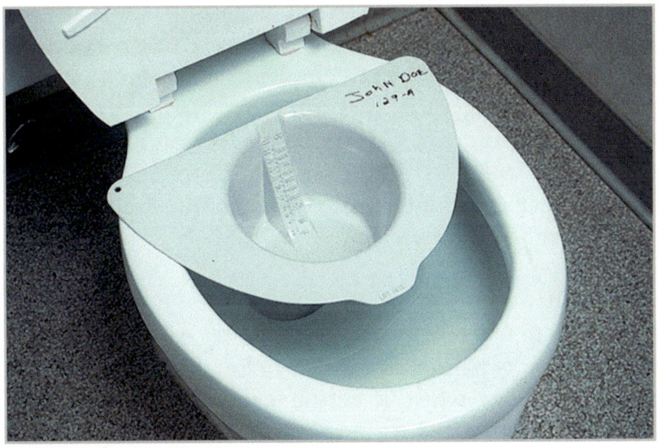

Fig. 12.55
A specimen pan is placed in the toilet for a stool specimen.

ASSISTING WITH URINARY ELIMINATION AND MANAGEMENT

After reading this section, you should be able to:

- be aware of the characteristics of normal urine
- understand the rules for normal urinary elimination
- know what to observe about urine
- understand the care required for urinary incontinence
- understand why catheters are used

- know how to care for persons with catheters
- understand the differences between straight catheters, indwelling catheters and uridomes
- understand basic concepts of bladder training
- know the rules for collecting and testing urine specimens
- understand the procedures described in this section.

Eliminating waste is a physical need. The respiratory, digestive, integumentary and urinary systems remove body wastes. The digestive system rids the body of solid wastes. The lungs remove carbon dioxide. Sweat contains water and other substances. Blood contains waste products from body cells burning food for energy. The urinary system removes waste products from the blood. It also maintains the body's water balance.

NORMAL URINATION

The healthy adult excretes about 1500 mL (millilitres) of urine a day. Factors affecting urine production include age, disease, the amount and kinds of fluid ingested, dietary salt, medications, body temperature and perspiration. Some substances increase urine production – coffee, tea, alcohol and some medications. A diet high in salt causes the body to retain water. When water is retained, less urine is produced.

Urination, **micturition** and **voiding** mean the process of emptying urine from the bladder. The amount of fluid ingested, personal habits and available toilet services affect frequency. So do activity, work and illness. People usually void at bedtime, after getting up and before meals. Some people void every 2–3 hours. The need to void at night disturbs sleep.

The accreditation standards require aged care services to provide care in a way that maintains the person's highest level of independence. The person's elimination needs are assessed. The care plan is developed to ensure that these needs are met.

Clients often need help with elimination. Some need help getting to the toilet, and others use bedpans, urinals or commodes. Follow the rules in Box 12.8 and the person's care plan.

Observations

Normal urine is pale yellow, straw-coloured or amber. It is clear with no particles. A faint odour is normal. Observe urine for colour, clarity, odour, amount and particles.

Some foods affect urine colour. Red food dyes, beetroot, blackberries and rhubarb cause red-coloured urine. Carrots and sweet potatoes cause bright yellow urine. Certain medications change urine colour. Asparagus causes a urine odour.

Ask your supervisor or nurse to observe urine that looks or smells abnormal. Report complaints of urgency, burning on urination or dysuria. **Dysuria** means painful or difficult (*dys*) urination (*uria*). Urinary tract infection is a common cause. Also report any of the problems listed in Table 12.1. The nurse uses the information for the nursing process to plan appropriate care.

BOX 12.8
Maintaining normal urinary elimination

- Use clean techniques.
- Follow Standard Precautions.
- Provide fluids. Follow the instructions in the care plan.
- Follow the person's normal voiding routines and habits. Check with the care plan.
- Help the person to the toilet when the request is made. Or provide the commode, bedpan or urinal. The need to void may be urgent.
- Help the person assume a normal position for voiding if possible. Women sit or squat; men stand.
- Warm the bedpan or urinal, if used.
- Cover the person for warmth and privacy.
- Provide for privacy. Pull the curtain around the bed, close room and bathroom doors and pull drapes or window shades. Leave the room if the person can be left alone.
- Tell the person that running water, flushing the toilet or playing music can mask voiding sounds. Voiding with others close by embarrasses some people.
- Stay nearby if the person is weak or unsteady.
- Place the call bell and toilet paper within reach.
- Allow enough time to void. Do not rush the person.
- Promote relaxation. Some people like to read.
- Run water in a nearby sink if the person cannot start the urine stream. Or place the person's fingers in warm water.
- Provide perineal care as needed.
- Assist with handwashing after voiding. Provide a washbasin, soap, washcloth and towel.
- Assist the person to the toilet or offer the bedpan, urinal or commode at regular times. Some people are embarrassed or are too weak to ask.

Bedpans

Bedpans are not often used, as clients are encouraged at all times to be as mobile as possible. However, there may be some occasions when a person cannot be out of bed. Women use bedpans for voiding and bowel movements. Men use them for bowel movements. Bedpans are made of plastic, stainless steel or disposable recycled cardboard.

Table 12.1
Common urinary elimination problems

Problem	Definition	Causes
Dysuria	Painful or difficult (*dys*) urination (*uria*)	Urinary tract infection, trauma, urinary tract obstruction
Haematuria	Blood (*haem*) in the urine (*uria*)	Kidney disease, urinary tract infection, trauma
Nocturia	Frequent urination (*uria*) at night (*noct*)	Excessive fluid intake, kidney disease, prostate disease
Oliguria	Scant amount (*olig*) of urine (*uria*), usually less than 500 mL in 24 hours	Inadequate fluid intake, shock, burns, kidney disease, heart failure
Polyuria	Abnormally large amounts (*poly*) of urine (*uria*)	Medications, excessive fluid intake, diabetes mellitus, hormone imbalance
Urinary frequency	Voiding at frequent intervals	Excessive fluid intake, bladder infections, pressure on the bladder, medications
Urinary incontinence	Inability to control the loss of urine from the bladder	Trauma, disease, urinary tract infections, reproductive or urinary tract surgeries, ageing, faecal impaction, constipation, not getting to the toilet in time, stress from exertion
Urinary urgency	The need to void immediately	Urinary tract infection, fear of incontinence, full bladder, stress

Stainless steel bedpans are often cold and should be warmed with water and dried before use.

A slipper pan has a thinner rim and is only about 1.25-cm deep at one end (Fig. 12.56). The small end is placed under the buttocks (Fig. 12.57). Slipper pans are used:

- by people with casts
- by people with limited back motion
- after a hip fracture.

CARING ABOUT CULTURE

Be aware that specific routines must be followed within some cultures in relation to elimination. Always check with your client how they manage their normal urinary elimination functions.

DELEGATION GUIDELINES

Bedpans

Before assisting a person with a bedpan, you need the following information from the care plan:

- the type of bedpan used – standard bedpan or slipper pan
- any position or activity limits
- whether the nurse needs to observe the results before disposing of the contents
- what observations to report and record:
  - urine colour, clarity and odour
  - amount
  - presence of particles
  - complaints of urgency, burning, dysuria or other problems.

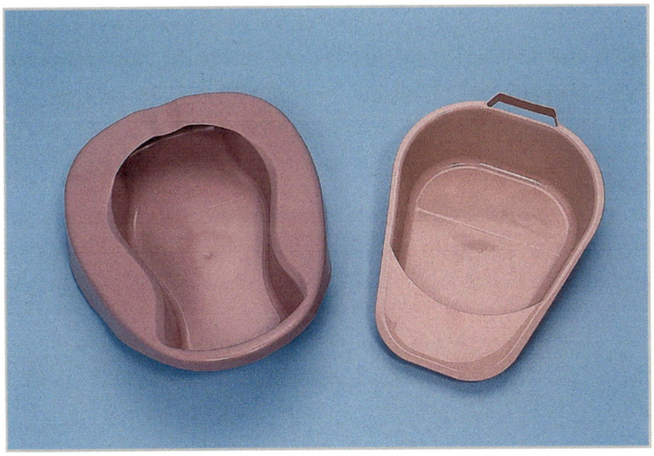

Fig. 12.56
Standard bedpan and slipper pan.

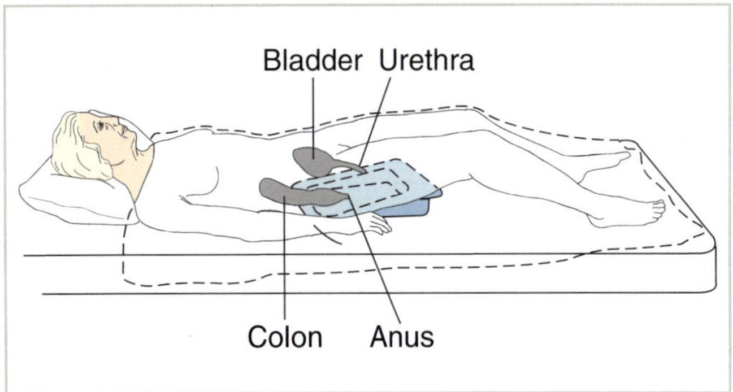

Fig. 12.57
A person positioned on a slipper pan. The smaller end is placed under the buttocks.

GIVING THE BEDPAN

Quality of life

Remember to respect the person's privacy while doing any procedure. Address the person by name and ensure they know your name.

Pre-procedure

1 Follow the delegation guidelines.
2 Provide for privacy.
3 Wash your hands.
4 Put on gloves.
5 Collect the following:
   - bedpan
   - bedpan cover
   - toilet paper.
6 Arrange equipment on the chair or bed.
7 Explain the procedure to the person.

Procedure

8 Warm and dry the bedpan if necessary.
9 Lower the bed rail near you if up.
10 Position the person supine. Raise the head of the bed slightly.
11 Fold the top linen and gown out of the way. Keep the lower body covered.
12 Ask the person to flex their knees and raise the buttocks by pushing against the mattress with their feet.
13 Slide your hand under the lower back and help raise the buttocks.
14 Slide the bedpan under the person (Fig. 12.58).
15 If the person cannot assist in getting on the bedpan:
   a Turn the person onto their side away from you.
   b Place the bedpan firmly against the buttocks (Fig. 12.59).
   c Push the bedpan down and towards the person.
   d Hold the bedpan securely. Turn the person onto their back.
   e Make sure the bedpan is centred under the person.
16 Cover the person.
17 Raise the head of the bed so the person is in a sitting position.
18 Make sure the person is correctly positioned on the bedpan (Fig. 12.60).
19 Raise the bed rail, if used.
20 Place the toilet paper and call bell within reach.
21 Ask the person to signal when done or when help is needed.
22 Remove the gloves. Wash your hands.
23 Leave the room and close the door.
24 Return when the person signals. Knock before entering.
25 Wash your hands and put on gloves.
26 Raise the bed for body mechanics. Lower the bed rail (if used) and the head of the bed.
27 Ask the person to raise their buttocks. Remove the bedpan. Or hold the bedpan and turn the person onto the side away from you.
28 Clean the genital area if the person cannot do so. Clean from front (urethra) to back (anus) with toilet paper. Use fresh tissue for each wipe. Provide perineal care if needed.
29 Cover the bedpan. Take it to the bathroom. Lower the bed and raise the bed rail (if used) before leaving the bedside.
30 Note the colour, amount and character of urine or faeces.
31 Use pan steriliser to empty and clean the bedpan.
32 Help the person with handwashing.
33 Remove the gloves. Wash your hands.
34 Provide for comfort.
35 Place the call bell within reach (if applicable).
36 Remove the screens from around the person.
37 Follow centre policy for soiled linen or place in client's laundry basket.
38 Wash your hands.
39 Report and record your observations.

SAFETY ALERT

Bedpans

Bedpan contents (urine and bowel movements) may contain blood and microbes. In addition, dirty bedpans provide an environment for microbes to live and grow. Follow Standard Precautions when handling bedpans and their contents and dispose in a safe manner as per organisational policy procedure. Thoroughly clean the bedpan after use.

Urinals

Men use a urinal to void (Fig. 12.61). Plastic urinals may have caps and hook-type handles. The urinal hooks onto the bed rail within the man's reach. He stands to use the urinal if possible. Or he sits on the side of the bed or lies in bed to use it. Some need support when standing. You may have to place and hold the urinal for some men.

After voiding, the cap is closed or a paper cover placed over the top. This prevents urine spills. Remind men to signal when urinals need emptying. Remind them not to place urinals on over-bed tables and bedside stands. The over-bed table is used for eating and as a work surface. Bedside stands are used for supplies and personal items. Table surfaces must not be contaminated with urine.

Some centres do not have bed rails on beds. Follow centre policy for where to place urinals.

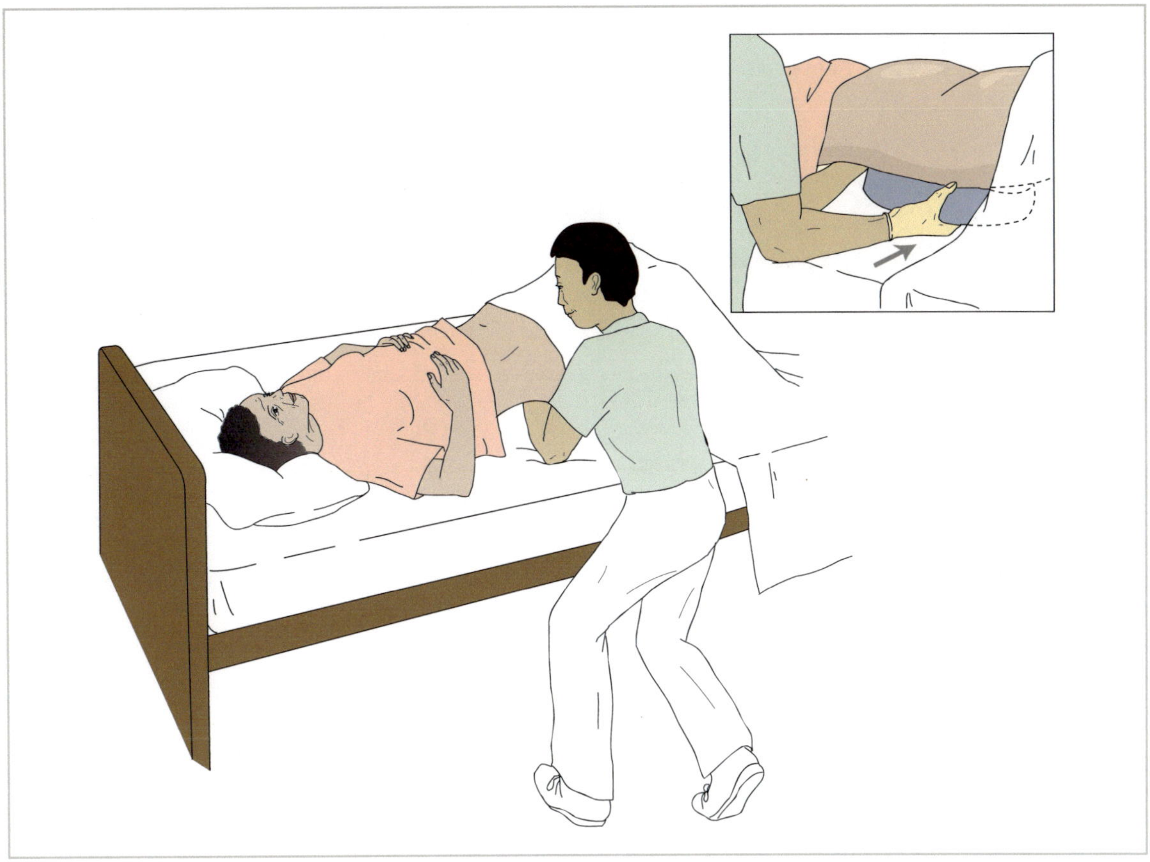

Fig. 12.58
The person raises their buttocks off the bed with help. The bedpan is slid under the person.

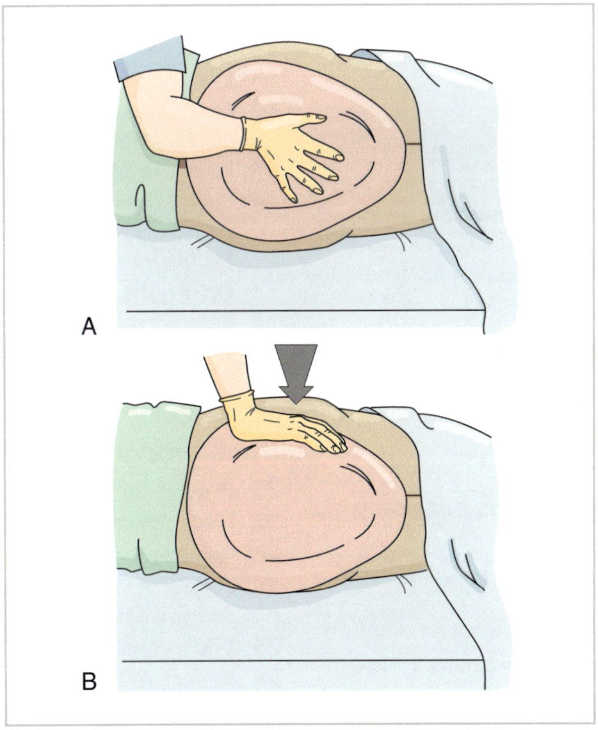

Fig. 12.59
Giving a bedpan.
A. Position the person on one side and place the bedpan firmly against their buttocks. **B.** Push downwards on the bedpan and towards the person.

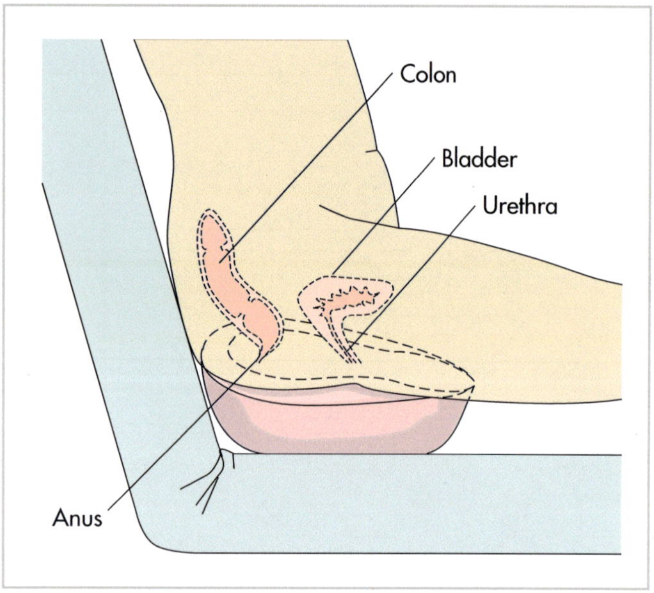

Fig. 12.60
The person is positioned on the bedpan so the urethra and anus are directly over the opening.

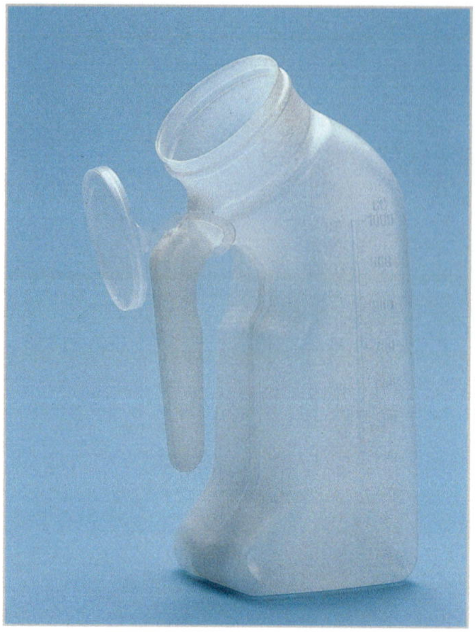

Fig. 12.61
A urinal.

GIVING THE URINAL

Quality of life

Remember to respect the person's privacy while doing any procedure. Address the person by name and ensure they know your name.

Pre-procedure

1 Follow the delegation guidelines.
2 Provide for privacy.
3 Determine whether the person will stand, sit or lie in bed.
4 Wash your hands and put on gloves.

Procedure

5 Give the person the urinal if he is in bed. Remind him to tilt the bottom down to prevent spills.
6 If he is going to stand:
   a Help him sit on the side of the bed.
   b Put non-skid footwear on him.
   c Help him stand. Provide support if he is unsteady.
   d Give him the urinal.
7 Position the urinal if necessary. Position his penis in the urinal if he cannot do so.
8 Provide for privacy.
9 Place the call bell within reach. Ask him to signal when done or when he needs help.
10 Remove the gloves and wash your hands.
11 Leave the room and close the door.
12 Return when he signals for you. Knock before entering.
13 Wash your hands and put on gloves.
14 Close the cap on the urinal or cover it with a paper cover. Take it to the bathroom.
15 Note the colour, amount and character of the urine.
16 Empty the urinal and rinse it with cold water. Clean it with a disinfectant or place it in the pan flusher if your facility has one.
17 Return the urinal to its proper place.
18 Remove soiled gloves. Wash your hands and put on clean gloves.
19 Assist with handwashing.
20 Remove the gloves. Wash your hands.

Post-procedure

21 Provide for comfort.
22 Place the call bell within reach (if applicable).
23 Remove the screens from around the person.
24 Follow centre policy for soiled linen or place in client's laundry basket.
25 Wash your hands.
26 Report and record your observations.

SAFETY ALERT

Urinals

Follow Standard Precautions when handling urinals and their contents. Empty them promptly to prevent odours and the spread of microbes, as a filled urinal spills easily, causing a safety hazard. Also, it is an unpleasant sight and a source of odour. Urinals are cleaned in the same way as bedpans.

DELEGATION GUIDELINES

Urinals

Before assisting a man with a urinal, you need the following information from the care plan:

- how the urinal is used – standing, sitting or lying in bed
- whether help is needed with placing or holding the urinal
- whether the man needs support to stand. If yes, how many staff members are needed
- whether the nurse needs to observe the urine before its disposal
- what observations to record and report:
  - urine colour, clarity and odour
  - amount
  - presence of particles
  - complaints of urgency, burning, dysuria or other problems.

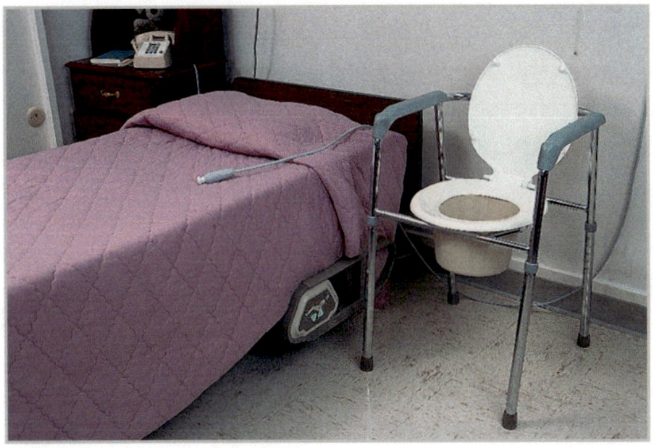

Fig. 12.62
The bedside commode has a toilet seat with a container. The container slides out from under the toilet seat for emptying.

Commodes

A commode is a chair or wheelchair with an opening for a bedpan or container (Fig. 12.62). People who are unable to walk to the toilet often use commodes. The commode allows a normal position for elimination. The commode arms and back provide support and help prevent falls.

Some commodes are wheeled into the bathroom and placed over the toilet. They provide privacy and safety for people who are unable to walk to the bathroom. They are also useful for those who cannot sit unsupported on the toilet. The container is removed if the commode is used with the toilet. Wheels are locked after the commode is positioned over the toilet.

DELEGATION GUIDELINES

Commodes

You need the following information from the care plan when assisting a person to use a commode:

- Is the commode used at the bedside or over the toilet?
- How much help does the person need?
- Can the person be left alone?
- Does the nurse need to observe urine or bowel movements?
- What observations to report and record:
  - urine colour, clarity and odour
  - amount
  - presence of particles
  - complaints of urgency, burning, dysuria or other problems.

HELPING A PERSON TO THE COMMODE

Quality of life

Remember to respect the person's privacy while doing any procedure. Address the person by name and ensure they know your name.

Pre-procedure

1. Follow the delegation guidelines.
2. Explain the procedure to the person.
3. Provide for privacy.
4. Wash your hands and put on gloves.
5. Collect the following:
   - commode
   - toilet paper
   - bath blanket.

Procedure

6. Bring the commode next to the bed. Remove the chair cushion and container lid.
7. Help the person sit on the side of the bed.
8. Help them put on a robe and non-skid footwear.

9 Assist the person to the commode. Use a transfer belt.
10 Cover the person with a bath blanket for warmth.
11 Place the toilet paper and call bell within reach.
12 Ask the person to signal when done or when help is needed. (Stay with the person if necessary. Be respectful. Provide as much privacy as possible.)
13 Remove the gloves and wash your hands.
14 Leave the room and close the door.
15 Return when the person signals. Knock before entering (if applicable).
16 Wash your hands and put on the gloves.
17 Help the person clean the genital area as needed. Remove the gloves and wash your hands.
18 Help the person back to bed. Remove the robe and footwear. Raise the bed rail, if used; follow the care plan.
19 Put on clean gloves. Remove and cover the commode container. Clean the commode.
20 Take the container to the bathroom.
21 Check urine and faeces for colour, amount and character.
22 Clean and disinfect the container.
23 Return the container to the commode. Return other supplies to their proper place.
24 Return the commode to its proper place.
25 Remove soiled gloves.
26 Wash your hands.
27 Assist the person with handwashing.

Post-procedure

28 Provide for comfort.
29 Place the call bell within reach (if applicable).
30 Remove the screens from around the person.
31 Follow centre policy for soiled linen or place in the client's laundry basket.
32 Wash your hands.
33 Report and record your observations.

URINARY INCONTINENCE

Urinary incontinence is the loss of bladder control. It may be temporary or permanent. The Australian Government has developed expected outcomes in relation to accreditation standards to ensure that clients receive the highest possible quality of care. Continence management is identified as an expected outcome in one of those standards.

There are several basic types of incontinence:

- *Stress incontinence* – urine leaks during exercise and certain movements. Urine loss is small (less than 50 mL). Often called dribbling, it occurs with laughing, sneezing, coughing, lifting or other activities. Late pregnancy and obesity are other causes. The problem is common in women. Pelvic muscles weaken from pregnancies and with ageing.
- *Urge incontinence* – there is loss of urine in response to a sudden, urgent need to void. The person cannot get to a toilet in time. **Urinary frequency**, **urinary urgency** and night-time voiding (**enuresis**) are common. Causes include urinary tract infections, nervous system disorders, bladder cancer and an enlarged prostate.
- *Overflow incontinence* – urine leaks when the bladder is too full. The person feels like the bladder is never completely empty. The person only dribbles or has a weak urine stream. Diabetes, an enlarged prostate and some medications are causes.
- *Functional incontinence* – the person has bladder control but cannot use the toilet in time. Immobility, restraints, unanswered call bells, no call bell within reach and not knowing where to find the toilet are causes. Therefore, it is difficult to remove clothing. Confusion and disorientation are other causes.
- *Reflex incontinence* – this is the loss of urine at certain intervals. Urine is lost when the bladder is full. The person does not feel the need to void. Nervous system disorders and injuries are common causes.

Sometimes incontinence results from intestinal, rectal and reproductive system surgery. More than one type of incontinence can be present. This is called mixed incontinence.

Incontinence is embarrassing. Clothing gets wet and odours develop. The person is uncomfortable. Skin irritation, breakdown and infection can occur. Falling is a risk when trying to get to the toilet quickly. Loss of independence, social isolation, decreased self-esteem and depression are common.

Caring for clients with incontinence will depend on the type of incontinence they have. Follow the care plan instructions. The care plan may include some of the measures in Box 12.9. Good skin care and dry garments and linen are essential. Following the rules for normal urination prevents incontinence in some people. Others need bladder training.

Caring for people with incontinence is stressful. They need frequent care. They may wet again immediately after providing skin care and changing wet garments and linens. Remember, incontinence is beyond the person's control. It is not something the person chooses to do. Be patient; the person's needs are great. It can be even more challenging for clients with dementia (see Box 12.10). The person has the right to be free from abuse, mistreatment and neglect. Kindness, empathy, understanding and patience are needed.

Incontinence products

Incontinence products help keep the person dry (Fig. 12.63). They generally have two layers of absorbent material and a waterproof back. Fluid passes through the first layer and is absorbed by the lower layer. These products assist with containing the fluid lost, maintaining skin integrity by drawing moisture away from the skin surface and improving quality

BOX 12.9
Management of a person with incontinence

- Record the person's voidings. This includes incontinent episodes and successful use of the toilet, commode, bedpan or urinal.
- Answer call bells promptly. The person may have an urgent need to void.
- Promote normal urinary elimination.
- Promote normal bowel elimination.
- Encourage voiding at scheduled intervals.
- Follow the person's bladder training program.
- Encourage the person to wear easy-to-remove clothing. Incontinence can occur while trying to deal with buttons, zippers and undergarments.
- Encourage the person to do pelvic muscle exercises as instructed by the nurse or physiotherapist.
- Help prevent urinary tract infections:
  - Encourage adequate fluid intake.
  - Encourage the person to wear cotton underpants.
  - Keep the perineal area clean.
- Decrease fluid intake before bedtime.
- Provide good skin care.
- Provide dry garments and linens.
- Observe for signs of skin breakdown.
- Use incontinence products as per the care plan.
- Follow the manufacturer's instructions when using incontinence products.
- Provide perineal care as needed. Remember to:
  - use a safe and comfortable water temperature
  - follow Standard Precautions
  - protect the person and dry garments and linen from the wet incontinence product
  - expose only the perineal area
  - wash, rinse and dry the perineal area and buttocks
  - remove wet incontinence products, garments and linen. Apply clean, dry ones.

BOX 12.10
Clients with dementia

Meeting the urinary elimination needs of people with dementia is often very stressful. These people may urinate in the wrong places. Rubbish bins, pot plants and heating vents are examples. Some remove incontinence products and throw them on the floor or in the toilet. Others resist your efforts to keep them clean and dry. They should be prompted regularly to go to the toilet to minimise the likelihood of urinating in the wrong places and to maintain their dignity. It is important that a history be taken from the family so that urinary habits are known to ensure maximisation of their independence. The health team must provide safe care for these people. The care plan lists needed measures. You may need a co-worker's help to keep the person clean and dry. If you have questions, ask the nurse for help.

Remember, everyone has the right to safe care. They also have the right to be treated with dignity and respect.

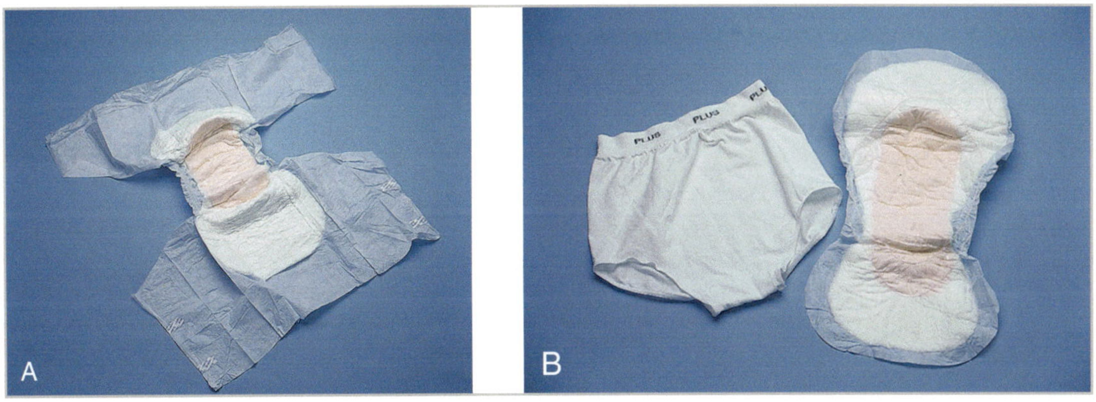

Fig. 12.63
Disposable garment protectors.
A. Complete incontinence brief. **B.** Pants liner and undergarment.

of life for the person. Incontinence products are varied and are designed to manage all degrees of urinary incontinence. Some consist of simple pads that can be placed inside the client's underwear, while others are larger and are worn in place of underwear.

For men who have minimal incontinence, small pouches with absorbent linings and waterproof exteriors that can be worn over the penis are available. These are held in place by the pressure of normal underwear.

Many care services and community care services will provide an assessment service to help your client determine which product is best for them. The client is assessed to ensure that the best products are used to meet the person's needs. Use these products according to centre procedures and your client's preferences.

When handling used or contaminated continence product, ensure that you follow all Standard Precautions and dispose of the products appropriately.

Catheters

Some clients may have catheters in situ. A **catheter** is a tube used to drain or inject fluid through a body opening. Inserted through the urethra into the bladder, a urinary catheter drains urine.

- A *straight catheter* drains the bladder and is removed.
- An *indwelling catheter* (retention or Foley catheter) is left in the bladder. Urine drains constantly into a drainage bag. A balloon near the tip is inflated after the catheter is inserted. The balloon prevents the catheter from slipping out of the bladder (Fig. 12.64). Tubing connects the catheter to the collection bag.

Usually only a doctor or a nurse can insert a catheter (**catheterisation**), as this must be done under strict aseptic conditions. Some people, especially those with long-term disabilities, will often perform self-catheterisation several times a day.

Some people are too weak or disabled to use the bedpan, commode or toilet. Dying people are an example. For them, catheters promote comfort and prevent incontinence. Catheters also protect wounds and pressure ulcers from contact with urine. They also allow for accurate urine measurement. However, they are a last resort for incontinence, as catheters do not treat the cause of incontinence.

In hospitals, catheters also have diagnostic uses. They are used to collect sterile urine specimens. Another test involves measuring the amount of urine left in the bladder (residual urine). The catheter is inserted after the person voids.

You will care for people with indwelling catheters. Follow the rules in Box 12.11 to promote comfort and safety.

SAFETY ALERT

Catheter care

Urine provides an environment for microbes. Also, urine may contain blood. Follow Standard Precautions.

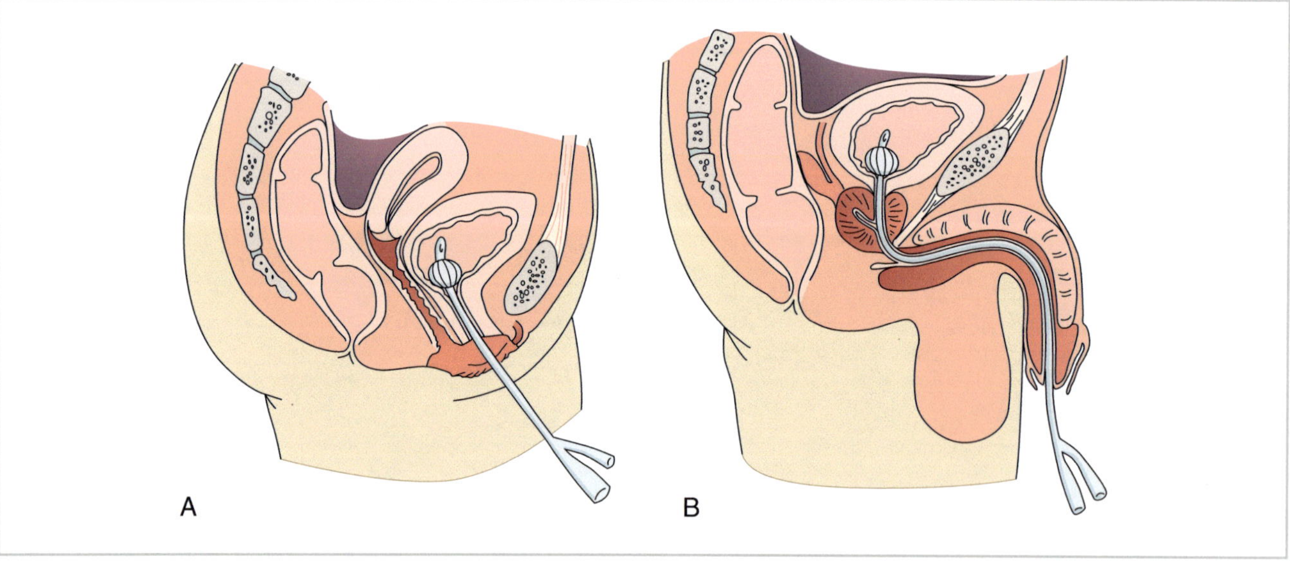

Fig. 12.64

Indwelling catheter.

A. Indwelling catheter in the female bladder. The inflated balloon at the top prevents the catheter from slipping out through the urethra. **B.** Indwelling catheter with the balloon inflated in the male bladder.

BOX 12.11
Caring for a person with an indwelling catheter

- Follow Standard Precautions.
- Allow urine to flow freely through the catheter and tubing. Tubing should not have kinks. The person should not lie on the tubing.
- Keep the catheter connected to the drainage tubing.
- Keep the drainage bag below the bladder. This prevents urine from flowing backwards into the bladder.
- Attach the drainage bag to the bed frame, to the back of a chair or to the lower part of an intravenous therapy pole. Never attach the drainage bag to the bed rail or other objects. Otherwise, the drainage bag is higher than the bladder when the bed rail is raised.
- Do not let the drainage bag rest on the floor. This can contaminate the system.
- Coil the drainage tubing on the bed. Secure it to the bottom bed sheet, but ensure facility policy is followed. Use a clip, tape or safety pin and rubber band. Tubing must not loop below the drainage bag.
- Secure the catheter to the inner thigh (Fig. 12.65). Or secure it to the man's abdomen. This prevents excess catheter movement and friction at the insertion site. Secure the catheter with tape or other devices as the nurse directs.
- Check for leaks. Check the site where the catheter connects to the drainage bag. Report leaks to the nurse at once.
- Give catheter care daily or twice a day. Some centres consider perineal care to be sufficient. Follow the care plan.
- Provide perineal care daily, after bowel movements and when vaginal drainage is present. Follow the care plan.
- Empty the drainage bag at the end of the shift or as the nurse directs. Measure and record the amount of urine (see 'Emptying a urinary drainage bag'). Report increases or decreases in the amount of urine.
- Use a separate measuring container for each person. This prevents the spread of microbes from one person to another.
- Do not let the drain on the drainage bag touch any surface.
- Report complaints to the nurse at once: pain, burning, the need to void or irritation. Also report the colour, clarity and odour of urine and the presence of particles (see Fig. 12.66).
- Encourage fluid intake, as instructed by the nurse.

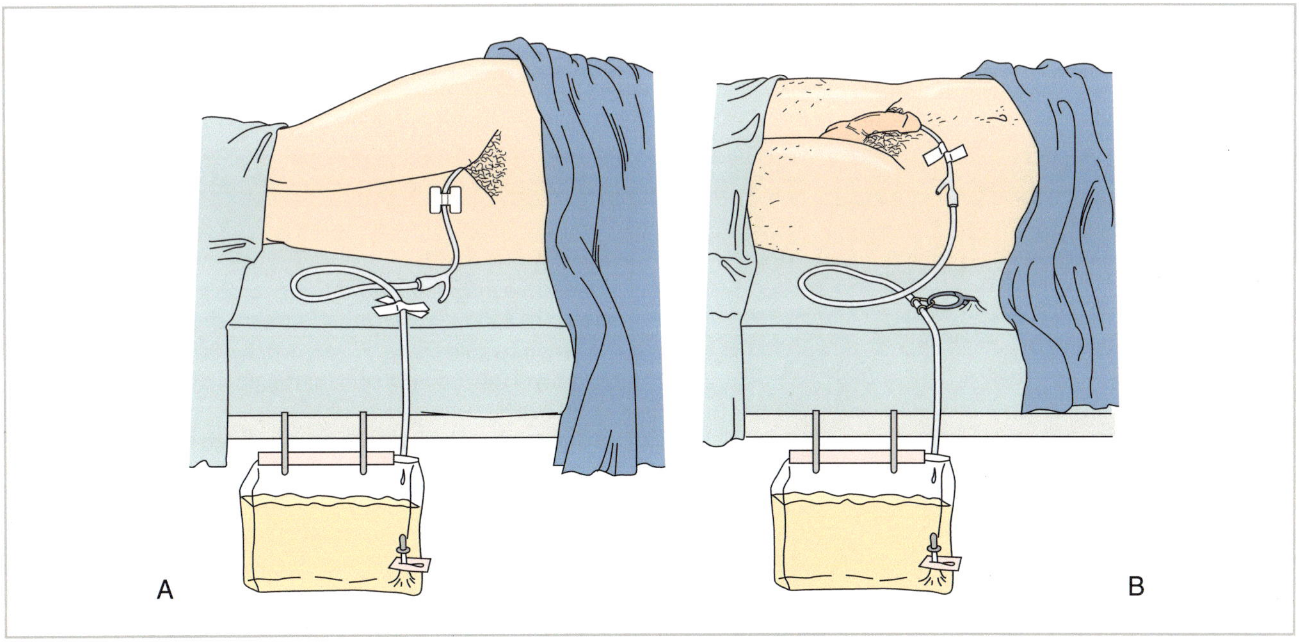

Fig. 12.65
Securing a catheter.
A. The drainage tube is coiled on the bed and secured to the bottom linen so urine flows freely. The catheter is taped to the inner thigh. Enough slack is left on the catheter to prevent friction at the urethra. **B.** The catheter is secured to the man's abdomen.

GIVING CATHETER CARE

Quality of life

Remember to respect the person's privacy while doing any procedure. Address the person by name and ensure they know your name.

Pre-procedure

1. Follow the delegation guidelines.
2. Explain the procedure to the person.
3. Wash your hands.
4. Collect the following:
   - items for perineal care
   - gloves
   - bed protector
   - bath blanket.
5. Call the person by name.
6. Provide for privacy.

Procedure

7. Put on the gloves.
8. Cover the person with a bath blanket. Fan-fold top linen to the foot of the bed.
9. Drape the person for perineal care.
10. Fold back the bath blanket to expose the genital area.
11. Ask client to flex knees and raise buttocks to place the bed protector under the buttocks.
12. Give perineal care.
13. Apply soap to a clean, wet washcloth.
14. Separate the labia (female). Or retract the foreskin (uncircumcised male) (Fig. 12.67). Check for crusts, abnormal drainage or secretions.
15. Hold the catheter near the meatus.
16. Clean catheter from the meatus down the catheter about 6 cm. Clean downwards, away from the meatus with one stroke (Fig. 12.68). Do not tug or pull on the catheter. Repeat as needed with a clean area of the washcloth. Use another clean washcloth if needed.
17. Rinse the catheter. Rinse from the meatus down the catheter about 6 cm. Rinse downwards, away from the meatus with one stroke. Do not tug or pull on the catheter. Repeat as needed with a clean area of the washcloth. Use a clean washcloth if needed.
18. Secure the catheter. Coil and secure tubing.
19. Remove the bed protector.
20. Cover the person. Remove the bath blanket.
21. Remove the gloves. Wash your hands.

Post-procedure

22. Provide for comfort.
23. Place the call bell within reach (if applicable).
24. Clean and return equipment to its proper place. Discard disposable items. (Wear gloves for this step.)
25. Remove the screens from around the person.
26. Follow centre policy for soiled linen or place in the client's laundry basket.
27. Wash your hands.
28. Report observations.

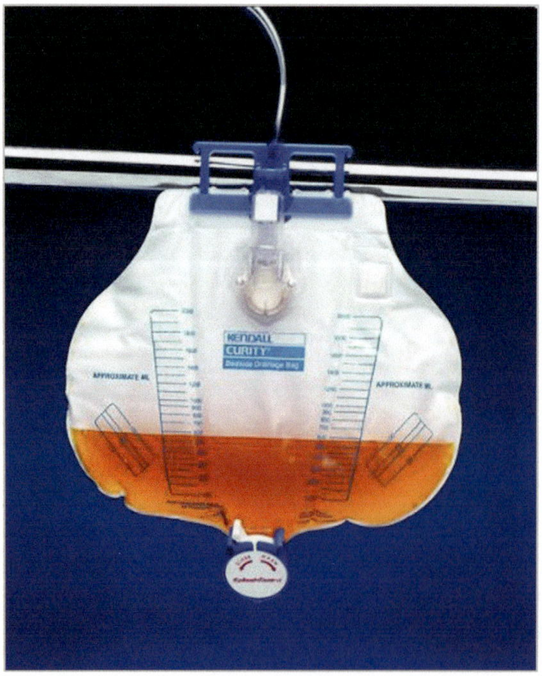

Fig. 12.66
A closed system urinary drainage bag.

DELEGATION GUIDELINES

Catheter care

The nurse may delegate catheter care to you. If so, you need the following information from the care plan:

- when to give catheter care – daily, twice a day, after bowel movements or when vaginal discharge is present
- where to secure the catheter – thigh or abdomen
- how to secure drainage tubing – clip, tape or safety pin and rubber band
- what observations to report and record:
  - complaints of pain, burning, irritation or the need to urinate
  - crusting, abnormal drainage or secretions
  - the colour, clarity and odour of urine
  - particles in the urine
  - drainage system leaks.

Drainage systems

A *closed drainage system* is used for indwelling catheters. Nothing can enter the system from the catheter to the

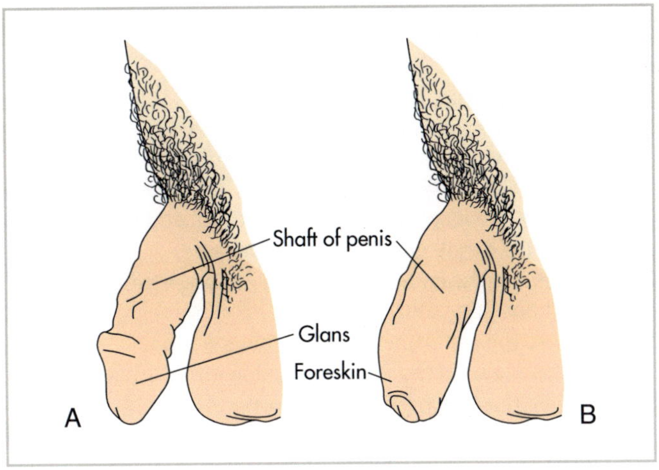

Fig. 12.67
A. Circumcised male. **B.** Uncircumcised male.

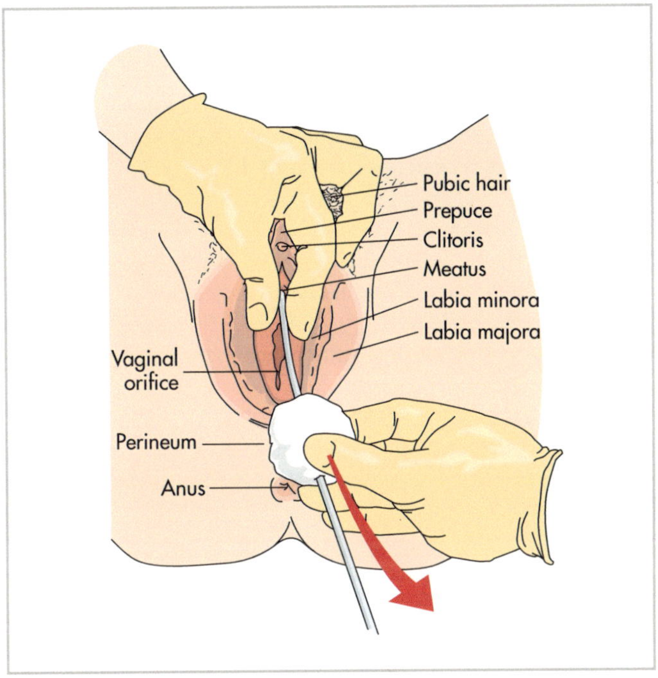

Fig. 12.68
The catheter is cleaned starting at the meatus. About 6 cm of the catheter is cleaned.

drainage bag. The urinary system is sterile, and infection can occur if microbes enter the drainage system. The microbes can travel up the tubing or catheter into the bladder and kidneys. A urinary tract infection can threaten health and life.

The drainage system involves tubing and a drainage bag. Tubing attaches at one end to the catheter. At the other end, it attaches to the drainage bag.

The bag hangs from the bed frame, chair or wheelchair. It must not touch the floor. The bag is kept lower than the person's bladder. Some people wear leg bags when up, as these are more discreet and can be hidden under trousers or a long skirt. The leg bag attaches to the thigh or calf.

Microbes can grow in urine. If the drainage bag is higher than the bladder, urine can flow back into the bladder. An infection can occur. Therefore, do not hang the drainage bag on a bed rail. When the bed rail is raised, the bag is higher than the bladder. When the person walks, the bag is held lower than the bladder.

Sometimes drainage systems are disconnected accidentally. If that happens, tell your supervisor or the nurse at once. Do not touch the ends of the catheter or tubing. Do the following:

- Wash your hands and put on gloves.
- Wipe the end of the tube with an antiseptic wipe.
- Wipe the end of the catheter with an antiseptic wipe. (Use separate wipes for the tube end and catheter end.)
- Do not put the ends down. Do not touch the ends after you clean them.
- Connect the tubing to the catheter.
- Discard the wipes into a biohazard plastic bag.
- Remove the gloves and wash your hands.

Leg bags are changed to drainage bags when the person is in bed. The *drainage bag* stays lower than bladder level. You will have to open the closed drainage system. You must prevent microbes from entering the system.

Drainage bags are emptied and urine measured:

- at the end of each shift
- when changing from a leg bag to a drainage bag
- when changing from a drainage bag to a leg bag
- when a leg bag is becoming full.

SAFETY ALERT

Drainage systems

Microbes can grow in urine. Urine can contain blood. Follow Standard Precautions.

CHANGING A LEG BAG TO A DRAINAGE BAG

Quality of life

Remember to respect the person's privacy while doing any procedure. Address the person by name and ensure they know your name.

Pre-procedure

1. Follow the delegation guidelines.
2. Explain the procedure to the person.
3. Wash your hands.
4. Collect the following:
   - gloves
   - drainage bag and tubing
   - antiseptic wipes
   - bed protector
   - sterile cap and plug
   - catheter clamp
   - paper towels
   - bedpan
   - bath blanket.
5. Arrange paper towels and equipment on the over-bed table.
6. Call the person by name.
7. Provide for privacy.

Procedure

8. Have the person sit on the side of the bed.
9. Put on the gloves.
10. Expose the catheter and leg bag.
11. Clamp the catheter (Fig. 12.69). This prevents urine from draining from the catheter into the drainage tubing.
12. Let urine drain from below the clamp site into the drainage tubing. This empties the lower end of the catheter.
13. Help the person lie down.
14. Raise the bed for body mechanics.
15. Cover the person with a bath blanket. Expose the catheter and leg bag.
16. Place the bed protector under the leg.
17. Open the antiseptic wipes. Set them on the paper towels. You will only need to use these if you accidentally contaminate the end of the catheter.
18. Open the package with the drainage bag and tubing.
19. Attach the drainage bag to the bed frame.
20. Disconnect the catheter from the drainage tubing. Do not let anything touch the ends.
21. Remove the cap from the new drainage tubing.
22. Insert the end of the drainage tubing into the catheter.
23. Remove the clamp from the catheter.
24. Loop drainage tubing on the bed. Secure tubing to the mattress.
25. Remove the leg bag. Place it in the bedpan.
26. Remove and discard the bed protector.
27. Cover the person. Remove the bath blanket.
28. Take the bedpan to the bathroom.
29. Remove the gloves. Wash your hands.

Post-procedure

30. Provide for comfort.
31. Place the call bell within reach (if applicable).
32. Lower the bed to its lowest position (if applicable).
33. Remove the screens from around the person.
34. Put on clean gloves. Discard disposable items.
35. Empty the drainage bag.
36. Discard the drainage tubing and bag following centre policy. Or clean the bag following centre policy.
37. Sanitise the bedpan.
38. Return the bedpan and other items to their proper place.
39. Remove the gloves. Wash your hands.
40. Report and record your observations.
41. Reverse the procedure to attach a leg bag to the catheter.

DELEGATION GUIDELINES

Drainage systems

Your delegated tasks may involve urinary drainage systems. If so, you need the following information from the care plan:

- when to empty the drainage bag
- what type of drainage bag the person uses
- when to switch drainage bags and leg bags
- whether you should clean or discard the drainage bag
- what observations to report:
  - the amount of urine measured
  - the colour, clarity and odour of urine
  - particles in the urine
  - complaints of pain, burning, irritation or the need to urinate
  - drainage system leaks.

DELEGATION GUIDELINES

Leg bags and drainage bags

Leg bags hold less than 1200 mL of urine. Most drainage bags hold at least 2000 mL of urine. Therefore, leg bags fill faster than drainage bags. You need to check leg bags often. Empty the leg bag if it is becoming full.

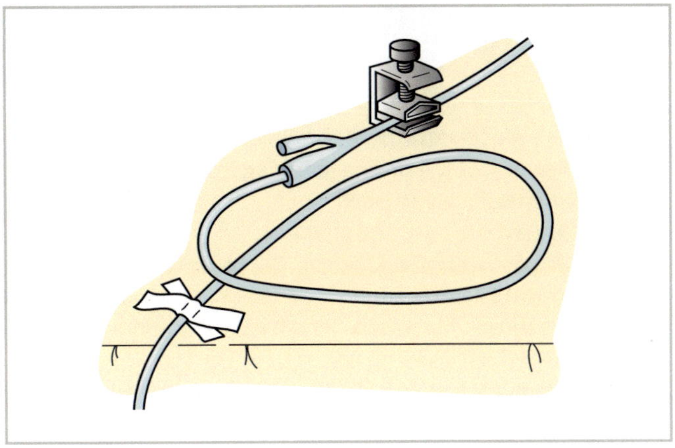

Fig. 12.69
The catheter is clamped. The clamped catheter prevents urine from draining out of the bladder. The clamp is applied to the catheter – not to the drainage tubing.

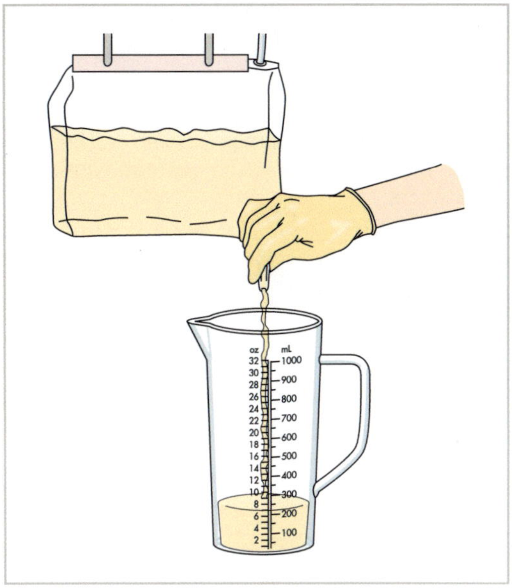

Fig. 12.70
The clamp on the drainage bag is opened. The drain is directed into the measuring container. The drain must not touch the inside of the container.

EMPTYING A URINARY DRAINAGE BAG

Quality of life

Remember to respect the person's privacy while doing any procedure. Address the person by name and ensure they know your name.

Pre-procedure

1 Follow the delegation guidelines.
2 Collect equipment:
   - graduated jug (measuring container)
   - gloves
   - paper towels.
3 Wash your hands.
4 Explain the procedure to the person.
5 Call the person by name.
6 Provide for privacy.

Procedure

7 Put on the gloves.
8 Place a paper towel on the floor. Place the measuring container on top of it.
9 Position the measuring container under the collection bag drain.
10 Open the clamp on the drain (Fig. 12.70).
11 Let all urine drain into the measuring container. Do not let the drain touch the measuring container.
12 Close and position the clamp.
13 Measure urine.
14 Remove and discard the paper towel.
15 Dispose of the urine.
16 Rinse the measuring container and dispose of the rinse.
17 Return the measuring container to its proper place.
18 Remove the gloves and wash your hands.
19 Record the time and amount on the intake and output (I&O) record.

Post-procedure

20 Remove the screens from around the person.
21 Report and record the amount and your other observations.

The uridome

Uridomes are sometimes used for incontinent men. They are also called external catheters or urinary sheaths. A uridome is a soft sheath that slides over the penis. Tubing connects the uridome and drainage bag. Many men use leg bags.

To apply a uridome, follow the manufacturer's instructions. Thoroughly wash the penis with soap and water. Then dry it before applying.

Adhesive tape secures the catheter in place. Use the adhesive tape packaged with the uridome. This tape has been designed by the manufacturer to suit the individual appliances. Never use other types of adhesive tape to secure uridomes or apply the tape too tightly, as blood flow to the penis can be cut off, injuring the penis.

APPLYING A URIDOME

Quality of life

Remember to respect the person's privacy while doing any procedure. Address the person by name and ensure they know your name.

Pre-procedure

1. Follow the delegation guidelines.
2. Explain the procedure to the person.
3. Wash your hands.
4. Collect the following:
   - uridome and tape
   - drainage bag or leg bag
   - cap for drainage bag
   - basin of warm water
   - soap
   - towel and washcloths
   - bath blanket
   - gloves
   - bed protector
   - paper towels.
5. Arrange paper towels and equipment on the over-bed table.
6. Provide for privacy.
7. Identify the person. Call the person by name.
8. Raise the bed for body mechanics (if applicable).

Procedure

9. Cover the person with a bath blanket. Lower top linen to the knees.
10. Ask the person to raise his buttocks off the bed. Or turn him onto his side away from you.
11. Slide the bed protector under his buttocks.
12. Have the person lower his buttocks. Or turn him onto his back.
13. Secure the drainage bag to the bed frame. Or have a leg bag ready. Close the drain.
14. Expose the genital area.
15. Put on the gloves.
16. Remove the uridome.
    a. Remove the tape. Roll the sheath off the penis.
    b. Disconnect the drainage tubing from the uridome. Cap the drainage tube.
    c. Discard the tape and uridome.
17. Provide perineal care. Observe the penis for skin breakdown or irritation.
18. Remove the protective backing from the uridome. This exposes the adhesive strip.
19. Hold the penis firmly. Roll the uridome onto the penis. Leave a 2.5 cm space between the penis and catheter end.
20. Secure the uridome with adhesive tape (Fig. 12.71). Apply tape in a spiral or as per manufacturer's guidelines. Do not apply tape completely around the penis.
21. Connect the uridome to the drainage tubing. Coil excess tubing on the bed. Or attach a leg bag (Fig. 12.72).
22. Remove the bed protector and gloves. Discard them. Wash your hands.
23. Cover the person. Remove the bath blanket.

Post-procedure

24. Provide for comfort.
25. Place the call bell within reach (if applicable).
26. Lower the bed to its lowest position (if applicable).
27. Remove the screens from around the person.
28. Wash your hands. Put on clean gloves.
29. Measure and record the amount of urine in the bag. Clean or discard the collection bag.
30. Discard disposable items.
31. Clean and return the washbasin and other equipment. Return items to their proper place.
32. Remove the gloves and wash your hands.
33. Report and record your observations.

SAFETY ALERT

Uridomes

If you are not familiar with the uridomes used by your client, ask your supervisor or the nurse to show you the correct application. Then ask to be observed when applying the uridome for the first time.

Remember, blood must be allowed to flow to the penis. Use the adhesive tape supplied. Apply it in a spiral fashion.

Microbes can grow in urine and urine may contain blood. Follow Standard Precautions.

DELEGATION GUIDELINES

Uridomes

Before applying or removing a uridome, you need the following information from the care plan:

- when to remove the uridome and apply a new one – daily or every few days
- whether the man uses a leg bag or standard drainage system
- what observations to report and record:
  - reddened or open areas on the penis
  - swelling of the penis
  - colour, clarity and odour of urine
  - particles in the urine.

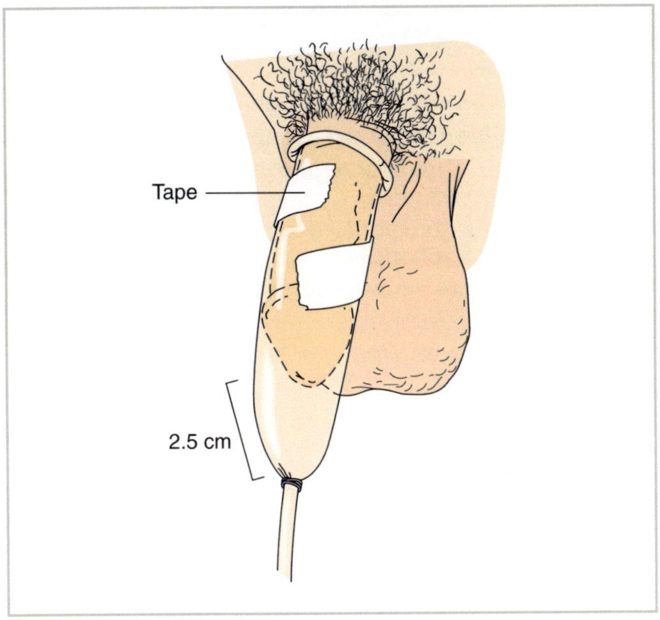

Fig. 12.71
A uridome applied to the penis. There is a 2.5 cm space between the penis and the end of the catheter. Tape is applied in a spiral fashion to secure the uridome to the penis.

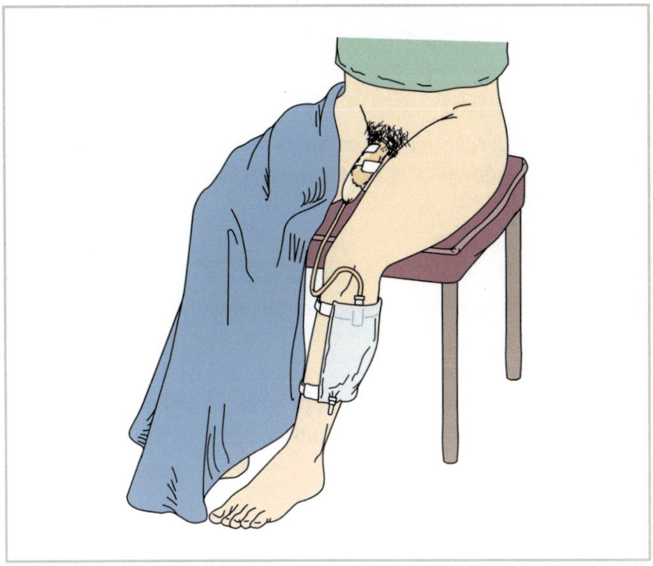

Fig. 12.72
A uridome attached to a leg bag.

Bladder training

Bladder training programs help some people with urinary incontinence. Some people need bladder training after removal of an indwelling catheter. The bladder training program is part of the care plan. Control of urination is the goal. Bladder control promotes comfort and quality of life. It also increases self-esteem. You assist with bladder training as directed by the nurse and the care plan.

Bladder training technique

The person uses the toilet, commode, bedpan or urinal at certain times. The person is given 15–20 minutes to start voiding. The rules for normal urination are followed. The normal position for voiding is assumed if possible. Privacy is important. Help the person relax and provide encouragement. These measures can help the person succeed.

COLLECTING URINE SPECIMENS

Urine specimens (samples) are collected for urine tests. Doctors use test results to diagnose or evaluate treatment. Follow the rules in Box 12.12 when collecting specimens.

The random urine specimen

The random urine specimen is used for urinalysis. No special measures are needed. It is collected at any time. Many people can collect the specimen themselves. Weak and very ill people need help.

BOX 12.12
Rules for collecting urine specimens

- Follow Standard Precautions.
- Use a clean container for each specimen.
- Use a container appropriate for the specimen.
- Label the container. Write the person's full name, room and bed number, date and time the specimen was collected. Some centres have pre-printed labels with this information. If pre-printed labels are used, place a label on the container.
- Do not touch the inside of the container or lid.
- Collect the specimen at the time specified.
- Ask the person not to have a bowel movement during specimen collection. The specimen must not contain faeces.
- Ask the person to put toilet paper in the toilet or waste bin. The specimen must not contain tissue.
- Make sure the requisition slip has the person's identifying information. The required test is marked.
- Take the specimen and requisition slip to the storage area. The specimen container should be placed in a plastic bag.

COLLECTING A RANDOM URINE SPECIMEN

Quality of life

Remember to respect the person's privacy while doing any procedure. Address the person by name and ensure they know your name.

Pre-procedure

1. Follow the delegation guidelines.
2. Explain the procedure to the person.
3. Wash your hands.
4. Collect the following:
   - bedpan and cover, urinal or specimen pan
   - specimen container and lid
   - label
   - gloves
   - plastic bag.

Procedure

5. Label the container.
6. Put the container and lid in the bathroom.
7. Identify the person. Call the person by name.
8. Provide for privacy.
9. Put on the gloves.
10. Ask the person to urinate in the receptacle. Remind them to put toilet paper into the waste bin or toilet. Toilet paper is not put into the bedpan or specimen pan.
11. Take the receptacle to the bathroom.
12. Measure urine if intake and output (I&O) is ordered.
13. Pour about 120 mL of urine into the specimen container. Dispose of excess urine.
14. Place the lid on the specimen container. Put the container in the plastic bag.
15. Clean and return the receptacle to its proper place.
16. Assist with handwashing.
17. Remove the gloves. Wash your hands.

Post-procedure

18. Provide for comfort.
19. Place the call bell within reach (if applicable).
20. Raise or lower bed rails. Follow the care plan.
21. Remove the screens from around the person.
22. Wash your hands.
23. Report and record your observations.
24. Take the specimen and the requisition slip to the storage area.

The midstream specimen

The midstream specimen is also called a clean-voided specimen or a clean-catch specimen. The perineal area is cleaned before collecting the specimen. This reduces the number of microbes in the urethral area. The person starts to void into a receptacle. Then the stream is stopped and a sterile specimen container positioned. The person voids into the container until the specimen is obtained.

Stopping the stream of urine is hard for many people. You may need to position and hold the specimen container in place after the person starts to void.

COLLECTING A MIDSTREAM SPECIMEN

Quality of life

Remember to respect the person's privacy while doing any procedure. Address the person by name and ensure they know your name.

Pre-procedure

1. Follow the delegation guidelines.
2. Explain the procedure to the person.
3. Wash your hands.
4. Collect the following:
   - label
   - water, washer and towel
   - disposable gloves
   - gloves
   - sterile specimen container
   - bedpan, urinal or commode if needed
   - plastic bag
   - supplies for perineal care.

Procedure

5. Label the container.
6. Call the person by name.
7. Provide for privacy.
8. Provide perineal care. Remove the gloves and wash your hands.
9. Put on the gloves.
10. Open the sterile specimen container. Do not touch the inside of the container or lid. Set the lid down so the inside is up.
11. For a female: clean the perineum with water.
    - a. Spread the labia with your thumb and index finger. Use your non-dominant hand. (This hand is now contaminated. It must not touch anything sterile.)
    - b. Clean down the urethral area from front to back. Use a clean part of the washer for each stroke.

c Keep the labia separated to collect the urine specimen.

12 For a male: clean the penis with the washer.

a Hold the penis with your non-dominant hand.

b Clean the penis, starting at the meatus. Clean in a circular motion.

c Keep holding the penis until the specimen is collected.

13 Ask the person to void into the toilet, bedpan, commode or urinal.

14 Pass the specimen container into the stream of urine. Keep the labia separated (Fig. 12.73).

15 Collect about 30–60 mL of urine.

16 Remove the specimen container before the person stops urinating.

17 Release the labia or penis.

18 Let the person finish voiding into the toilet, bedpan, commode or urinal.

19 Put the lid on the specimen container. Touch only the outside of the container or lid.

20 Wipe the outside of the container.

21 Place the container in a plastic bag.

22 Provide toilet paper after the person finishes voiding.

23 Remove and empty the bedpan, commode container or urinal.

24 Clean the bedpan, urinal or commode container and other items. Return equipment to its proper place.

25 Remove soiled gloves.

26 Wash your hands.

27 Assist with handwashing.

Post-procedure

28 Follow Post-procedure steps for 'Collecting a random urine specimen'.

SAFETY ALERT

Urine specimens

Microbes can grow in urine. Urine also may contain blood. Follow Standard Precautions.

DELEGATION GUIDELINES

Urine specimens

Before collecting a urine specimen, you need the following information from the nurse and care plan:

- the type of specimen needed
- what time to collect the specimen
- what special measures are needed
- whether you need to test the specimen
- what observations to report and record:
  - difficulty in obtaining the specimen
  - colour, clarity and odour of urine
  - particles in the urine
  - complaints of pain, burning, urgency, dysuria or other problems.

TESTING URINE

You may be asked to do simple urine tests. You can test for pH, glucose, ketones and blood using reagent strips. The doctor orders the type and frequency of urine tests.

Testing pH

Urine pH measures whether the urine is acidic or alkaline. Changes in normal pH (4.6–8.0) occur from illness, foods and medications. A routine urine specimen is needed.

Testing for glucose and ketones

In diabetes mellitus, the pancreas does not secrete enough insulin, or any insulin. The body needs insulin to use sugar for energy. If not used, sugar builds up in the blood. Some sugar appears in the urine. **Glucosuria**, or glycosuria, means sugar (*glucos*, *glycos*) in the urine (*uria*). The diabetic person may also have **acetone** (**ketone bodies**) in the urine. These appear in urine from the rapid breakdown of fat for energy. The body uses fat for energy if it cannot use sugar. Urine is also tested for ketones. Although many diabetics test their blood for levels of glucose, urine may also be tested.

Testing for blood

Injury and disease can cause blood (*haem*) to appear in the urine (*uria*). This is called **haematuria**. Sometimes blood is visible in the urine. At other times, it is unseen (*occult*). A routine urine specimen is needed.

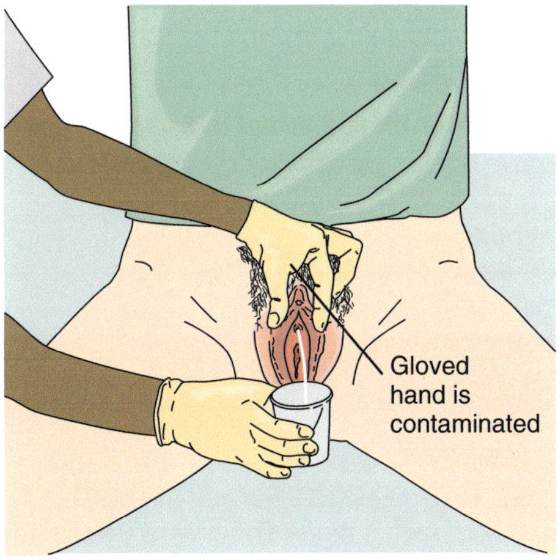

Fig. 12.73
The labia are separated to collect a midstream specimen.

USING REAGENT STRIPS

Reagent strips have sections that change colour when they react with urine. To use a reagent strip, dip the strip into urine. Then compare the strip to the colour chart on the bottle (Fig. 12.74). The nurse gives you instructions for the urine test ordered.

TESTING URINE WITH REAGENT STRIPS

Quality of life

Remember to respect the person's privacy while doing any procedure. Address the person by name and ensure they know your name.

Pre-procedure

1 Follow the delegation guidelines.
2 Check that the reagent strips are not out of date.
3 Explain the procedure to the person.
4 Wash your hands.
5 Call the person by name.

Procedure

6 Put on the gloves.
7 Collect the following:
   - urine specimen
   - reagent strip as ordered
   - gloves.
8 Remove a strip from the bottle. Put the cap on the bottle at once. It must be on tight.
9 Dip the strip test areas into the urine.
10 Remove the strip after the correct amount of time. See the manufacturer's instructions.
11 Tap the strip gently against the container. This removes excess urine.
12 Hold the test strip in a horizontal position.
13 Wait the required amount of time. See the manufacturer's instructions.
14 Compare the strip with the colour chart on the bottle. Read the results.
15 Discard disposable items and the specimen.

Post-procedure

16 Clean and return equipment to its proper place.
17 Remove the gloves and wash your hands.
18 Report and record the results and other observations.

SAFETY ALERT

Using reagent strips

When using reagent strips, read and follow the manufacturer's instructions. Otherwise, you could get the wrong result. The doctor uses the test results in diagnosing and treating the person. A wrong result could lead to serious harm.

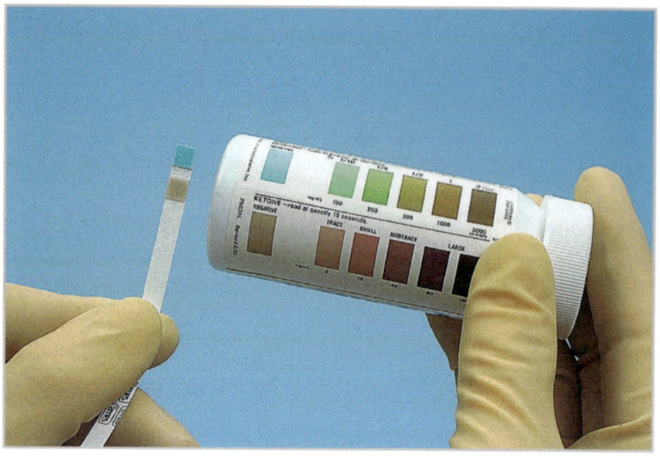

Fig. 12.74
Reagent strip for sugar and ketones.

SAFETY ALERT

Testing urine

You must be accurate when testing urine. Promptly report the results to the nurse. Ordered medications may depend on test results.

Microbes can grow in urine. Urine also may contain blood. Follow Standard Precautions.

DELEGATION GUIDELINES

Testing urine

When testing urine is a delegated task, you need the following information from the care plan:

- which test is needed
- what equipment to use
- when to test the urine
- specific instructions for the test ordered
- whether the nurse wants to observe the results of each test
- what observations to report and record:
  - test results
  - difficulty obtaining the specimen
  - colour, clarity and odour of urine
  - particles in the urine
  - complaints of pain, burning, urgency, dysuria or other problems.

QUALITY OF LIFE

People usually do not void in front of others. Unfortunately, illness, disease and ageing can affect this very private act. Clients often depend on the nursing staff to assist with elimination needs. Some are very weak and disabled. They cannot use the toilet, commode, bedpan or urinal alone.

You must protect the person's privacy. Pull privacy curtains and close doors, shades and drapes. If you must stay in the room, allow as much privacy as possible. Stand just outside the bathroom door in case the person needs you. Or stand on the other side of the privacy curtain if safe to do so.

The nurse will help you with ways to protect the person's privacy.

Privacy and confidentiality are important for people who are incontinent. Incontinence is embarrassing. It affects the person's pride, dignity and self-esteem. Only those involved in the person's care need to know about the incontinence. Patience and understanding are important. Incontinence is not something the person wants or chooses.

ASSISTING WITH WOUND CARE

After reading this section, you should be able to:

- define the key terms listed in this section
- identify clients at risk of skin tears and pressure injury
- understand what causes skin tears and how to prevent them
- recognise the signs, symptoms and causes of pressure injury
- know how to prevent pressure injury
- identify the pressure points in the basic bed and sitting positions
- know the causes of circulatory ulcers and how to prevent them
- understand the process, types and complications of wound healing
- know what to observe about wounds and wound drainage
- understand the rules for applying basic dressings
- know how to meet the basic needs of clients with wounds
- perform the procedures described in this section.

The skin is the body's first line of defence. It protects the body from microbes, which cause infection. Providing good skin care is one of your most important tasks as a carer. Box 12.13 lists the common causes of skin breakdown. Older and disabled clients are at great risk of skin breakdown as their skin is easily injured.

A **wound** is a break in the skin or mucous membrane, and is a portal of entry for microbes. Wounds result from many causes. A surgical incision leaves a wound. Wounds often result from **trauma**, such as an accident or violent act that injures the skin, mucous membranes, bones or internal organs. Falls, vehicle accidents, gunshots, stabbings and other violent acts are sources of trauma. **Pressure ulcers** are wounds that occur from poor skin care and immobility. Circulatory ulcers are caused by decreased blood flow through the arteries and veins.

You must prevent skin injury and give good skin care. When injury does occur, infection is a major threat. Wound care involves preventing infection and further injury to the wound and nearby tissues.

The care plan will describe how to keep the client's skin healthy. Some services have a skin care team to manage all skin problems. Team members may include a registered nurse, a physiotherapist and a dietitian.

TYPES OF WOUNDS

Wounds are described in many ways (Box 12.14). The following wounds are common:

- **abrasion** – a partial-thickness wound caused by the scraping away or rubbing of the skin

BOX 12.13
Common causes of skin breakdown

- Age-related changes in the skin
- Dryness
- Fragile and weak capillaries
- General thinning of the skin
- Loss of fatty layer under the skin
- Decreased sense of touch, heat and cold
- Decreased mobility
- Sitting in a chair or lying in bed most or all of the day
- Chronic diseases (diabetes, high blood pressure)
- Diseases that decrease circulation
- Poor nutrition
- Poor hydration
- Incontinence
- Moisture in dark areas of the body (skin folds, under breasts and perineal areas)
- Poor care of fingernails or toenails
- Friction and shearing

BOX 12.14
Types of wounds

Intentional and unintentional wounds

- **Intentional wounds** – are created for therapy; for example, surgical incisions, and venepunctures for starting intravenous therapy or for collecting blood specimens.
- **Unintentional wounds** – result from trauma (falls, vehicle accidents, gunshots, stabbings and other violent acts).

Open and closed wounds

- **Open wound** – when the skin or mucous membrane is broken. Intentional and most unintentional wounds are open.
- **Closed wound** – tissues are injured but the skin is not broken (bruises, twists and sprains).

Clean and dirty wounds

- **Clean wound** – is not infected. Microbes have not entered the wound. Closed wounds are usually clean. Therefore, they are intentional wounds created under surgically aseptic conditions. The urinary, respiratory and gastrointestinal systems are not entered.
- **Clean-contaminated wound** – occurs from the surgical entry of the urinary, reproductive, respiratory or gastrointestinal system. These systems are not sterile and contain normal flora.
- **Contaminated wound** – has a high risk of infection. Unintentional wounds are generally contaminated. Wound contamination also occurs from breaks in surgical asepsis and spillage of intestinal contents. Tissues may show signs of inflammation.
- **Infected wound (dirty wound)** – contains large amounts of bacteria and shows signs of infection. Examples include old wounds, surgical incisions into infected areas and traumatic injuries that rupture the bowel.
- **Chronic wound** – one that does not heal easily. Pressure ulcers and circulatory ulcers are examples.

Partial- and full-thickness wounds (describe wound depth)

- **Partial-thickness wound** – the dermis and epidermis of the skin are broken.
- **Full-thickness wound** – the dermis, epidermis and subcutaneous tissue are penetrated. Muscle and bone may be involved.

- **contusion** – a closed wound caused by a blow to the body (a **bruise**)
- **incision** – an open wound with clean, straight edges; usually intentionally produced with a sharp instrument
- **laceration** – an open wound with torn tissues and jagged edges
- **penetrating wound** – an open wound in which the skin and underlying tissues are pierced

BOX 12.15
Skin tear classification system

- Category 1a – A skin tear where the edges **can** be realigned to the normal anatomical position (without undue stretching) and the skin or flap colour **is not** pale, dusky or darkened.
- Category 1b – A skin tear where the edges **can** be realigned to the normal anatomical position (without undue stretching) and the skin or flap colour **is** pale, dusky or darkened.
- Category 2a – A skin tear where the edges **cannot** be realigned to the normal anatomical position and the skin flap colour **is not** pale, dusky or darkened.
- Category 2b – A skin tear where the edges **cannot** be realigned to the normal anatomical position and the skin or flap colour **is** pale, dusky or darkened.
- Category 3 – A skin tear where the skin flap is completely absent.

Silver Chain & Curtin University of Technology (2010). Skin Tear Audit Research (STAR) Classification system. Online 7 March 2021. Available: baynav.bopdhb.govt.nz/media/1480/skin-tear-classification-tool.pdf

- **puncture wound** – an open wound made by a sharp object; entry into the skin and underlying tissues may be intentional or unintentional.

SKIN TEARS

A **skin tear** is a break or rip in the skin. The epidermis (top skin layer) separates from the underlying tissue. The hands, arms and lower legs are common sites for skin tears. Many older clients have very thin and fragile skin, and even slight pressure can cause a skin tear.

A classification system for skin tears has been developed and is outlined in Box 12.15.

Causes

Skin tears are caused by friction, shearing, pulling or direct pressure on the skin. A skin tear can occur by bumping a hand, arm or leg on any hard surface. Beds, bed rails, chairs, wheelchair foot pedals and tables are dangers. You can cause a skin tear by holding onto a client's arm or leg too tightly. Be careful when moving, repositioning, or transferring the client. Bathing, dressing and other tasks can cause skin tears. So can pulling buttons or zippers across fragile skin.

Skin tears are painful and are a portal of entry for microbes. Tell the registered nurse at once if you cause or find a skin tear.

Clients at risk

Clients at risk of skin tears:

- require moderate assistance to complete help in moving
- the elderly
- have poor nutrition
- have poor hydration
- have altered mental awareness (see Box 12.16)
- are very thin.

BOX 12.16
Clients with dementia

Some clients are confused and may resist care. They often move quickly and without warning or pull away from you during care. Some may try to hit or kick staff members. These sudden movements can cause skin tears.

If a client resists care, ask the nurse for help. Never force care on a client. Always follow the care plan.

BOX 12.17
Measures to prevent skin tears

Follow the care plan for moving, lifting, repositioning, transferring, dressing and bathing the client.

- Keep the skin moisturised. Follow the care plan.
- Offer fluids. Follow the care plan.
- Dress and undress the client carefully.
- Dress the client in soft clothing with long sleeves and long pants. Tracksuits are an example.
- Keep your fingernails short and smoothly filed.
- Keep the client's fingernails short and smoothly filed. Report long and rough toenails to the nurse.
- Do not wear rings with large or raised stones.
- Follow the safety rules when moving and transferring the client to and from bed and wheelchair.
- Prevent friction and shearing during lifting, moving, transfers and repositioning.
- Use a slide sheet to move and turn the client in bed.
- Use pillows to support arms and legs. Follow the care plan.
- Be patient and stay calm when the client is confused, agitated or resists care.
- Pad bed rails and wheelchair arms, foot pedals and leg supports. Follow the care plan.
- Provide good lighting. It helps prevent the client from bumping into furniture, walls and equipment.

Prevention and treatment

Giving careful and safe care helps prevent skin tears and further injury. Follow the measures in Box 12.17.

The doctor and the nurse or skin care team direct skin tear treatment. Dressings may be ordered, as some dressings protect the skin from injury. They also help the healing process. Follow the care plan and the nurse's instructions.

PRESSURE INJURY (ULCER)

A **pressure injury** is any injury caused by unrelieved pressure. It usually occurs over a bony prominence. A bony prominence is an area where the bone sticks out or projects out from the flat surface of the body. The shoulder blades, elbows, hips, sacrum, knees, ankles, heels and toes are bony prominences (Fig. 12.75).

Causes

Pressure, friction, and shearing are common causes of skin breakdown and pressure injury. Other factors include breaks in the skin, poor circulation to an area, moisture, dry skin and irritation by urine and faeces.

Pressure occurs when the skin over a bony area is squeezed between hard surfaces. The bone is one hard surface; the other is usually the mattress or chair seat. Squeezing or pressure prevents blood flow to the skin and underlying tissues. Lack of blood flow means oxygen and nutrients cannot get to the cells. Therefore, the skin and tissues die (Fig. 12.76).

Friction scrapes the skin. An open area, the scrape, is a portal of entry for microbes. The open area needs to heal, so a good blood supply is needed. Infection is prevented so that healing can occur. A poor blood supply or an infection can lead to a pressure ulcer.

Shearing is when the skin sticks to a surface (usually the bed or chair) and deeper tissues move downwards. Shearing occurs when the client slides down in the bed or chair. As blood vessels and tissues are damaged, blood flow to the area is reduced.

Clients at risk

Clients at risk of pressure injury are those who:

- are confined to bed or a chair
- require moderate to complete help in moving
- have loss of bowel or bladder control
- have poor nutrition
- have poor fluid balance
- have altered mental awareness
- have problems sensing pain or pressure
- have circulatory problems
- are elderly
- are obese or very thin.

Signs of pressure injury

The first sign of a pressure injury is pale skin or a reddened area. Colour changes may be hard to notice in clients with dark skin. The client may complain of pain, burning or tingling in the area, although some do not feel anything unusual. Pressure injuries occur in stages (Fig. 12.77). Box 12.18 describes the pressure injury stages.

BOX 12.18
Stages of pressure injury

Stage 1: The skin is red. The colour does not return to normal when the skin is relieved of pressure.
Stage 2: The skin cracks, blisters or peels. There may be a shallow crater.
Stage 3: The skin is gone. Underlying tissues are exposed. The exposed tissue is damaged. There may be drainage from the area.
Stage 4: Muscle and bone are exposed and damaged. Drainage is likely.

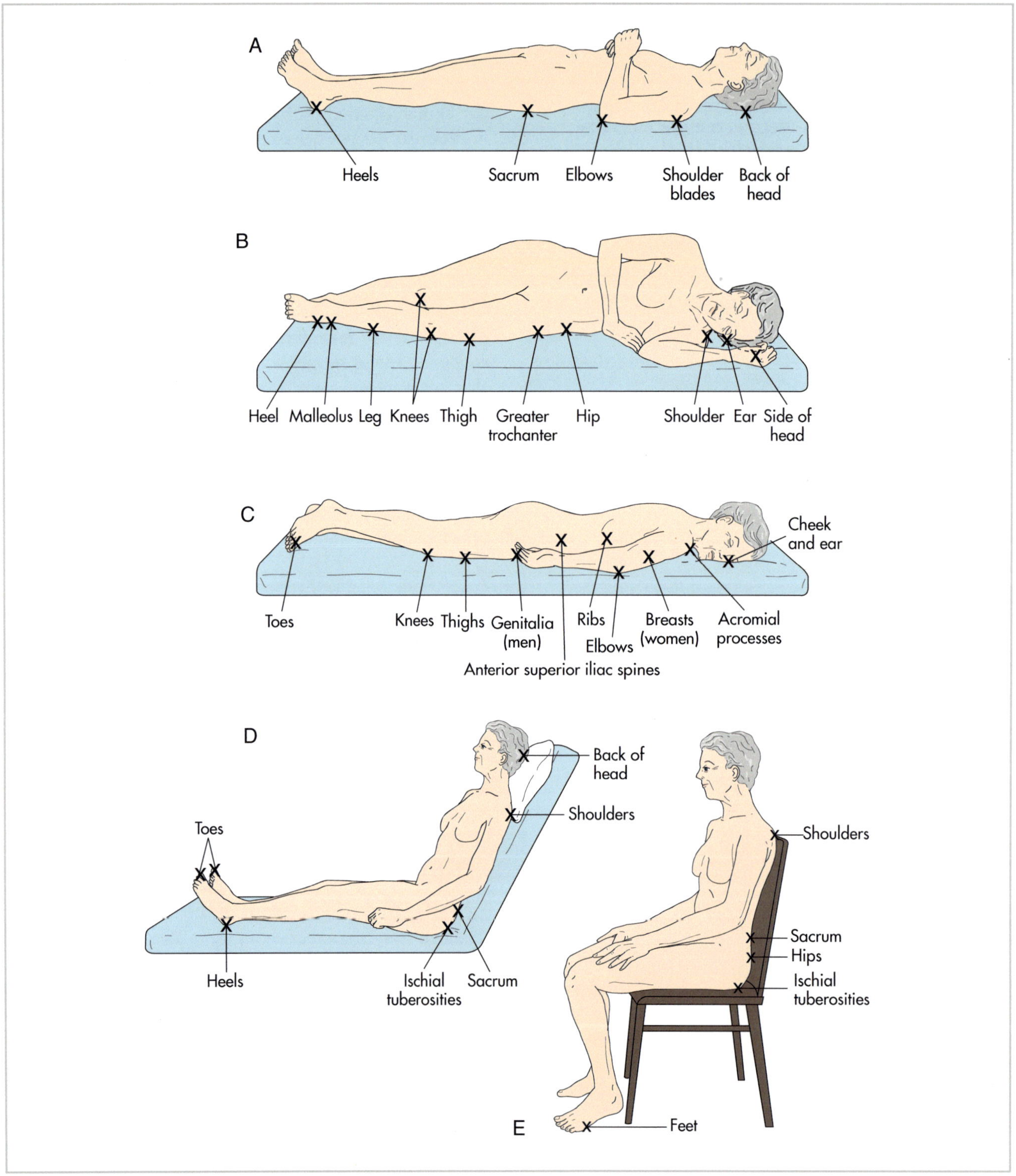

Fig. 12.75

Pressure points.

A. The supine position. **B.** The lateral position. **C.** The prone position. **D.** Fowler's position. **E.** The sitting position.

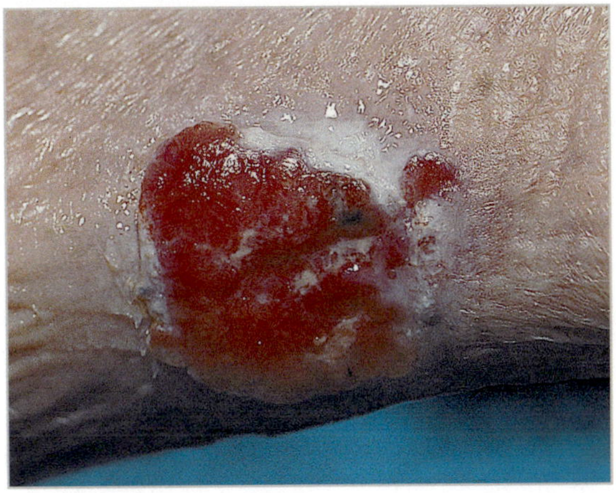

Fig. 12.76
A pressure ulcer.

Sites

Pressure injuries usually occur over bony areas, which are called pressure points. This is because they bear the weight of the body in a certain position. Pressure from body weight can reduce the blood supply to the area.

In obese people, pressure injury can occur in areas where skin is in contact with skin. Common sites are between abdominal folds, the legs, the buttocks and underneath the breasts, as friction occurs in these areas.

Clients who spend a lot of time in bed are at risk of pressure ulcers on the ears. This is from the pressure of the ear on the mattress when the person is in the side-lying position.

Prevention and treatment

Preventing pressure ulcers is much easier than trying to heal them. Good care, cleanliness and skin care are essential.

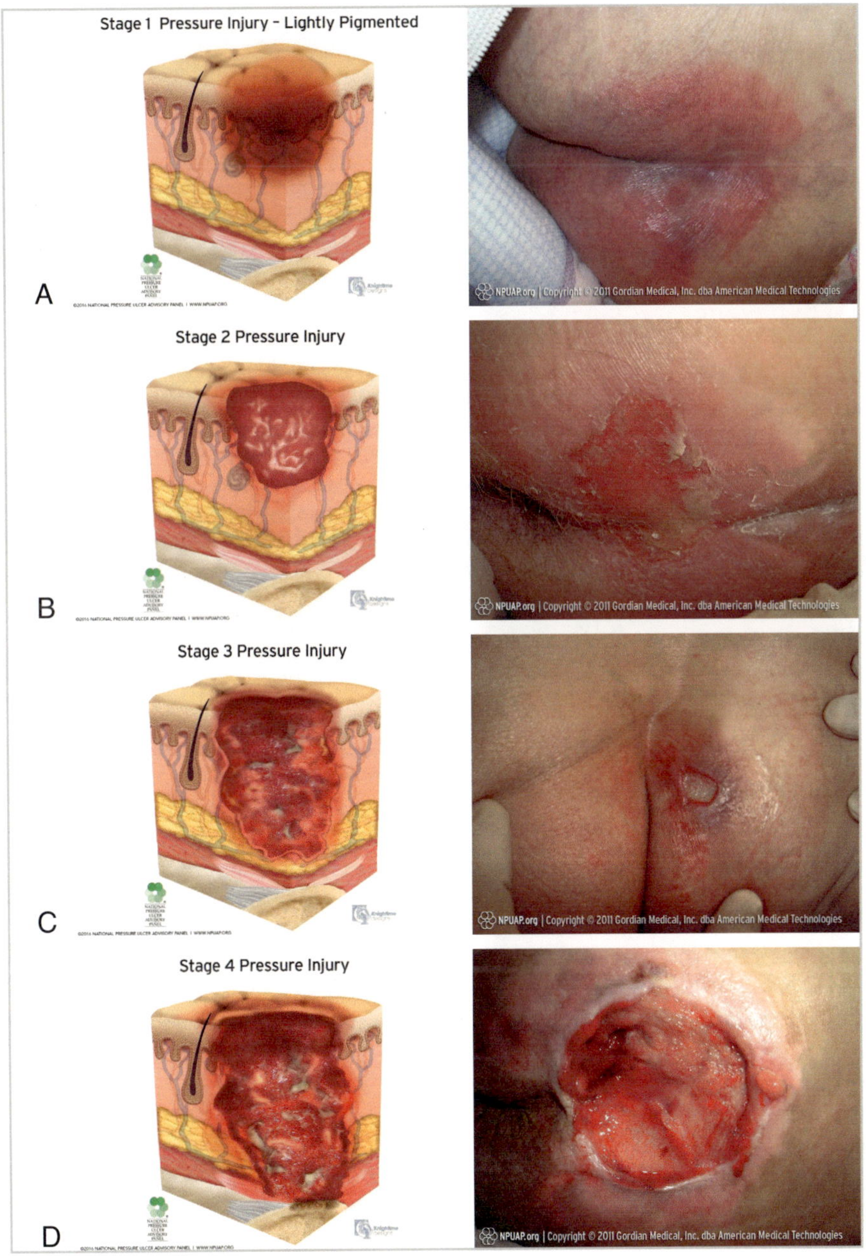

Fig. 12.77
Stages of pressure ulcers. **A.** Stage 1. **B.** Stage 2. **C.** Stage 3. **D.** Stage 4.

The measures in Box 12.19 help prevent skin breakdown and pressure ulcers. A care plan is developed by the aged care team to prevent pressure ulcers for each client at risk. You must know and follow the care plan.

Any client at risk of pressure ulcers is placed on a surface that reduces or relieves pressure. Such surfaces include foam, air, alternating air, gel or water mattresses. The aged care team decides on the best surface for the client.

The doctor and aged care team directs pressure ulcer treatment. Wound care products, medications, treatments and special equipment help promote healing. The nurse and care plan will detail the processes and products to be used. The following protective devices are often ordered, as they prevent and treat pressure ulcers and other types of skin breakdown.

- *Bed cradle* – this is a metal frame placed on the bed and over the client (Fig. 12.79).
- Top linen is brought over the cradle to prevent pressure on the legs and feet. Top linen is tucked in at the bottom of the mattress and mitred. It is also tucked under both sides of the mattress. This protects the client from air draughts and chilling.
- *Elbow protectors* – these are made of foam rubber or sheepskin. They fit the shape of the elbow (Fig. 12.80). Some have straps to secure them in place. Friction is prevented between the bed and the elbow.
- *Heel elevators* – pillows or special cushions raise the heels off the bed. Special braces and splints also keep pressure away from the heels.
- *Flotation pads* – flotation pads or cushions (Fig. 12.81) are like water beds. They are used for chairs and wheelchairs and are made of a gel-like substance. The outer case is heavy plastic. The pad is placed in a pillowcase or special cover, as this prevents the plastic from touching the skin.
- *Gel or fluid mattress* – a number of different types of mattresses or overlays are filled with gel or fluid substances that support a client and reduce pressure points.
- *Eggshell mattress* – this is a foam pad that looks like an egg carton and is placed on top of the regular mattress (Fig. 12.82). The peaks in the mattress distribute the client's weight more evenly. The eggshell mattress is put in a special cover that protects against moisture and soiling. Only a bottom sheet is used over the eggshell mattress and cover. No other bottom linen is used. (This mattress is not used as much now, as gel, fluid and air flotation mattresses are more effective.)
- *Pressure-relieving mattress* – this is an air flotation mattress (Fig. 12.83) that alternates pressure on various parts of the body. This ensures that there is little pressure on bony parts and body weight is distributed evenly. Place the mattress on the bed or over the existing mattress, depending on the manufacturer's instructions.
- *Other equipment* – trochanter rolls, footboards and pillows are also used.

BOX 12.19
Measures to prevent ulcers

- Follow the repositioning schedule in the client's care plan.
- Position the client according to the care plan. Use pillows for support as instructed by the nurse. The 30-degree lateral position is recommended (Fig. 12.78).
- Prevent shearing and friction during lifting, moving, transferring and repositioning procedures.
- Do not raise the head of the bed more than 30 degrees. This prevents shearing. Follow the care plan.
- Provide good skin care. The skin is clean and dry after bathing. The skin is free of moisture from urine, faeces, sweat and wound drainage.
- Minimise skin exposure to moisture. Check incontinent clients often. Also, check clients who perspire heavily and those with wound drainage. Change linen and clothing as needed. Provide good skin care.
- Check with the nurse before using soap. Soap can dry and irritate the skin.
- Apply a moisturiser to dry areas – the hands, elbows, legs, ankles and heels. The nurse tells you what to use and where to apply it.
- Give a gentle back massage when repositioning the client. Do not massage bony areas.
- Keep linen clean, dry and wrinkle-free.
- If a powder is to be used where skin touches skin, only use corn starch. This should never be applied to the perineal areas.
- Do not irritate the skin. Daily showers are no longer advocated as this merely dries out the skin and ordinary soap usually alters the skin's normal pH, further compromising skin integrity. Avoid scrubbing or rubbing when bathing or drying the client.
- Do not massage pressure points. Never rub or massage reddened areas.
- Use pillows and blankets to prevent skin from being in contact with skin. They also reduce moisture and friction.
- Keep the heels off the bed. Use pillows or other devices as directed. Place the pillows or devices under the lower legs from mid-calf to the ankles.
- Use protective devices as the nurse and care plan direct.
- Remind clients sitting in chairs to shift their positions frequently. This decreases pressure on bony points.
- Report signs of skin breakdown or pressure ulcers at once. Record your observations according to the facility's policy.

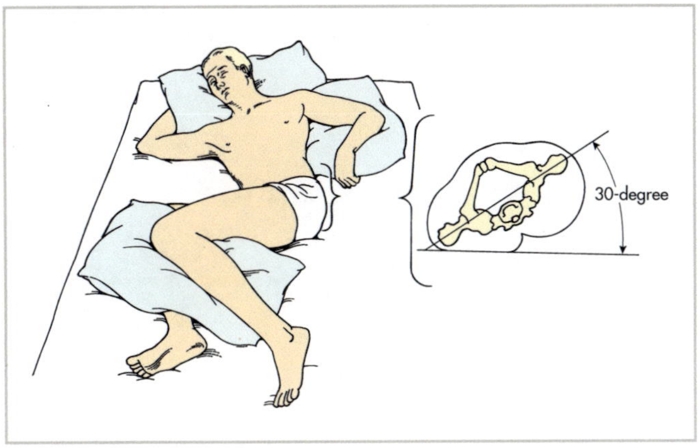

Fig. 12.78
The 30-degree lateral position. Pillows are placed under the head, shoulder and leg. This position inclines (lifts up) the hip to avoid pressure on the hip. The client does not lie on the hip as in the side-lying position.

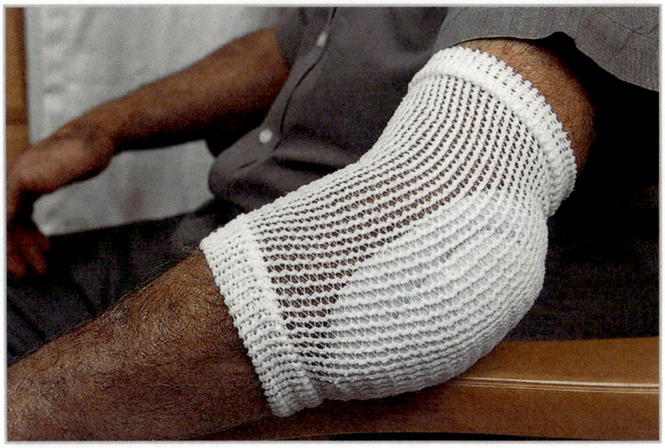

Fig. 12.80
Elbow protector.

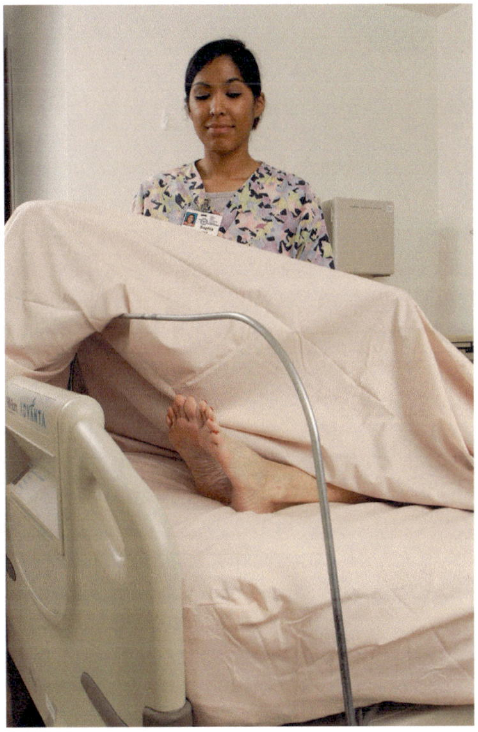

Fig. 12.79
Bed cradle.

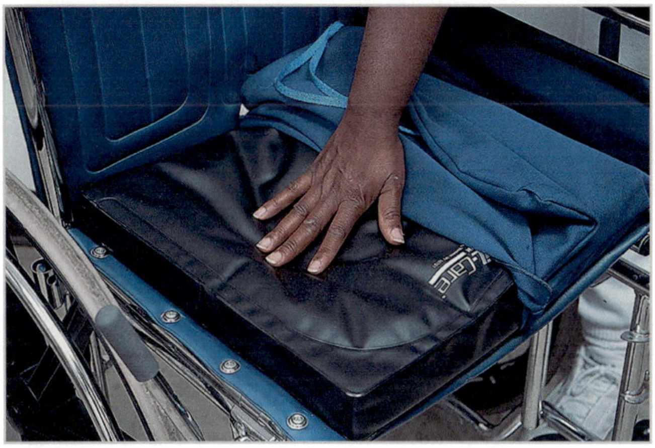

Fig. 12.81
Flotation pad.

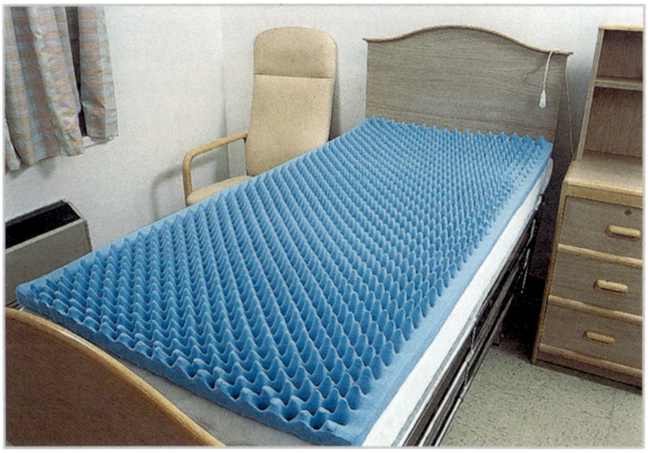

Fig. 12.82
Eggshell mattress.

LEG AND FOOT ULCERS

Some diseases affect blood flow to and from the legs and feet. They can cause pain, open wounds and oedema. **Oedema** is swelling caused by fluid collecting in tissues. Infection and **gangrene** can result from the open wound and poor circulation. Gangrene is a condition in which there is death of tissue.

The client needs special skin care. The doctor and aged care team direct the client's care and the nurse uses the nursing process (client-centred care) to identify and meet

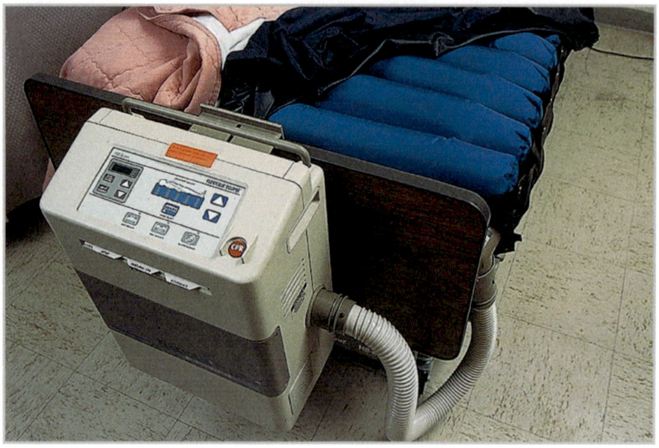

Fig. 12.83
Pressure-relieving mattress.

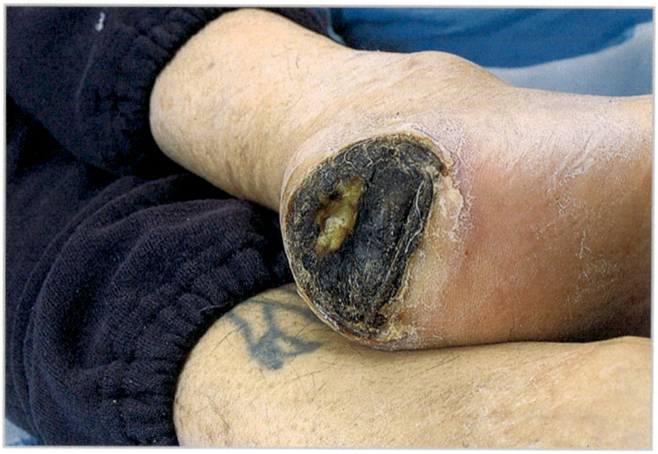

Fig. 12.84
Stasis ulcer.

the client's needs. Preventing skin breakdown on the legs and feet is very important.

Circulatory ulcers

Circulatory ulcers (**vascular ulcers**) are open wounds on the lower legs and feet caused by decreased blood flow through arteries or veins. Older clients with diseases affecting the blood vessels are at risk of these ulcers on the legs and feet. These wounds are often painful and hard to heal.

Stasis ulcers

Stasis ulcers (**venous ulcers**) are open wounds on the lower legs and feet caused by poor blood return through the veins (Fig. 12.84). If the valves in the leg veins do not close well, the blood is not able to be pumped through them back to the heart normally. This causes blood and fluid to collect in the legs and feet. Oedema occurs in the legs and feet, and small veins in the skin can rupture. Remember, haemoglobin gives blood its red colour. When veins rupture, haemoglobin enters the tissues and causes the skin to turn brown and become dry, leathery and hard. Itching is common.

The heels and inner aspect of the ankles are common sites for stasis ulcers. They can occur from skin injury. Scratching is a common cause, or the ulcers can occur spontaneously.

Stasis ulcers are painful and make walking difficult. As they are open wounds, they weep fluid, and infection is a great risk. Healing may be very slow.

Causes

Some chronic diseases cause blood and fluid to collect in the legs and feet. The skin is easily injured and heals slowly. Even a small injury may lead to an ulcer. Factors such as obesity, inactivity, long periods with the legs crossed and pressure under the knees can make the problem worse.

Risk factors

Risk factors for stasis ulcers include:

- history of blood clots
- history of varicose veins
- decreased mobility
- obesity
- leg or foot injury
- advanced age
- surgery on bones and joints of the legs
- **phlebitis** (inflammation [*itis*] of a vein [*phleb*]).

Prevention and treatment

Preventing skin breakdown caused by poor venous circulation is very important. Stasis ulcers are hard to heal. Box 12.20 lists measures that help prevent stasis ulcers. They may be part of the client's care plan.

Clients at risk require professional foot care. Corns and calluses are treated and the client's toenails are only cut by foot-care professionals. The doctor may order medications to treat infection and to decrease swelling. Medicated leg wrappings and other wound care products are often ordered. So is equipment used for pressure ulcers.

Help prevent further injury by not bumping the client's legs or feet. Carefully move, lift, reposition and transfer the client.

The doctor may order elastic support stockings, which promote comfort and circulation by providing support and pressure to the veins. The stockings also promote healing and prevent injury. Elastic stockings must be applied correctly, otherwise severe discomfort, skin irritation and circulatory problems may occur.

Elastic stockings

Clients with circulatory disorders, heart disease and those on bed rest are at risk of blood clots. A blood clot is called a **thrombus**. Elastic stockings help prevent blood clots (thrombi) forming.

Blood clots can form if blood flow is sluggish. They tend to form in deep leg veins (Fig. 12.85A). A thrombus can break loose and travel through the bloodstream and become an embolus. An embolus is a blood clot that travels through the vascular system until it lodges in a distant vessel (Fig. 12.85B). An **embolus** from a vein can lodge in

BOX 12.20
Measures to prevent stasis ulcers

- Apply elastic stockings according to the care plan.
- Remind the client not to sit with legs crossed.
- Do not use elastic or rubber band type of garters to hold socks or stockings in place.
- Do not dress the client in tight clothing.
- Provide good skin care daily. Clean and dry between the toes. Remember to inform the nurse in charge if a podiatry referral is necessary.
- Avoid injury to legs and feet.
- Keep linen clean, dry and wrinkle-free.
- Follow the care plan for walking and exercise. This increases venous blood flow.
- Reposition the client frequently. Follow the care plan.
- Elevate the legs according to the care plan.
- Have the client wear comfortable socks and shoes.
- Do not irritate the skin. Avoid scrubbing or rubbing when bathing or drying the client.
- Avoid massaging over pressure points. Never rub or massage reddened areas.
- Keep the heels off the bed. Use pillows or other devices as instructed by the nurse. Place the pillows or devices under the lower legs from mid-calf to the ankles.
- Use protective devices as the nurse directs. Follow the care plan.
- Report signs of skin breakdown, stasis ulcers or pressure ulcers at once.

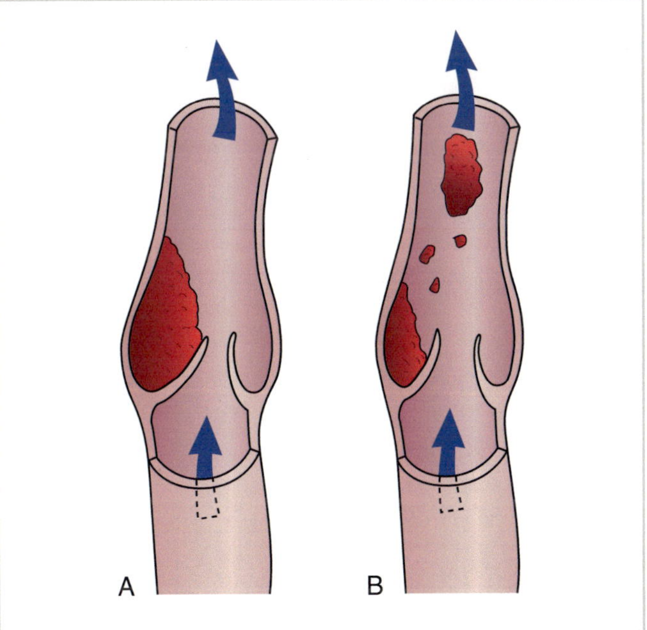

Fig. 12.85
A. A blood clot has formed on the wall of a vein. The arrows show the direction of blood flow. **B.** Part of the thrombus has broken off and become an embolus. An embolus will travel in the bloodstream until it lodges in a distant vessel.

the lungs (pulmonary embolus) and can cause severe respiratory problems and death.

Elastic stockings are also known as *anti-embolism* or *anti-embolic* (AE) *stockings*. The elastic exerts pressure on the veins, which promotes venous blood flow to the heart.

Most stockings have an opening near the toes. Others have an opening in the top or bottom of the foot. The opening is used to check circulation, skin colour and temperature.

Stockings come in thigh-high or knee-high lengths. The nurse or physiotherapist measures the client for the correct size. They are applied in the morning before the client gets out of bed, as the legs can swell from sitting or standing. Stockings are difficult to put on when legs are swollen. They are removed every 8 hours for 30 minutes or according to the care plan. The client lies in bed while they are off. This prevents the legs from swelling.

The client usually has two pairs of stockings. One pair is washed while the client wears the other pair. Wash the stockings by hand with a mild soap and hang to dry.

Follow these rules when applying elastic bandages:

- Use the correct length and width.
- Position the limb in good alignment.
- Face the client during the procedure.
- Expose fingers or toes if possible. This allows circulation checks.
- Apply the bandage with firm, even pressure.
- Check the colour and temperature of the extremity every hour.
- Reapply a loose, wrinkled, moist or soiled bandage.

DELEGATION GUIDELINES

Elastic stockings

Before you apply elastic stockings, you need the following information from the nurse and care plan:

- what size stockings to use (small, medium or large)
- what length stocking is ordered: thigh-high or knee-high
- when to remove and reapply them
- observations to report and record:
  - when you applied the stockings
  - skin colour and skin temperature
  - leg and foot swelling
  - signs of skin breakdown
  - complaints of pain, tingling or numbness
  - when you removed the stockings and for how long
  - when you reapplied the stockings
  - when you washed the stockings.

SAFETY ALERT

Elastic stockings

Stockings should not have twists, creases or wrinkles after you apply them. Twists can affect circulation. Creases and wrinkles can cause skin breakdown.

APPLYING ELASTIC STOCKINGS

Quality of life

Remember to respect the person's privacy while doing any procedure. Address the person by name and ensure they know your name.

Pre-procedure

1 Follow the delegation guidelines.
2 Explain the procedure to the client.
3 Wash your hands.
4 Obtain elastic stockings in the correct size and length.
5 Identify the client.
6 Ensure privacy.
7 Raise the bed for body mechanics (if applicable).

Procedure

8 Lower the bed rail near you if it is up (if applicable).
9 Position the client in the supine position.
10 Expose the legs. Fan-fold top linen towards the client's thighs.
11 Turn the stocking inside out down to the heel (Fig. 12.86).
12 Slip the foot of the stocking over the toes, foot and heel.
13 Grasp the stocking top. Slip it over the foot and heel. Pull it up the leg. It turns right side out as it is pulled up. The stocking is even and snug.
14 Remove twists, creases or wrinkles.
15 Repeat steps 11 to 14 for the other leg.

Post-procedure

16 Cover the client.
17 Provide for comfort.
18 Lower the bed (if applicable).
19 Remove the screens from around the client.
20 Wash hands.
21 Report and record your observations.

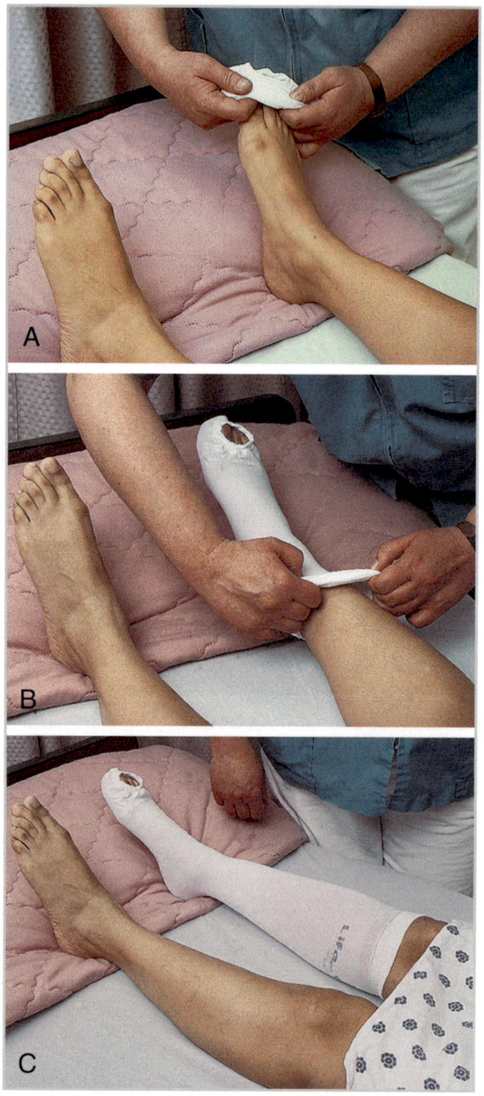

Fig. 12.86
Applying elastic stockings.
A. The stocking is turned inside out down to the heel. **B.** The stocking is slipped over toes, foot and heel. **C.** The stocking turns right side out as it is pulled up over the leg.

DELEGATION GUIDELINES

Elastic bandages

Before applying an elastic bandage, you need the following information from the nurse and the plan:

- where to apply the bandage
- what width and length to use
- when to remove the bandage and for how long
- what to do if the bandage is wet or soiled
- observations to report and record:
  - when you applied the bandage
  - skin colour and temperature
  - leg and foot swelling
  - signs of skin breakdown
  - complaints of pain, itching, tingling or numbness
  - when you removed the bandage and for how long
  - when you reapplied the bandage.

APPLYING ELASTIC BANDAGES

Quality of life

Remember to respect the person's privacy while doing any procedure. Address the person by name and ensure they know your name.

Pre-procedure

1 Follow the delegation guidelines.
2 Explain the procedure to the client.
3 Wash your hands.
4 Collect the following:
   - elastic bandage as directed by the nurse
   - tape (unless the bandage has Velcro).
5 Ensure privacy.
6 Raise the bed for body mechanics (if applicable).

Procedure

7 Lower the bed rail near you if it is up (if applicable).
8 Help the client to a comfortable position. Expose the part you will bandage.
9 Make sure the area is clean and dry.
10 Hold the bandage so that the roll is up. The loose end is on the bottom.
11 Apply the bandage to the smallest part of the wrist, foot, ankle or knee.
12 Make two circular turns around the part.
13 Make overlapping spiral turns in an upward direction. Each turn overlaps about two-thirds of the previous turn.
14 Apply the bandage smoothly with firm, even pressure. It is not tight.
15 Secure the bandage in place with tape.
16 Check the fingers or toes for coldness or cyanosis (bluish colour). Ask about pain, itching, numbness or tingling. Remove the bandage if any are noted. Report your observations to the nurse.

Post-procedure

17 Provide for comfort.
18 Place the call bell within reach (if applicable).
19 Lower the bed (if applicable).
20 Remove the screens from around the client.
21 Wash your hands.
22 Report and record your observations.

SAFETY ALERT

Elastic bandages

Elastic bandages must be firm and snug; however, they must not be tight. A tight bandage can affect circulation. Some aged care services do not allow carers to apply elastic bandages. Be familiar with your facility's policy.

Arterial ulcers

Arterial ulcers are open wounds on the lower legs and feet, caused by poor arterial blood flow. The leg and foot may feel cold and look blue or shiny. The ulcer is often painful during rest. The pain is usually worse at night.

Causes and risk factors

Arterial ulcers are caused by diseases or injuries that decrease arterial blood flow to the legs and feet. High blood pressure and diabetes are common causes. So are narrowed arteries from ageing. Smoking is another risk factor.

Elastic bandages

Elastic bandages have the same purpose as elastic stockings. They provide support and reduce swelling from injuries. They also hold dressings in place. They are applied to the upper or lower extremities. Clients with varicose veins may need elastic bandages. Varicose veins sit under the skin and are dilated (wide) and bulging (Fig. 12.87).

The bandage is applied from the lower (distal) part of the extremity to the top (proximal) part. The care plan will detail what area to bandage. Elastic bandages are removed every 8 hours for 30 minutes.

Sites

Arterial ulcers are found:

- between the toes
- on the tops of the toes
- on the outer side of the ankle
- on the heels (common sites in clients on bed rest)
- on pressure sites from shoes that fit poorly.

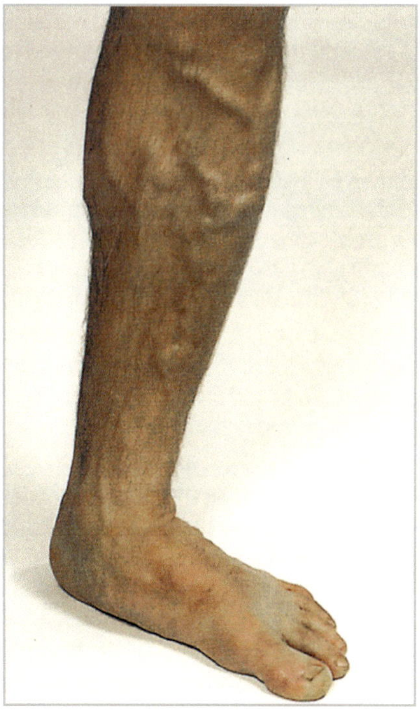

Fig. 12.87
Varicose veins.

BOX 12.21
Measures to prevent arterial ulcers

- No smoking.
- Remind clients not to sit with legs crossed.
- Avoid exposure to the cold.
- Do not use elastic or rubber band type of garters to hold socks and stockings in place.
- Make sure shoes fit well.
- Keep feet clean and dry.
- Keep pressure off heels and other bony points.
- Keep pressure from under the knees.
- Check the client's legs and feet daily. Report changes in skin colour or breaks in the skin to the nurse.
- Avoid massaging over pressure points. Never rub or massage reddened areas.
- Use protective devices as the nurse directs. Follow the care plan.

Prevention and treatment

Box 12.21 lists preventive measures required for arterial ulcers. The client's care plan gives instructions for foot care.

Clients at risk require professional foot care. Corns and calluses are treated and the person's toenails are only cut by foot-care professionals.

The doctor treats the disease process that caused the problem. Medication can be used to control oedema and pain. Medication may also be prescribed to clean and dress wounds. Exercise and walking schedules are ordered.

Check with the nurse before giving care to clients with leg and foot wounds. Be very careful not to cause further injury, and always follow the care plan.

QUALITY OF LIFE

Clients have the right to care that promotes healthy skin and prevents skin breakdown. A care plan is developed for each client, and this must address the need for skin care. Sometimes special skin care products, protective devices and stockings or bandages are needed. It is important to keep the client's skin healthy.

The skin is the body's first line of defence against changes in the environment. The skin is kept clean and intact. This promotes comfort and prevents infection. Providing good skin care is an important part of your job. Older clients require special skin care as their skin is thin and frail.

Clients who spend a lot of time in bed or in chairs are at risk of skin breakdown and pressure ulcers. They are also at risk of thrombi (blood clots).

Many clients have poor arterial or venous circulation and are at risk of open wounds on the lower legs and feet. You must follow the client's care plan. Be very careful not to injure the skin during care.

Wounds result from surgery, trauma, pressure and circulatory problems. Many factors affect wound healing. These include wound type and location. The client's age, general health, nutrition and lifestyle are other factors. Wounds cause pain and discomfort. Basic needs are affected. You must treat the client with dignity and respect.

WOUND HEALING

The healing process has four phases:

1. *Haemostasis* – the first stage of wound healing, when bleeding stops.
2. *Inflammatory phase* (day 1 to 3) – bleeding stops. A scab forms over the wound, preventing microbes from entering the wound. Blood supply to the wound increases, which brings nutrients and healing substances. Signs and symptoms of inflammation appear with blood increase: redness, swelling heat, warmth and pain. Loss of function may occur.
3. *Proliferative phase* (day 3 to 21) – 'proliferate' means to multiply rapidly. Tissue cells multiply to repair the wound.
4. *Maturation phase* (day 21 to 1–2 years) – the scar gains strength. The red, raised scar becomes thin and pale.

Types of wound healing

- The healing occurs through primary intention, secondary intention or tertiary intention. With *primary intention* (first intention, primary closure) the wound is closed. Sutures (stitches), staples, clips, special glue or adhesive strips hold the wound edges together.
- *Secondary intention* (second intention) is used for contaminated and infected wounds. Wounds are cleaned and dead tissue removed. Wound edges are not brought together and the wound gapes. Healing occurs naturally. However, healing takes longer and leaves a larger scar. The risk of infection is great.
- *Tertiary intention* (third intention, delayed intention) involves leaving the wound open and closing it later. It combines secondary and primary intention. Infection and poor circulation are common reasons for tertiary intention.

Complications

Many factors affect healing and increase the risk of complications (Box 12.22). The type of wound is one factor. Other factors include the client's age, general health, nutrition and lifestyle.

- Good circulation is important. Age, smoking, circulatory disease and diabetes all affect circulation. Some

BOX 12.22
Complications affecting wound healing

- **Infection** – wound contamination can occur during or after injury. Trauma often causes contaminated wounds. Surgical wounds can be contaminated during or after surgery. An infected wound appears inflamed (reddened) and has drainage. The wound is painful and tender. The client has a fever.
- **Dehiscence** – the separation of the wound layers. Separation may involve the skin layer or underlying tissues. Abdominal wounds are commonly affected. Coughing, vomiting and abdominal distension place stress on the wound. The client often describes the sensation of the wound popping open.
- **Evisceration** – the separation of the wound along with the protrusion of abdominal organs. Causes are the same as for dehiscence. Dehiscence and evisceration are surgical emergencies. Tell the nurse at once if they happen. The nurse covers the wound with large sterile dressings saturated with sterile saline. Help prepare the client for emergency transport to hospital.

medications, including anticoagulants, may prolong bleeding.

- Good nutrition is needed, and protein is needed for tissue growth and repair.
- Infection is a risk for clients with immune system changes and for those taking antibiotics. Specific antibiotics kill certain pathogens. In doing so, an environment may be created that allows other pathogens to grow and multiply.

Wound drainage

During the healing process, doctors and nurses observe the wound and its drainage. They observe for healing and complications. Box 12.23 lists wound observations.

During injury and the inflammatory phase of wound healing, fluid and cells escape from the tissues. The amount of drainage may be small or large. The amount depends on wound size and location. Bleeding and infection also affect the amount and kind of drainage. Wound drainage is observed and measured.

- **Serous drainage** – clear, watery fluid. The fluid in a blister is serous. Serous comes from the word serum. *Serum* is the clean, thin, fluid portion of blood. Serum does not contain blood cells or platelets.
- **Sanguineous drainage** – bloody drainage. *Sanguineous* comes from the Latin word sanguis. It means blood. The amount and colour of sanguineous drainage is important. Haemorrhage is suspected when large amounts are present. Bright drainage means fresh bleeding. Older bleeding is darker.
- **Serosanguineous drainage** – thin, watery drainage (sero) that is blood-tinged (sanguineous).
- **Purulent drainage** – thick drainage that is green, yellow or brown.

BOX 12.23
Wound observations

Wound location

- Multiple wounds may exist from surgery or trauma.

Wound size and depth (measure in centimetres)

- Size: measured from top to bottom and side to side (Fig. 12.88).
- Depth: (1) A sterile swab is inserted inside the deepest part of the wound. (2) The swab is removed and the distance on the swab measured. Only the nurse measures wound depth.
- Use the same ruler to measure the wound.

Wound appearance

- Is the wound red and swollen?
- Is the area around the wound warm to touch?
- Are sutures, staples or clips intact or broken?
- Are wound edges closed or separated? Did the wound break open?

Drainage

- Is the drainage serous, sanguineous, serosanguineous or purulent (Fig. 12.89)?
- What is the amount of drainage?

Odour

- Does the wound or drainage have an odour?

Surrounding skin

- Is surrounding skin intact?
- What is the colour of surrounding skin?
- Are surrounding tissues swollen?

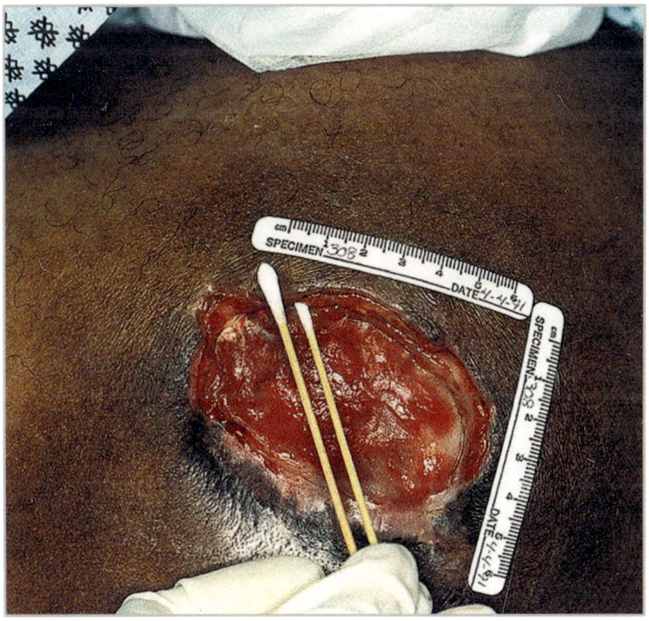

Fig. 12.88
The size and depth of this pressure ulcer are measured.

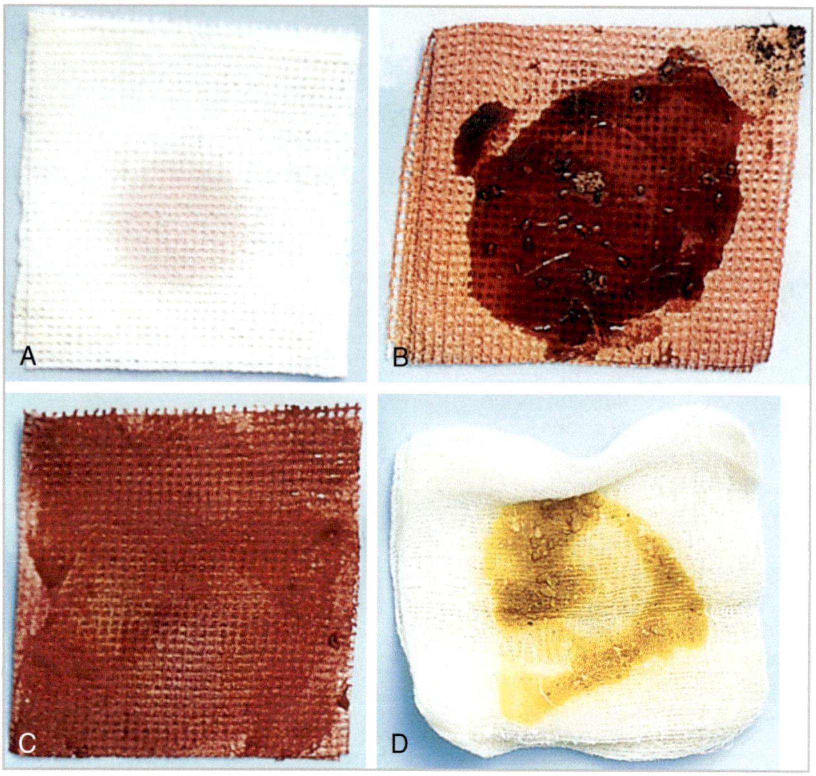

Fig. 12.89
Wound drainage.
A. Serous drainage. **B.** Sanguineous drainage. **C.** Serosanguineous drainage. **D.** Purulent drainage.

For healing to occur, drainage must leave the wound. If drainage is trapped inside the wound, the underlying tissues swell. The wound may heal at the skin level, but the underlying tissues do not close. Infection and other complications can occur.

When large amounts of drainage are expected, the doctor inserts a drain. A Penrose drain (Fig. 12.90) is a rubber tube that drains onto a dressing. It opens onto the dressing, therefore it is an open drain. Microbes can enter the drain and wound.

Closed drainage systems prevent microbes from entering the wound. A drain is placed in the wound and attached to suction. The Haemovac and Belovac systems are examples. Other systems used depend on wound type, size and location.

It is the nurse's role to undertake management of these wounds. However, you will be expected to report relevant observations.

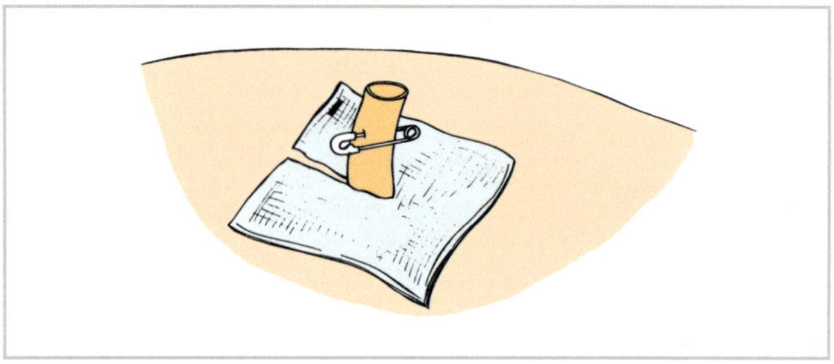

Fig. 12.90
Penrose drain. The safety pin prevents the drain from slipping into the wound.

DRESSINGS

Wound dressings have many functions:
- they protect wounds from injury and microbes
- they absorb drainage
- they clean wounds
- they promote comfort
- they provide a moist environment for wound healing
- when bleeding is a problem, pressure dressings help control bleeding.

Dressing type and size depend on many factors. These include the type of wound, its size and location and the amount of drainage. Infection is a factor. The dressing's function and the frequency of dressing changes are other factors. The doctor and nurse choose the best type of dressing for each wound.

Types of dressings

Dressings are described by the material used and application method. There are many dressing products and you must ask the nurse which type of dressing to use. Follow

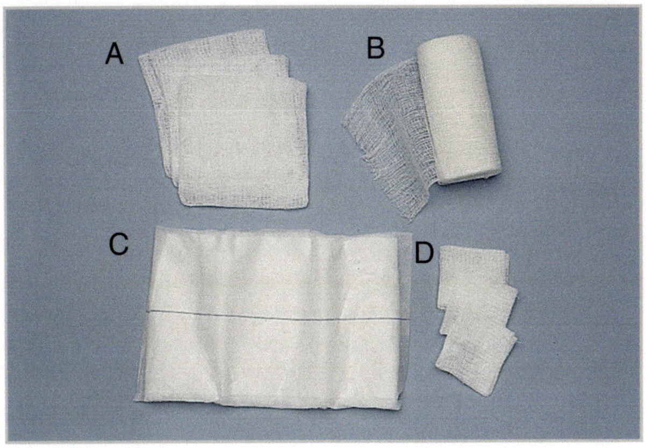

Fig. 12.91
Gauze dressings.
A. 12 cm × 12 cm. **B.** Gauze roll. **C.** Abdominal pad. **D.** 5 cm × 5 cm.

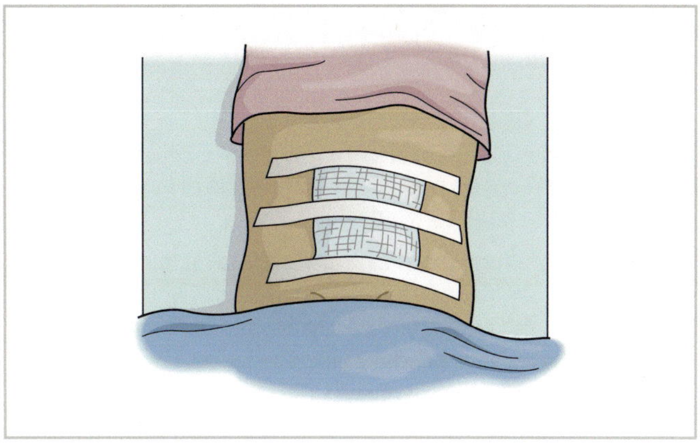

Fig. 12.92
Tape is applied at the top, middle and bottom of the dressing. The tape extends several centimetres beyond each side of the dressing.

the manufacturer's instructions when using dressings. The following are common dressings:

- tulle gras dressings
- gauze dressing (Fig. 12.91)
- Steri-strips (for skin closure)
- foam dressings
- calcium alginate dressings
- hydrocolloid dressings
- hydro gel dressings
- gel sheets
- non-adherent/non-absorbent dressings
- transparent adhesive film – this dressing should only be used as a secondary dressing; do not use on skin tears.

Some of these dressings contain special agents to promote wound healing. If you assist with the dressing change, the nurse will explain its use to you.

Securing dressings

Dressings must be secure over wounds. If the dressing is dislodged, microbes can enter the wound and drainage can escape. Dressings are either self-adhesive or held in place with tape. Some clients are allergic to adhesive tape. Paper and plastic tapes usually do not cause allergic reactions. Elastic tape allows movement of the body part.

Tape is applied to secure the top, middle and bottom of the dressing (Fig. 12.92). The tape extends several centimetres beyond each side of the dressing. The tape must not circle the entire body part. If swelling occurs, circulation to the part is impaired.

Applying dressings

The nurse may ask you to assist with dressing changes, as some aged care services allow carers to apply simple, dry, non-sterile dressings to simple wounds. Box 12.24 lists the rules for applying non-sterile dressings.

BOX 12.24
Rules for applying non-sterile dressing

- Collect needed supplies and equipment before you begin.
- Control your non-verbal communication and body language. Wound odours, appearance and drainage may be unpleasant. Do not communicate your thoughts and reactions to the client.
- Remove dressings so that the client cannot see the soiled side. The drainage and its odour may upset the client.
- Do not force the client to look at the wound. A wound can affect body image and self-esteem. The nurse helps the client deal with the wound.
- Remove tape by pulling it towards the wound.
- Remove dressings gently, in the shower under running water if possible. This is especially important if the dressing has stuck to the wound and will help prevent damage to the wound or surrounding skin on removal. It is not necessary to cleanse a wound using a dressing pack unless the wound is of an acute surgical nature or it is infected.
- Observe the wound and report your observations to the nurse.

SAFETY ALERT

Applying dressings

Contact with blood, body fluids, secretions or excretions is likely. Practise Standard Precautions and follow infection control principles. Wear personal protective equipment (PPE) as necessary.

DELEGATION GUIDELINES

Applying dressings

Some services allow carers to apply simple, dry non-sterile dressings; others do not. Always check the organisational policy prior to commencement.

When you are requested to apply a dressing, make sure that:

- you have the necessary education and training
- you review the procedure with the nurse
- a nurse is available to answer questions and to supervise you.

If the above conditions are met, you need the following information from the nurse before applying a dressing:

- when to change the dressing
- what dressing products to use
- how to secure the dressing
- the type of tape to be used
- what observations to report and record:
  - a red or swollen wound
  - an area around the wound that is warm to touch
  - wound edges are closed or separated
  - a wound that has broken open
  - drainage appearance: clear, bloody or watery and blood-tinged; thick and green, yellow or brown
  - the amount of drainage
  - wound or drainage odour
  - intactness and colour of surrounding skin
  - swelling of surrounding tissues.

APPLYING A DRY, NON-STERILE DRESSING

Quality of life

Remember to respect the person's privacy while doing any procedure. Address the person by name and ensure they know your name.

Pre-procedure

1. Follow the delegation guidelines.
2. Explain to the client what you are going to do. If possible, remove the dressing in the shower under running water.
3. Provide for the client's fluid and elimination needs.
4. Wash your hands.
5. Collect needed supplies and equipment:
   - gloves
   - protective equipment for the client as needed
   - tape
   - dressings as directed by the nurse
   - scissors
   - plastic bag
   - sheet to cover the client.
6. Identify the client.
7. Ensure privacy.
8. Arrange your work area.
9. Raise the bed for body mechanics (if applicable).

Procedure

10. Lower the bed rail near you, if it is up (if applicable).
11. Help the client into a comfortable position.
12. Cover the client with a sheet. Fan-fold top linen to the foot of the bed.
13. Expose the affected body part.
14. Make a cuff on the plastic bag. Place it within reach.
15. Put on a gown and mask if needed.
16. Put on the gloves.
17. Remove soiled dressing, if not already removed in the shower. Adhesive remover wipes will help remove sticky dressings.
18. Observe the wound and drainage.
19. Remove the gloves. Place them in the bag.
20. Wash your hands.
21. Put on clean gloves.
22. Open the dressings.
23. Cut the length of tape needed.
24. Apply dressings as directed by the nurse.
25. Secure the dressings in place.
26. Remove your gloves. Place them in the bag.
27. Wash your hands.

Post-procedure

28. Provide for comfort.
29. Cover the client and remove the bath blanket.
30. Place the call bell within reach (if applicable).
31. Lower the bed to its lowest position (if applicable).
32. Remove the screens from around the client (if applicable).
33. Discard supplies into the bag. Tie the bag closed.
34. Dispose of the bag according to facility policy.
35. Clean your work surface. Follow infection control principles.
36. Wash your hands.
37. Report and record your observations.

MEETING BASIC NEEDS

A wound can affect the client's basic needs. However, it is only one part of the client's care. The wound causes pain and discomfort, which can affect breathing and moving. Turning, repositioning and walking may also be painful. Handle the client gently. Sometimes the client may require pain medication before care is given. Always allow pain medication to take effect before giving care.

Good nutrition is needed for healing. However, pain and discomfort can affect appetite. So can odours from wound drainage. Remove soiled dressings promptly from the room and use room deodorisers as directed. Keep drainage containers out of the client's sight. Tell the nurse if the client has a taste for certain foods or drinks.

Infection is always a threat. Follow Standard Precautions and infection control principles. Carefully observe the wound and observe for signs and symptoms of infection.

Delayed healing is a risk for clients who are older, obese or have poor nutrition. Poor circulation and diabetes also affect healing. These conditions are also risk factors for infection. Many fears affect safety and security needs. The client fears scarring, disfigurement, delayed healing, infection and the wound opening up.

The wound may be large or small and may be clearly seen if on the face, arms or legs. Clothing can hide some wounds. Wound drainage may have odours. The wound may be disfiguring and may even affect the client's sense of sexuality. Amputation of a finger, hand, arm, toe, foot or leg can affect function and daily activities. Eye injuries can affect vision. Abdominal trauma and surgery can affect eating and elimination.

Whatever the wound's location, size or function, the person's body image is affected. Love and belonging and self-esteem needs are affected. You must be sensitive to the client's feelings. The client may be sad and tearful or angry and hostile. Adjustment may be difficult and rehabilitation necessary. Be gentle and kind, give thoughtful care and practise good communication. Other aged care team members – therapists, social workers, psychiatrists, pastoral care workers and the clergy – may be involved in the client's care.

ASSISTING WITH IDENTIFYING AND MANAGING PAIN

After reading this section, you should be able to:

- identify four types of pain
- understand why pain is a personal experience, and the factors that affect pain
- describe the signs and symptoms of pain
- understand the caring measures that relieve pain.

To be in **discomfort** or **pain** means to ache, hurt or be sore. It is unpleasant. Comfort and discomfort are subjective. That is, you cannot see, hear, touch or smell comfort or discomfort. You must rely on what the person says. Always report complaints of pain to your supervisor. Pain is personal and differs for each person. What 'hurts' to one person may 'ache' to another. What one person calls 'sore', another may call 'aching'. If a person complains of pain or discomfort, then the person *has* pain or discomfort. You must believe the person. You cannot see, hear, feel or smell the person's pain.

Pain is a warning from the body. It means there is tissue damage. Pain often causes the person to seek healthcare.

TYPES OF PAIN

There are different types of pain. Doctors will use the type of pain to help them diagnose a condition.

- **Acute pain** is felt suddenly from injury, disease, trauma or surgery. There is tissue damage. Acute pain lasts a short time, usually less than 6 months. It lessens with healing.
- **Chronic pain** lasts longer than 6 months. The pain is constant or occurs off and on. Chronic pain remains long after healing. Arthritis and cancer are common causes.
- **Radiating pain** is felt at the site of tissue damage and in nearby areas. Pain from a heart attack is often felt in the left chest, left jaw, left shoulder and left arm. Gallbladder disease can cause pain in the right upper abdomen, the back and the right shoulder (Fig. 12.93).
- **Phantom pain** is felt in a body part that is no longer there. A person who has had a leg amputated may still feel leg pain.

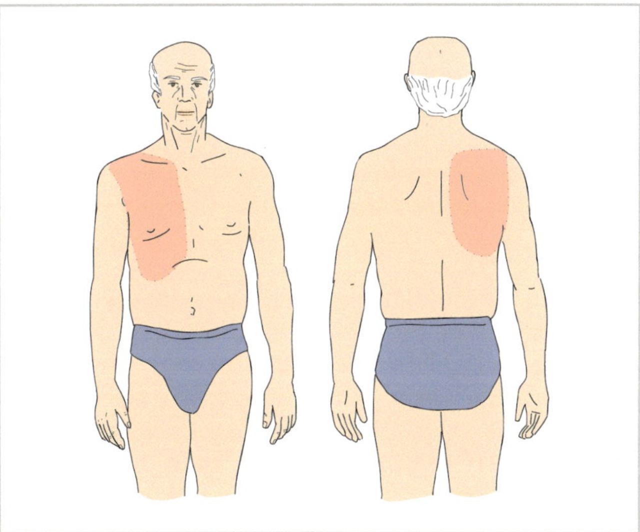

Fig. 12.93
Gallbladder pain radiates to the right upper abdomen, the back and the right shoulder.

FACTORS AFFECTING PAIN

A person may handle pain well on one occasion and poorly on the next occasion. Many factors affect the way a person reacts to pain.

Past experience

We learn from experiences, as these help us know what to do or what to expect. Whether it is going to school, driving a car, taking a test, shopping, having a baby or caring for children, the past prepares us for similar events at another time. We also learn from the experiences of family and friends.

The experience of previous pain – its cause, how long it lasted and whether relief occurred – all affect the person's current response to pain. Knowing what to expect can help or hinder how the person handles pain.

Pain can also cause fear and anxiety, which makes the pain much worse.

Anxiety

Anxiety relates to feelings of fear, dread, worry and concern. The person is uneasy and tense, and they may feel troubled or threatened. Sometimes it is just a feeling that something is wrong, but the person does not know what or why.

Pain and anxiety are related. Pain can cause anxiety, and anxiety increases how much pain the person feels. Reducing anxiety will, therefore, help lessen pain. For example, if an older person is having pain in the mornings in their joints, they will be advised that this may be caused by an existing condition, such as rheumatoid arthritis. They could also be advised that warmth, gentle movement and a mild painkiller will ease the pain. This person then knows the cause of the pain and what to expect. This helps reduce anxiety and therefore the amount of pain felt.

Rest and sleep

Rest and **sleep** restore energy. They reduce body demands and help the body repair itself. Lack of needed rest and sleep affects our thinking and our ability to cope with daily life. A person's sleep and rest needs increase with illness and injury. Pain seems worse when the person is tired or restless, as the person tends to focus on their pain when tired and unable to rest or sleep.

Attention

The more a person thinks about the pain, the worse it seems. Sometimes, pain is so severe that it is all the person can think about. Even mild pain can seem worse if the person thinks about it all the time. Pain, therefore, often seems worse at night, as activity is less and it is quiet. There are no visitors, the radio or television is often off and others are asleep. When unable to sleep, the person has time to think about the pain.

Personal and family duties

Personal and family duties affect pain responses. Often pain is ignored when there are children to care for. Some people will go to work with pain. Others will deny their pain if they fear a serious illness. Therefore, pain can interfere with a job, going to school, caring for children or any other activities of daily living.

The value and meaning of pain

People will sometimes ignore pain for various reasons. For some, acknowledging pain can be a sign of weakness. For others, ignoring pain may be an attempt to not acknowledge a serious illness or a need for painful tests and treatment.

For some people, pain means not having to work or assume daily routines, as it is used to avoid certain people or things. Sometimes pain can be used as a way to attract attention, as some people like being doted on and pampered. The person values and needs such attention.

Support from others

Dealing with pain is often easier when family and friends offer comfort and support. For example, the pain of childbirth is easier when a loving partner gives support and encouragement. Children will also manage pain much better when comforted by a caring parent or family member. The use of touch by a valued person is very comforting. Even just knowing that somebody is close by can help a great deal.

Some people do not have caring family or friends and need to manage their pain alone. However, being alone can increase anxiety, as the person has more time to think about the pain. Facing pain alone can be hard, especially for the older person.

Culture

Culture affects pain responses. In some cultures, the person in pain is stoic. To be stoic means to show no reaction to joy, sorrow, pleasure or pain. In other cultures, strong verbal and non-verbal reactions to pain are shown.

Considering a person's culture in the care planning process is a requirement of the Aged Care Accreditation Standard 3.8. Non-English-speaking people may have problems describing their pain. The carer must know how they demonstrate pain. If necessary, someone must be available to interpret the person's needs, as all people have the right to be comfortable and as pain-free as possible.

Age/illness

Some diseases cause decreased pain sensations, and the person may not feel pain or the severity of the pain. The person is, therefore, at risk of undetected disease or injury. Pain occurs with tissue damage and is an alert to illness or injury. If pain is not felt, the person does not know to seek healthcare.

Some older people have many painful health problems. As chronic pain may mask new pain, older people may ignore or deny new pain as they may think it relates to a known health problem. Like other adults, older people often deny or ignore pain because of what it may mean.

BOX 12.25
Clients with dementia

People with dementia may not be able to tell you about their pain. Changes in their usual behaviour may signal pain. A person who normally moans and groans may become quiet and withdrawn. A person who is friendly and outgoing may become agitated and aggressive. Someone who is non-verbal and quiet may become restless and cry easily. Loss of appetite can also signal pain.

Report any changes in a person's usual behaviour to your supervisor. All people have the right to correct pain management. The Aged Care Accreditation Standard 2.8 states that 'All consumers are as free as possible from pain'.

As thinking and reasoning are affected in some older people, such as those with dementia, they sometimes cannot verbally communicate pain (see Box 12.25). Care staff must be alert for the signs of pain.

SIGNS AND SYMPTOMS OF PAIN

You cannot see, hear, feel or smell the person's pain. You must rely on what the person says. Promptly report any information you collect about pain. Use the person's exact words. The following information is required to assess the person's pain.

- *Location* – Where is the pain? Ask the person to point to the area of pain (Fig. 12.94). Pain can radiate. Ask the person if the pain is anywhere else and to point to those areas.
- *Onset and duration* – When did the pain start? How long has it lasted?
- *Intensity* – Does the person complain of mild, moderate or severe pain? Ask the person to rate the pain from 1 to 10, with 10 the most severe pain.
- *Description* – Ask the person to describe the pain. Box 12.26 lists some words used to describe pain. Write down what the person says. Use the person's words when reporting and recording.
- *Factors causing pain* – These are called precipitating factors. To precipitate means to cause. Such factors include moving or turning in bed, coughing or deep breathing and exercise. Ask what the person was doing before the pain started and when it started.
- *Vital signs* – What are the person's pulse, respiration and blood pressure? Increases in these vital signs often occur with pain.
- *Other signs and symptoms* – Does the person have other symptoms: dizziness, nausea, vomiting, weakness, numbness or tingling, or others? Box 12.27 lists the signs and symptoms that often occur with pain.

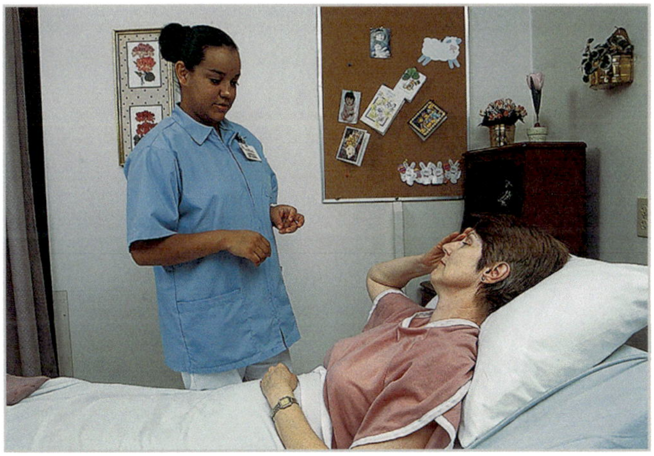

Fig. 12.94
The person points to the area of pain.

BOX 12.26
Words used to describe pain

- Aching
- Pressure
- Burning
- Sharp
- Cramping
- Sore
- Crushing
- Squeezing
- Dull
- Stabbing
- Gnawing
- Throbbing
- Knife-like
- Vice-like
- Piercing

BOX 12.27
Signs and symptoms of pain

Body responses

- Excess sweating (diaphoresis)
- Increased pulse, respiration and blood pressure
- Nausea
- Pale skin (pallor)
- Vomiting

Behaviours

- Changes in speech: slow or rapid; loud or quiet
- Crying
- Gasping
- Grimacing
- Groaning
- Grunting
- Holding the affected body part (splinting)
- Irritability
- Maintaining one position; refusing to move
- Moaning
- Quietness
- Restlessness
- Rubbing
- Screaming

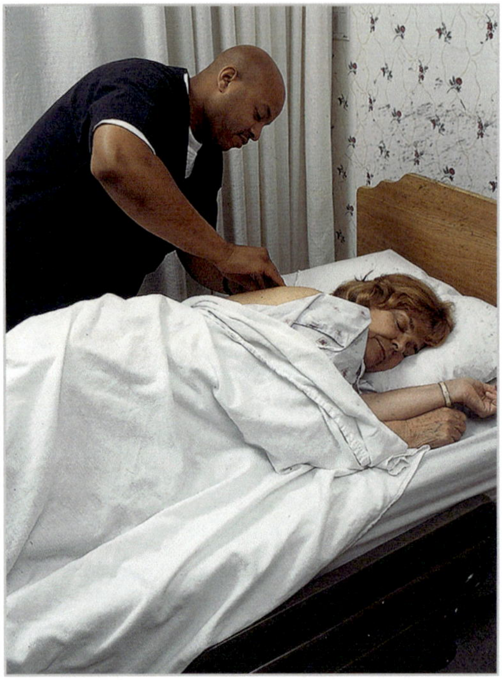

Fig. 12.95
Measures are implemented to relieve pain. The person is positioned in good alignment, with pillows for comfort. The room is darkened. Blankets provide warmth. A back massage provides touch and promotes relaxation.

BOX 12.28
Measures to promote comfort and relieve pain

- Position the person in good alignment. Use pillows for support (see Fig. 12.95).
- Keep bed linen tight and wrinkle-free.
- Make sure the person does not lie on drainage tubes.
- Assist with elimination needs.
- Provide blankets for warmth and to prevent chilling.
- Use correct lifting, moving and turning procedures.
- Wait 30 minutes after pain medications are given before giving care.
- Give a back massage.
- Provide soft music to distract the person.
- Use touch to provide comfort.
- Allow family and friends at the bedside as requested by the person.
- Avoid sudden or jarring movements of the bed or chair.
- Handle the person gently.
- Practise safety measures if the person takes strong pain medications or sedatives:
  - Keep the bed in the low position.
  - Check on the person every 12–15 minutes.
  - Provide help when the person is up.
  - Apply warm or cold applications as directed by your supervisor.
  - Provide a calm, quiet, darkened setting.

PAIN-RELIEVING MEASURES

Although mild analgesics, such as paracetamol, are often used for pain relief, some people are prescribed other specific pain-relieving medications by their doctors. It is sometimes the carer's role to assist the person with these medications as they are required and as per legislative requirements.

Other non-medicinal measures are often used (Fig. 12.95). These include distraction, relaxation and guided imagery. Nurses and physiotherapists and occupational and diversional therapists may assist with these measures. If asked to assist, they will tell you what to do. Although a few of these techniques are outlined here, more techniques are discussed elsewhere in this text (Box 12.28).

Complementary measures in pain management

Complementary therapies are treatments that are used alongside traditional treatment modalities in managing pain. They can include the following:

- **Distraction** – changing the person's centre of attention. Attention is moved away from the pain. Music, games, singing, praying, watching television and needlework can distract attention.
- **Relaxation** – to help the person feel free from mental or physical stress. This state reduces pain and anxiety. The person is taught relaxation methods. They are taught to breathe deeply and slowly and to contract and relax muscle groups. A comfortable position is important. So is a quiet room.
- **Guided imagery** – creating and focusing on an image. The person is asked to create a pleasant scene. This is noted on the care plan, so all staff use the same image with the person. A calm, soft voice is used to help the person focus on the image. Soft music, a blanket for warmth and a darkened room may help. The person is coached to focus on the image and then to practise relaxation exercises.

ASSISTING WITH FEEDING AND DRINKING

After reading this section, you should be able to:

- be aware of factors that affect eating and nutrition
- understand the purpose of special diets
- understand ways to provide better nutrition to the aged person
- recognise the signs and symptoms of dysphagia

- recognise the signs, symptoms and precautions relating to aspiration
- be aware of the fluid requirements for adults
- know what to do when a person has special fluid orders
- understand the purpose of intake and output records
- know what to count as fluid intake
- know how to assist with food and fluid needs
- be aware of the purpose, methods and comfort measures for enteral nutrition.

Food and water are physical needs that are necessary for life. The amount and quality of foods and fluids in the diet affect our physical and mental well-being. Older and disabled people may have special dietary needs. Poor diet and poor eating habits:

- increase the risk of infection
- increase the risk of chronic diseases
- cause chronic illnesses to become worse
- cause healing problems
- cause changes in physical and mental function, increasing the risk of accidents and injuries.

Eating and drinking provide pleasure (Fig. 12.96). They are often a part of social times with family and friends. A friendly, social setting for meals is important. It is important to remember that eating should be enjoyed and that it may be one of the few pleasures for older people. People may eat poorly when eating alone or in an unpleasant setting.

Many factors affect people's dietary practices. They include culture, finances and personal choice. Dietary practices also include selecting, preparing and serving food. The health team considers these factors when planning to meet the person's nutrition needs.

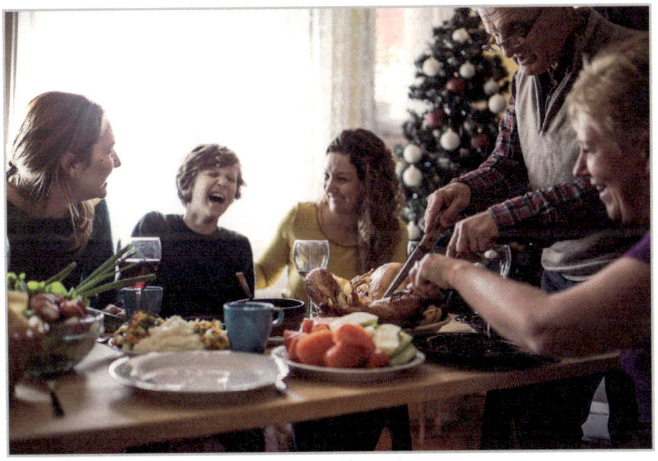

Fig. 12.96
Meals are enjoyed when shared with family and friends.

BASIC NUTRITION

Although nutrition is discussed elsewhere within this text in greater detail, a basic summary is presented here. **Nutrition** is the many processes involved in the ingestion, digestion, absorption and use of foods and fluids by the body. Good nutrition is needed for growth, healing and body functions. A well-balanced diet and correct kilojoule intake are needed. A high-fat and high-kilojoule diet causes weight gain and obesity. Weight loss occurs with a low-kilojoule diet.

Foods and fluids contain nutrients. A **nutrient** is a substance that is ingested, digested, absorbed and used by the body. Nutrients are grouped into fats, proteins, carbohydrates, vitamins and minerals.

Fats, proteins and carbohydrates give the body fuel for energy. The amount of energy provided by a nutrient is measured in kilojoules. A **kilojoule** is the amount of energy produced when the body burns food. More information about nutrition can be found in Chapter 13.

CARING ABOUT CULTURE

Food practices vary between religious groups and are often an important part of religious observance.

- *Christianity* – religious preference varies from faith to faith. Variations of fasting are observed by Roman Catholics on holy days such as Good Friday and during Lent. A majority of Seventh Day Adventists don't eat meat or dairy products. Mormons avoid coffee and alcohol.
- *Judaism* – can be liberal or Orthodox, depending on the degree of adherence to Jewish Law. Kosher food is permitted, and 'unclean' foods, such as pork and shellfish, are forbidden. Food preparation and consumption rules can be strict.
- *Islam* – prohibited foods are called *haram* and are believed to make the Creator deaf to a Muslim who eats them. This list can include pork, alcohol, bread products made with dried yeast and caffeinated drinks. Many Muslims choose to fast on certain days and during religious holidays.
- *Hinduism* – Hindus do not eat meat and often avoid foods that may have caused pain to animals. Many Hindus believe that food contains energy, such as sound waves, and can literally believe the saying 'You are what you eat'. Many Hindus fast, depending on their caste or social status.
- *Buddhism* – the dietary rules of Buddhism vary according to country and which branch of Buddhism is being practised. Some avoid meat and dairy products, others avoid only beef. Some Buddhists practise fasting, while others fast for religious festivals.

Source: Encyclopedia.com (2019). Religion and dietary practices. Online 30 Sept 2021. Available: www.encyclopedia.com/food/news-wires-white-papers-and-books/religion-and-dietary-practices

FACTORS AFFECTING THE NUTRITIONAL STATUS OF OLDER PEOPLE

A number of factors can affect the nutritional status of older people. These include physical, social, emotional and metabolic (the way the body utilises food) factors. Physical factors include:

- loss of teeth, poorly fitting dentures or mouth pain
- rigidity of eating habits, as people may choose food that is more familiar to them
- a decreased amount of food consumed, which may lead to nutritional deficiencies
- physical difficulty with eating, such as arthritic hands or the inability to use one side of the body
- limited financial resources to provide a healthy, balanced diet
- changes in the way food tastes
- changes in the gastrointestinal system – swallowing may become more difficult
- medical conditions, such as stroke, dementia or other nervous system disorders
- dulling of taste and smell
- a decreased appetite
- decreased metabolism
- decrease in the amount of digestive juices secreted – this makes fried and fatty foods hard to digest, and may cause indigestion.

Dry, fried and fatty foods should be avoided to assist swallowing and digestion. Good oral hygiene and denture care improve taste. Some people have to avoid high-fibre foods, which are needed for bowel elimination. High-fibre foods are hard to chew and can irritate the intestines; examples include apricots, celery and fruits and vegetables with skins and seeds. Foods providing soft bulk are often ordered for people with chewing problems or constipation. These foods include wholegrain cereals and cooked fruits and vegetables.

Older people need fewer kilojoules than younger people do. This is because their energy and activity levels are lower. Foods that contain calcium help prevent musculoskeletal changes. Protein is needed for tissue growth and repair. However, the diets of some older people may lack protein. High-protein foods are often expensive to buy.

Social factors include:

- different routines of times of meal (e.g. many traditional Italian and Spanish families do not have their evening meal until midnight)
- changes to social interactions: whether a person is used to eating alone or at a local club. They may find it difficult eating alone after the loss of a spouse, or eating within a communal setting if admitted to an aged care facility after living alone for some time.
- Emotional factors can include:
  - depression
  - feelings of isolation
  - sense of loss of control over their personal food and mealtime choices.
- Metabolic factors can include:
  - decreased overall metabolic rate
  - increased need for calcium and vitamins C and A
  - decreased peristalsis time, which may increase the incidence of constipation.

An understanding of these issues will allow for better care for the older person.

Meeting a client's nutritional needs requires a team approach. The doctor, dietitian, nurse, speech–language pathologist, occupational therapist and carer are involved. With the participation of the client, they develop and administer a nutritional care plan. The client is always part of this team, with their individual likes, dislikes and lifelong habits being considered. Sometimes the person's family is involved.

Culture

Culture influences dietary practices, food choices and food preparation. Frying, baking, smoking and roasting food, using sauces and spices or even eating raw food can be a core component of individual cultural practices.

Religion

Selecting, preparing and eating food often involves religious practices. A person may follow all, some or none of the dietary practices of their faith. You must always respect these practices and work to ensure that they are maintained. Sometimes there is a need to involve the family or religious organisations to ensure that appropriate food is selected, prepared and served.

Finances

Many people have a limited income and may often buy cheaper carbohydrate foods. Their diets often lack protein and certain vitamins and minerals. If the client is living at home, a referral to a local dietitian may be required to help them identify how to shop and select appropriate foods on a limited budget. If the client receives meals on wheels, they are then assured of at least one nutritious meal per day.

Appetite

Appetite relates to the desire for food. When hungry, a person seeks food and will eat until their appetite is satisfied. Aromas and thoughts of food can stimulate the appetite. However, loss of appetite (**anorexia**) can occur. Causes include illness, medications, unpleasant thoughts or sights, anxiety, pain and depression. Decreased senses of taste and smell cause loss of appetite in older people. Within some aged care services, staff may cook high-aroma food on portable grills in the living areas. Aromas from foods such as meat and pikelets cooked in this way will often stimulate salivation and a desire to eat.

Personal choice

Food likes and dislikes are personal and begin in childhood. They are influenced by food served in the home. As children grow older, they try new foods at school and social

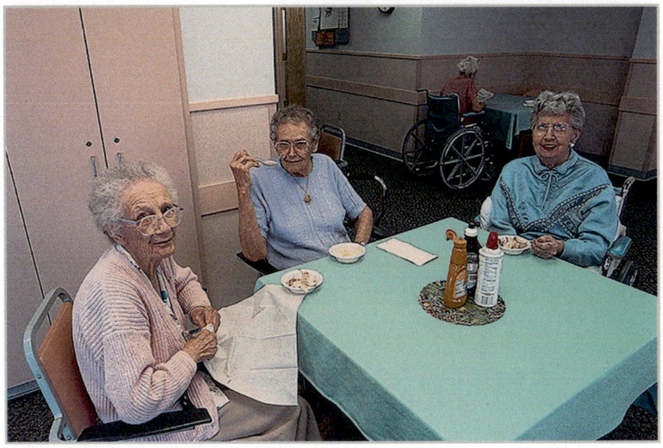

Fig. 12.97
Clients enjoying a meal together.

events. Food choices also depend on how it looks, how it is prepared, how it smells and its ingredients. Usually a person's food likes expand with age and social experiences.

Body reactions affect food choices. People usually avoid foods that cause allergic reactions. They also avoid foods that cause nausea, vomiting, diarrhoea, indigestion, gas or headaches.

Consumer care services must serve balanced meals with clients often selecting from food menus (Fig. 12.97). Some centres involve client groups in planning special meals. They often plan meals for holidays and birthdays, picnics, pizza parties and barbecues. Remember, clients have the right to personal choice.

Illness

Appetite usually decreases during illness and recovery from injuries. However, the person's nutritional needs increase at these times. The body must fight infection, heal tissue and replace lost blood cells. Nutrients lost through vomiting and diarrhoea need to be replaced. Some diseases and medications cause a sore mouth, making eating painful. Tooth loss or poor-fitting dentures affect chewing. Protein foods (the meat group) may be hard to chew.

DIETARY REQUIREMENTS

Upon admission to a care facility, each client should be assessed to ensure that:

- personal and cultural preferences are met
- special dietary needs are met
- food allergies and intolerances are noted
- special requirements for feeding equipment are provided for
- chewing or swallowing difficulties are provided for
- a current nutritional assessment is made.

To stimulate the client's appetite and to provide mealtime pleasure, food should be:

- nourishing and good to taste, well-seasoned and not too salty or too sweet
- appetising and attractive, with an appealing aroma
- served at the correct temperature – hot food should be served hot, cold food should be served cold
- served promptly, otherwise hot food cools down and cold food warms up
- prepared to meet each person's needs – some people need food cut, ground or chopped; others have special diets ordered by the doctor
- served three times a day; a bedtime snack is also offered
- served with any special eating equipment and utensils that are needed (Fig. 12.98).

Disease or injury can affect the hands, wrists and arms. Adaptive equipment lets the person eat independently and the speech–language pathologist and occupational therapist teach the person how to use the item. Make sure the person has necessary equipment at mealtimes.

SPECIAL DIETS

Doctors may order special eating plans for a nutritional deficiency or a disease (Table 12.2). They also order them for weight control or to eliminate or reduce certain substances in the diet. The doctor, nurses and dietitian work together to meet the person's nutritional needs. They consider the need for dietary changes, personal choices, religion, culture and eating problems. They also consider food allergies and sensitivities. The nurse and dietitian teach the person and family about the eating plan.

General diet, regular diet and house diet mean no dietary limits or changes. People with diabetes or diseases of the heart, kidneys, gallbladder, liver, stomach or intestines often need special diets. People with wounds or pressure ulcers need high-protein diets for healing. Older or disabled people may have bran added to their diets, as it provides fibre for bowel elimination. Allergies, excess weight and other disorders also require special diets.

Sometimes changes in food texture are needed. A dysphagia diet is ordered for a person who has difficulty swallowing. Food thickness is changed to meet the person's needs. Other people need their food pureed.

The sodium-controlled diet and dysphagia diet are often ordered. So is diabetes meal planning. These are described in detail below.

The sodium-controlled diet

The average amount of sodium in the daily diet is 3000–5000 milligrams (mg). The body needs no more than 2400 mg. Healthy people excrete excess sodium in the urine. However, heart and kidney diseases cause the body to retain the extra sodium, as do some medications.

Heart, liver and kidney disease, hypertension (high blood pressure) and certain medications often require a sodium-controlled diet. Sodium causes the body to retain water. If there is too much sodium, the body retains more water. This makes the body tissues swell with water. There is excess fluid in the blood vessels, and so the heart has to work harder. In other words, the workload of the heart increases. With heart disease, the extra workload can cause serious problems or death.

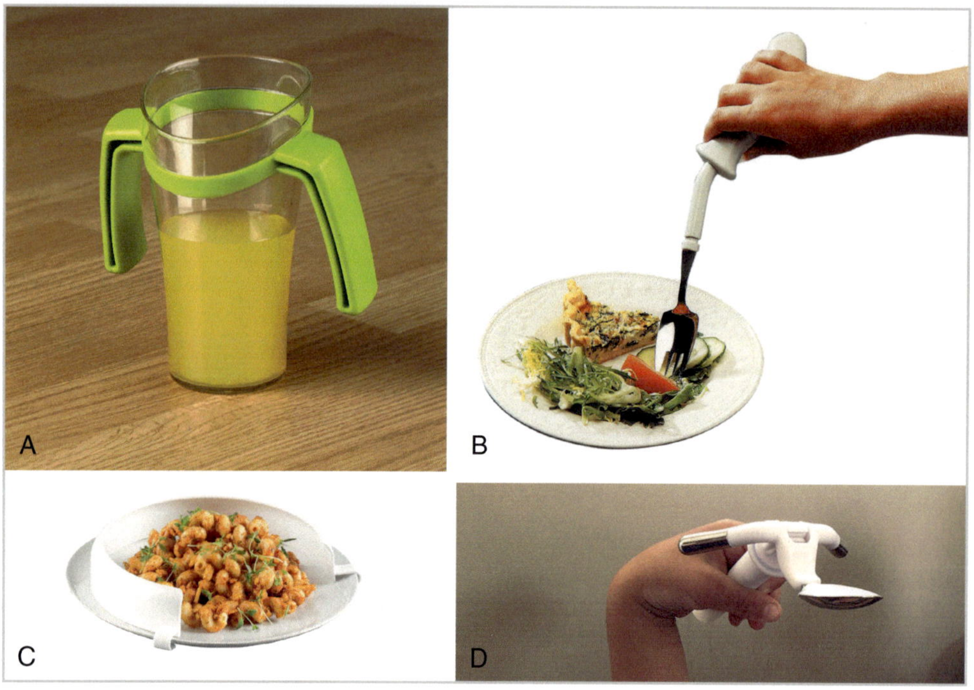

Fig. 12.98
Eating utensils for people with special needs.
A. Glass or cup holder. **B.** The curved fork fits over the hand. The rounded plate helps keep food on the plate. Special grips and swivel handles are helpful for some people. **C.** Plate guards help keep food on the plate. **D.** Knives with rounded blades are rocked back and forth to cut food. The person does not need a fork in one hand and a knife in the other.

Table 12.2
Special diets

Diet	Use	Foods allowed
Clear-liquid – foods that are liquid at body temperature and that leave small amounts of a residue; non-irritating and non-gas-forming	Postoperatively, acute illness, infection, nausea and vomiting, and in preparation for gastrointestinal examination	Water, tea and coffee (without milk or cream); carbonated beverages; jelly; clear fruit juices (apple, grape and cranberry); fat-free clear broth; hard lollies, sugar and icy poles/iced sweets
Full-liquid – foods are liquid at room temperature or melt at body temperature	Advance from clear-liquid diet postoperatively; for stomach irritation, fever and nausea and vomiting; and for people unable to chew, swallow or digest solid foods	Foods on the clear-liquid diet; custard; eggnog; strained soups; strained fruit and vegetable juices; milk and milkshakes; strained, cooked cereals; plain ice cream and jelly; pudding; yoghurt
Mechanical soft – semi-solid foods that are easily digested	Advance from full-liquid diets; chewing difficulties, gastrointestinal disorders and infections	All liquids; eggs (not fried); broiled, baked or roasted meat, fish or poultry that is chopped, ground or shredded; mild cheeses (e.g. cheddar cheese, cream cheese, cottage cheese); strained fruit juices; refined bread (no crust) and crackers; cooked cereal; cooked or pureed vegetables; cooked or canned fruit without skin or seeds; pudding; plain cakes and soft biscuits without fruit or nuts
Fibre and residue restricted – food that leaves a small amount of residue in the colon	Diseases of the colon and diarrhoea	Coffee, tea, milk, carbonated beverages, strained fruit juices; refined bread and crackers; creamed and refined cereal; rice; cottage and cream cheese; eggs (not fried); plain puddings and cakes; custard; jelly and ice cream; strained vegetable juices; canned or cooked fruit without skin or seeds; potatoes (not fried); strained cooked vegetables; plain pasta; no raw fruits and vegetables

Table 12.2
Special diets *continued*

Diet	Use	Foods allowed
High-fibre – foods that increase the amount of residue and fibre in the colon to stimulate peristalsis	Constipation and gastrointestinal disorders	All fruits and vegetables; whole wheat bread; wholegrain cereals; fried foods; wholegrain rice; milk, cream, butter and cheese; meats; nuts
Bland – foods that are mechanically and chemically non-irritating and low in roughage; foods served at moderate temperatures; no strong spices or condiments	Ulcers, gallbladder disorders and some intestinal disorders; after abdominal surgery	Lean meats; white bread; creamed and refined cereals; cream or cottage cheese; jelly, plain puddings, cakes and biscuits; eggs (not fried); butter and cream; canned fruits and vegetables without skin and seeds; strained fruit juices; potatoes (not fried); pastas and rice; strained or soft cooked carrots, peas, beets, spinach, squash and asparagus tips; creamed soups from allowed vegetables; no fried foods
High-kilojoule – kilojoule intake is increased to about 3000–4000 per day; includes three full meals and between-meal snacks	Weight gain and some thyroid imbalances	Dietary increases in all foods; large portions of a regular diet with three between-meal snacks
Kilojoule-controlled – provides adequate nutrients while controlling kilojoules to promote weight loss and reduction of body fat	Weight reduction	Foods low in fats and carbohydrates and lean meats; avoid butter, cream, rice, gravies, salad oils, noodles, cakes, pastries, carbonated and alcoholic beverages, lollies, potato chips and similar foods
High-iron – foods that are high in iron	Anaemia; following blood loss; for women during the reproductive years	Liver and other organ meats; lean meats; egg yolks; shellfish; dried fruits; dried beans; green leafy vegetables; lima beans; peanut butter; enriched breads and cereals
Fat-controlled (low cholesterol) – foods low in fat and foods prepared without adding fat	Heart disease, gallbladder disease, disorders of fat digestion, liver disease, diseases of the pancreas	Skim milk or buttermilk; cottage cheese and non-fat or low-fat cheese (no other cheeses allowed); jelly; fruit; lean meat, poultry and fish (baked, broiled or roasted); fat-free broth; soups made with skim milk; margarine; rice, pasta, breads and cereals; vegetables; potatoes; fat-free egg substitutes
High-protein – aids and promotes tissue healing	For burns, high fever, infection and some liver diseases	Meat, milk, eggs, cheese, fish, poultry; breads and cereals; beans and green leafy vegetables
Sodium-controlled – a certain amount of sodium is allowed	Heart disease, fluid retention, liver disease and some kidney diseases	Fruits and vegetables and unsalted butter are allowed; adding salt at the table is not allowed; highly salted foods and foods high in sodium are not allowed; the use of salt during cooking may be restricted
Diabetes meal planning – the same amount of carbohydrates, protein and fat are eaten at the same time each day	Diabetes mellitus	Determined by nutritional and energy requirements

Sodium control decreases the amount of sodium in the body, so the body retains less water. Less water in the tissues and blood vessels reduces the heart's workload.

The doctor orders the amount of restriction:

- *2000–3000 mg sodium diet* – called the low-salt or no added salt diet. Sodium control is mild. All high-sodium foods are omitted (Box 12.29). A small amount of salt is used in cooking. Salt is not added to foods at the table.
- *1200 mg sodium diet* – sodium control is moderate. Food is cooked without salt. Foods high in sodium are omitted. Vegetables high in sodium are restricted in amount. Salt-free products, such as salt-free bread, are used. Diet planning is needed.

Diabetes meal planning

Diabetes meal planning is for people who have diabetes mellitus. Diabetes mellitus is a chronic disease resulting from a lack of insulin or poor usage of insulin by the body. Insulin is produced by the pancreas; it lets the body use sugar. Without enough insulin, glucose builds up in the bloodstream. It is not used by cells for energy. Diabetes is usually treated with insulin or other medications, diet and exercise.

The dietitian and the person develop a meal plan. Consistency is important. The meal involves:

- the person's food preferences – likes and dislikes, eating habits, mealtimes, culture and lifestyle; it may be

BOX 12.29
High-sodium foods

Bread, cereal/rice and pasta group
Salted crackers
Baking powder biscuits
Muffins
Pretzels
Quick breads (corn bread, nut bread)
Pancakes
Waffles
Instant cooked cereal
Processed bran cereals
Noodle mixes
Corn chips and bread, other salted snacks

Vegetables and legumes group
Sauerkraut
Tomato juice
Vegetable juice
Vegetables in creams or sauces
Frozen vegetables processed with salt or sodium
Bloody Mary mixes
Potato chips, French fries
Instant potatoes
Pickles
Relishes

Fruit group
No restrictions

Milk, yoghurt and cheese group
Buttermilk
Cheese
Commercial dips made with sour cream

Meat, poultry, fish, dry beans, eggs and nuts group
Bacon
Ham
Sausage
Salt pork
Luncheon meats
Corned or chopped beef
Organ meats
Shellfish
Sardines
Herring
Anchovies
Caviar
Kosher meats
Canned tuna
Canned salmon
Mackerel
Salted nuts or seeds
Peanut butter

Fats, oils and sweets
Salad dressings
Mayonnaise
Baked desserts

Other
Mineral water
Club soda
Canned soups
Stock cubes
Dried soup mixes
Olives
Salted popcorn
Frozen or canned dinners
Salt
Baking powder
Baking soda
Celery, onion, garlic and other seasoning salts
Meat tenderisers
Worcestershire sauce
Soy sauce
Mustard
Tomato sauce
Horseradish
Sauces: chilli, tomato, steak, barbecue

necessary to limit amounts or change the way food is prepared
- the kilojoules needed and the glycaemic index of foods – the same amount of carbohydrates, protein and fat are eaten each day.
- eating meals and snacks at regular times.

Meal and snack times are the same each day. You must serve the person's meals and snacks on time, as the person eats at regular times to maintain a certain blood sugar level.

Always check the tray to see what has been eaten. Tell the nurse what the person did and did not eat. If not all food is eaten, a between-meal supplement is needed. The supplement makes up for what the person did not eat at the meal. The amount of insulin given also depends on daily food intake. Always tell the nurse about changes in the person's eating habits.

DELEGATION GUIDELINES

Preparing for meals
Before preparing a person for a meal, you need the following information from the nurse and care plan:
- how much help the person needs
- where the person will eat – dining area or room
- what the person uses for elimination – toilet, commode, bedpan, urinal or specimen pan
- what type of oral hygiene the person needs
- how to position the person – in bed or in a chair
- whether the person wears glasses or hearing aids
- how the person gets to the dining area – by self or with help
- whether the person uses a wheelchair, walker or cane.

The texture-modified diet

The texture-modified diet (Box 12.30) is for people who have difficulty swallowing. At times this may include the addition of food thickeners. **Dysphagia** means difficulty (*dys*) swallowing (*phagia*). Food thickness is changed to meet the person's needs. The doctor, speech–language pathologist, occupational therapist, dietitian and nurse choose the right food thickness.

A *slow swallow* means the person has difficulty getting enough food and fluids for good nutrition and hydration. An *unsafe swallow* means that food enters the airway (aspiration). Aspiration is breathing fluid or an object into the lungs.

Often you will feed people with dysphagia. To promote these people's safety, you must:

- know the signs and symptoms of dysphagia
- position the person's head and neck correctly – follow the care plan
- feed the person according to the care plan and swallow guide
- follow aspiration precautions
- report changes in how the person eats
- report choking, coughing or difficulty breathing during or after meals. Also report abnormal breathing or respiratory sounds at once.

FLUID BALANCE

We need water to live. Death can result from too much or too little water. You ingest water through fluids and foods and lose water through urine and faeces. Water is also lost through the skin (perspiration) and the lungs (expiration).

Fluid balance is needed for health. The amount of fluid taken in and the amount lost must be equal. If fluid intake exceeds fluid output (the amount lost), our tissues swell with water. This is called oedema. Oedema is common in people with heart and kidney diseases. **Dehydration** is a decrease in the amount of water in body tissues. It occurs when fluid output is greater than intake. Common causes are poor fluid intake, vomiting, diarrhoea, bleeding, excess sweating and increased urine production.

BOX 12.30
Texture-modified diet

- *Puree* – no lumps; mounds on a plate. May be thick, like mashed potatoes.
- *Thickened liquid* – no lumps; puree with milk, gravy or broth to the thickness of baby food peaches. In some foods, food is pureed and thickener added as needed (e.g. many fruits). Does not mound significantly on a plate. May be called creamy or sauce. Stir before serving if the food settles. A spoon is used (baby food consistency). Cannot be drunk from a glass. Served in a bowl.
- *Medium thick* – the thickness of nectar (does not hold its shape). Stir just before serving. (Some beverages of this thickness do not look very thick.)
- *Extra thick* – the thickness of honey. Mounds a bit on a spoon, but drinkable from a cup. Stir before serving.
- *Yoghurt-like consistency* – the thickness of yoghurt; holds its shape. Served with a spoon.

Normal requirements

An adult needs 1500 mL of water daily to survive. About 2000–2500 mL of fluid per day is needed for normal fluid balance. Water requirements increase with hot weather, exercise, fever, illness and excess fluid loss. Older people may have a decreased sense of thirst. Their bodies need water, but they may not feel thirsty. You need to offer water often. Some people have special fluid orders.

Special orders

The doctor may order the amount of fluid that a person can have during a 24-hour period. This is done to maintain fluid balance. In the care plan, common orders are:

- *Encourage fluids* – the person needs to drink an increased amount of fluid. The order states the amount to ingest. Intake records are kept. The person is given a variety of fluids allowed on the diet. Fluids are kept within the person's reach. They are served at the correct temperature. Fluids are offered regularly to people who cannot feed themselves.
- *Restrict fluids* – fluids are restricted to a certain amount. They are offered in small amounts and in small containers. The water jug is removed from the room or kept out of sight. Intake records are kept. The person needs frequent oral hygiene, to help keep the mucous membranes of the mouth moist.
- *Nothing by mouth* (*NBM*) – the person cannot eat or drink anything. NBM is the abbreviation for 'nothing by mouth' or 'nil by mouth'. NBM is often ordered for some laboratory tests or X-ray procedures and in treating certain illnesses.

  People who are tube-fed may be NBM. An NBM sign is posted above the bed. The water jug and glass are removed. Frequent oral hygiene is important, but the person must not swallow any fluid.
- *Thickened liquids* – all fluids are thickened. The thickness depends on the person's ability to swallow. Thickening is added before fluids are served or commercial fluids are used, which are already thickened.

Intake and output records

The doctor or nurse may order fluid *intake and output (I&O) measurements*. This means keeping I&O records. These are used to evaluate fluid balance and kidney function. They help in evaluating and planning medical treatment. They are also kept when the person has special fluid orders.

All fluids taken by mouth are measured and recorded – water, milk, coffee, tea, juices, soups and soft drinks. So are soft and semi-solid foods, such as ice cream, custard, pudding, creamed cereals, jelly and icy poles or iced sweets. The nurse measures and records intravenous fluids and tube feedings. Output includes urine, vomitus, diarrhoea and wound drainage.

Measuring intake and output

Intake and output are measured in millilitres (mL) or in cubic centimetres (cc). These metric system measurements are equal in amount.

You need to know the serving size of the bowls, dishes, cups, jugs, glasses and other containers. The information may be on the I&O record.

A measuring container or **graduated jug** is used to measure fluids, including leftover fluids, urine, vomitus and drainage from suction. It is marked in fluid ounces and in millilitres (Fig. 12.99). Plastic urinals and kidney basins often have amount marks.

An I&O record is kept. When intake or output is measured, the amount is recorded in the correct column (Fig. 12.100). Amounts are totalled at the end of the shift and totals are recorded in the person's chart. They are also shared during the end-of-shift report.

The purpose of measuring input and output, and how to help with this, are explained to the person. Some people measure and record their intake. The urinal, commode, bedpan or specimen pan is used for voiding. Remind the person not to void in the toilet. Also remind the person not to put toilet tissue into the container.

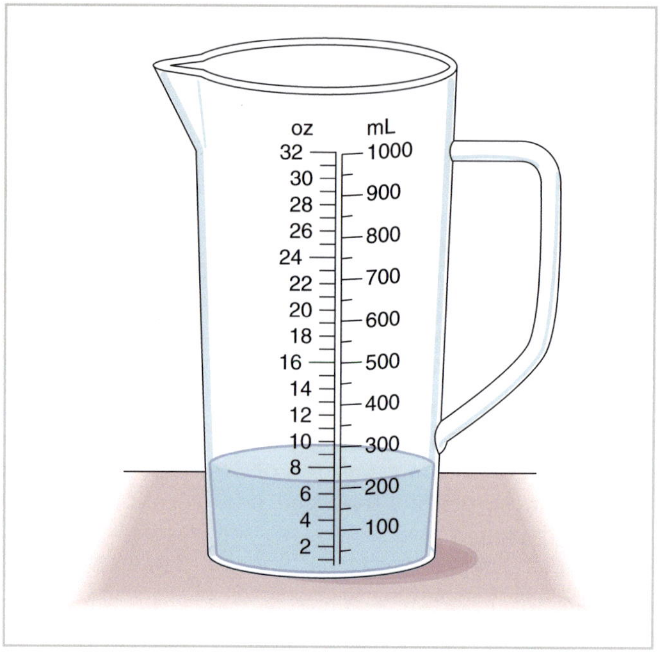

Fig. 12.99
A measuring container marked in millilitres and fluid ounces.

DELEGATION GUIDELINES

Intake and output

You need the following information from the nurse and the care plan when delegated I&O measurements:

- Does the person have special fluid orders (e.g. encourage fluids, restrict fluids or NBM)?
- When to report measurements (e.g. hourly or end of shift)?
- What does the person use for voiding (e.g. urinal, bedpan, commode or specimen pan)?
- Does the person have a catheter?

MEASURING INTAKE AND OUTPUT

Quality of life

Remember to respect the person's privacy while doing any procedure. Address the person by name and ensure they know your name.

Pre-procedure

1. Follow the delegation guidelines.
2. Explain the procedure to the person.
3. Wash your hands.
4. Collect the following:
   - intake and output (I&O) record
   - measuring container
   - gloves.

Procedure

5. Put on gloves and protective eyewear.
6. Measure intake as follows:
   a. Pour liquid remaining in a container into the measuring container.
   b. Measure the amount at eye level. Keep the container level.
   c. Check the amount of the serving on the I&O record.
   d. Subtract the remaining amount from the full serving amount. Record the amount.
   e. Repeat steps 6a–d for each liquid.
   f. Add the amounts from each liquid together.
   g. Record the amount and time on the I&O record.
7. Measure output as follows:
   a. Pour fluid into the measuring container. Avoid spills and splashes.
   b. Measure the amount at eye level. Keep the container level.
8. Dispose of fluid in the toilet. Avoid splashes.
9. Rinse the measuring container. Discard rinse into the toilet. Return the measuring container to its proper place.
10. Clean and rinse the bedpan, urinal, emesis basin or other drainage container. Discard the rinse into the toilet. Return the item to its proper place.
11. Remove the protective apparel and wash your hands.
12. Record the amount on the I&O record.

Post-procedure

13. Report and record your observations.

FLUID BALANCE CHART

Name ______ Room No. ______ Ward ______

Intake from previous day ______ Estimated fluid requirements/24 hrs ______

Outputut from previous day ______ Estimated K requirements/24 hrs ______

Balance ______ Estimated Nz requirements/24 hrs ______

Body weight ______ Yellow jug Yes/No

DATE	INTAKE						OUTPUT				
15/6/22	Oral		IV/SC		Other		Urine	Vomit	Tube	Other	Total
TIME	mL	Fluid	mL	Fluid	mL	Nature of flud	mL	mL	mL	mL	
2400-0100							150				
0100-0200								150			
0200-0300											
0300-0400											
0400-0500											
0500-0600											
0600-0700	125						200				
0700-0800											
8-hour subtotal	125						350	150			
0800-0900	400						250				
0900-1000	100										
1000-1100											
1100-1200											
1200-1300	400						250				
1300-1400											
1400-1500	200										
1500-1600											
8-hour subtotal	1100						500				
1600-1700							270				
1700-1800	350										
1800-1900	50										
1900-2000	200										
2000-2100							400				
2100-2200											
2200-2300											
2300-2400											
8-hour subtotal	600						670				
24-hour Total	1825						1520	150			

310' Marie Mills

Form No. MF36722 (Rev. 5/97) *MFI*

Fig. 12.100

An intake and output record and charting sample.

FOOD, FLUIDS AND THE SOCIAL ENVIRONMENT

Weakness, illness and confusion affect our appetite and ability to eat. So do unpleasant odours, sights and sounds. Uncomfortable positions, the need for oral hygiene or the need to eliminate also affect appetite.

Some clients are alert and oriented. They enjoy being together for meals. Some like to eat in their rooms. Others are confused and noisy at mealtimes. Some people are incontinent or have other odour problems. Some are too weak or ill to leave their rooms for meals. Services have dining programs to meet these different needs:

- *Social dining* – people eat in a dining room with four or six people at a table. Tables have tablecloths or placemats. Food is served as in a restaurant. This program is for people who are oriented and can feed themselves. Sometimes quietly confused people are included. They should be able to feed themselves and not disrupt others.

- *Family dining* – this is like social dining, except that food is served in bowls and on platters. Clients serve themselves as they would at home.
- *Assistive dining* – the assistive dining room usually has dining tables or other furniture. People who need assistance with eating still get to benefit from social contact with other clients. Carers provide the client with whatever assistance is required. Food is served promptly at the correct temperature.
- *Low-stimulation dining* – this program prevents distractions during meals. The aged care team decides on the best place for each person to sit. Some centres have dining areas where clients can dine with guests. The person can have a family meal with a spouse, children, grandchildren, family or friends. They can celebrate holidays, birthdays, anniversaries or other special events. The dietary department provides the meal or the guests bring it. If food is supplied by visitors or family it must be registered with the facility and must comply with organisational standards.

Preparing for meals

Comfort is important during meals. The setting must be free of unpleasant sights, sounds and odours. Clients must be properly prepared. They may need to visit the toilet and have oral care attended to. Persons who are incontinent need to be clean and dry. Clients need dentures, glasses and hearing aids in place. To increase mealtime enjoyment and comfort, remove unpleasant equipment from the room. Help clients assume a comfortable position.

DELEGATION GUIDELINES

Serving meal trays

Before serving a meal tray, you need the following information from the nurse and the care plan:

- What adaptive equipment does the person use?
- How much help does the person need with opening cartons, cutting food or buttering bread?
- Is the person's intake and output measured?
- Are kilojoule counts done?

PREPARING THE PERSON FOR A MEAL

Quality of life

Remember to respect the person's privacy while doing any procedure. Address the person by name and ensure they know your name.

Pre-procedure

1. Follow the delegation guidelines.
2. Explain to the person that it is mealtime.
3. Wash your hands.
4. Collect the following:
   - equipment for oral hygiene
   - bedpan, urinal or commode and toilet tissue
   - washbasin
   - soap
   - washcloth
   - towel
   - gloves.
5. Provide for privacy.

Procedure

6. Make sure the person's glasses and hearing aids are in place.
7. Assist with oral hygiene. Make sure dentures are in place.
8. Assist with elimination. Make sure the incontinent person is clean and dry.
9. Help the person with handwashing.
10. Do the following if the person is to eat in bed:
    - a Raise the head of the bed to a comfortable sitting position.
    - b Clean the table. Adjust it in front of the person.
    - c Place the call bell within reach.
    - d Remove the screens from around the person.
11. Do the following if the person is to sit in a chair:
    - a Position the person in a chair or wheelchair.
    - b Remove items from the over-bed table. Clean the table.
    - c Adjust the over-bed table in front of the person.
    - d Place the call bell within reach.
    - e Remove the screens from around the person.
12. Assist the person to the correct dining area. Follow centre procedures for dining programs.

Post-procedure

13. Return to the room.
14. Clean and return equipment to its proper place. Wear gloves for this step.
15. Straighten the room. Eliminate unpleasant noise, odours or equipment.
16. Wash your hands.

SAFETY ALERT

Preparing for meals

Preparing the person for meals involves helping with oral hygiene and elimination. It is also important to ensure the client is positioned in a safe position to ensure they can easily chew and swallow their food; otherwise they can be at risk of choking. Follow Standard Precautions. Also follow Standard Precautions when cleaning equipment and the room.

Meal trays are served after clients are prepared for meals. Trays are served promptly, with containers that keep food hot or cold. Food should be at the desired temperature when the person receives it.

Serve trays in the order assigned by the health team. Clients seated at a table are served at the same time. If a tray is not served within 15 minutes, recheck the food temperature. If not at the right temperature, get another tray. Temperature guides and food thermometers are in dining rooms. Some centres allow reheating of hot foods in a microwave oven.

SERVING A MEAL TRAY

Quality of life

Remember to respect the person's privacy while doing any procedure. Address the person by name and ensure they know your name.

Pre-procedure

1. Follow the delegation guidelines.
2. Wash your hands.

Procedure

3. Make sure the tray is complete. Check items on the tray with the dietary card. Make sure adaptive equipment is included.
4. Call the person by name.
5. Place the tray within the person's reach. Adjust the over-bed table as needed.
6. Remove food covers. Open cartons, cut meat and butter bread as needed.
7. Place the serviette, clothes protector, adaptive equipment and cutlery within reach.
8. Measure and record intake if ordered. Note the amount and type of foods eaten.
9. Check for and remove any food in the mouth (pocketing). Wear gloves.
10. Remove the tray.
11. Clean spills and change soiled linen.
12. Help the person to bed if indicated.

Post-procedure

13. Assist with oral hygiene and with handwashing.
14. Provide for comfort.
15. Remove the gloves and wash your hands.
16. Place the call bell within reach.
17. Raise or lower bed rails. Follow the care plan.
18. Follow centre policy for soiled linen.
19. Wash your hands.
20. Report and record your observations.

Feeding the person

Weakness, paralysis, casts, confusion and other limits can make self-feeding impossible. Serve food and fluids in the order the person prefers. Offer fluids during the meal, as these help the person chew and swallow.

Spoons are used because they are less likely to cause injury. The spoon should be only one-third full. A portion of this size is easy to chew and swallow. Some people need smaller portions. Follow the person's care plan.

People who need to be fed are often angry, humiliated and embarrassed. Some are depressed, resentful or refuse to eat. Let them do as much as possible. Some can manage 'finger foods' (bread, biscuits and crackers). If strong enough, let them hold milk or juice glasses (never hot drinks). Never exceed the limits ordered by the doctor. Provide support and encourage them to try, even if food is spilled.

A person with a vision impairment is often very aware of food aromas. They may know what food is being served. Always tell the person what is on the tray. When feeding a visually impaired person, describe what you are offering. For people who feed themselves, describe the foods and fluids and their place on the tray. Use the numbers on a clock to describe the location of foods (Fig. 12.101).

Many people pray before eating. Allow time and privacy for prayer. This shows that you respect and care about the person.

Meals provide social contact with others (Fig. 12.102). Engage the person in pleasant conversation. However, allow for chewing and swallowing. Also, sit facing the person. Sitting is more relaxing. It shows the person that you have time for them. Standing communicates non-verbally that you are in a hurry. By facing the person, you can see how well they are eating. You can also see if the person has problems swallowing.

Between-meal nourishments

Many special diets involve between-meal nourishments. Common nourishments are crackers, milk, juice, a milkshake, cake,

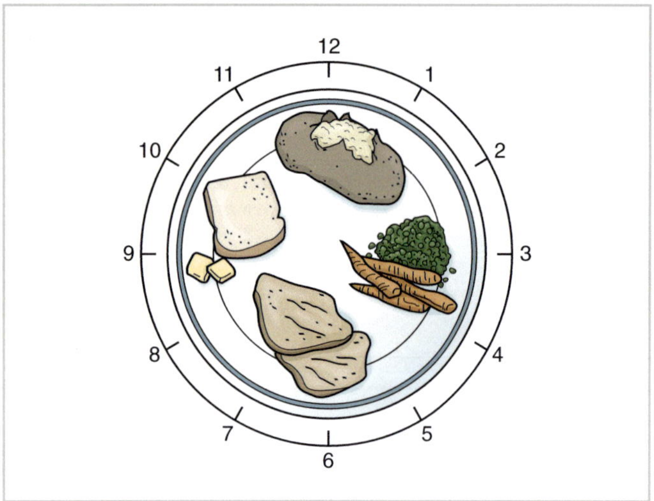

Fig. 12.101
The numbers on a clock are used to help a person with a vision impairment locate food.

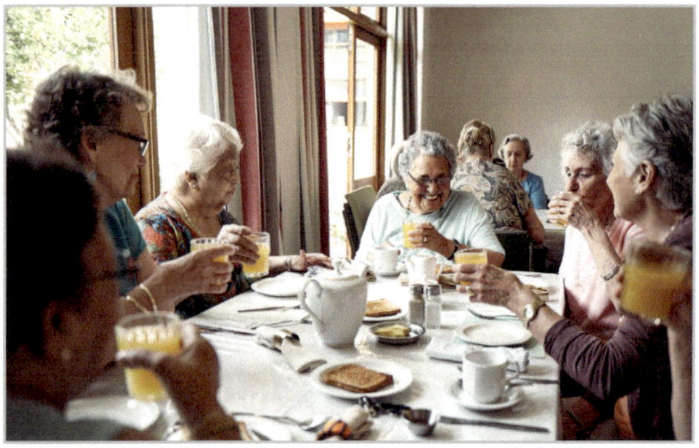

Fig. 12.102
Clients enjoy a pleasant meal in the dining room.

wafers, a sandwich, jelly and custard. Serve nourishments when they arrive in the nursing unit. Clients who are confused or who expend a lot of energy wandering may need extra attention to their nutritional needs. If you notice a client is losing weight, make sure you notify your team leader. The client may need special assistance. Provide needed eating utensils, a straw and a napkin. Follow the same considerations and procedures for serving meal trays and feeding people.

Providing drinking water

Clients need fresh drinking water each shift. They also need water whenever the jug is empty. Before providing water, ask the nurse about any special orders. Follow centre procedure for providing fresh drinking water. Research shows that many people in aged care services are dehydrated. Over time this can lead to further health problems for the individual, so it is important to make sure people have adequate water and that they are able to access this water (e.g. it is placed within reach with a clean cup available). Offer water on a regular basis, especially in warm weather, to those clients who may not be drinking enough or who tend to forget to drink.

FEEDING A PERSON

Quality of life

Remember to respect the person's privacy while doing any procedure. Address the person by name and ensure they know your name.

Pre-procedure

1 Follow the delegation guidelines.
2 Explain the procedure to the person.
3 Wash your hands.
4 Position the person in a sitting position.
5 Get the tray. Place it on the over-bed table or dining table.

Procedure

6 Call the person by name.
7 Drape a serviette across the person's chest and under the chin.
8 Tell the person what foods and fluids are on the tray.
9 Prepare the food for eating. Season food as the person prefers and is allowed by the care plan.
10 Serve foods in the order the person prefers. Alternate between solid and liquid foods. Use a spoon for safety. Allow enough time for chewing. Do not rush the person.
11 Use straws for liquids if the person cannot drink out of a glass or cup. Have one straw for each liquid. Provide short straws for weak persons.
12 Follow the swallow guide and care plan if the person has dysphagia. (Some people with dysphagia do not use straws.) Give thickened liquid with a spoon.
13 Converse with the person in a pleasant manner.
14 Encourage the person to eat as much as possible.
15 Wipe the person's mouth with a napkin as needed.
16 Note how much and which foods were eaten.
17 Measure and record intake if ordered.
18 Remove the tray.
19 Take the person back to their room.
20 Assist with oral hygiene and handwashing. (Wear gloves for this step.)
21 Remove and dispose of gloves.
22 Wash your hands.

Post-procedure

23 Provide for comfort.
24 Place the call bell within reach.
25 Wash your hands.
26 Report and record your observations.

DELEGATION GUIDELINES

Feeding a person

Feeding clients is a task commonly done by carers. Before feeding a person, you need the following information from the care plan:

- Why does the person need help?
- How much help does the person need? Can the person manage finger foods?
- What are the person's activity limits?
- What are the person's dietary restrictions?
- What size portion should the person be fed (e.g. spoonful or less)?
- Does the person have dysphagia? If so, what safety measures are needed?
- What observations to report and record:
  - the amount and kind of food eaten
  - complaints of nausea or dysphagia
  - signs of aspiration.

QUALITY OF LIFE

Nutrition and fluid balance are important for quality of life.

The right to personal choice is important in meeting food and fluid needs. Everyone has a lifetime of food likes and dislikes. These do not change when in a consumer care facility. Food preferences may relate to religion or culture. With the person's help, the dietitian plans healthy meals that include personal choices. Clients may tell you that they like or want certain foods. Share this information with the nurse.

People with dementia may require special measures to meet their nutritional needs, and most particularly with hydration. You must be patient and offer frequent sips of water. Provide a quiet and calm dining experience. Remember, all people have the right to be treated with dignity and respect.

Sometimes family and friends bring food from home. This helps the person's love and belonging needs. Sometimes the centre cannot provide all the person's food preferences. It usually pleases clients when family and friends bring favourite foods. Holidays have food traditions. Holidays mean more when lifelong family traditions are shared. Many families and friends bring food as gifts. The nurse needs to know when the person receives food. The food must not interfere with a special diet.

Standard 3.2.1 of the Food Safety Standards requires aged care services to develop a food safety program. These are to be developed based on the HACCP (Hazard Analysis and Critical Control Point) system, which identifies potential hazards. The HACCP system requires that food be served correctly:

- Hot food must be hot. Cold food must be cold.
- Meals must be served promptly. If there is a delay in serving a tray, get a new tray of food from the dietary department. Tell the person why the meal was delayed.
- Provide any needed help with eating. This includes providing any special equipment or eating utensils.

Source: Food Standards Australia and New Zealand (2021). Food Safety Programs: Standard 3.2.1. Online 7 March 2021. Available: www.foodstandards.gov.au

FOCUS ON COMMUNITY CARE

When assisting your client with their nutritional and dietary needs, you need to always consider their individual needs and desires. If you are required to undertake their grocery shopping, the client will give you a list of their grocery needs. Always check which brand of product they prefer, rather than purchasing the brand that you usually buy. It is important to always consider your client's ethnicity, culture and religious requirements and preferences. When preparing foods, ask your client how they wish them to be prepared and presented. In some cultures certain foods should never be presented alongside or even cooked with others. If you are required to assist in meal planning, ensure that the client directs you. The digestive system of some clients is affected considerably by their disability. This may mean that they have some restrictions in their diet.

ENTERAL NUTRITION

Many people cannot eat or drink because of illness, surgery or injury. The doctor orders other methods to meet their food and fluid needs. People who cannot chew or swallow often require enteral nutrition. **Enteral nutrition** is giving nutrients through the gastrointestinal tract (enteral). A nurse gives a formula through a feeding tube. (**Gavage** is another term for tube feeding.)

A **nasogastric (NG) tube** is inserted through the nose (*naso*) into the stomach (*gastro*) (Fig. 12.103). A doctor or a registered nurse performs the procedure.

A **gastrostomy** is a surgically created opening (*stomy*) in the stomach (*gastro*) (Fig. 12.104). A **percutaneous endoscopic gastrostomy (PEG) tube** is inserted with an endoscope. An endoscope is a lighted instrument (*scope*). It lets the doctor see inside a body cavity or organ (*endo*). With an endoscope, the doctor can see inside the stomach. The doctor inserts the endoscope through the person's mouth

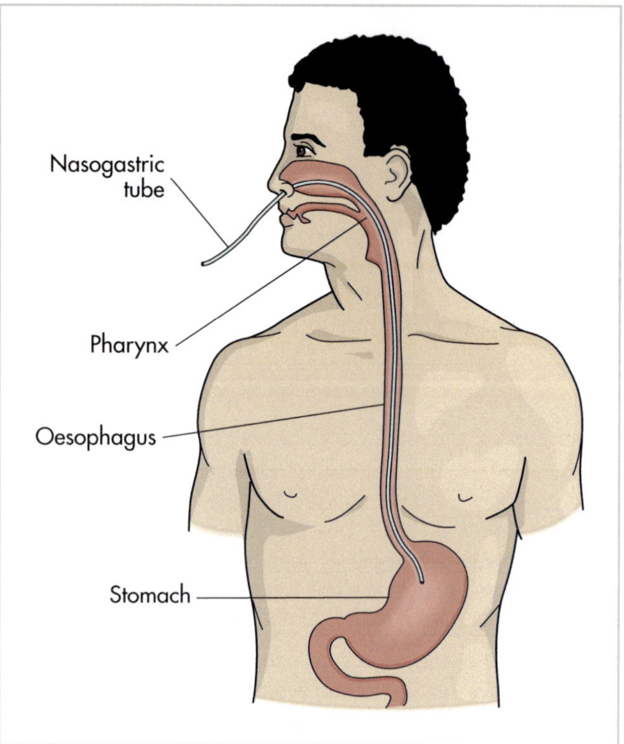

Fig. 12.103
A nasogastric tube is inserted through the nose and oesophagus into the stomach.

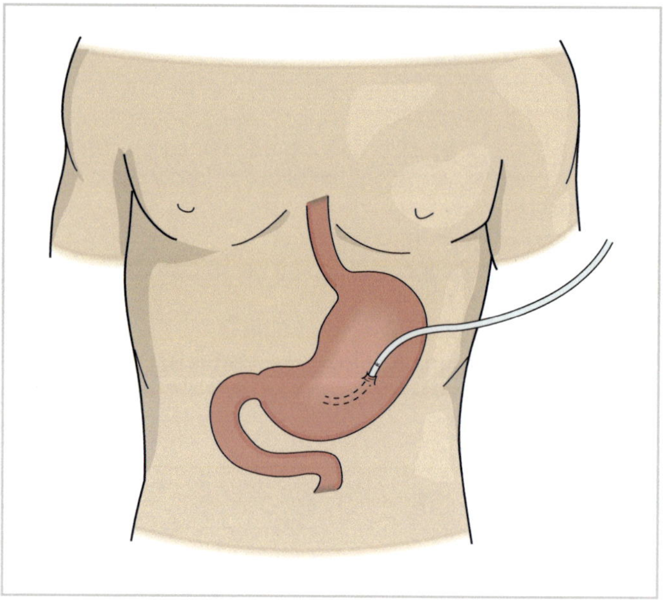

Fig. 12.104
A gastrostomy tube.

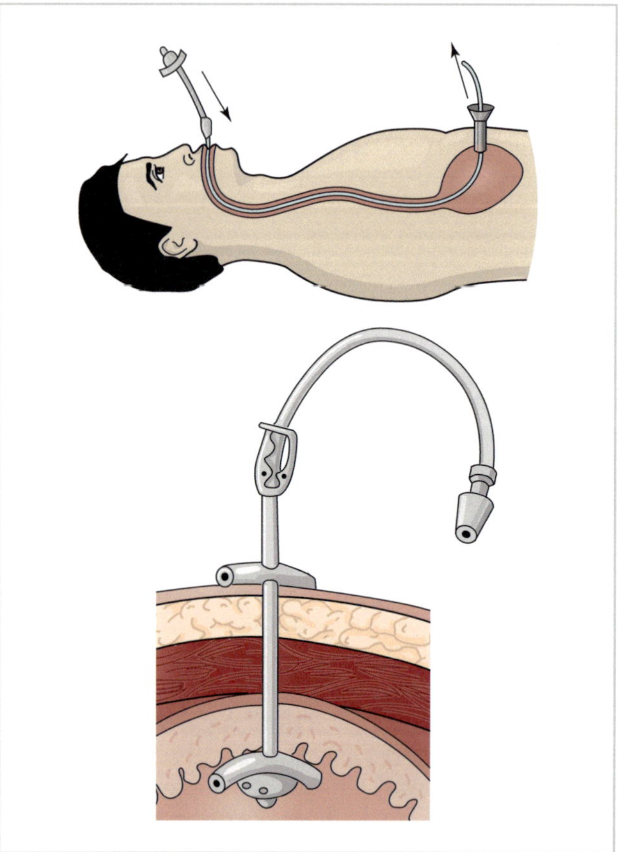

Fig. 12.105
A percutaneous endoscopic gastrostomy (PEG).

and oesophagus and into the stomach. A stab or puncture wound (*stomy*) is made through (*per*) the skin (*cutaneous*) and into the stomach (*gastro*). A tube is inserted into the stomach through the stab wound (Fig. 12.105).

A feeding tube is used when food cannot pass normally from the mouth into the oesophagus and then into the stomach. Cancer of the head, neck or oesophagus is a common cause. So is trauma or surgery to the face, mouth, head or neck. Coma is another reason for tube feeding, and so is dysphagia caused by paralysis. Some people with dementia no longer know how to eat. They may require tube feedings.

Gastrostomy, **jejunostomy** and PEG feedings are used for long-term enteral nutrition. The ostomy can be temporary or permanent.

Formulas

The doctor orders the type and amount of formula. Most formulas contain protein, carbohydrates, fat, vitamins and minerals. Commercial formulas are common. Sometimes the dietary department prepares the formula.

Scheduled and continuous feeding

Scheduled or continuous feedings are ordered. Scheduled feedings are usually given four times a day with a syringe or feeding bag (Fig. 12.106). Usually about 400 mL is given over 20 minutes. The amount and rate are like eating a regular meal.

Continuous feedings require electronic feeding pumps (Fig. 12.107). Formula is given at room temperature. Cold fluids can cause cramping. Sometimes, continuous feedings are kept cold with ice chips around the container. Microbes

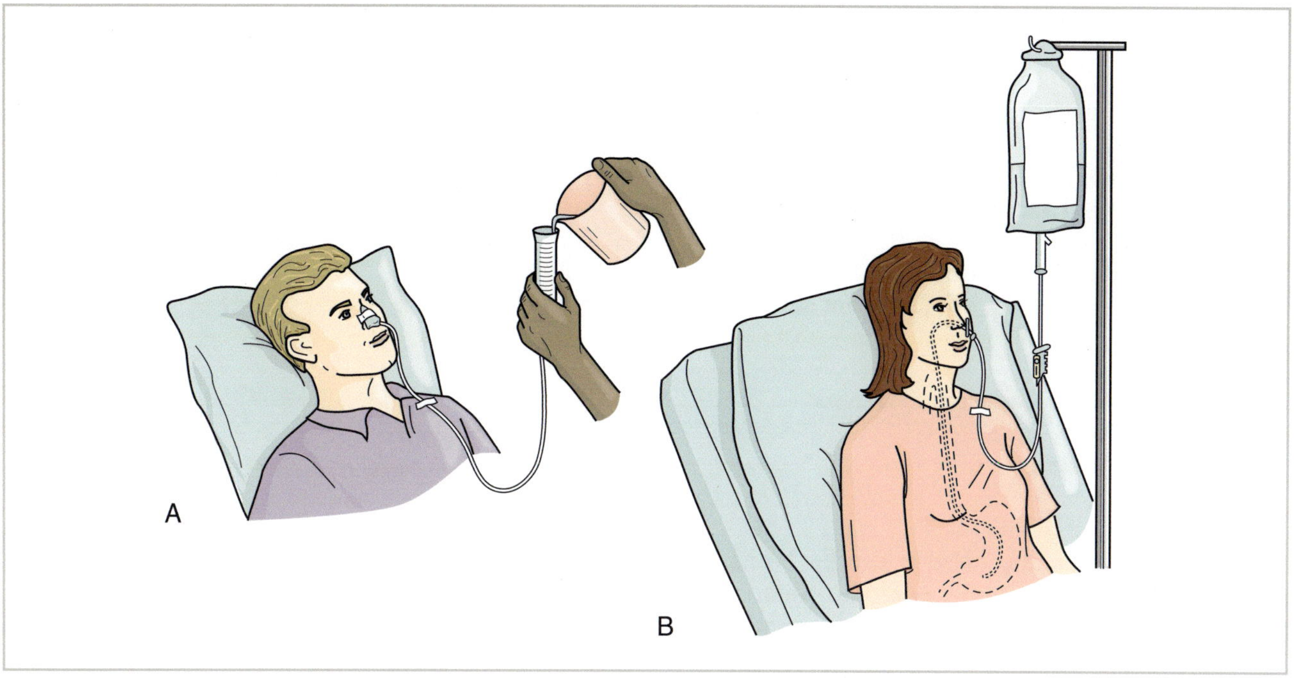

Fig. 12.106
A. Tube feeding is given with a jug. **B.** Formula drips from a feeding bag into the feeding tube.

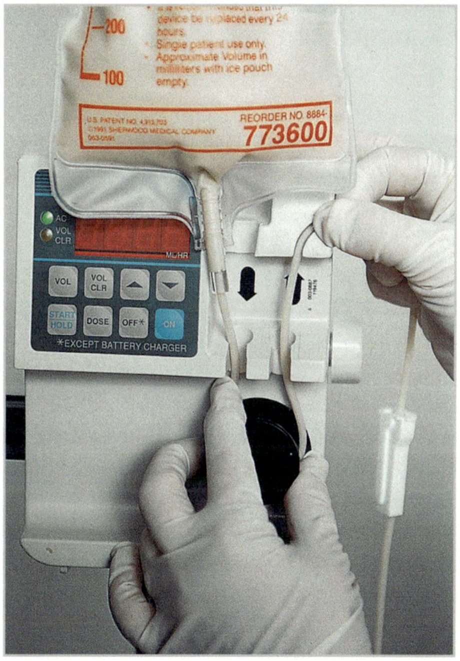

Fig. 12.107
Feeding pump.

grow in warm formula. The formula warms to room temperature as it drips from the bag and passes through the connecting tubing to the feeding tube. The nurse adds formula every 3–4 hours.

Preventing aspiration

Aspiration is a major risk of nasogastric tubes. Remember, aspiration is the breathing of fluid or an object into the lungs. It can cause pneumonia and death. These tubes are passed through the oesophagus, then into the stomach or small intestine. During insertion, the tube can slip into the airway. This causes aspiration. An X-ray, taken after the tube is inserted, is the best way to determine tube placement.

After insertion, the tube can move out of place from coughing, sneezing, vomiting, suctioning or poor positioning. It can move from the stomach or intestines into the oesophagus and then into the airway. Therefore, the nurse checks tube placement before every scheduled tube feeding. With continuous tube feedings, the nurse checks tube placement every 4–8 hours. To do so, the nurse attaches a syringe to the tube and removes gastrointestinal secretions. Then the nurse measures the pH of the secretions.

Aspiration also occurs from regurgitation. **Regurgitation** is the backward flow of food from the stomach into the mouth. This can occur with nasogastric, gastrostomy and PEG tubes. Delayed stomach emptying and overfeeding are common causes. To prevent regurgitation:

- position the person in semi-Fowler's position
- have the person remain in this position for at least 1 hour after the feeding – this promotes movement of the formula through the gastrointestinal system and prevents aspiration
- avoid the left side-lying position – this position prevents the stomach from emptying.

Remember that during digestion, food slowly passes from the stomach to the small intestine. The stomach handles larger amounts of food at one time than does the small intestine.

Observations

Aspiration is a major risk of tube feeding. Other risks include diarrhoea, constipation and delayed stomach emptying.

When a person is receiving a tube feeding, report the following to the nurse at once:

- nausea
- discomfort during the tube feeding
- vomiting
- diarrhoea
- distended (enlarged and swollen) abdomen
- coughing
- complaints of indigestion or heartburn
- redness, swelling, drainage, odour or pain at the ostomy site
- elevated temperature
- signs and symptoms of respiratory distress
- increased pulse rate
- complaints of flatulence.

Comfort measures

The person with a feeding tube is usually NBM. Dry mouth, dry lips and sore throat cause discomfort. Some people are allowed hard lollies or gum. The person needs frequent oral hygiene, lubricant for the lips and mouth rinses. The nose and nostrils are cleaned every 4–8 hours. Give needed care as directed by the nurse and the care plan.

Feeding tubes (except gastrostomy and PEG tubes) can irritate and cause pressure on the nose. Sometimes they alter the shape of the nostrils. Securing the tube helps prevent these problems. Tape or a tube holder secures the tube to the nose (Fig. 12.108). Tube holders have foam cushions that prevent pressure on the nose. There is no need for re-taping, which irritates the nose. The tube is also secured to the person's upper garment. Loop a rubber band around the tube. Then pin the rubber band to the garment with a safety pin. Alternatively, tape the tube to the garment. Follow centre policy for securing the tube to the garment.

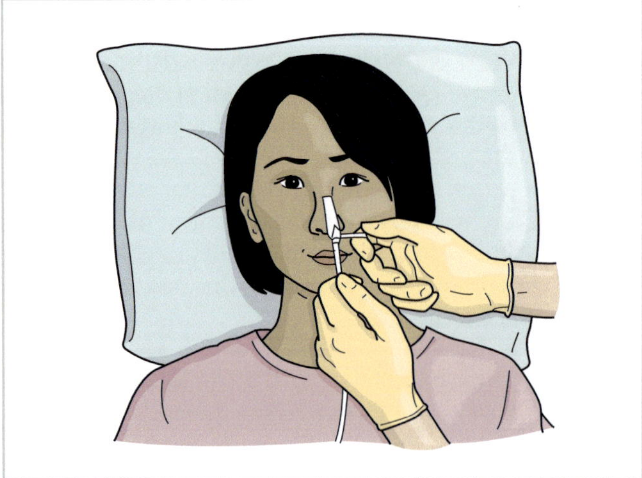

Fig. 12.108
The feeding tube is taped to the nose.

ASSISTING WITH EXERCISE AND ACTIVITY

After reading this section, you should be able to:

- understand the purpose of bed rest
- know how to prevent the complications of bed rest
- be aware of the devices used to support and maintain body alignment
- know how to perform range-of-motion exercises
- know how to help a person walk
- understand the purpose of four walking aids
- know how to help a person who is falling
- perform the procedures described in this section.

Exercise is one of the keys to physical and mental health and to a sense of wellbeing. Exercise, even in limited amounts, can help prevent muscle atrophy and the other complications of bed rest.

Most people can move about and function without help. Ageing, illness, surgery, injury and pain can cause weakness and some activity limits; some people are in bed for a long time; some are paralysed; some disorders are progressive. They cause decreases in activity. Examples include arthritis and nervous system and muscular disorders. Inactivity, whether mild or severe, affects every body system. It also affects mental wellbeing. Clients with dementia can find the notion of exercise and activity threatening (Box 12.31).

Muscle atrophy is the loss of muscle strength from inactivity. When not active, older people lose muscle tone quickly. Each person is encouraged to be as active as possible. The care plan tells you about the person's activity level and what exercises to perform.

BOX 12.31
Clients with dementia

People with dementia may resist exercise and activity. They do not understand what is happening and may fear harm. They may become agitated and combative. Some cry out for help. Do not force the person to exercise or take part in activities. Stay calm and ask your supervisor or nurse for help. Follow the care plan.

To help promote exercise and activity, you need to understand:

- bed rest
- how to prevent complications from bed rest
- how to help with exercise.

BED REST

Doctors will sometimes order bed rest to treat a health problem. At other times it is used if the person's condition changes. You must know the activities allowed for each person. The care plan has this information. Check with your supervisor or the nurse if you have questions. Generally, bed rest is ordered:

- to reduce physical activity
- to reduce pain
- to encourage rest
- to regain strength
- to promote healing
- as a safety measure (e.g. for the comatose client).

The following types of bed rest are common:

- *bed rest* – some activities of daily living (ADLs) are allowed, such as self-feeding, oral hygiene, bathing, shaving and hair care
- *strict bed rest* – everything is done for the person – no unassisted ADLs are allowed
- *bed rest with commode privileges* – the person can use the bedside commode for elimination
- *bed rest with bathroom privileges* (*bed rest with BRP*) – the person can use the bathroom for elimination.

Always check with the care plan to see what bed rest means for each person.

Complications of bed rest

Many older clients were brought up in an era when bed rest was an important part of illness and old age. They may, therefore, often want to spend time in bed. Bed rest and lack of exercise and activity can cause serious complications. Every system is affected. Pressure ulcers, constipation and faecal impaction can result. Urinary tract infections and renal calculi (kidney stones) can occur. So can blood clots (thrombi) and pneumonia (infection of the lung).

The musculoskeletal system is affected. A **contracture** is the lack of joint mobility caused by abnormal shortening of a muscle. The contracted muscle is fixed into position, is deformed and cannot stretch (Fig. 12.109). Common sites are the fingers, wrists, elbows, toes, ankles, knees and hips. Contractures also occur in the neck and spine. The person is permanently deformed and disabled. **Atrophy** is the decrease in size or the wasting away of tissue. Muscle atrophy is a decrease in size or a wasting away of muscle (Fig. 12.110). These complications must be prevented to maintain normal movement.

Orthostatic hypotension and blood clots occur in the cardiovascular system. Orthostatic hypotension is a drop in (*hypo*) blood pressure when the person stands (*ortho* and *static*). When a person moves from lying or sitting to a standing position, the blood pressure drops. The person feels dizzy and weak and sees spots before their eyes. Syncope can occur. **Syncope** (fainting) is a brief loss of consciousness (from the Greek word *synkoptein*, meaning to cut short). Orthostatic hypotension is also called **postural hypotension** (postural relates to posture or standing).

Box 12.32 lists the measures that prevent orthostatic hypotension. Slowly changing positions is key.

Good care practices prevent complications from bed rest. Positioning in good alignment, range-of-motion (ROM)

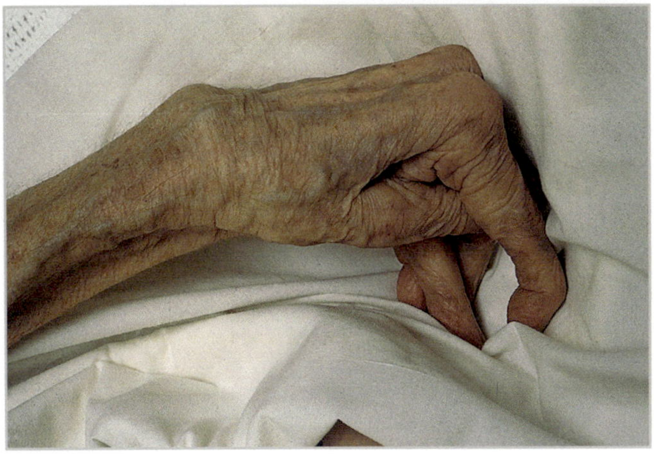

Fig. 12.109
A contracture.

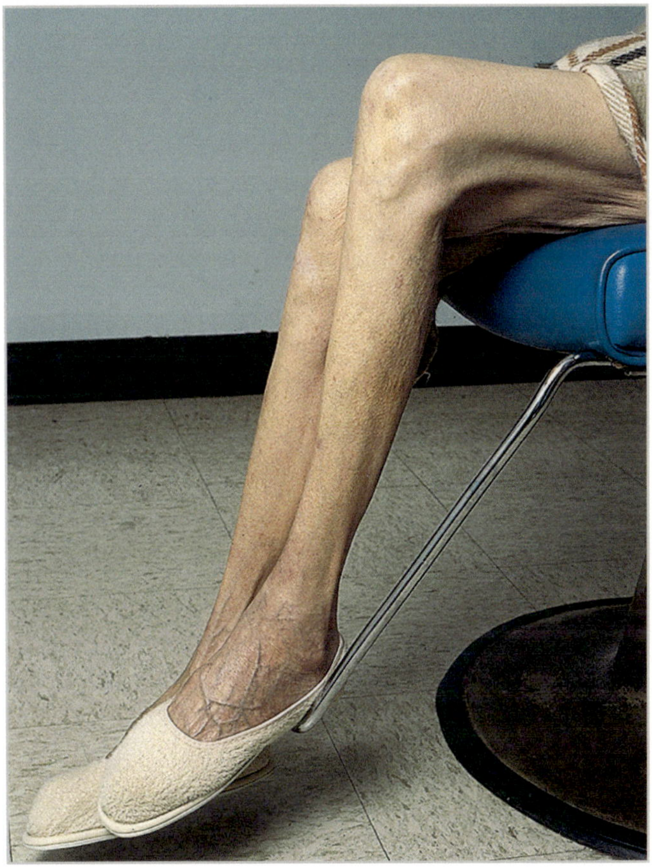

Fig. 12.110
Muscle atrophy.

BOX 12.32
Preventing orthostatic hypotension

- Position the person in Fowler's position. Raise the head of the bed slowly.
  - Ask the person about weakness, dizziness or spots before the eyes. Lower the head of the bed if symptoms occur.
  - Keep the person in Fowler's position for a short while. Ask about weakness, dizziness or spots before the eyes.
- Help the person sit on the side of the bed.
  - Ask about weakness, dizziness or spots before the eyes. Help the person to Fowler's position if symptoms occur.
- Have the person sit on the side of the bed for a short while.
- Help the person stand.
  - Ask about weakness, dizziness or spots before the eyes. Help the person sit on the side of the bed if any symptoms occur.
  - Help the person sit in a chair or walk as directed by the nurse.
  - Ask about weakness, dizziness or spots before the eyes. If the person is walking, help them to sit if symptoms occur.
- Report blood pressure, pulse and respirations to the nurse. Also report other symptoms or complaints. If any weakness, dizziness or spots before the eyes occur at any stage, assist the person into a sitting or lying position and call the nurse immediately.

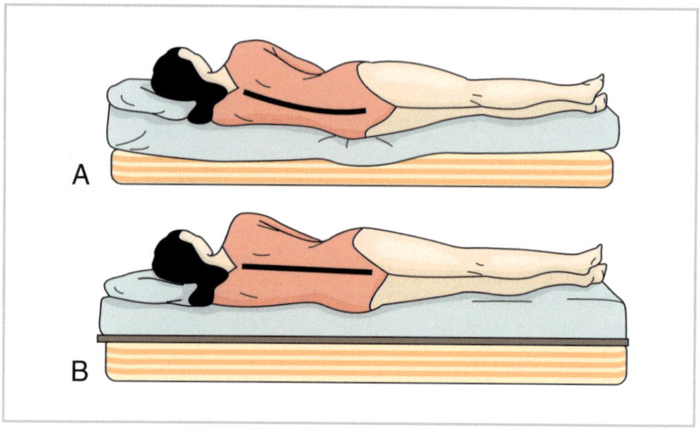

Fig. 12.111
A. The mattress sags without bed boards. **B.** Bed boards are under the mattress. No sagging occurs.

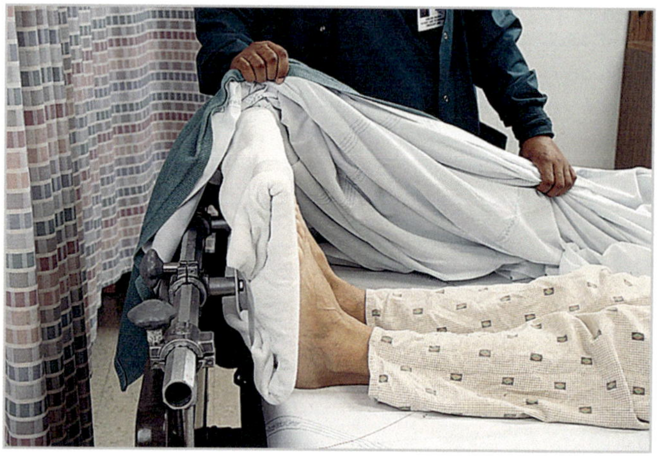

Fig. 12.112
Footboard. Feet are flush with the board to keep them in normal alignment.

exercises and frequent position changes are important measures. These are part of the care plan.

Positioning

Correct body alignment and positioning are important. Supportive devices are often used to support and maintain the person in a certain position:

- *Bed boards* – may be placed under the mattress if it sags and does not provide sufficient support. They prevent the mattress from sagging (Fig. 12.111). They are usually made of plywood and covered with canvas or other material. There are two sections so the head of the bed can be raised. One section is for the head of the bed, the other is for the foot of the bed.
- *Footboard* – this is placed at the foot of the mattress (Fig. 12.112). It prevents plantar flexion, which can lead to footdrop. In **plantar flexion**, the foot (plantar) is bent (flexion). **Footdrop** is when the foot falls down at the ankle (permanent plantar flexion). The footboard is placed so the soles of the feet are flush against it. The feet are in good alignment, as when standing. A footboard also serves as a bed cradle. It keeps the top linen off the feet.
- *Trochanter roll* – prevents the hips and legs from turning outwards (**external rotation**) (Fig. 12.113). A bath blanket is folded to the desired length and rolled up. The loose end is placed under the person from the hip to the knee. Then the roll is tucked alongside the body. Pillows or sandbags also keep the hips and knees in alignment.
- *Hand roll or handgrip* – prevents contractures of the thumb, fingers and wrist (Fig. 12.114). Foam rubber sponges, rubber balls and finger cushions (Fig. 12.115) are also used.
- Splints – keep the wrist, thumb and fingers in normal position (Fig. 12.116). They are usually secured in place with Velcro. Some have foam padding.

EXERCISE

Exercise helps prevent contractures, muscle atrophy and other complications of bed rest (Box 12.33). Some exercise occurs with ADLs and when turning and moving in bed without help. Other exercises are needed for muscles and joints.

Range-of-motion exercises

The **range of motion (ROM)** of a joint is the movement of that joint to the extent possible without causing pain.

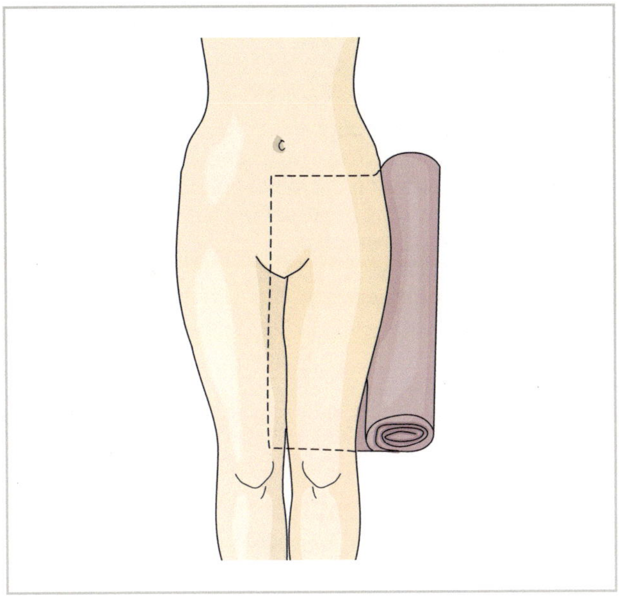

Fig. 12.113
Trochanter roll made from a bath blanket.
It extends from the hip to the knee.

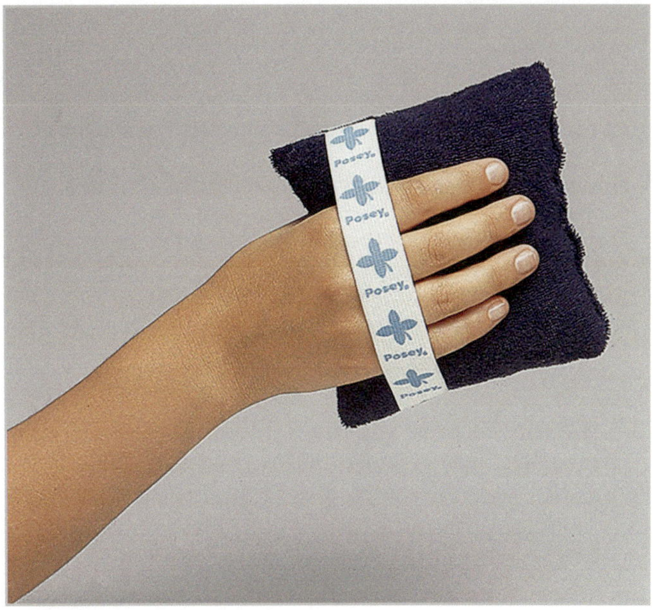

Fig. 12.114
Hand grip.

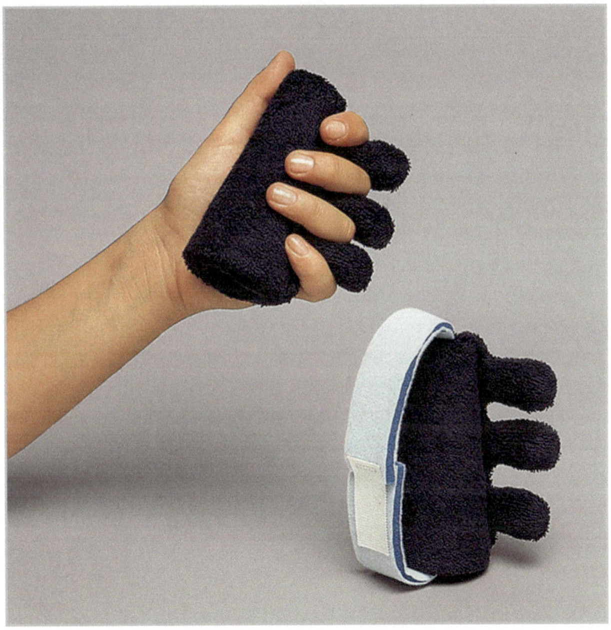

Fig. 12.115
Finger cushion.

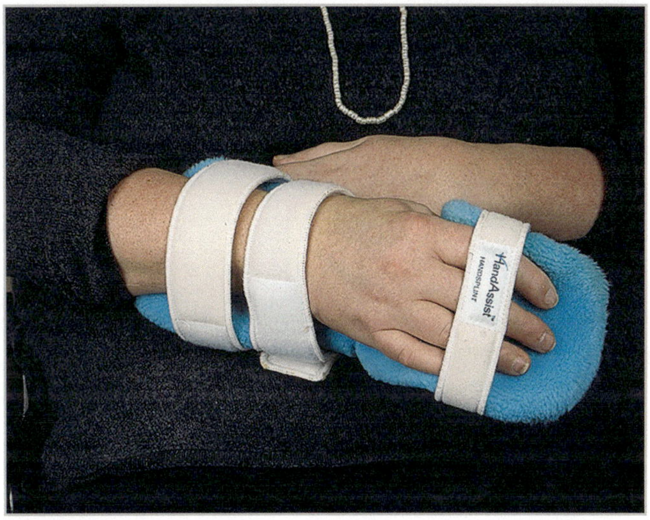

Fig. 12.116
Splint.

ROM exercises move the joints through their complete range of motion. They are usually done at least twice a day:

- *active ROM exercises* – are done by the person
- *passive ROM exercises* – someone moves the joints through their range of motion
- *active–assistive ROM exercises* – the person does the exercises with some help. Bathing, hair care, eating, reaching and walking all involve joint movements. People on bed-rest may need more frequent ROM exercises. So may those who have lost mobility from illness or injury.

BOX 12.33
Focus on rehabilitation

The person works closely with physiotherapists and occupational therapists to improve strength and endurance. Care plan goals for both exercise and ambulation may change daily. The goal is to improve the person's independence. The health team works with the person to meet rehabilitation goals. Follow the care plan carefully. Aged Care Accreditation Standard 2.14 states: 'Optimum levels of mobility and dexterity are achieved for all consumers'.

BOX 12.34
Joint movements

Abduction – moving a body part away from the midline of the body
Adduction – moving a body part towards the midline of the body
Dorsiflexion – bending the toes and foot up at the ankle
Extension – straightening a body part
External rotation – turning the joint outwards
Flexion – bending a body part
Hyperextension – excessive straightening of a body part
Internal rotation – turning the joint inwards
Plantar flexion – bending the foot down at the ankle
Pronation – turning downwards
Rotation – turning the joint
Supination – turning upwards

The doctor or nurse may order ROM exercises.

Prevention may involve ROM exercises. Sometimes splints and braces are used. Box 12.34 lists the terms typically used for different types of joint movements.

DELEGATION GUIDELINES

Range-of-motion exercises

Assisting with exercise is part of your job. When delegated ROM exercises, you need the following information from the nurse and the care plan:

- the kind of ROM exercises ordered – active, passive or active–assistive
- which joints to exercise
- how often the exercises are done
- how many times to repeat each exercise
- what to report and record:
  - the time the exercises were performed
  - the joints exercised
  - the number of times the exercises were performed on each joint
  - complaints of pain, or signs of stiffness or spasm
  - the degree to which the person took part in the exercises.

SAFETY ALERT

Range-of-motion exercises

ROM exercises can cause injury if not done properly. Practise the rules in Box 12.35 when performing or assisting with ROM exercises.

BOX 12.35
Performing range-of-motion exercises

- Exercise only the joints the nurse tells you to exercise.
- Expose only the body part being exercised.
- Use good body mechanics.
- Support the part being exercised.
- Move the joint slowly, smoothly and gently.
- Do not force a joint beyond its present range of motion or to the point of pain.
- Perform ROM exercises to the neck only if allowed by centre policy. In some centres, only physiotherapists or occupational therapists do neck exercises. This is because of the danger of neck injuries.

PERFORMING RANGE-OF-MOTION EXERCISES

Quality of life

Remember to respect the person's privacy while doing any procedure. Address the person by name and ensure they know your name.

Pre-procedure

1. Follow the delegation guidelines.
2. Identify the person. Speak to the person by name.
3. Explain the procedure to the person.
4. Wash your hands.
5. Obtain a bath blanket.
6. Provide for privacy.

Procedure

7. Lower the bed rail near you (if applicable).
8. Position the person supine.
9. Cover the person with a bath blanket. Fan-fold top linen to the foot of the bed.
10. Exercise the neck if allowed by the centre and if the nurse instructs you to (Fig. 12.117).
    a. Place your hands over the person's ears to support the head. Support the jaws with your fingers.

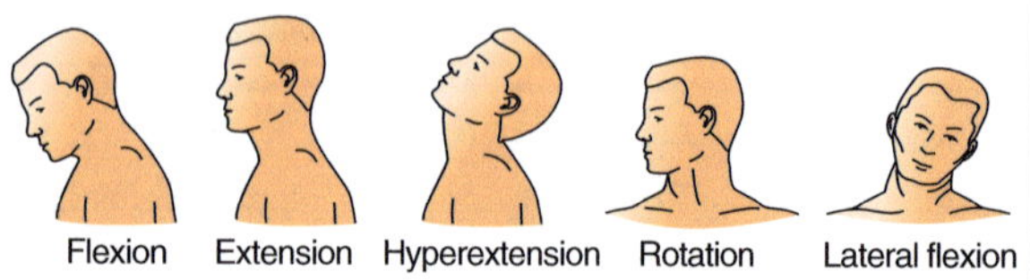

Fig. 12.117
ROM exercises for the neck.

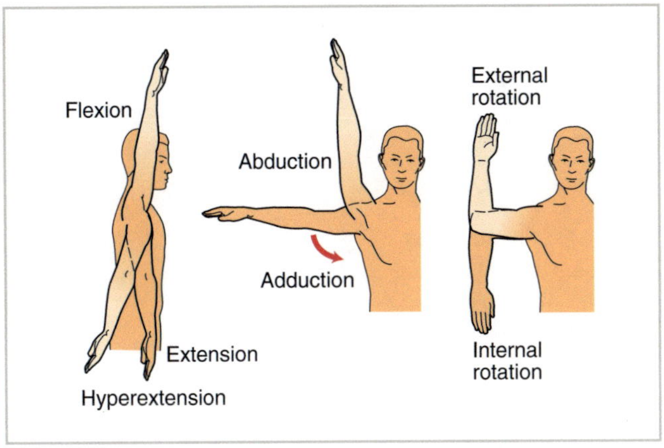

Fig. 12.118
ROM exercises for the shoulder.

- b Flexion – bring the head forwards. The chin touches the chest.
- c Extension – straighten the head.
- d Hyperextension – bring the head backwards until the chin points up.
- e Rotation – turn the head from side to side.
- f Lateral flexion – move the head to the right and to the left.
- g Repeat flexion, extension, hyperextension, rotation and lateral flexion five times – or the number of times stated on the care plan.

11 Exercise the shoulder (Fig. 12.118).
- a Grasp the wrist with one hand. Grasp the elbow with your other hand.
- b Flexion – raise the arm straight in front and over the head.
- c Extension – bring the arm down to the side.
- d Hyperextension – move the arm behind the body. (Do this if the person sits in a straight-backed chair or is standing.)
- e Abduction – move the straight arm away from the side of the body.
- f Adduction – move the straight arm to the side of the body.
- g Internal rotation – bend the elbow. Place it at the same level as the shoulder. Move the forearm down towards the body.
- h External rotation – move the forearm towards the head.
- i Repeat flexion, extension, hyperextension, abduction, adduction and internal and external rotation five times – or the number of times stated on the care plan.

12 Exercise the elbow (Fig. 12.119).
- a Grasp the person's wrist with one hand. Grasp the elbow with your other hand.
- b Flexion – bend the arm so the same-side shoulder is touched.
- c Extension – straighten the arm.
- d Repeat flexion and extension five times – or the number of times stated on the care plan.

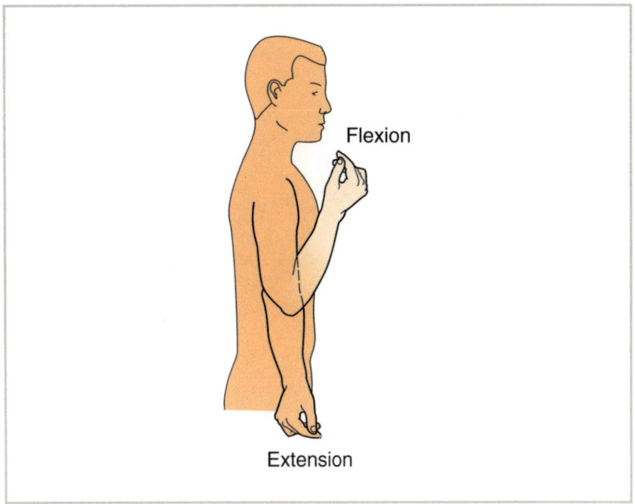

Fig. 12.119
ROM exercises for the elbow.

13 Exercise the forearm (Fig. 12.120).
- a Pronation – turn the hand so the palm is down.
- b Supination – turn the hand so the palm is up.
- c Repeat pronation and supination five times – or the number of times stated on the care plan.

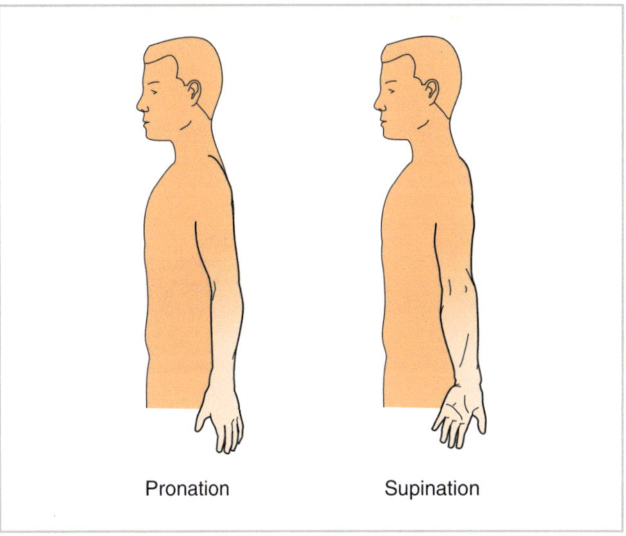

Fig. 12.120
ROM exercises for the forearm.

14 Exercise the wrist (Fig. 12.121).
- a Hold the wrist with both of your hands.
- b Flexion – bend the hand down.
- c Extension – straighten the hand.
- d Hyperextension – bend the hand back.
- e Radial flexion – turn the hand towards the thumb.
- f Ulnar flexion – turn the hand towards the little finger.
- g Repeat flexion, extension, hyperextension and radial and ulnar flexion five times – or the number of times stated on the care plan.

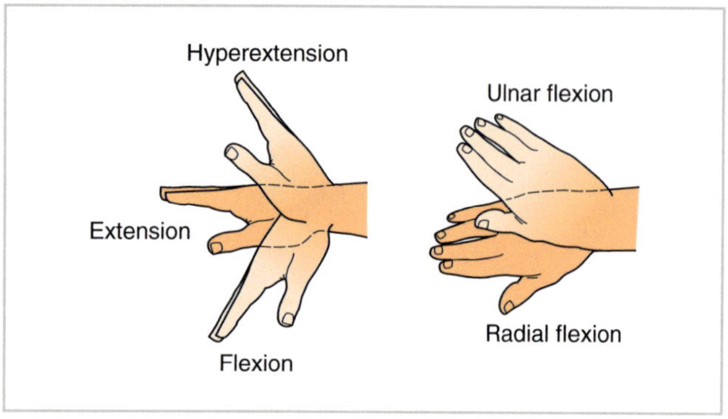

Fig. 12.121
ROM exercises for the wrist.

15 Exercise the thumb (Fig. 12.122).

- **a** Hold the person's hand with one hand. Hold the thumb with your other hand.
- **b** Abduction – move the thumb out from the inner part of the index finger.
- **c** Adduction – move the thumb back next to the index finger.
- **d** Opposition – touch each fingertip with the thumb.
- **e** Flexion – bend the thumb into the hand.
- **f** Extension – move the thumb out to the side of the fingers.
- **g** Repeat abduction, adduction, opposition, flexion and extension five times – or the number of times stated on the care plan.

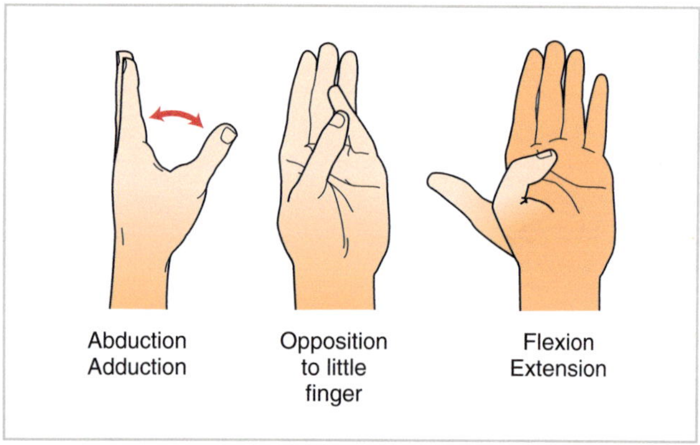

Fig. 12.122
ROM exercises for the thumb.

16 Exercise the fingers (Fig. 12.123).

- **a** Abduction – spread the fingers and the thumb apart.
- **b** Adduction – bring the fingers and thumb together.
- **c** Extension – straighten the fingers so the fingers, hand and arm are straight.
- **d** Flexion – make a fist.
- **e** Repeat abduction, adduction, extension and flexion five times – or the number of times stated on the care plan.

17 Exercise the hip (Fig. 12.124).

- **a** Support the leg. Place one hand under the knee. Place your other hand under the ankle.

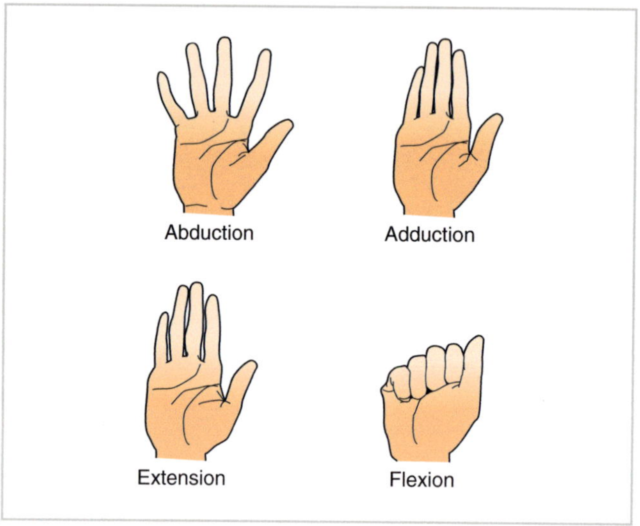

Fig. 12.123
ROM exercises for the fingers.

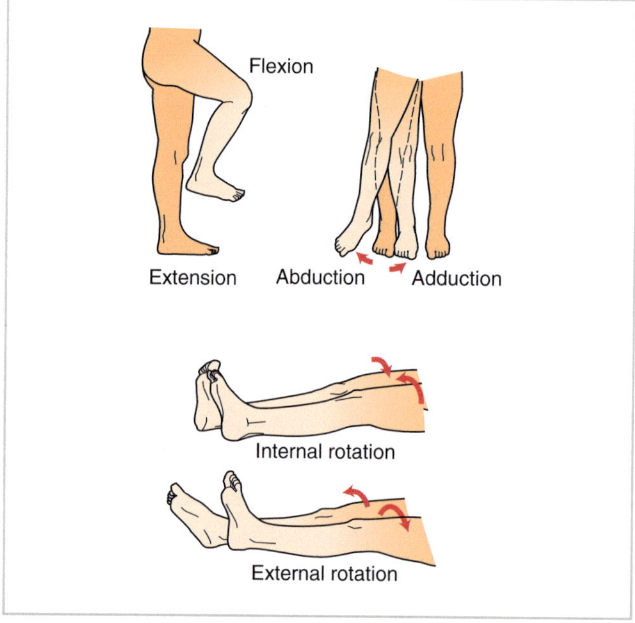

Fig. 12.124
ROM exercises for the hip.

- **b** Flexion – raise the leg.
- **c** Extension – straighten the leg.
- **d** Abduction – move the leg away from the body.
- **e** Adduction – move the leg towards the other leg.
- **f** Internal rotation – turn the leg inwards.
- **g** External rotation – turn the leg outwards.
- **h** Repeat flexion, extension, abduction, adduction, and internal and external rotation five times – or the number of times stated on the care plan.

18 Exercise the knee (Fig. 12.125).

- **a** Support the knee. Place one hand under the knee. Place your other hand under the ankle.
- **b** Flexion – bend the leg.

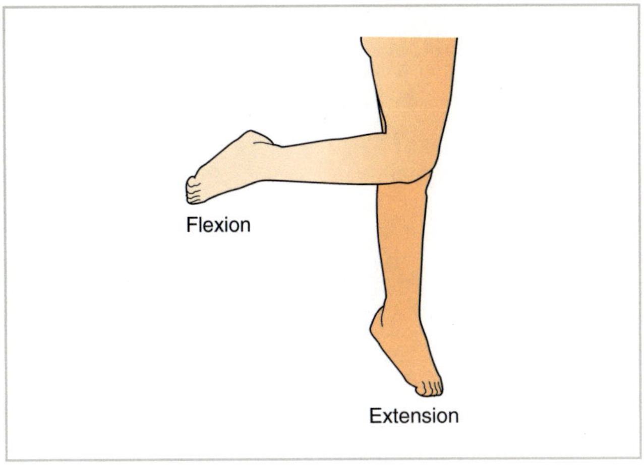

Fig. 12.125
ROM exercises for the knee.

c Extension – straighten the leg.
d Repeat flexion and extension of the knee five times – or the number of times stated on the care plan.

19 Exercise the ankle (Fig. 12.126).
a Support the foot and ankle. Place one hand under the foot. Place your other hand under the ankle.
b Dorsiflexion – pull the foot forwards. Push down on the heel at the same time.
c Plantar flexion – turn the foot down. Or point the toes.
d Repeat dorsiflexion and plantar flexion five times – or the number of times stated on the care plan.

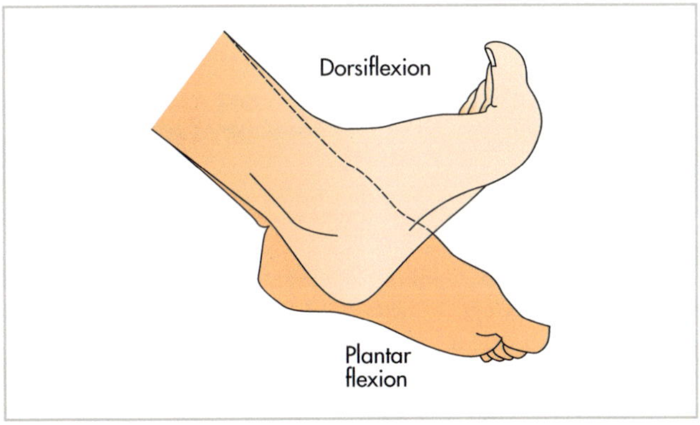

Fig. 12.126
ROM exercises for the ankle.

20 Exercise the foot (Fig. 12.127).
a Continue to support the foot and ankle.
b Pronation – turn the outside of the foot up and the inside down.
c Supination – turn the inside of the foot up and the outside down.
d Repeat pronation and supination five times – or the number of times stated on the care plan.

21 Exercise the toes (Fig. 12.128).
a Flexion – curl the toes.
b Extension – straighten the toes.

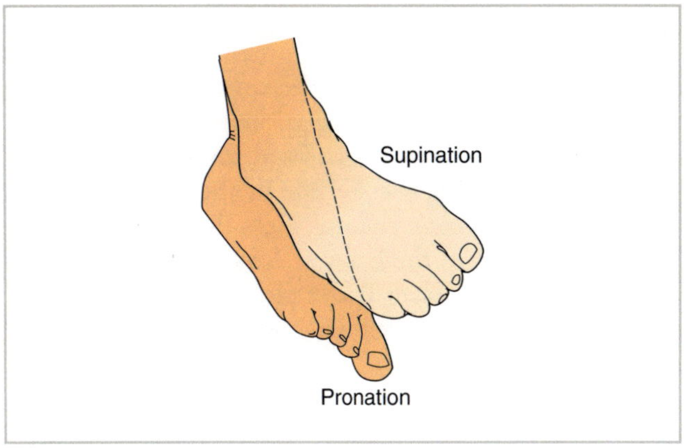

Fig. 12.127
ROM exercises for the foot.

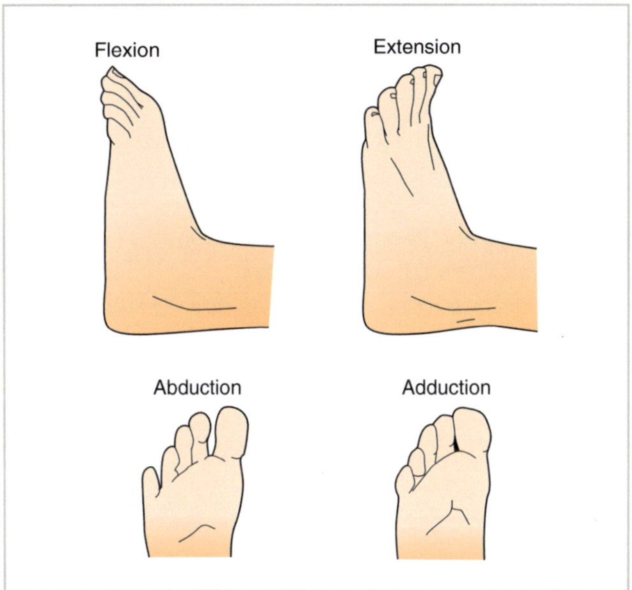

Fig. 12.128
ROM exercises for the toes.

c Abduction – spread the toes apart.
d Adduction – pull the toes together.
e Repeat flexion, extension, abduction and adduction five times – or the number of times stated on the care plan.

22 Cover the leg. Raise the bed rail, if used.
23 Go to the other side. Lower the bed rail near you if up.
24 Repeat steps 11 to 22.

Post-procedure

25 Provide for comfort.
26 Cover the person. Remove the bath blanket.
27 Raise or lower bed rails. Follow the care plan.
28 Lower the bed to its lowest level.
29 Place the call bell within reach.
30 Remove the screens from around the person.
31 Return the bath blanket to its proper place.
32 Wash and dry your hands.
33 Report and record your observations.

AMBULATION

Walking regularly helps prevent muscular atrophy. Many people need help walking. Some become strong enough to walk alone. Others will always need help.

After bed rest, activity is increased slowly and in steps. The first step is sitting on the side of the bed (dangling). Sitting in a bedside chair follows. Next the person walks in the room and then in the hallway. **Ambulation**, the act of walking, is not a problem if complications are prevented. Proper positioning and exercise prevent contractures and muscle atrophy.

Some people are weak and unsteady from inactivity, illness or injury. Some people who use wheelchairs can walk with help. Help them walk according to the care plan.

Use a walking belt if the person is weak or unsteady (Fig. 12.129). The person also uses handrails along the wall. Always check the person for orthostatic hypotension.

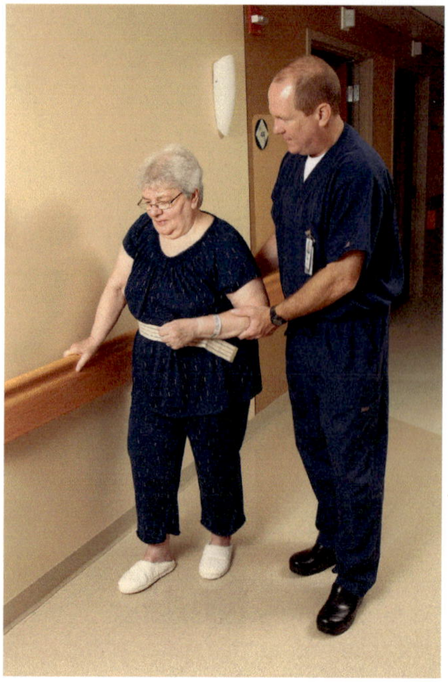

Fig. 12.129
Assist with ambulation by walking at the person's side. Use a walking belt for the person's safety.

DELEGATION GUIDELINES

Ambulation

Before helping with ambulation, you need the following information from the nurse and the care plan:

- how much help the person needs
- whether the person uses a cane, walker or crutches
- areas of weakness – right arm or leg, left arm or leg
- how far to walk the person
- what observations to report and record:
  - how well the person tolerated the activity
  - complaints of pain or discomfort
  - the distance walked.

BOX 12.36
Clients with dementia

A confused person may not understand why they cannot move or get up after a fall. Forcing a person not to move may injure the person and you. You may need to let the person move about. This is for their safety and your own. Stay calm and protect the person from injury. Talk to the person in a quiet and soothing voice until someone can assist you. Never use force or hold a person down.

THE FALLING PERSON

A person may start to fall when standing or walking. The person may be weak, light-headed or dizzy. Fainting may occur. Falling may be due to slipping or sliding on spills, waxed floors, throw rugs or improper shoes.

Do not try to prevent the fall. You could injure yourself and the person while twisting and straining to stop the fall. Balance is lost as a person falls. If you try to prevent the fall, you could lose your balance. Both you and the person could fall, or you could cause the other person to fall. Head, hip and knee injuries could occur.

If a person starts to fall, ease them to the floor. This lets you control the direction of the fall. You can also protect the person's head. Do not let the person move or get up before the nurse checks for injuries. Clients with dementia may be confused as to why they cannot get up again (Box 12.36). Calmly explain that a nurse will check for serious injuries, such as broken bones. An incident report is completed after all falls. The nurse may ask you to help fill out the incident report.

HELPING THE PERSON TO WALK

Quality of life

Remember to respect the person's privacy while doing any procedure. Address the person by name and ensure they know your name.

Pre-procedure

1. Follow the delegation guidelines.
2. Explain the procedure to the person.
3. Wash your hands.
4. Collect the following:
   - robe and non-slip shoes
   - paper or sheet to protect bottom linen
   - walking belt.
5. Speak to the person by name.
6. Provide for privacy.

Procedure

7 Lower the bed to its lowest position. Lock the bed wheels. Lower the bed rail (if used).
8 Fan-fold top linen to the foot of the bed.
9 Place the paper or sheet under the person's feet. This protects the bottom sheet from the shoes. Put the shoes on the person.
10 Help the person to dangle.
11 Help the person put on the robe.
12 Apply the walking belt. (See 'Applying a walking belt', p. 57).
13 Help the person stand. Grasp the walking belt on each side, or place your arms under the person's arms around to the shoulder blades.
14 Stand at the person's side while they gain their balance. Hold the belt at the side and back. Or have one arm around the back to support them.
15 Encourage the person to stand erect with their head up and back straight.
16 Help the person walk. Walk to the side and slightly behind the person. Provide support with the walking belt, or have one arm around the back to support the person.
17 Encourage the person to walk normally. The heel strikes the floor first. Discourage shuffling, sliding or walking on tiptoes.
18 Walk the required distance if the person can tolerate the activity. Do not rush the person.
19 Help the person return to bed.
20 Lower the head of the bed. Help the person to the centre of the bed.

Post-procedure

21 Remove footwear. Remove the paper or sheet over the bottom sheet.
22 Provide for comfort. Cover the person.
23 Place the call bell within reach.
24 Return the robe and footwear to their proper place.
25 Remove the screens from around the person.
26 Wash and dry your hands.
27 Report and record your observations (Fig. 12.130)

HELPING THE FALLING PERSON

Procedure

1 Stand with your feet apart. Keep your back straight.
2 Bring the person close to your body as quickly as possible. Use the walking belt. Or wrap your arms around the person's waist. You can also hold the person under the arms (Fig. 12.131).
3 Move your leg so the person's buttocks rest on it. Move the leg near the person.
4 Lower the person to the floor. The person slides down your leg to the floor. Bend at your hips and knees as you lower the person.
5 Call a nurse to check the person. Stay with the person.
6 Help the nurse return the person to bed. Get other staff to help as needed.
7 Report the following to the nurse:
  - How the fall occurred
  - How far the person walked
  - How activity was tolerated before the fall
  - Complaints before the fall
  - How much help the person needed while walking.
8 Complete an incident report.

Date	Time	
7/8/22	1000	Ambulated 10 metres in the hallway with assist of one and use of a
		gait belt. Reminded x3 not to shuffle feet. Showed no signs of
		distress or discomfort. Denies feeling dizzy, lightheaded, or weak.
		No c/o pain. Assisted to recliner chair and elevated feet after
		ambulation. BP=132/84 (L) arm sitting. P=76 regular rate and rhythm.
		R=20 and unlaboured. Call bell and water placed within reach.
		Adam Aims, EN

Fig. 12.130
Charting sample

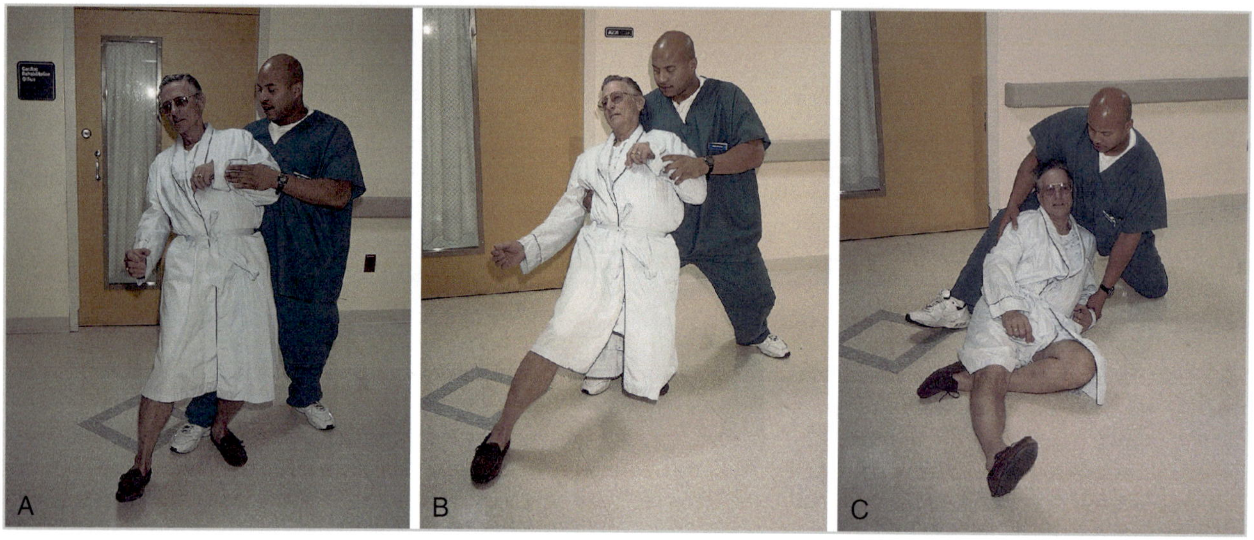

Fig. 12.131

A. The falling person is supported. **B.** The person's buttocks rest on the carer's leg. **C.** The person is eased to the floor on the carer's leg.

WALKING AIDS

Walking aids support the body. Older people often need walkers or canes for safety. The doctor, physiotherapist or nurse orders them. The need is temporary or permanent. The type ordered depends on the person's condition, amount of support needed and type of disability. The physiotherapist or nurse measures and teaches the person to use the device.

Crutches

Crutches are used when the person cannot use one leg, or when one or both legs need to gain strength. Some people with permanent leg weakness can use crutches. They usually use *Lofstrand* or *double-adjustable forearm crutches* (Fig. 12.132). *Axillary crutches* extend from the underarm (*axilla*) to the ground (Fig. 12.133).

- The person learns to crutch walk, climb up and down stairs and sit and stand. Safety is important. The person on crutches is at risk of falls. Follow these safety measures:
  - Check the crutch tips. They must not be worn down or wet. Replace worn crutch tips. Dry wet tips with a towel or paper towels.
  - Check crutches for flaws. Check wooden crutches for cracks and metal crutches for bends. All bolts must be tight.
  - Street shoes are worn. They must be flat and have non-skid soles.

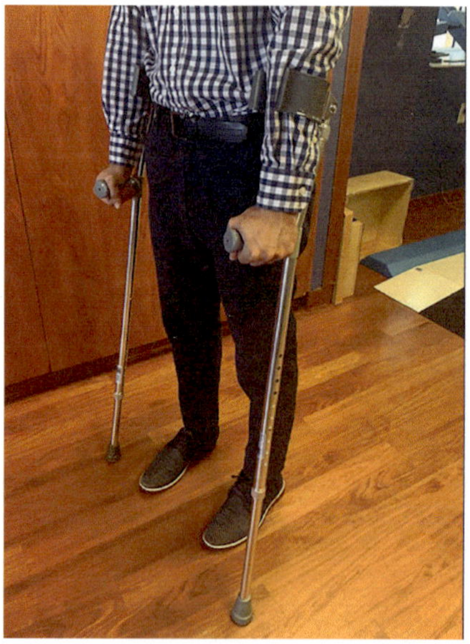

Fig. 12.132

Lofstrand or double-adjustable forearm crutches.

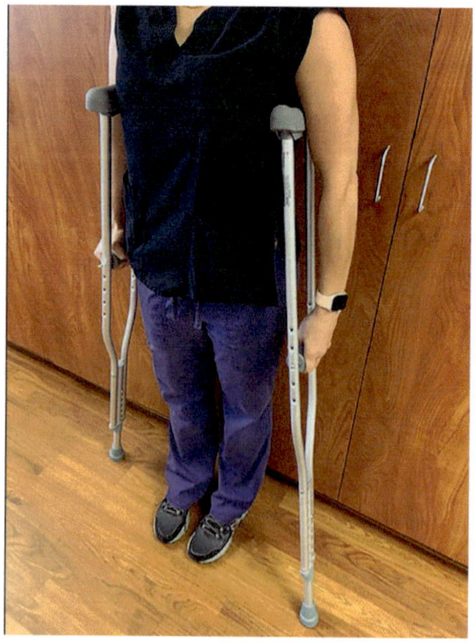

Fig. 12.133

Axillary crutches.

    - Clothes must fit well. Loose clothes may get caught between the crutches and underarms. Loose clothes can also hang forwards and block the person's view of the feet and crutch tips.
    - Practise safety measures to prevent falls.
    - Keep the crutches within the person's reach. Put them by the person's chair or against a wall.
- Know which crutch gait the person uses:
    - four-point gait (Fig. 12.134)
    - three-point gait (Fig. 12.135)
    - two-point gait (Fig. 12.136)
    - swing-to gait (Fig. 12.137)
    - swing-through gait (Fig. 12.138).

Canes

A cane is used for weakness on one side of the body. It helps provide balance and support. There are single-tip and four-point (quad) canes (Fig. 12.139). A cane is held on the strong side of the body. (If the left leg is weak, the cane is held in the right hand.) Four-point canes give more support than single-tip canes; however, they are harder to move.

The cane tip sits about 15–20 cm from the side of the foot. It is about 15–20 cm in front of the foot on the strong

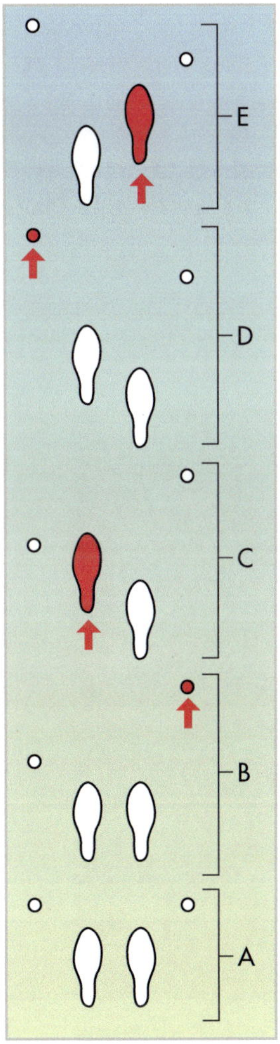

Fig. 12.134
The four-point gait.
The person uses both legs. The right crutch is moved forwards and then the left foot. Then the left crutch is moved forwards followed by the right foot.

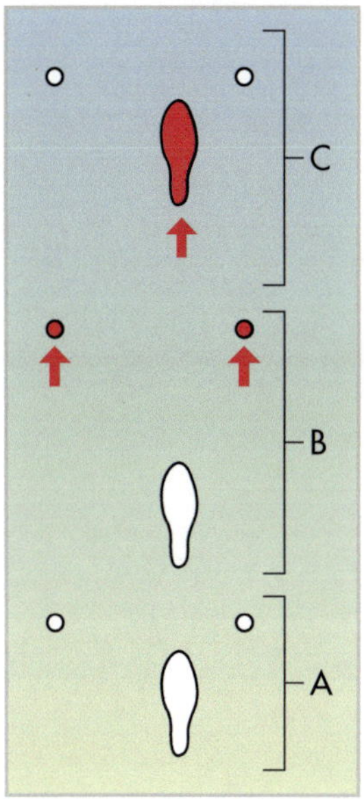

Fig. 12.135
The three-point gait.
One leg is used. Both crutches are moved forwards. Then the good foot is moved forwards.

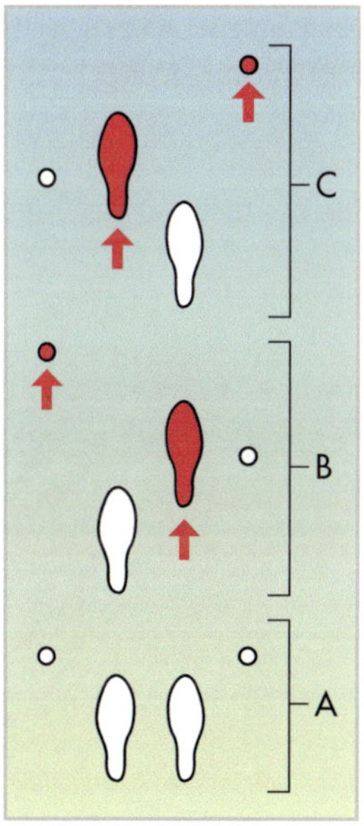

Fig. 12.136
The two-point gait.
The person bears some weight on each foot. The left crutch and right foot are moved forwards at the same time. Then the right crutch and left foot are moved forwards.

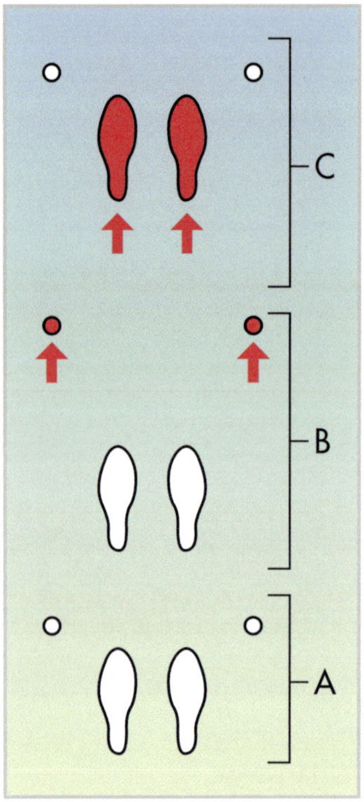

Fig. 12.137
Swing-to gait.
The person bears some weight on each leg. Both crutches are moved forwards. Then the person lifts both legs and swings to the crutches.

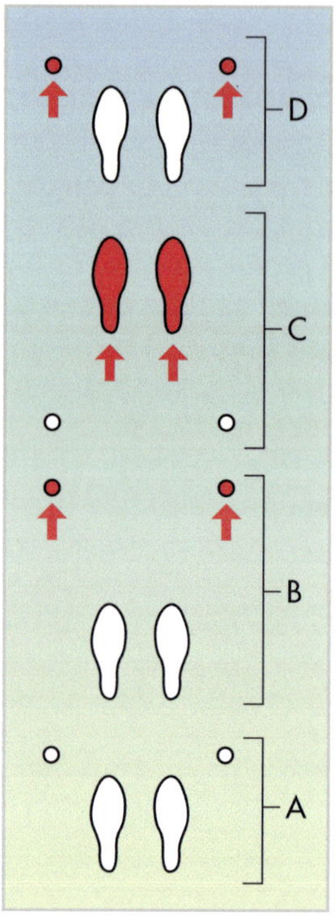

Fig. 12.138
Swing-through gait.
The person bears some weight on each leg. Both crutches are moved forwards. Then the person lifts both legs and swings through the crutches.

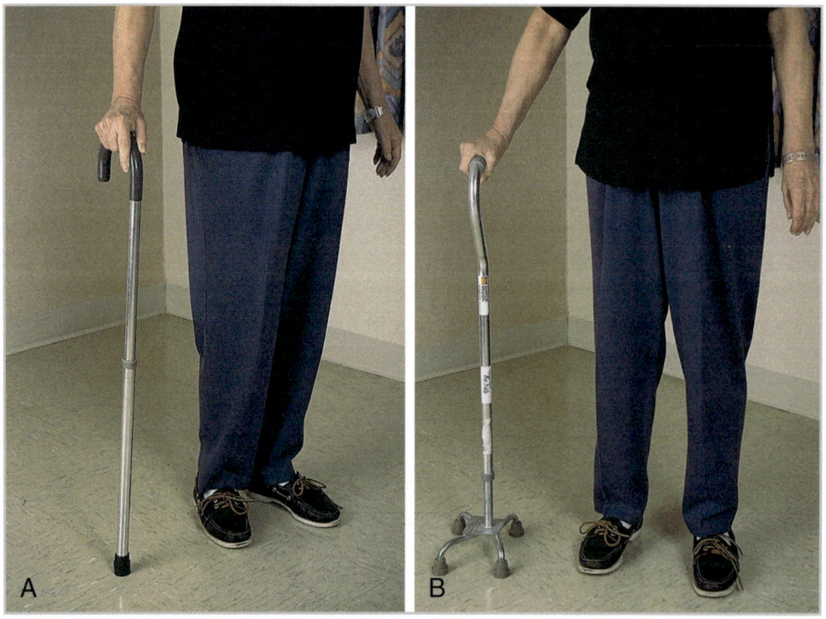

Fig. 12.139
A. Single-tip cane. **B.** Four-point cane.

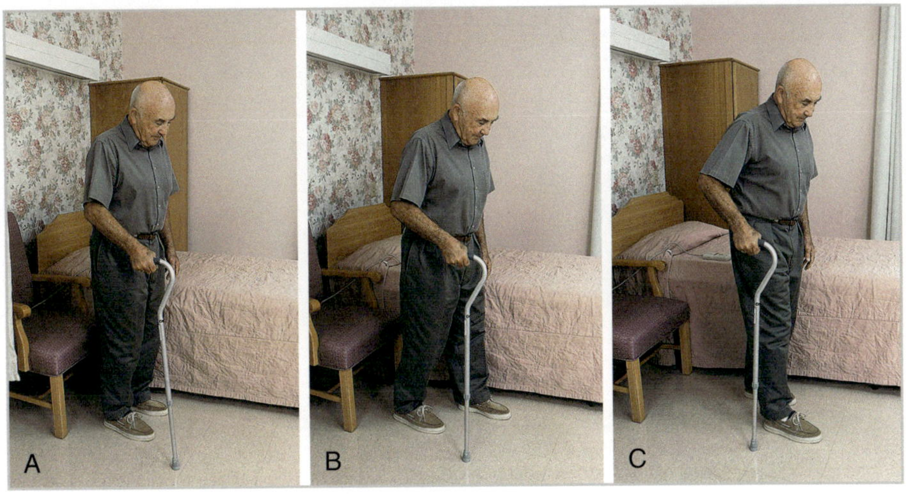

Fig. 12.140
Walking with a cane.
A. The cane is moved forwards about 15–20 cm. **B.** The leg opposite the cane (weak leg) is brought forwards, so it is even with the cane. **C.** The leg on the cane side (strong side) is moved ahead of the cane and the weak leg.

side. The grip is level with the hip. The person walks as follows:

1 The cane is moved forwards 15–20 cm (Fig. 12.140a).
2 The weak leg (opposite the cane) is moved forwards, so it is even with the cane (Fig. 12.140b).
3 The strong leg is brought forwards and ahead of the cane and the weak leg (Fig. 12.140c).

Walkers

A walker is a four-point walking aid (Fig. 12.141). It gives more support than a cane. Many people feel safer and more secure with walkers than with canes. There are many kinds of walkers. The *standard walker* is picked up and moved about 15–20 cm in front of the person. The person then moves the weak leg and foot and then the strong leg and foot up to the walker (Fig. 12.142).

Some people use a *wheeled walker* (Fig. 12.143). They have wheels on the front legs and rubber tips on the back legs. The person pushes the walker ahead about 15–20 cm and then walks up to it. Rubber tips on the back legs prevent the walker from moving while the person is walking or standing. Some have a braking action when weight is applied to the walker's back legs.

Baskets, pouches and trays attach to the walker. The attachment is used for needed items, which allows more independence. The attachment also frees the hands to grip the walker.

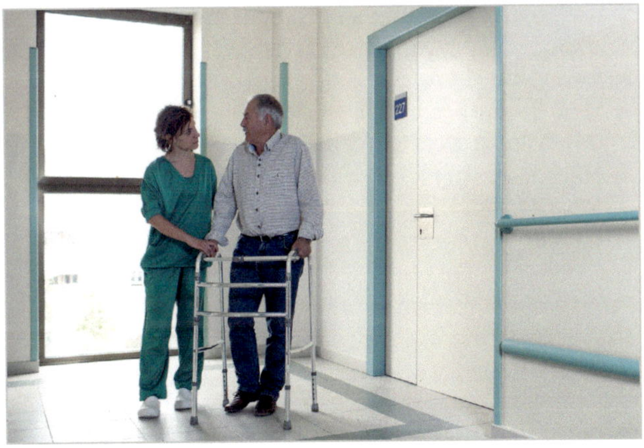

Fig. 12.141
A walker.

Braces

A brace supports a weak body part. It also prevents or corrects a deformity or prevents movement of a joint. Metal, plastic or leather is used for braces. A brace is applied over the ankle, knee or back. An ankle–foot orthosis (AFO) is placed in the shoe (Fig. 12.144). Then the foot is inserted. The device is secured in place with a Velcro strap. This type of brace is common after a stroke.

Skin and bony points under braces are kept clean and dry, to prevent skin breakdown. Report redness or signs of skin breakdown to the nurse at once. Also report complaints of pain or discomfort.

You must assess the skin under braces at every shift. The care plan tells you when to apply and remove braces.

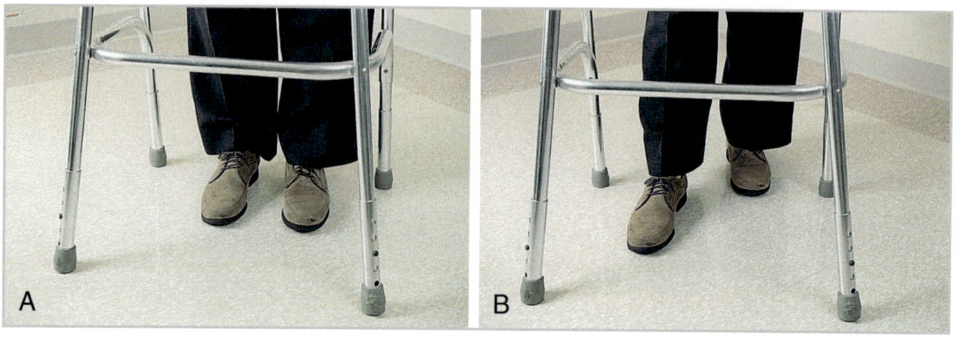

Fig. 12.142
Walking with a walker.
A. The walker is moved about 15 cm in front of the person. **B.** Both feet are moved up to the walker.

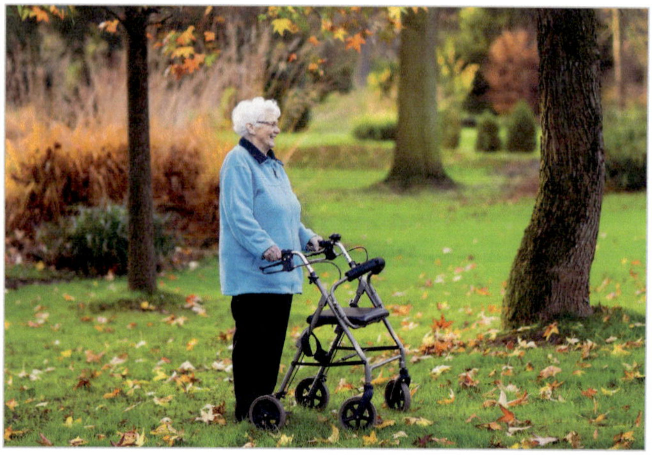

Fig. 12.143
A wheeled walker.

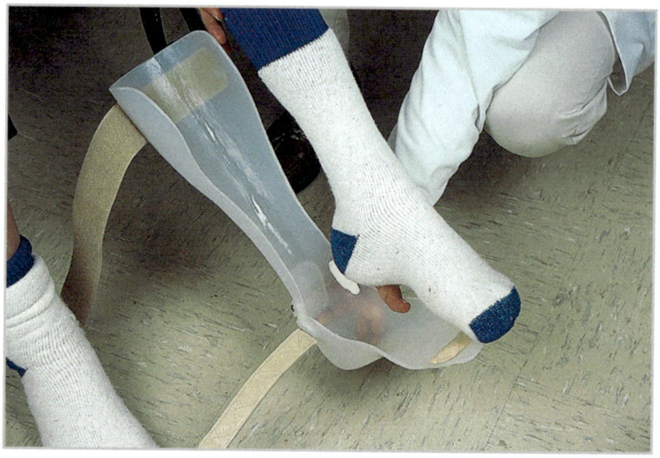

Fig. 12.144
Ankle-foot orthosis (AFO).

FOCUS ON COMMUNITY CARE

For various reasons, the older person or the person with a disability may be socially isolated within their home. There are, however, many opportunities for people within the community to participate in recreational and social activities. Often your client may be unaware of these opportunities. Always bring advice about these activities to your client's notice, and determine whether your client would like to be involved. If they are agreeable, seek advice from your supervisor on how you can assist your client to attend these activities. There are a number of groups who will transport older people and those with disabilities to such events. Some local councils give concessions to older people for travel in taxis. Discuss these options with your client, their family and your supervisor.

ACCREDITATION

You are working in residential or home care and accreditors are at your service. Can you answer the following questions?

- How do you ensure the dignity of those you care for, when doing activities of daily living?
- How do you personalise the care you provide to those you care for?
- How do you ensure the privacy of those you care for?

REVIEW QUESTIONS

Circle the BEST answer:

1 Which of the following is not a type of pain?
   a Acute
   b Chronic
   c Radiating
   d Pulsating

2 How often should an older person in an aged care facility be bathed?
   a Every day
   b Every second day
   c As per their personal preferences
   d Twice a day

3 Which of the following factors can affect the nutritional status of a person?
   a physical, social, emotional and metabolic
   b diet, taste, portion size, activity
   c physical, social, emotional, but NOT metabolic
   d diet, taste, activity, but NOT portion size

4 Which of the following is the recommended water temperature to use when bathing a person?
   a 36°–38°C
   b 43°–46°C
   c 38°–42°C
   d 34°–36°C

5 Perineal care involves cleaning:
   a around the ears
   b the mouth and nose
   c the genital and anal areas
   d the hands and feet

6 Which of the following is deemed a 'normal' bowel evacuation routine?
   a Once a day
   b Twice a day
   c Once every 2 or 3 days
   d All of the above

7 Which of the following groups are permitted to catheterise a person?
   a Personal carers and enrolled/registered nurses
   b Any person who has had specific training in the workplace
   c Qualified nurses and doctors only
   d The senior person on duty at the time

Circle T if the statement is true, or F is the statement is false:

8 T / F You should never place the feet of a person on a bowl of water as it is far too difficult to dry between the toes.

9 T / F If a person is unable to be showered or bathed, their hair should be cut short to minimise dirty hair and scalp infections.

10 T / F Always pull back the foreskin of a non-circumcised male to clean underneath.

Answers to these questions are on p. 454.

References

Food Standards Australia and New Zealand (2021). Food Safety Programs: Standard 3.2.1. Online 7 March 2021. Available: www.foodstandards.gov.au

Lewis SM, Heitkemper MM & Dirkson SR (2014). Medical–surgical nursing: assessment and management of clinical problems. 10th edn. Mosby, St Louis.

McGiger JN & Davidhizar RE (2016). Transcultural nursing: assessment and intervention. 7th edn. Mosby, St Louis.

SA Dental Association (2009). Better oral health in consumer care. Final report. Australian Government. Online 7 March 2021. Available: www.sahealth.sa.gov.au

Silver Chain & Curtin University of Technology (2010). Skin Tear Audit Research (STAR) Classification system. Online 7 March 2021. Available: https://baynav.bopdhb.govt.nz/media/1480/skin-tear-classification-tool.pdf

CHAPTER 13
Promoting and maintaining health and wellness

By Margaret Webb and Karen Scott

AFTER READING THIS CHAPTER, YOU SHOULD BE ABLE TO:

- define the key terms listed in this chapter
- identify improved nutritional choices
- identify the importance of recreational activities
- maintain fitness levels
- understand the value of body work
- identify a number of complementary therapies and their role in enhancing wellbeing.
- understand the importance of providing comfort in enhancing wellbeing
- understand the importance of promoting quality sleep.

Key terms

body work: Any therapeutic technique that involves working with the human body in a form involving manipulative therapy, such as massage

circadian rhythm: Daily rhythm based on a 24-hour cycle; the day–night cycle or body rhythm

comfort: A state of wellbeing; the person has no physical or emotional pain and is calm and at peace

complementary therapies: Practices and products that are not generally considered to be part of conventional medicine

enuresis: Urinary incontinence in bed at night

homeopathy: Based on the principle of 'like cures like', remedies are chosen that would cause symptoms in large doses, but in small doses trigger the body to use its own process of healing

insomnia: A chronic condition in which the person cannot sleep or stay asleep for the entire night

naturopathy: A system of healing that aims to provide holistic or whole body healthcare by drawing on treatment methods from several traditional systems of medicine

non-REM (NREM) sleep: The phase of sleep when there is no rapid eye movement (REM) sleep

phytotherapy: Herbal medicine

proprioceptive devices: Pieces of equipment designed to balance the abdominal and back muscles

relaxation: Being free from mental or physical stress

REM sleep: The phase of sleep when there is rapid eye movement (REM)

rest: A state of calmness, ease and relaxation, free from anxiety and stress

sleep: A state of unconsciousness, reduced voluntary muscle activity and lowered metabolism

Promoting and maintaining wellness for the older person does not need to be dependent on medical or pharmacological measures only. When caring for the older person there are a considerable number of non-clinical measures that can be undertaken or promoted to ensure that the older person maintains optimum health and wellbeing. This chapter discusses some of these measures.

NUTRITION

Although basic nutrition has been discussed elsewhere in this text, this chapter will provide more detail on understanding and improving nutritional status. Improving basic nutrition for the older person will considerably improve not only their physical, but also their psychological wellbeing.

> Let food be thy medicine and medicine be thy food.
> – Hippocrates, father of medicine, 431 BC

The above, famous statement by Hippocrates is still relevant today. A diet with a variety of fruits, vegetables and unprocessed whole foods, has properties that benefit and promote health, wellbeing and longevity. It is well known that a less than optimum diet compromises general health and immunity. Therefore, maintaining a healthy and nutritious diet is vital, especially for the older person. A Mediterranean diet has been found to be beneficial for general health and there is some evidence that it gives protection against dementia.

Diet

The simplest complementary additions to health and wellbeing for the ageing population are eating well, regular exercise, enjoying sunshine, drinking fresh water and keeping active. As people age, the appetite can decrease. With a decrease in nutritional intake, the flow-on effect will be a reduction in available nutrients for the body, so it is important to maintain a healthy balanced diet with adequate nutrient intake (Box 13.1).

Unfortunately, major changes, such as the loss of a partner or changes in health, may influence food choices for the older person. Often this is accompanied by a lack of desire to cook.

Understanding how a person's body changes later in life makes it easier to manage health and support the person nutritionally.

Salivary gland atrophy

Often the salivary glands begin to shrink as a person gets older and a reduction in saliva will lead to a dry mouth, making certain foods more difficult to eat and less enjoyable. One of the simplest remedies is to drink more water. It is common for younger people to carry a sports bottle, but this is less common in the ageing population unless they are physically active.

BOX 13.1
Dietary guidelines for Australians

- Aim for fitness
- Aim for a healthy weight
- Be physically active each day
- Build a healthy base
- Let *The Guide to Healthy Eating* guide your food choices
- Choose a variety of fruits and vegetables daily. Keep food safe to eat.
- Choose sensibly
- Choose a diet low in saturated fat and cholesterol, and moderate in total fat.
- Choose beverages and foods that moderate your intake of sugars.
- Choose and prepare foods with less salt.
- If you drink alcoholic beverages, do so in moderation.

Many seniors have been led to believe that drinking tea and coffee provides adequate sources of water. This is not entirely correct. Although they will lead to an overall gain in hydration, tea and coffee contain caffeine, a powerful diuretic that can cause a loss of minerals. Although tap water is readily available, better options are often filtered water, spring water, alkaline or energised water. The body needs both minerals and water to stay hydrated, so adding a pinch of sea salt to water will replace some lost minerals and replenish fluid in the body. However, adding salt to an older person's intake can lead to health issues if they have kidney or heart disease. Always seek advice before doing this.

Signs of dehydration include:

- allergies
- cramps in arms and legs
- constipation or hard stools
- dark coloured, pungent urine
- dry mouth or lips
- dry skin
- fatigue
- headaches
- loss of elasticity of skin
- low energy and weakness
- restlessness.

Foods that are high in water include raw vegetables and fruits, such as:

- broccoli
- cabbage
- carrots
- cantaloupe (rock melon)
- peaches
- strawberries
- watermelon
- cucumber
- celery

- green leafy vegetables
- lettuce.

Essential fats are also beneficial for salivary atrophy. Including food sources of omega-3 in the diet will help to support essential fat intake.

These are available in:

- fish, including blue mackerel, salmon, sardines, tuna
- chia seeds, linseeds and walnuts
- healthy cooking oils, including grape seed and coconut oils
- olive oil for low-heat cooking and as salad dressing.

Loss of taste

With the change in taste sensation, many people resort to using table salt to add flavour to meals. High dietary salt intake is recognised as one of the leading risks to cardiovascular health in the world as it increases blood pressure in adults and children (Cogswell et al 2016).

Try to reduce salt intake where possible. The addition of fresh and dried herbs and spices is another healthy way to add flavour to meals.

Ill-fitting dentures

Acrylic dentures move around and can cause painful ulcers to form. Pain causes changes to the bite, which will affect food choices, particularly leading to the choice of less nutritious, softer foods.

Dentures need to be checked annually to prevent permanent damage and collapsed facial muscles from occurring.

Loose dentures can lead to:

- cracked and sore corners of the mouth
- a change in bite or clicking jaw
- dull headache or pain around the ear
- impaired hearing.

Decreased secretion of stomach acid

Stomach acid begins to diminish from age 35. Stress, eating on the run and taking antacid medications will lead to poor stomach acid. This will affect absorption of calcium, iron and vitamin B_{12}, which will impact on bones and teeth, blood and oxygenation, as well as nervous system function. A simple remedy to enhance hydrochloric acid is to drink apple cider, vinegar or lemon juice in water. However, if the older person has a history of gastrointestinal ulceration, these options may cause discomfort due to their acidic nature.

Foods to include

Pawpaw and pineapple contain enzymes that enhance digestion. Add pawpaw to breakfast grains and, if tolerated, pineapple can be enjoyed as a juice, on its own or in fruit salad.

Fibre

The fibre present in fresh fruit, vegetables, legumes, nuts, seeds and whole grains is fundamental to health of the ageing population. For many, these foods have been the normal choice throughout life, as it is only in the last few decades that Australians have taken to eating fast food. This is more the case for the younger generations.

The Australian Guide to Healthy Eating

A snapshot for healthy eating can be found within *The Australian Guide to Healthy Eating* (Fig. 13.1). It promotes wise food choices and divides foods into six food groups:

1. Bread, cereal, rice and pasta
2. Vegetables, legumes
3. Fruits
4. Milk, yoghurt and cheese
5. Meat, poultry, fish, dry beans, eggs and nuts
6. Fats, oils and sweets.

Serving recommendations

Bread, cereal, rice and pasta group

This group allows the most servings: 4–9 servings a day (Box 13.2).

The high-fibre content in fresh food aids detoxification, which is beneficial for promoting healthy and regular bowel function. The natural fibre content has many health benefits, including lowering blood cholesterol. The group that is particularly beneficial are the whole grains. This includes wheat, rice, corn, barley, buckwheat, millet, oats and

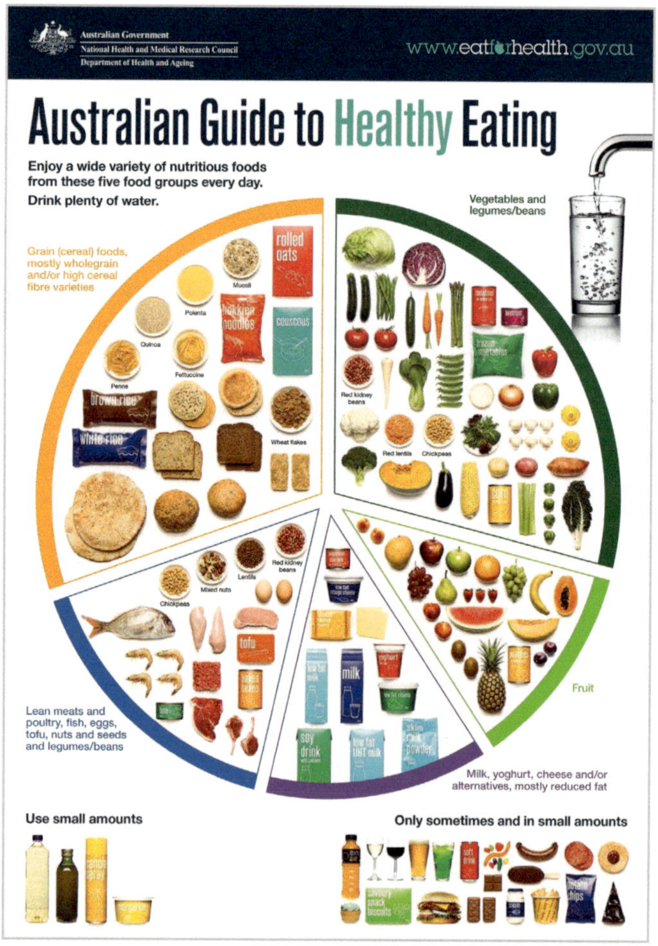

Fig. 13.1

The Australian Guide to Healthy Eating.

BOX 13.2
Serving sizes

Bread, cereal, rice and pasta group (4–9 servings daily)
1 slice of bread = 1 serving
1 cup of ready-to-eat cereal = 1 serving
½ cup of cooked cereal, rice or pasta = 1 serving

Vegetable and legumes group (4–5 servings daily)
1 cup raw leafy vegetables = 1 serving
½ cup other cooked or chopped raw vegetables = 1 serving
¼ cup vegetable juice = 1 serving

Fruit group (2–3 servings daily)
1 medium apple, orange, banana or pear = 1 serving
½ cup chopped, cooked or canned fruit = 1 serving
¾ cup fruit juice = 1 serving

Milk, yoghurt and cheese group (2–3 servings daily)
1 cup of milk or yoghurt = 1 serving

Meat, poultry, fish, dry beans, eggs and nuts group (1–2 servings daily)
½ cup cooked dry beans = 1 serving
1 egg = 1 serving
2 tablespoons peanut butter = 1 serving
⅓ cup of nuts = 1 serving

Fats, oils and sweets group
Use sparingly

quinoa, all rich in cholesterol-lowering soluble fibre. Soluble fibre lowers low density lipoproteins, or LDLs, known as 'bad cholesterol'. There is approximately 3 g of soluble fibre in ¼ cup of raw oats (cooked in water). Research shows that a high-fibre diet containing foods such as oats can reduce cholesterol and is a good source of nutrition (McRae 2017).

Vegetable and legume group

Vegetables are rich in vitamins A and C, minerals and phytochemicals (plant chemicals), including beta-carotene, vitamins C and E, magnesium, zinc, phosphorus and folic acid. The health-promoting nutrients in vegetables feed and nourish the body, promote healthy immune function and contribute to the prevention of heart disease, stroke and hypertension. The inclusion of raw or lightly steamed vegetables, such as salads and stir fries, at lunch and/or dinner will be a nourishing addition of healthy carbohydrates to the diet. Many varieties of vegetables can be eaten, including dark green and yellow vegetables, tomatoes, potatoes and vegetable juices. Legumes include dried peas, beans, lentils and chickpeas. These not only provide nutrients, but also water and fibre to help maintain bowel health. A person needs four to five vegetable servings a day.

Fruit group

Fruits contain some sugar and are low in fat. A person needs two to three servings of fruit daily.

Fruits provide carbohydrates, vitamins A and C, potassium and other minerals. Fresh fruits and juices are best. Frozen or canned fruits should be unsweetened. Sweetened or syrupy juices are high in sugar and kilojoules.

Milk, yoghurt and cheese group

This group is high in protein, carbohydrates, fat, calcium and riboflavin. A person needs two to three servings daily. Children and breastfeeding mothers need three servings a day.

Skim milk has less fat than whole milk. Cheeses made with skim milk, low-fat or non-fat yoghurt and frozen milk (rather than ice cream) are low in fat.

Meat, poultry, fish, dry beans, eggs and nuts group

This food group is high in protein, fat, iron and thiamine. It has more fat than the milk, fruit, vegetable and bread groups. A person needs one to two servings a day (Fig. 13.2). Serving size is important. Culture, appetite, personal choice and the recipe affect serving size.

Wise food choices lower fat intake and kilojoules. Fish and shellfish are low in fat. Chicken and turkey have less fat than veal, beef, pork and lamb. Skinless chicken and turkey are even lower in fat. Veal is lower in fat than beef. Use lean cuts of beef and pork. Egg yolks have more fat than egg whites. Cold water fish is rich in omega-3 fatty acids. Omega-3 and polyunsaturated fatty acids (PUFAs) are known to enhance brain function and aid concentration, which is ideal for enhancing memory in the ageing brain (Luchtman & Song 2013). The oils in fish are also beneficial for cardiovascular and skin health. Taken as a supplement, omega-3 can work as a potent anti-inflammatory, and can improve symptoms of arthritis and other degenerative conditions, helping to alleviate joint stiffness of osteoarthritis.

Raw, unsalted nuts and seeds, cooked legumes and beans are high in nutrients, fibre and plant-based amino acids

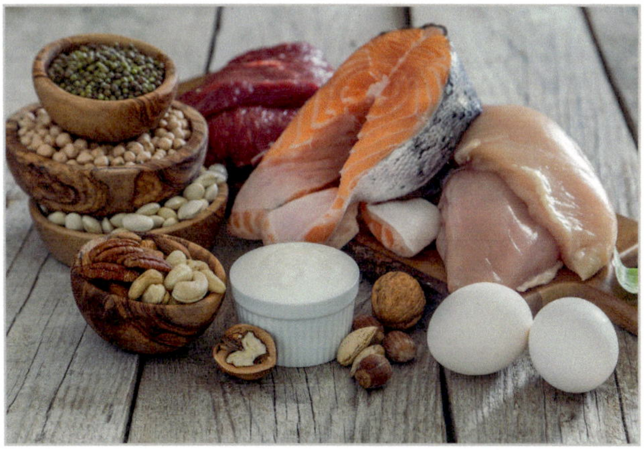

Fig. 13.2
One to two servings a day are needed from this food group.

(protein), provide good oils and are filling! The healthy fats in nuts and seeds slow down digestion, making the eater feel full and satisfied for longer. As nuts and seeds are a low sugar snack, a small handful will help to balance blood sugar levels, which may be beneficial for those with conditions such as diabetes.

Fats, oils and sweets group

Fats, oils and sweets (foods with added sugar) are high in kilojoules and have few nutrients. Use them sparingly and as little as possible. This group includes cooking oils, shortening, butter, margarine, salad dressing, soft drinks, sour cream, cream cheese and frosting. All lollies, most desserts (biscuits, cakes, pies and ice cream), jelly and jam, syrup and alcohol are included.

Buying low-fat or non-fat foods is preferable to buying full fat content foods. Food labels show fat content.

NUTRIENTS

No one food or food group has every essential nutrient. A well-balanced diet has servings from the five food groups in the 'pie' of *The Guide to Healthy Eating*. It ensures an adequate intake of the essential nutrients.

- *Protein* – this is the most important nutrient. It is needed for tissue growth and repair. Sources include meat, fish, poultry, eggs, milk and milk products, cereals, beans, peas and nuts.
- *Carbohydrates* – provide energy and fibre for bowel elimination. They are found in fruits, vegetables, breads, cereals and sugar. Carbohydrates break down into sugars during digestion. The sugars are absorbed into the bloodstream. The fibre is not digested. It provides the bulky part of chyme for elimination.
- *Fats* – provide energy. They also add flavour to food and help the body use certain vitamins. Sources include meats, lard, butter, shortening, salad and vegetable oils, milk, cheese, egg yolks and nuts. Dietary fat not needed by the body is stored as body fat (adipose tissue).
- *Vitamins* – are needed for certain body functions. They do not provide kilojoules. The body stores vitamins A, D, E and K. Vitamin C and the B complex vitamins are not stored. They must be ingested daily. A lack of a certain vitamin results in signs and symptoms of an illness. See Table 13.1 for the sources and major functions of common vitamins.
- *Minerals* – are used for many body processes, such as bone and tooth formation, nerve and muscle function and fluid balance. Table 13.2 lists the major functions and sources of common minerals.

Table 13.1
Functions and sources of common vitamins

Vitamin	Major functions	Sources
Vitamin A	Growth, vision, healthy hair, skin and mucous membranes, resistance to infection	Liver, spinach, green leafy and yellow vegetables, yellow fruits, fish liver oils, egg yolk, butter, cream and whole milk
Vitamin B_1 (thiamine)	Muscle tone, nerve function, digestion, appetite, normal elimination, carbohydrate use	Pork, fish, poultry, eggs, liver, breads, pastas, cereals, oatmeal, potatoes, peas, beans, soybeans, peanuts
Vitamin B_2 (riboflavin)	Growth, healthy eyes, protein and carbohydrate metabolism, healthy skin and mucous membranes	Milk and milk products, liver, green leafy vegetables, eggs, breads and cereals
Vitamin B_3 (niacin)	Protein, fat and carbohydrate metabolism, nervous system function, appetite, digestive system function	Meat, pork, liver, fish, peanuts, breads and cereals, green vegetables, dairy products
Vitamin B_{12}	Formation of red blood cells, protein metabolism, nervous system functioning	Liver, meats, poultry, fish, eggs, milk, cheese
Folic acid	Formation of red blood cells, functioning of the intestines, protein metabolism	Liver, meats, fish, poultry, green leafy vegetables, whole grains
Vitamin C (ascorbic acid)	Formation of substances that hold tissues together; healthy blood vessels, skin, gums, bones and teeth; wound healing; prevention of bleeding; resistance to infection	Citrus fruits, tomatoes, potatoes, cabbage
Vitamin D	Absorption and metabolism of calcium and phosphorus; healthy bones	Fish liver oils, milk, butter, liver, exposure to sunlight
Vitamin E	Normal reproduction, formation of red blood cells, muscle function	Vegetable oils, milk, eggs, meats, cereals, green leafy vegetables
Vitamin K	Blood clotting	Liver, green leafy vegetables, egg yolk, cheese

Table 13.2
Functions and sources of common minerals

Mineral	Major functions	Sources
Calcium	Formation of teeth and bones, blood clotting, muscle contraction, heart function, nerve function	Milk and milk products, green leafy vegetables, whole grains, egg yolks, dried peas and beans, nuts
Phosphorus	Formation of bones and teeth; use of proteins, fats and carbohydrates; nerve and muscle function	Meat, fish, poultry, milk and milk products, nuts, egg yolks, dried beans and peas
Iron	Allows red blood cells to carry oxygen	Liver, meat, eggs, green leafy vegetables, breads and cereals, dried peas and beans, nuts
Iodine	Thyroid gland function, growth and metabolism	Iodised salt, seafood and shellfish
Sodium	Fluid balance, nerve and muscle function	Almost all foods
Potassium	Nerve function, muscle contraction, heart function	Fruits, vegetables, cereals, meats, dried peas and beans

RECREATIONAL ACTIVITIES

Recreational activities are important for an older person's physical and psychological wellbeing. Joints and muscles are exercised and circulation is stimulated. Recreational activities are also social events and are mentally stimulating. A good activity program improves a person's quality of life.

These activities must meet each person's interests and physical, mental and psychosocial needs. Bingo, movies, dances, exercise groups, shopping trips, museum trips, concerts and guest speakers are common. Some centres have gardening activities.

The right to personal choice is protected. Wellbeing is promoted when the person attends activities of personal choice. The person is not forced to do things that are not of interest to them.

Clients may need help getting to an activity. Some need help taking part in them. You must assist as needed.

Activity ideas are always welcome. Clients may share ideas or provide information about their favourite pastimes. Share these with the aged care team.

Fitness

Quite often as people age, they stop moving. Retirement age is from 60–70 years of age and unfortunately many people do not just retire from work; to a certain extent they may also retire from life. Sometimes the person who was quite vibrant and active often becomes an 'old person' rapidly, as their muscle mass declines from their new stay-at-home routine, for example, watching television. Having an age-specific exercise routine in place for older people is important. Often a simple increase in time spent walking will have significant effects. Within aged care facilities and in community aged care programs, physiotherapists and allied health professionals, such as exercise physiologists and diversional therapists, will often develop programs of gentle exercises that encourage movement.

Chronic diseases, including diabetes, cancer and heart disease, are steadily rising in the ageing population. Exercise is a crucial part of longevity promotion, disease prevention and wellness promotion. A fitness professional is the best person to provide guidance and design a personal program with suitable exercises. Continuing fitness from midlife may be associated with the reduction of morbidity in older age. Box 13.3 discusses some of the exercise options available.

BODY WORK

Massage

Regular **body work**, such as massage, will help improve blood flow to neck, shoulders and hips. Massage can be an extremely beneficial addition in promoting wellness for the older person.

The benefits include:

- better posture
- improved range of motion
- increased joint flexibility
- reduced muscular tension
- decreased incidence of headaches
- stress relief
- pain reduction
- alleviation of muscle aches
- relief of tension headaches
- mental and physical fatigue reduction
- enhanced sense of wellbeing
- improved blood circulation and lymphatic flow
- general pain relief.

There are many forms of therapeutic massage suitable to the ageing population. Refer to Box 13.4 for further details.

BOX 13.3
Fitness programs suitable for the older client

Proprioceptive devices

Proprioceptive devices include fit ball, Bosu ball and balance boards. Exercising with these devices leads to improvements in core strength and stability, balance, coordination and agility, by building up the core muscles including the abdominals, lower back and spine. Progressive exercises build strength and fitness of all muscles, including the pelvic floor, aiding those with incontinence.

Water aerobics

There are a number of benefits of water exercise, including an increased sense of wellbeing. There is no stress from pressure on the joints, making it ideal for those suffering chronic pain conditions. This type of workout improves cardiorespiratory health through weightless aerobic exercises in water.

Weight-bearing exercise

Functional body weight exercises are performed by using the individual's own body weight. Exercises may include squats; lunges; push-ups against the wall or floor, depending on fitness; pelvic floor raises; isometric exercises, such as the plank, to work core muscles; low mass work with dumbbells and medicine balls, as well as seated-rows with light weights.

Resistance bands

The use of resistance bands is a form of slow controlled exercise that forces the muscles to work against tension provided by an elastic band. Bands provide resistance without using weights and build or maintain lean muscle mass. Resistance exercise also increases muscle strength, prevents bone loss and can provide a good cardiovascular workout when done with high repetitions.

BOX 13.4
Massage therapy modalities

Aromatherapy

Aromatherapy massage is done with the addition of pure essential oils to the cold pressed massage oil. Individual oils are chosen to suit the person being treated, including blends for relaxation, muscle and joint pain, skin rashes, improving circulation and more. Oils are extracted from different parts of plants (leaves, flowers, bark, fruit, etc).

Some common oils and uses in massage include:

- *frankincense:* for calming the mind, to overcome stress, for ageing and dry skin
- *lavender:* for relaxation and high blood pressure
- *peppermint:* refreshing and cooling on the skin
- *sandalwood:* for relaxation, rehydration of dry skin
- *wintergreen:* pain relief – often included in creams for aches and pains
- *ylang ylang:* mood elevator, for anxiety and tension.

Hot stone

For stress relief and to soothe muscle tension, hot stone massage is performed with the use of smooth warmed stones placed on specific points of the body. The heat penetrates deep into the tissues, improving circulation, soothing the nervous system, relaxing muscles and calming body and mind.

Lymphatic drainage

This is a very gentle massage technique performed by light touch and gentle strokes to stimulate lymphatic flow. There are numerous health benefits from lymphatic massage, including:

- helping the body eliminate waste and toxins
- boosting the immune system; particularly good for those prone to regular colds and flu
- improving circulation; beneficial for puffiness or swelling – oedema

It is advisable to drink plenty of water after lymphatic drainage.

Reflexology

Reflexology is a therapeutic massage commonly performed on the feet or hands. It works on the principle that reflex areas on the hands and feet correspond to the whole body, including the organs, glands and systems. Gentle massage stimulation of these reflexes can have a number of benefits, including:

- relief from stress and tension
- improving circulation and lymphatic flow
- encouraging elimination of waste
- promotion of wellbeing.

Remedial

Remedial massage is especially beneficial for focusing on problem areas, to help correct imbalances and chronic aches and pains. The therapist will use a variety of massage techniques of varying pressure to holistically address issues, including:

- arthritic discomfort
- headaches
- neck, back and shoulder complaints
- frozen shoulder.

Swedish

The most soothing of all the massage techniques, Swedish massage is done with long flowing strokes, the pressure just enough to elicit a relaxation response. Deep circular movements help to increase blood flow and circulation and break down scar tissue. This is the original 'feel good' massage!

Complementary therapies

There are a number of other natural therapies, frequently referred to as **complementary therapies**, that will improve wellness in the older person. These natural therapies include:

- acupuncture
- naturopathy
- herbal medicine
- homeopathy
- music therapy
- pet therapy
- aromatherapy.

Acupuncture

Acupuncture can help to restore balance by rebuilding the body's Qi (Chi), or vital energy flow. An acupuncturist identifies imbalances and blockages in energy lines, known as meridians, and inserts ultra-fine sterile needles into specific acupuncture points. This is done to re-establish the free flow of energy, restore balance and trigger the body's natural responses to health and healing.

Many older people taking combinations of medication for various ailments, including pain and chronic disease, find relief from symptoms with periodic acupuncture treatments. An elderly person's quality of life can be improved in many ways, including:

- improvement in pain and bodily functions
- relief from headaches and migraines
- tenderness and discomfort post-surgery.

Naturopathy

Naturopathy is a holistic system of healing that recognises the body's innate ability to heal itself. Treatment includes individualised dietary changes, supplemental and herbal prescriptions to nourish the body and enable the body's processes of self-healing to restore balance and promote health. The naturopath initially takes an hour to gather the medical history and design an individualised treatment plan to treat acute and chronic conditions, followed by periodic consultations for reassessment and ongoing support.

Remedies and lifestyle recommendations are chosen not only to provide symptomatic relief, but also to help treat the cause of ill health. Naturopaths prescribe natural or traditional medicines to promote natural healing of the body for numerous conditions, including:

- allergies, including food allergies; intolerances and sensitivities
- arthritic conditions, including osteoarthritis, rheumatoid arthritis; conditions causing pain, swelling and joint stiffness
- asthma, bronchial and respiratory ailments
- chronic fatigue syndrome; depression
- digestive complaints such as irritable bowel syndrome and ulcers; constipation
- general immunity for cold and flu
- hypertension (high blood pressure) and hypotension (low blood pressure)
- menstrual and menopausal problems; fertility and infertility
- migraine and headache
- skin conditions, such as eczema, dermatitis and psoriasis.

Herbal medicine

Herbal medicine, also known as **phytotherapy**, is the use of plant remedies to prevent and treat ill health. A herbalist or naturopathic practitioner prescribes herbal tinctures, herbal supplements and preparations made from plants with medicinal properties. Some of the most commonly used herbal supplements include echinacea and St John's wort, ginkgo, garlic, saw palmetto, ginseng, goldenseal, valerian, chamomile, feverfew, ginger, evening primrose and milk thistle. However, it is important to be alert to the interactions of some of these supplements with prescribed medications.

Homeopathy

Based on the principle of like cures like, **homeopathy** means that remedies chosen would cause symptoms in large doses, but in small doses trigger the body to use its own process of healing. Homeopathic remedies come from many kinds of sources, including animal, vegetable, mineral and electromagnetic. It is used in many German hospitals to assist healing and in some UK hospitals.

Homeopathy can be considered for almost any type of ill health, including:

- allergies, hay fever, sinus, respiratory conditions
- headaches and migraines
- musculoskeletal conditions and pain, strains and bruising
- gastrointestinal upsets, diarrhoea and nausea
- conditions of chronic pain.

Some complementary therapies do not require the specialist skills of a qualified practitioner, but can be undertaken by the aged care team. They are often inexpensive and relatively easy to use. These include music therapy, pet therapy and aromatherapy.

Music therapy

The use of music therapy has been linked to a reduction in pain, especially for the older person suffering from arthritic pain. In addition to reducing pain, music also gives older adults a sense of control when they are permitted to choose the type of music to listen to and when they are able to play the music when they wish. It may also reduce behavioural symptoms for those suffering from Alzheimer's dementia.

Pet therapy

Touching, holding or being with animals can reduce feelings of loneliness, particularly in individuals who have a history of emotional intimacy with pets. In addition, animal-assisted therapy provides motivational, recreational and socialisation benefits and decreases behavioural symptoms in older adults with dementia.

Aromatherapy

Vaporising essential oils produces fragrances that can effectively minimise any clinical or bodily smells that may pervade the aged care environment. Other claimed uses include pain and anxiety reduction, enhancement of energy and short-term memory and to promote a feeling of relaxation.

Some of the more commonly used essential oils include:

- lavender – for calming and anxiety reduction, insomnia and for general aches and pains
- peppermint – for improving digestion
- tea tree – for improving respiratory disorders
- rosemary – for improving mental stimulation.

COMFORT

Comfort, rest and sleep are needed for wellbeing. The need for comfort is closely associated with the ability to achieve adequate rest and sleep. The total person – the physical, emotional, social, psychological and spiritual – is affected by comfort, rest and sleep problems.

Rest and sleep restore our energy and wellbeing. Illness and injury increase the need for rest and sleep, because the body needs more energy for healing and repair. When a person is ill or injured, more energy than normal is needed to perform daily functions. The carer's role is to implement measures that will ensure the client's needs for rest are met and that sources of discomfort, mental and physical, are prevented or at least minimised. These measures include the maintenance of a wrinkle-free and clean bed to rest and sleep in.

Comfort is a state of wellbeing. There is no physical or emotional pain and the person is calm and at peace. Age, illness and activity affect comfort. So do temperature, ventilation, noise, odours and lighting. These factors are controlled to meet the person's needs.

Comfort, rest and sleep are needed for physical, emotional and psychological wellbeing. Rooms are designed and equipped for comfort.

Accepted means of maintaining comfort include:

- no more than four people in a room
- a curtain around the bed for privacy
- a bed of the proper height and size for the person
- a clean, comfortable mattress
- linen that suits the weather and climate
- a clean and orderly room
- an odour-free room
- room temperature at an acceptable level
- an acceptable noise level
- adequate ventilation and room humidity
- appropriate lighting.

REST

Rest means being calm, at ease and relaxed. The person is free of anxiety or stress. Rest may involve inactivity or doing things that are calming and promote **relaxation**. Examples include reading, listening to music, watching television, needlework and prayer. Some people do activities such as gardening, baking, golfing, walking or woodworking to promote calmness and ease.

You can promote rest by meeting the person's physical needs. Thirst, hunger and elimination needs can affect rest. So can pain or discomfort. A comfortable position and good body alignment are important. A quiet setting promotes rest, as does a comfortable bed. Directions on how to prepare a bed for rest and sleep are included later in this chapter. Some people rest more easily in a clean, neat and uncluttered room.

The person must feel safe from falling or other injuries. If available, a call bell should be within reach. Understanding the reasons for care also helps the person feel safe. So does knowing how care is given. That is why you always explain procedures before doing them.

Many people have rituals or routines before they can rest. These may include:

- going to the bathroom, brushing teeth and washing the face and hands
- praying
- having a snack or beverage
- locking doors or making sure loved ones are safe at home
- getting a certain blanket.

Always follow the individual's routines and rituals whenever possible.

Love and belonging promote rest. Visits or calls from family and friends may relax the person. A pet can also be a comfort (Fig. 13.3). The person knows that others care and are concerned. Reading cards and letters can also help the person relax and rest (Fig. 13.4).

The feeling of being loved and belonging to the group has a positive effect on the wellbeing of the person and boosts their self-esteem. This can encourage the person to actively participate in hygiene and grooming and social activities. Good grooming and hygiene help people feel good about themselves.

Ill or injured people need to rest more often. Some rest during or after a procedure. For example, a bath or getting dressed tires Mr Garrison. Therefore, he needs to rest before undertaking any further activities. Some people need a

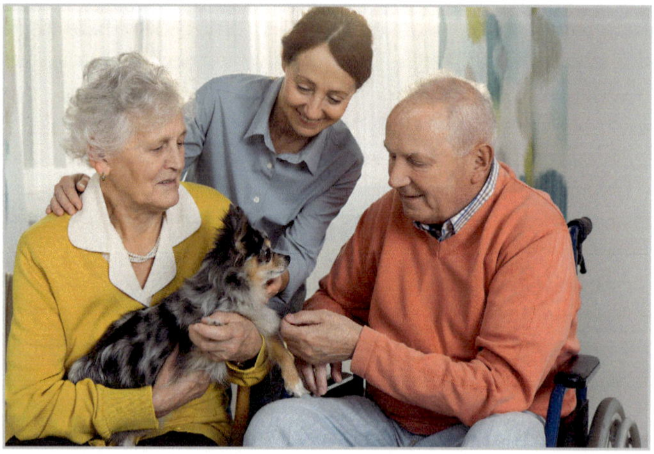

Fig. 13.3
A comforting pet can promote rest.

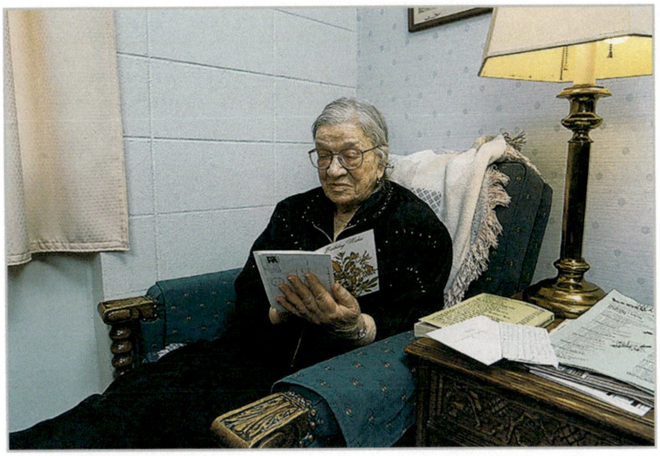

Fig. 13.4
Reading cards and letters from family and friends can help the client relax and rest.

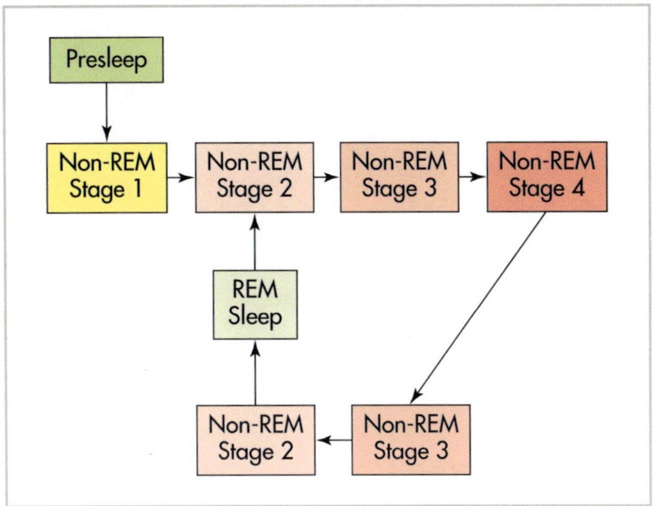

Fig. 13.5
Adult sleep cycle.

few hours for even basic hygiene and grooming. Others need to rest after meals. Do not push the person beyond his or her limits and allow rest periods when needed. Never rush the person.

SLEEP

Sleep is a state of unconsciousness, reduced voluntary muscle activity and lowered metabolism. An unconscious person is unaware of the environment. He or she cannot respond to people and things in the environment. During sleep, there are no voluntary arm or leg movements. Metabolism is the burning of food and energy for use by the body. Less energy is needed during sleep. Thus, metabolism is reduced during sleep. The sleep state is temporary. Sleep is a basic need and it lets the mind and body rest. The body saves energy and body functions slow. Vital signs are lower than when awake. Tissue healing and repair occur. Sleep lowers stress, tension and anxiety. It refreshes and renews the person. The person regains energy and mental alertness. The person thinks and functions better after sleep.

Circadian rhythm

Sleep is part of our **circadian rhythm** (*circa* means about, *dies* means day). Circadian rhythm is a daily rhythm based on a 24-hour cycle. It is called the day–night cycle or body rhythm and it affects functioning. Some people function better in the morning. They are more alert, active and think and react better. Others do better in the evening.

Circadian rhythm includes a sleep–wake cycle. The person's biological clock signals when to sleep and when to wake up. You sleep and wake up at certain times. That is part of your biological clock. Disease and illness often interfere with a person's circadian rhythm and the sleep–wake cycle. Sleep problems occur easily.

Many people work evening and night shifts. Their bodies must adjust to changes in the sleep–wake cycle.

Sleep cycle

There are two phases of sleep (Fig. 13.5):

- non-rapid eye movement phase – this is called **non-REM (NREM) sleep**. NREM sleep has four stages. Sleep goes from light to deep as the person moves through the four stages.
- Rapid eye movement (REM) phase – this is called **REM sleep**. In REM sleep, the person is hard to rouse (wake). Mental restoration occurs in this phase. It is also thought that the events and problems of the day before are reviewed and the person prepares for the next day.

Box 13.5 shows the stages of NREM and REM sleep. There are usually four to six cycles of NREM and REM sleep during 7–8 hours of sleep. Stage 1 of NREM sleep is usually not repeated.

Sleep requirements

Sleep needs vary for each age group. The amount needed decreases with age (see Table 13.3). Infants need more sleep than toddlers; toddlers need more sleep than preschool children; school-age children need more sleep than teenagers. Older people need less sleep than middle-aged adults.

Factors affecting sleep

Many factors affect the amount and quality of sleep. Quality relates to how well the person sleeps. It involves getting needed amounts of NREM and REM sleep.

- *Illness* – increases the need for sleep. However, the signs and symptoms of illness interfere with sleep. They include pain, nausea, vomiting, coughing, difficulty breathing, diarrhoea, frequent voiding and itching. Treatments and therapies can also interfere with sleep. Often people are woken up for treatments or medications. The emotional effects of illness affect sleep. These include fear, anxiety and worry.
- *Nutrition* – sleep needs increase with weight gain and decrease with weight loss. Some foods affect sleep. Those

BOX 13.5
The sleep cycle

Stage 1: NREM sleep
- Lightest sleep level
- Lasts a few minutes
- Gradual decrease in vital signs
- Gradual lowering of metabolism
- Person feels drowsy and relaxed
- Person easily roused
- Daydreaming feeling after being roused

Stage 2: NREM sleep
- Sound sleep
- Relaxation increases
- Still easy to rouse
- Lasts 10–20 minutes
- Body functions continue to slow

Stage 3: NREM sleep
- First stages of deep sleep
- Hard to rouse the person
- Person rarely moves
- Muscles relax completely
- Vital signs decrease
- Lasts 15–30 minutes

Stage 4: NREM sleep
- Deepest stage of sleep
- Hard to rouse the person
- Body rests and is restored
- Vital signs much lower than when awake
- Lasts about 15–30 minutes
- Sleepwalking and **enuresis** (urinary incontinence in bed at night) may occur

REM sleep
- Vivid, full-colour dreaming
- Usually starts 50–90 minutes after sleep has begun
- Rapid eye movements
- Blood pressure, pulse and respiration may fluctuate
- Voluntary muscles are relaxed
- Mental restoration occurs
- Hard to rouse the person
- Lasts about 20 minutes

Source: Modified from Crisp, Douglas, Robeiro et al (2017). Potter and Perry's fundamentals of nursing, 5th edn. Elsevier, Sydney.

Table 13.3
Average sleep requirements

Age group	Hours per day
Newborns (birth to 4 weeks)	14–18
Infants (4 weeks to 1 year)	12–15
Toddlers (1–2 years)	11–14
Preschoolers (3–5 years)	10–13
Middle and late childhood (5–12 years)	9–11
Adolescents (12–18 years)	8–10
Young adults (18–40 years)	7–9
Middle-aged adults (40–65 years)	7–9
Older adults (65 years and older)	7–8

Source: National Sleep Foundation (2015). Sleep duration recommendations

with caffeine (chocolate, coffee, tea and cola) prevent sleep. The protein l-tryptophan tends to help sleep and is found in milk, cheese and beef.

- *Exercise* – improves health and fitness. Exercise requires energy. People usually feel good after exercising. Eventually they tire. Being tired helps them sleep well. Exercise before bedtime interferes with sleep. It causes the release of substances into the bloodstream that stimulate the body. Therefore, exercise should be avoided in the 2 hours before bedtime.
- *Environment* – people adjust to their usual sleep settings. They get used to such things as the bed, pillows, noises, lighting and sleeping partner. Any change in the usual setting can affect the amount and quality of sleep.
- *Medications and other substances* – sleeping pills promote sleep. Medications for anxiety, depression and pain may cause the person to sleep. However, these medications and sleeping pills reduce the length of REM sleep. Mental restoration occurs during REM sleep. Behavioural problems and sleep deprivation can occur. Alcohol is a medication and causes drowsiness and sleep. However, it interferes with REM sleep. Those under the influence of alcohol may awaken during sleep. Difficulty returning to sleep is common. Some medications contain caffeine, which is a stimulant and prevents sleep. Caffeine is also found in coffee, tea, chocolate and cola. The side-effects of some medications can disrupt sleep. These include frequent voiding and nightmares.
- *Lifestyle changes* – these relate to a person's daily routines and way of living. Work, school, play and social events are all part of lifestyle. Travel, holidays and social events often affect sleep and wake times. Children usually stay up later during school holidays and may sleep later, too. If work hours change, sleep hours may change. Such changes affect sleep–wake cycles and the circadian rhythm. Moving into residential care or assisted care accommodation can result in altered sleep patterns.

- *Emotional problems* – fear, worry, depression and anxiety affect sleep. Causes include work, personal or family problems. Loss of a loved one or friend is another cause. Money problems are stressful. People may have problems falling asleep or may awaken often. Some have problems getting back to sleep.

Sleep disorders

Sleep disorders involve repeated sleep problems. The amount and quality of sleep are affected. Sleep disorders can affect a person's lifestyle. Box 13.6 lists the signs and symptoms that occur.

Insomnia is a chronic condition in which the person cannot fall asleep or stay asleep the entire night. There are three forms of insomnia:

- The person cannot fall asleep.
- The person cannot stay asleep.
- The person wakes early and cannot get back to sleep.

Emotional problems are a common cause of insomnia. The fear of dying during sleep is another cause. Some people are afraid of not waking up. This may occur with heart disease or when told of a terminal illness. The fear of not being able to sleep is another cause. The physical and emotional discomforts of illness can also cause insomnia.

The care plan will outline measures to promote sleep. Emotional or physical problems causing insomnia are also treated.

Sleep deprivation

With sleep deprivation, the amount and quality of sleep are decreased. Sleep is interrupted and NREM and REM sleep stages are not completed. Illness, pain and hospital care are common causes. The signs and symptoms of sleep disorders may occur.

Sleepwalking

A person who sleepwalks leaves the bed and walks about. They are not aware of sleepwalking. He or she does not remember the event on awakening. Children sleepwalk more than adults. The event may last 3–4 minutes or longer.

Stress, fatigue and some medications are common causes. If you are caring for someone who sleepwalks, you need to protect them from injury, as falling is a high risk. Guide sleepwalkers back to bed. As they startle easily, wake them up gently.

Promoting sleep

The carer assesses the person's sleep patterns. Report any of the signs and symptoms of sleep disorders listed in Box 13.6. Measures are planned to promote sleep (Box 13.7). Report

BOX 13.6
Signs and symptoms of sleep disorders

- Hand tremors
- Slowed responses to questions, conversations or situations
- Reduced word memory; problems finding the right word
- Decreased reasoning and judgement
- Irregular pulse
- Red, puffy eyes
- Dark circles under the eyes
- Moodiness; mood swings
- Disorientation
- Irritability
- Fatigue
- Sleepiness
- Agitation
- Restlessness
- Decreased attention
- Hallucinations
- Coordination problems
- Slurred speech

BOX 13.7
Measures to promote sleep

- Organise care for uninterrupted rest.
- Avoid physical activity before bedtime.
- Encourage the person to avoid business or family matters before bedtime.
- Allow a flexible bedtime. Bedtime is when the person is tired and fatigued – not a certain clock time.
- Provide a comfortable room temperature.
- Let the person take a warm bath or shower.
- Provide a bedtime snack (milk).
- Avoid caffeine (coffee, tea, cola and chocolate).
- Avoid alcoholic drinks.
- Have the person void before going to bed.
- Make sure incontinent people are clean and dry.
- Follow bedtime rituals.
- Make sure the person wears loose-fitting nightwear.
- Provide for warmth (blankets, socks) for those who tend to get cold.
- Reduce noise.
- Darken the room – close shades, blinds and the privacy curtain. Shut off or dim the lights. Dim lights in hallways.
- Make sure linen is clean, dry and wrinkle-free.
- Position the person in good alignment.
- Support body parts as ordered.
- Make sure the person is in a comfortable position.
- Give a back massage.
- Implement measures to relieve pain.
- Let the person read.
- Let the person listen to music.
- Let the person watch television.
- Assist with relaxation exercises as ordered.
- Sit and talk with the person.

to your supervisor your observations about how the person slept. This helps them evaluate whether the goal of a regular sleep pattern was met.

Many people have rituals and routines before bedtime. These are often important to the person. These include some of those rituals and routines as described for rest. Always remember, it is the person's choice when to nap or go to bed, and the measures that promote comfort, rest and sleep. Always follow the person's wishes.

Check linen for crumbs after meals and remove them. Change linen whenever it becomes wet, soiled or damp.

When you are handling linen and making beds, always use safe handling practices and hold linen away from your body and clothing. Never shake linen in the air, as shaking it spreads microbes. Clean linen is always placed on a clean surface, such as a chair or table, and never placed on the floor. Never put dirty linen on the floor.

Clients with dementia

Sleep problems are common in people with Alzheimer's disease and other dementias. Night wandering is common. Restlessness and confusion often increase at night. This increases the risk of falls. It often helps to quietly and calmly direct the person to his or her room. Allowing night-time wandering in a safe and supervised setting is the best approach for some people. Follow the care plan.

FOCUS ON COMMUNITY CARE

When caring for a client within their home, you may be responsible for assisting them to prepare for bed at night. Always ask your client what their bedtime routine is and follow this. Ensure that items such as uridomes are applied securely, because if they leak or come off during the night your client may have to stay in a wet bed until help arrives the next day. Not only can this result in skin breakdown and damage, but also considerable discomfort, both physical and emotional, for your client.

Once your client is in bed, there will be times when they are unable to move or get out of it until a carer arrives the following morning to assist them to get up. It is your responsibility to ensure that not only are they safely positioned and have all their needs attended to, but that you have also secured their home well before you leave. Always check lights, electrical appliances, windows and doors. Ensure that they have appropriate emergency call devices accessible.

QUALITY OF LIFE

Comfort, rest and sleep are needed for quality of life and wellbeing. Aged Care Accreditation Standards require care strategies that promote comfort, rest and sleep. These relate to the bed, mattress, room temperature, noise level, lighting, linen, odours and the number of people in each room. The right to personal choice and taking part in planning care also promote comfort, rest and sleep.

Clients have the right to have their pain assessed and managed. Untreated pain decreases quality of life. You must report signs and symptoms of pain. This helps the nurse meet the person's needs.

CASE STUDY

Mina Chowdry lives by herself within the community in her own home. Her family is becoming increasingly concerned about her tiredness, lethargy and lack of willingness to do anything requiring any effort. She used to enjoy going to her grandchildren's sports days and concerts, but nowadays she says that 'she just doesn't have the energy to do so'. Her daughter contacted her GP about their worries. He sent his practice nurse to see her, who conducted an assessment. Mina admitted to not eating well at all and was just making jam sandwiches for most of her meals. Her fluid intake was also limited to just a few cups of tea during the day. She also advised the nurse that it hurt her to eat as her dentures moved around when she chewed. Meals on Wheels was immediately organised for Mina, providing her with a substantial and nutritious meal once a day. Her family bought her some water bottles, which Mina was able to fill and carry round the house with her. She also went to see her dental prosthetist, who remoulded her dentures so that they no longer moved around.

Within a few weeks Mina had improved considerably and her family were pleased to see her taking an interest in her home and grandchildren once again.

The regular meals, increased fluid intake and better-fitting dentures all contributed to her being able to achieve a better nutritional status. This subsequently improved both her physical and her psychological wellbeing.

ACCREDITATION

You are working in residential or home care and accreditors are at your service. Can you answer the following questions?

- How can you support a resident or client to get a well-balanced diet?
- How can you ensure residents or clients have access to recreational and social activities?

REVIEW QUESTIONS

Circle the best answer:

1 Salivary gland atrophy is:
  a a purely voluntary activity
  b as secretion of saliva increases, the pH changes
  c a normal consequence of ageing often causing a reduction in saliva
  d an increase in saliva production

2 The signs of dehydration are:
  a cramps in arms and legs
  b constipation
  c low energy and restlessness
  d All of the above

3 Stomach acid:
  a is affected by stress and some medications
  b is necessary for adequate digestion and nutrient absorption
  c may be supported with apple cider vinegar and lemon juice
  d All of the above

4 A healthy diet is based on:
  a low fat, artificially sweetened and processed foods
  b high animal protein, high fat and low carbohydrate
  c grapefruit, yoghurt and cabbage soup
  d vegetables, whole grains, nuts, seeds, legumes and lean protein

5 Soluble and insoluble fibre:
  a are present in fresh fruit, vegetables, legumes, nuts, seeds and whole grains
  b aid detoxification, regulate bowel functions and lower cholesterol
  c are not present in meat, dairy and fat
  d All of the above

6 A fitness program can benefit healthy ageing by:
  a improving pelvic floor strength
  b increasing blood flow and oxygen to the tissues
  c decreasing the risk of chronic disease
  d All of the above

7 Physical fitness:
  a is not advised during ageing as it increases the risk of a heart attack
  b promotes longevity and disease prevention
  c can increase the risk of osteoporosis
  d can be achieved by watching TV

8 Massage can:
  a increase blood circulation and sense of wellbeing
  b rapidly increase the ageing process
  c should be avoided by the elderly as it may damage skin
  d is only beneficial when pain is experienced during a treatment

9 Aromatherapy massage:
  a as performed with the addition of fragrant oils made from synthetic means
  b has therapeutic benefits including mood elevation, increased circulation and pain relief
  c is performed with the use of stones
  d follows meridians and uses ultra fine needles

10 A naturopath:
  a prescribes supplements, herbal tinctures, diet and lifestyle
  b individualises programs according to clients' particular needs
  c promotes the body's own natural healing processes
  d All of the above

Answers to these questions are on p. 454.

Acknowledgement

The authors would like to acknowledge the work of Leonie Macdonald, who contributed to the previous editions of this text.

Further reading

Ball EL, Owen-Booth B, Gray A et al (2020). Aromatherapy in dementia. Cochrane Database. Online 27 March 2021. 19 October 2017. Available: https://pubmed.ncbi.nlm.nih.gov/32813272/

Campbell NR, Johnson JA, Campbell TS (2012). Sodium consumption: an individual's choice? International Journal of Hypertension. Epub. doi: 10.1155/2012/860954 Online 27 March 2021. Available: www.hindawi.com/journals/ijht/2012/860954/cta

References

Cogswell ME, Mugavero K, Bowman BA et al (2016). Dietary sodium and cardiovascular disease risk – measurement matters. New England Journal of Medicine 75(6):580–586.

Luchtman DW & Song C (2013). Cognitive enhancement by omega-3 fatty acids from childhood to old age: Findings from animal and clinical studies. Neuropharmacology 64:550–565.

McRae MP (2017). Dietary fiber is beneficial for the prevention of cardiovascular disease: an umbrella review of meta-analyses. Journal of Chiropractic Medicine 16(4):289–299.

CHAPTER 14
Working with older clients with dementia

By Margaret Webb

AFTER READING THIS CHAPTER, YOU SHOULD BE ABLE TO:

- define the key terms listed in this chapter
- understand the causes of confusion
- know the procedures that help people who are confused
- understand the causes of delirium and how it is different to dementia
- describe at least three types of dementia
- describe the signs, symptoms and behaviours of dementias
- describe the features of Alzheimer's disease
- describe the care required by the person with dementia
- explain the effects that dementia can have on the family
- explain the importance of good communication with the person with dementia and their family
- explain how various techniques, such as reminiscence and redirection, can assist a person with dementia
- know how to promote quality of life for people with dementia.

Key terms

Alzheimer's disease: The most common form of dementia; a progressive degenerative condition that attacks the brain

behavioural psychological symptoms of dementia (BPSD): Used to describe a broad range of psychological reactions, psychiatric symptoms and behaviours occurring in people with any form of dementia

care-giver burden: Negative physical or psychosocial effects experienced by a person as a direct result of looking after someone in need of care; often seen in family members caring for their loved one at home when no or limited support services are used

cognition: The process of thinking, learning and remembering. This includes the ability to plan, manipulate information, start and end activities and recognise errors

delirium: A temporary state of acute mental confusion

delusion: A false belief

dementia: A progressive decline of cognitive and social function caused by changes in the brain

dementia-friendly community: A community that assists people with dementia to remain included through consideration of physical and social factors and education of health providers

dementia with Lewy bodies (DLB): A type of dementia characterised by Lewy bodies, microscopic protein deposits that develop within the nerve cells involved in thinking, memory and motor control

diversional therapy: Participation in leisure-type activities that promote a feeling of wellbeing or positive experience based on the person's interests

hallucination: Seeing, hearing or feeling something that is not real

person-centred care: An approach recognising that caring for a person with dementia needs to be approached holistically, recognising the *person* with dementia, their values, beliefs and preferences, rather than a biomedical approach emphasising the effects of dementia

redirection: The redirection of thoughts that are causing distress to something more pleasant and acceptable

reminiscence: The act of remembering and reflecting on previous life experiences, especially those with a personal significance

spatial perception: The ability to evaluate how things are arranged in space and recognise their relations in the environment, for example, the space between a cup and table when putting the cup down on it

sundowning: Signs, symptoms and behaviours of a person with dementia that usually increase as the sun goes down; however, it can also occur at other times

validation: Similar to redirection where painful or distressing emotions are redirected to less distressing thoughts; however, there is also validation or recognition of the emotions being experienced

Confusion and dementia are not a natural progression of growing older. Most older people will never experience the effects of dementia; however, as the general population is getting older there is a marked increase in the number of people experiencing dementia. For those who develop dementia or have a loved one who has developed dementia, the trauma can be significant. This chapter reviews the functions of the brain and causes of confusion, delirium and dementia. It also provides insight on how the carer can assist people with dementia and their families to promote continuation of a good quality of life and to minimise traumatic behaviours.

BOX 14.1
Changes in the nervous system from ageing

- Brain cells are lost
- Nerve conduction slows
- Response and reaction times are slower
- Reflexes are slower
- Vision and hearing decrease
- Taste and smell decrease
- Touch and sensitivity to pain decrease
- Blood flow to the brain is reduced
- Sleep patterns change
- Memory span becomes shorter
- Minor forgetfulness occurs
- Dizziness can occur

THE BRAIN

The brain is an extremely complex organ, made up of several pieces, including portions of the brain called lobes (Fig. 14.1).

There are four main lobes:

- the *frontal lobe* – located at the *front* of the brain, is associated with reasoning, motor skills, higher level **cognition** and expressive language. Damage to the frontal lobe can lead to changes in sexual habits, socialisation and attention, as well as increased risk-taking
- the *parietal lobe* – located in the *middle* section of the brain is associated with processing sensory information, such as pressure, touch and pain. It is essential to the processing of the body's senses. Damage to the parietal lobe can result in problems with verbal memory, an impaired ability to control eye gaze and problems with language
- the *temporal lobe* – located on the *bottom* section of the brain. This lobe is important for interpreting sounds and the language we hear. The hippocampus is also located in the temporal lobe, which is why this portion of the brain is also heavily associated with the formation of memories. Damage to the temporal lobe can lead to problems with memory, speech perception and language skills
- the *occipital lobe* – located at the *back* of the brain, is associated with interpreting visual stimuli and information. Damage to this lobe can cause visual problems, such as difficulty recognising objects, an inability to identify colours and trouble recognising words.

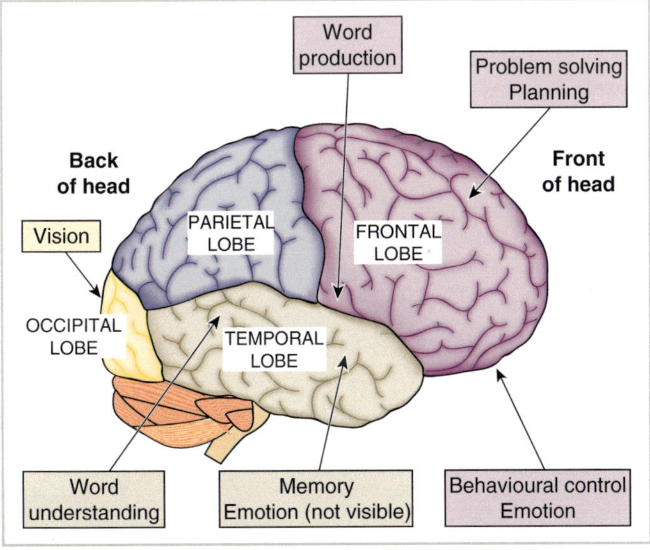

Fig. 14.1
The four lobes of the brain – frontal, parietal, temporal and occipital.

If one part of the brain is damaged, it will depend on where the damage has occurred to determine the effects it will have on the person.

Changes in the brain and nervous system occur naturally with ageing (Box 14.1); however, significant damage to the brain is not part of normal ageing.

Significant changes to the brain generally occur due to injury or disease. Certain diseases affect the brain, causing changes that can affect cognitive function. Cognitive function involves the process of thinking, learning and remembering. This includes the ability to plan, manipulate information, start and end activities and recognise errors. It also involves judgement and consequent behaviours.

While minor cognitive decline may occur in an ageing person, significant cognitive decline is *not* a normal part of the ageing process. Significant cognitive decline generally shows up in a person as confusion. However, there are a variety of causes of confusion, which we will look at now.

CONFUSION

Confusion has many causes and is often reversible. Several diseases, infections, hearing and vision loss, side-effects of medications and brain injury are just some of the possible causes of confusion. When a person is confused they may not know the time or place or recognise people. General forgetfulness, such as misplacing the keys, is normal; forgetting what you use keys for is not.

BOX 14.2
Caring for the confused person

If you are caring for a confused person in the community (i.e. their own home), the risks are different from those who live in a residential service. Essentially, residential services provide 24-hour care and/or supervision, which is pivotal to reducing risks for the client. The client's personal safety should always be paramount when providing care, whether they are in a facility or the community. Remember that you are perfectly placed to ensure the benefits outweigh the risks if the client remains in their own home. The following information may assist you to deliver appropriate care for a confused client, irrespective of the setting.

- Follow the person's care plan.
- Ensure the safety of the person and yourself.
- Face the person. Speak clearly and slowly.
- Call the person by their preferred name every time you are in contact with them.
- State your name. Show your name tag.
- Inform the person of the date, time and place each morning. Repeat as needed during the course of the day, but do it tactfully, for example: 'This morning is going so quickly, it's 11.30 already. We'll be getting ready for lunch soon.'
- Explain what you are going to do and why. Give clear, simple directions and answers to questions.
- Ask clear and simple questions. Give the person time to respond.
- Keep calendars and clocks with large numbers in the person's room, and in common rooms and other public areas (Fig. 14.2). Remind the person of holidays, birthdays and special events.
- Have the person wear glasses and hearing aids if needed.
- Use touch to communicate, unless this causes aggravation or resistance. Place familiar objects and pictures within the person's view.
- Provide newspapers, magazines, television and radio; however, you must be selective when supplying a TV, as many programs can increase confusion; for example, news programs jump from one story to another very quickly. In addition, there can be upsetting stories during the news or in newspapers, which the person with dementia may believe has a direct impact on them. This will lead to distress and increased confusion. Be selective with programs: a person who is 80 years old is unlikely to appreciate the latest rap or rock music program. Read to the person if appropriate, again keeping in mind that you need to avoid articles that may cause distress.
- Discuss current events with the person (see caution in previous point). Weather, football and other sports are generally good conversation topics that they can participate in, particularly if it is an area of interest they had when they were younger.
- Maintain the day–night cycle. Open curtains, shades and drapes during the day. Close them at night. Use a nightlight at night. The person wears normal clothes during the day, not sleepwear.
- Provide a calm, relaxed and peaceful setting. Prevent loud noises, rushing and congested hallways and dining rooms.
- Follow the person's usual routine. Meals, bathing, exercise, television and other activities have a schedule. This promotes a sense of order and what to expect.
- Break tasks down into small steps when helping the person.
- Do not rearrange furniture or the person's belongings.
- Encourage the person to take part in self-care. Be consistent.

Acute confusion (delirium) occurs suddenly. It is usually temporary. Causes include infection, such as a urine infection; illness, particularly if it causes dehydration; injury; some medications; and side-effects from anaesthesia during surgery. Treatment is aimed at the cause, and, if successful, once the cause is treated – for example, a person with a urine infection has treatment to get rid of the infection – the confusion disappears and the person returns to normal cognitive function at the level they were before the infection. Regardless of the cause of confusion, the carer must meet the person's physical and safety needs (see Box 14.2).

DELIRIUM

Delirium is a state of temporary but acute mental confusion. The onset is sudden. It is common in older people with acute or chronic illnesses. Infections, heart and lung conditions and poor nutrition are common causes. So are hormone disorders and hypoglycaemia (low blood glucose levels). Alcohol and many medications can cause delirium.

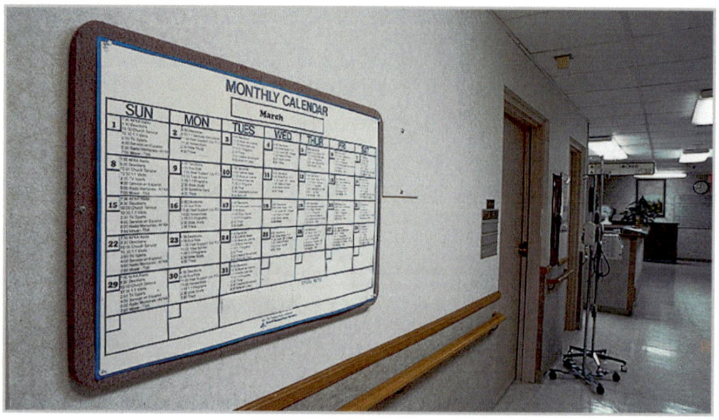

Fig. 14.2
A large calendar can help people who are confused.

Delirium has a short course, from a few hours to weeks, rarely longer than a month. It is usually worse at night.

Delirium signals physical illness in an older person and in those with dementia. It is recognised as an emergency as it can lead to permanent brain damage if undetected. It is very important that the cause is found and treated. Signs and symptoms of delirium include:

- anxiety
- disorientation to time and place, and sometimes to person
- tremors
- hallucinations
- delusions
- attention problems
- fluctuating level of consciousness
- sleep problems
- memory problems.

The rate of onset and often no previous history of confusion are major indicators that the person is suffering from delirium, not dementia.

DEPRESSION

Depression is the most common mental health problem in older people and is often overlooked as many people see its signs and symptoms as part of the normal ageing process. A correct diagnosis is needed for proper treatment. Otherwise, the person and family suffer unnecessary emotional, physical, social and financial discomfort. Depression, ageing and some medication side-effects have similar signs and symptoms. They may include:

- sadness
- inactivity
- lack of desire to socialise, leading to withdrawal
- difficulty thinking
- difficulty concentrating
- reluctance to make decisions
- problems sleeping
- changes in appetite
- fatigue
- agitation
- feelings of despair
- recurrent thoughts of death.

Depression, although frequently overlooked in older people, needs to be taken very seriously. In fact, in previous studies it has been demonstrated that the highest rate of suicide belonged to males over the age of 65 years.

Confusion caused by major physical changes in the brain cannot be cured, although some measures can improve function.

DEMENTIA

Some key statistics for Australia relating to dementia:

- Dementia is the second leading cause of death of Australians (AIHW 2021).
- In 2016 dementia became the leading cause of death of Australian women, surpassing heart disease which has been the leading cause of death for both men and women since the early 20th century. In 2019, dementia remained the leading cause of death for women, and the second leading cause of death for men. Overall, it accounted for 14,919 deaths (AIHW 2021).
- Females account for 64.5% of all dementia-related deaths.
- In 2021, there are an estimated 472,000 Australians living with dementia. Without a medical breakthrough, the number of people with dementia is expected to increase to 590,000 by 2028 and 1,076,000 by 2058 (Dementia Australia 2018, 2021).
- Currently an estimated 250 people are joining the population with dementia each day. The number of new cases of dementia will increase to 318 people per day by 2025 and more than 650 people by 2056 (Brown et al 2017).
- Three in 10 people over the age of 85 and almost one in 10 people over 65 have dementia (Scott et al 2019).
- In 2021, there were an estimated 28,300 people with younger onset dementia, expected to rise to 29,350 people by 2028 and 41,250 people by 2058 (Dementia Australia 2018).
- An average of 36 people died per day where dementia was the underlying cause of death in 2016. Of the 13,126 people that lost their lives, 8,447 were female (ABS 2017).
- In 2021, it is estimated that almost 1.6 million people in Australia are involved in the care of someone living with dementia (Dementia Australia 2018, 2021).

Some key statistics for New Zealand from Alzheimers New Zealand (2021):

- In New Zealand there are currently 70,000 people living with dementia. It is anticipated this figure will rise to 170,000 by 2050.
- The total financial cost of dementia on the health system in 2021was estimated at $2.5 billion.
- A total of 1 million hours of unpaid care are spent per week caring for people with dementia.
- Dementia also has a significant impact on the family/whānau and friends of people with the condition. A survey conducted in 2017 indicated that four out of five New Zealanders knows or has known someone with dementia.

The World Health Organisation (WHO) estimates that around 50 million people have dementia worldwide, with nearly 60 per cent living in low- and middle-income countries (WHO 2021). Every year, there are nearly 10 million new cases. The estimated proportion of the general population aged 60 and over with dementia at a given time is between 5 and 8 per cent. The total number of people with dementia is projected to reach 82 million in 2030 and 152 million in 2050. Much of this increase is attributable to the rising numbers of people with dementia living in low- and middle-income countries.

Dementia is one of a large group of illnesses that cause a progressive decline in mental and social functioning, due to abnormal changes in the brain.

According to the WHO (2021):

> Dementia is a syndrome – usually of a chronic or progressive nature – in which there is deterioration in

cognitive function (i.e. the ability to process thought) beyond what might be expected from normal ageing. It affects memory, thinking, orientation, comprehension, calculation, learning capacity, language and judgement. Consciousness is not affected. The impairment in cognitive function is commonly accompanied, and occasionally preceded, by deterioration in emotional control, social behaviour or motivation.

Dementia is *not* a normal part of ageing. Older people do not all have dementia, and while only a small number of older people are affected, the numbers are increasing with the ageing population. Dementia occurs in both men and women; however, as women live longer than men, there are more women with dementia. Dementia:

- is an organic brain condition
- is not a psychiatric illness
- is not a deliberate act for attention
- does not consist of deliberate disruptive behaviours.

There are over 100 causes of dementia. This chapter will explore some of the most common types, those being vascular dementia, Lewy bodies dementia (LBD), frontotemporal dementia, Korsakoff syndrome, younger onset dementia, Parkinson's disease, Huntington's disease and Alzheimer's disease. Some (not all) types and causes of dementia are listed in Box 14.3. Dementia is often used as the 'umbrella term' when referring to the conditions that cause it (Fig. 14.3).

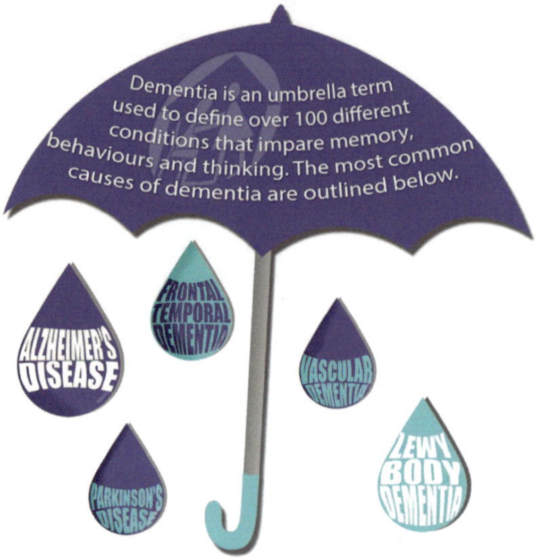

Fig. 14.3
The dementia umbrella.

Dementia may also be a symptom that develops in the later stages of some illnesses; for example, many people with Parkinson's disease may go on to develop dementia, but not everyone with Parkinson's will get dementia. A person can experience more than one type of dementia at the same time. The type and severity of symptoms will vary depending on the type of dementia and the stage of the condition. For example, a person with mild dementia might only experience one or two symptoms that have a relatively minor impact on day-to-day living, while a person in the late stages of dementia might experience many symptoms and require 24-hour care.

Alzheimer's disease is the most common type of dementia and is discussed in further detail later in the chapter.

BOX 14.3
Types and causes of dementia

- Alcohol-related dementia and Korsakoff syndrome; alcohol has a toxic effect on brain cells
- AIDS-related dementia
- Alzheimer's disease, the most common form of dementia
- Dementia with Lewy bodies – tiny protein deposits in nerve cells
- Frontal lobe dementia (including Pick's disease, a rare brain disorder)
- Huntington's disease, a nervous system condition
- Vascular dementia – diseased blood vessels (vascular) in the brain; also called multi-infarct dementia, the second most common type of dementia
- Parkinson's disease
- Trauma and head injury
- A combination of two or more of the above

OVERVIEW OF DEMENTIA TYPES

VASCULAR DEMENTIA

Vascular dementia (VaD) is the second most common dementia, accounting for around 15–20 per cent of all cases (Dementia Australia 2020c). It occurs through a reduced blood supply to the brain, usually caused by a stroke or other conditions that can interfere with the blood supply of the brain, such as arteriosclerosis, blocked arteries, blood clots or haemorrhage within the brain. The interruption to the blood supply leaves an area of damage called an *infarct*. Vascular dementia may occur on its own or may also be experienced with Alzheimer's disease.

People with vascular dementia display symptoms based on where the damage is located in the brain. If the damage is large, such as a large bleed or blood clot in the brain, one-sided weakness in the body may also be noted. If the right side of the body is weak, this will indicate the left side of the brain has been affected (due to the crossover of nerves at the base of the brain) and vice versa. Night-time wandering and depression are commonly seen in a person with vascular dementia.

Multi-infarct dementia is another term for vascular dementia, but rather than being caused by a large bleed or clot, it is caused by damage to the smaller blood vessels of the brain. This is sometimes described as a 'mini stroke' or transient ischaemic attack (TIA). In this situation there may be no obvious physical disability to indicate blood vessel damage to the brain, although it can usually be seen on specific brain scans.

As it is difficult to tell what part of the brain will be affected by vascular dementia, the symptoms are related specifically to the lobe that experiences damage.

Lewy body dementia

Dementia with Lewy bodies (DLB) accounts for around 15 per cent of all dementia, and is associated with Lewy bodies, which are abnormal brain cells. Each case of DLB is as individual as the person living with it. Different people will show different combinations of symptoms. At present, a diagnosis of DLB can only be confirmed by autopsy, but a careful clinical evaluation of the patient and their symptoms can, in many cases, form the basis for making a reasonably confident lifetime diagnosis. The photograph in Fig. 14.4 is of a slide of brain cells showing a Lewy body. Lewy bodies are microscopic protein deposits that develop within the nerve cells involved in thinking, memory and motor control. They are named after Dr Friedrich Lewy, who first described them under the microscope in 1912. It is not yet known whether the Lewy bodies are the cause or effect of degeneration of brain cells, but they are thought to be the result of the problems with a protein, alpha-synuclein. They are present in the brains of people with DLB and Parkinson's disease. Lewy bodies are associated with the death of brain cells and subsequent deterioration of the brain.

One of the big differences between a person with Parkinson's disease and DLB is the location of the Lewy bodies in the brain. In Parkinson's disease they are found mainly in the mid-brain (above the medulla oblongata and pons), whereas in DLB they are more widely distributed throughout the cerebral cortex (throughout the lobes). Clinically, DLB closely resembles the dementia typically associated with Parkinson's. If the physical symptoms precede the cognitive symptoms by one year, a diagnosis of Parkinson's will be made; if the onset of cognitive symptoms precedes or starts at the same time as the physical symptoms start, it is considered to be DLB.

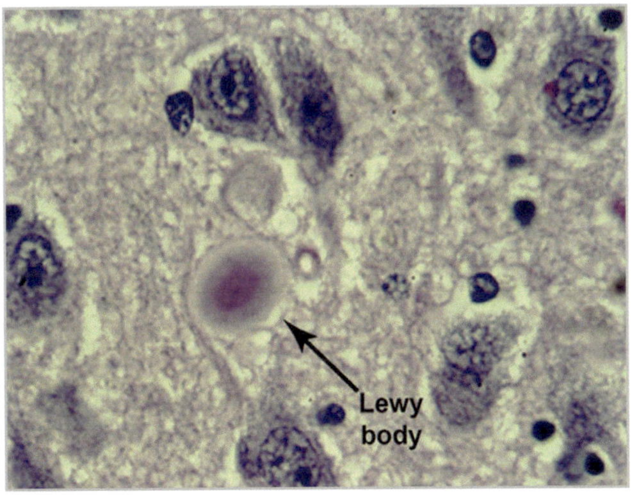

Fig. 14.4
Lewy bodies in the brain

DLB shares mental symptoms with Alzheimer's disease, such as confusion and loss of memory, and motor symptoms, such as gait and slow movement, with Parkinson's disease. For that reason it is often misdiagnosed. Accurate diagnosis is essential for successful treatment of the disease: people with DLB are characteristically highly sensitive to certain drugs, which can worsen unpleasant symptoms or even be fatal.

However, it is generally accepted that a diagnosis of DLB can be made if the person presents with fluctuating states of consciousness, visual hallucinations and/or spontaneous Parkinsonism in addition to accepted dementia symptoms. These presenting symptoms can affect the person significantly or be identified as minor changes. For example, fluctuating states of consciousness can occur suddenly and last for a few moments or even days. Although two-thirds of people experience visual hallucinations, there is no pattern as to whether they are pleasant or threatening. However, if Parkinsonism symptoms are present, they are generally significant. These usually include the motor difficulties of someone with Parkinson's disease: slow movement (bradykinesia), greater difficulty in walking, rigidity and falls. Often the person may suffer from a sudden drop in blood pressure upon standing, characterised by becoming dizzy or falling just after standing up. They may also develop difficulty in swallowing, incontinence or constipation (The Lewy Body Society 2017).

Parkinson's disease

Parkinson's disease is NOT a dementia; however, as identified above, many people with Parkinson's disease that has developed in later life are at high risk of developing dementia similar to DLB. Fifty to 80 per cent of those with Parkinson's disease eventually experience dementia as their disease progresses (Alzheimer's Association 2021). This is a progressive disorder of the central nervous system that results from loss of the neurotransmitter dopamine in the brain. It is characterised by tremors, stiffness in the limbs and joints, speech impediments and difficulty in initiating physical movements. A shuffling style of walking with limited arm movement and a stooped posture are common in people with Parkinson's disease.

Huntington's disease

Similar to Parkinson's disease, people with Huntington's disease are at a high risk of developing dementia, but not everyone who has Huntington's disease will develop dementia. Huntington's disease is an inherited condition in which nerve cells in the brain break down over time.

Frontotemporal dementia

Frontotemporal dementia, also known as frontal lobe dementia and previously known as Pick's disease, is caused by degeneration of nerve cells in the frontal and temporal lobes of the brain. It accounts for approximately 5 to 10 per cent of dementia cases and is common in younger groups, developing between the ages of 45 and 65 years (The Australian Frontotemporal Dementia Association 2020). People usually live between 2 and 10 years after diagnosis, although some people have lived for 20 years with it. Damage to these areas produces symptoms that separate this type of dementia from other types.

Frontotemporal dementia can also occur with Parkinsonian symptoms. These include involuntary tremor, muscular stiffness and mobility difficulties due to slow movements.

There are two main types of frontotemporal dementia, depending on the area of the brain that is most affected. Behavioural variant frontotemporal dementia occurs when mostly the frontal lobe is affected, producing behavioural and personality changes. For example, the person may display a lack of emotional warmth, apathy, altered eating behaviours, selfishness, sexually inappropriate behaviours and irritability and compulsive behaviours. The person is generally unaware about the changes in behaviour.

The second type, semantic dementia, occurs when it is mainly the temporal lobe that is affected. As a result, the person experiences a decline in language where the meaning of words are affected Commonly the initial complaint is of being unable to remember words, including people's names, but as the disease progresses people see a loss of spontaneous speech. Speech comprehension, reading and spelling become affected and eventually as the disease progresses to the frontal lobe behavioural changes occur.

Standard dementia screening tools may not be effective in diagnosis of frontotemporal lobe dementia, especially as people with this type of dementia do not experience as much memory loss as those with Alzheimer's Disease. They also usually know where they are and are able to recall information about the past and present. Even in late stages, people with frontotemporal lobe dementia can coordinate themselves to negotiate their surroundings and remain oriented; this is very different to someone with Alzheimer's disease.

Younger onset dementia

Younger onset dementia, previously known as early onset dementia, refers to dementia in people aged less than 65 years; however, dementia has been diagnosed in people in their 30s, 40s and 50s. Familial Alzheimer's disease, a tendency to inherit Alzheimer's disease, although unusual, has been recognised in younger onset dementia. Other more frequently encountered types of dementias in those who have early onset dementia include frontotemporal lobe dementia, vascular dementia, dementia with Lewy bodies (DLB) and alcohol-related dementia (Korsakoff dementia).

The duration between symptom onset and diagnosis of early onset dementia has been found to be on average 1.6 years longer than for those diagnosed with later onset dementia (de Vugt & Verhey 2013). Young age and being diagnosed with frontotemporal dementia were related to increases in the time to diagnosis. Subjects with vascular dementia experienced shorter time to diagnosis (de Vugt & Verhey 2013). However, overall younger onset dementia is generally not diagnosed as early as it is in older people, as there is no expectation in the general and health communities that dementia occurs in younger people. The delay in referral and diagnosis can lead to significant family and relationship difficulties. Additionally, there is also a lack of specialist advice and support after a diagnosis of early onset dementia, which adds to feelings of distress and isolation for both the person and their family (Hayo 2015).

Korsakoff dementia

Alcohol-related dementia is a form of dementia related to the excessive drinking of alcohol. This affects memory, learning and other mental functions. Korsakoff syndrome and Wernicke/Korsakoff syndrome are particular forms of alcohol-related brain injury that may be related to alcohol-related dementia. It is currently suspected that the damage to the brain is caused by a lack of thiamine (vitamin B_1) and/or direct toxicity of alcohol on the brain cells. It is thought that in the early stages the damage may be reversed when the person with the dementia is treated with thiamine supplements; however, this is not always successful.

Although the symptoms of dementia are similar whatever a person's age, younger people with dementia have additional issues. They may:

- be in work at the time of diagnosis
- have dependent children still living at home
- have significant financial commitments
- be physically fit, but behave in ways that other people find different or unusual
- be more aware of their disease in the early stages
- find it hard to accept and cope with losing skills at such a young age
- find it difficult to access information, support and services for younger people with dementia
- have a carer who is still in fulltime employment.

Often the person with early onset dementia has frontotemporal dementia or DLB, both of which can present with more changed behaviours.

ALZHEIMER'S DISEASE

Alzheimer's disease, the most common form of dementia, is a progressive, degenerative condition that attacks the brain. Brain cells that control intellectual and social functioning are damaged by plaques, thought to be a result of protein build-up. These then cause tangles (technically known as neurofibrillary tangles) within the brain cells (Fig. 14.5).

Alzheimer's disease generally follows a similar pattern of progression through the lobes in the brain for each person. Considering the functions of the lobes in the

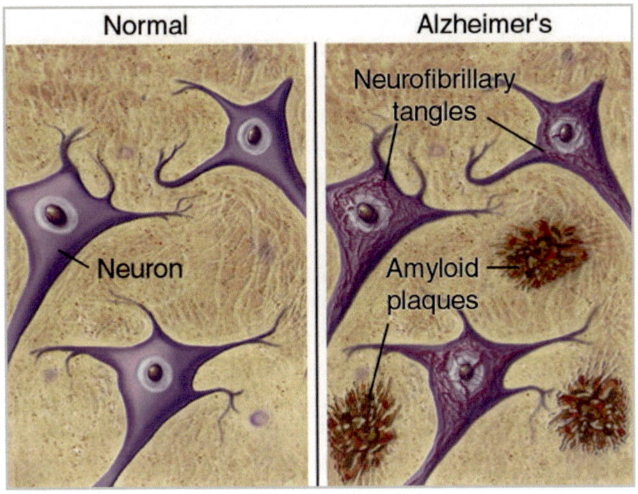

Fig. 14.5
Changes to the brain in Alzheimer's disease

brain (see Fig. 14.1), it is obvious that the lobes that are affected reflect the signs and symptoms of Alzheimer's disease. For example, as the temporal lobes area is affected, the person may lose the ability to process sensory input; for example, a light touch may feel painful or they might not realise how hot water is and scald themselves. Once the frontal lobes are affected, mood, judgement, behaviours and self-control are affected. Recognising this helps the carer to understand that the actions displayed by people with Alzheimer's, or any dementia, are generally a direct result of the damage to the brain. In fact, people with dementia usually do not have the planning abilities it would take to undertake a deliberate act of annoyance. This can also provide the family with reassurance.

Signs of Alzheimer's

The person has problems with work and everyday functions. Problems with family and social relationships occur. There is a steady decline in memory and mental function. The condition is gradual in onset, usually developing over several years. Some people aged in their 40s or 50s have Alzheimer's disease, although it usually occurs after the age of 65. It is often diagnosed around the age of 80. The cause is unknown. However, a family history of Alzheimer's disease and Down syndrome are risk factors.

The classic sign of Alzheimer's disease is gradual loss of short-term memory. Other early signs include (Box 14.4):

- problems finding or speaking the right word
- not recognising objects
- forgetting how to use simple, everyday things (like a pencil)
- forgetting to turn off the stove, close windows or lock doors
- mood and personality changes
- agitation
- poor judgement (may cause odd behaviour).

BOX 14.4
Signs and symptoms of Alzheimer's disease

The person:

- forgets recent events
- forgets simple directions
- forgets conversations
- forgets appointments
- forgets names (including family members)
- forgets the names of everyday things (clock, radio, television, etc)
- forgets words
- substitutes unusual words and names for what is forgotten
- loses their train of thought
- speaks in a native language
- curses or swears
- misplaces things
- puts things in odd places
- has problems managing finances
- gives away large amounts of money
- does not recognise or understand numbers
- has difficulty following conversations
- has problems reading
- has problems writing
- becomes lost in familiar settings
- forgets where they are
- does not know how to get back home
- wanders from home
- cannot tell or understand the time
- cannot tell or understand dates
- cannot solve everyday problems (iron is left on, hotplate on stove left on, food is left burning on the stove, etc)
- cannot perform everyday tasks (dressing, bathing, brushing teeth, etc)
- distrusts others
- is stubborn
- withdraws socially
- is restless
- becomes suspicious
- becomes fearful
- does not want to do things
- sleeps more than usual.

Alzheimer's disease affects a person's ability to perform complex and simple tasks. Problems with complex tasks appear first. The person has problems using the telephone, driving, managing money, planning meals and working. Over time, problems occur with simple tasks; these include bathing, dressing, eating, using the toilet and walking.

As mentioned earlier, Alzheimer's disease is caused by the formation of tangles in the brain and usually progresses through the brain in a similar pattern. Although signs and symptoms vary from person to person, and become more severe with each stage, they will generally move in the same pattern of progression within the brain. A person's abilities may vary from day to day, becoming worse in times of stress, fatigue or ill health. It is a progressive and irreversible disease that ends in death.

Regardless of the type of dementia, it is essential that a medical diagnosis be obtained at an early stage, when symptoms first appear, to ensure that a person with a treatable condition is diagnosed and treated correctly. Early warning signs include:

- recent memory loss that affects job skills
- problems with common tasks (e.g. dressing, cooking, driving)
- problems with language; forgetting simple words
- getting lost in familiar places
- misplacing things and putting things in odd places (e.g. putting a watch in the oven)
- personality changes
- poor or decreased judgement (e.g. crossing a busy road without looking to see if there is any traffic)
- loss of interest in life.

BEHAVIOURAL AND PSYCHOLOGICAL SYMPTOMS OF DEMENTIA (BPSD)

Behavioural and psychological symptoms of dementia (BPSD) is a term used to describe a broad range of psychological reactions, psychiatric symptoms and behaviours occurring in people with any form of dementia. Examples include:

- personality alterations
- misidentifications
- delusions
- hallucinations
- mood symptoms (depression, anxiety, euphoria, apathy)
- disorders of 'neuro-vegetative' function (sleep, appetite, sexual expression)
- changed behaviours ('agitation', excessive motor activity, repetitive movements, restlessness, noisiness).

It is imperative you remember that these are caused by the effects of dementia. They are not deliberate, calculated acts to obtain attention from someone.

Wandering

The person with dementia is frequently not oriented to person, time or place. They may wander away and not find their way back. Wandering may be by foot, car, bicycle or other means. They may be with you one moment and gone the next. The person's judgement is poor. They cannot tell what is safe or dangerous. Life-threatening accidents are great risks. They can walk into traffic or into a nearby river, lake, ocean or the bush. If they are not properly dressed, heat or cold exposure is a risk.

Wandering may have no cause, or the person may be looking for something or someone: the bathroom, the bedroom, a child, a partner. Pain, medication side-effects, stress, restlessness and anxiety are possible causes. Frequently being able to identify the cause prevents wandering; for example, if someone is looking for the toilet and you take them to a toilet they can recognise and use, they will become comfortable and no longer need to wander.

Hallucinations

A **hallucination** is seeing, hearing or feeling something that is not real. The person's senses are dulled. They may see animals, insects or people that are not present. Some hear voices. They may feel bugs crawling or feel that they are being touched. Sometimes the problem is caused by impaired vision or hearing. The person needs to wear glasses and hearing aids, as prescribed. Many medications given to elderly people can produce hallucinations as a side-effect, so it is important that they are always reported to allow appropriate staff to follow it up with the doctor.

Delusions

Delusions are false beliefs. People with dementia may think they are some other person.

Some believe they are in jail, are being killed or are being attacked. A person may believe that the carer is someone else. Many other false beliefs can occur. Often these can result from something they have seen on television or overheard and misinterpreted in someone else's conversation.

Agitation and restlessness

The person may pace, hit or yell. Common causes are pain or discomfort, anxiety, lack of sleep and too much or too little stimulation. Hunger and the need to eliminate are also causes. A calm, quiet setting helps calm the person. So does meeting basic needs.

Carers can cause these behaviours. A carer may rush the person or be impatient. They may send mixed verbal and non-verbal messages. Carers always need to look at how their behaviour affects others, as well as potential triggers in the environment. Never try and force the person to do something they are reluctant to do.

Aggression and combativeness

Aggressive and combative behaviours include hitting, pinching, grabbing, biting or swearing. They may result from agitation and restlessness and can frighten others. Sometimes these behaviours are part of the person's personality. Pain, fatigue, too much stimulation, carer stress and feeling lost or abandoned may also be causes. The behaviours can occur during care measures (bathing, dressing) that upset or frighten the person. Always follow the person's care plan. However, your own safety is also important and if you are working with a client who has aggressive behaviour, try and strategically place yourself in the area so that you can exit easily if required.

Keep in mind that due to short-term memory loss it is possible at times for you to leave the room/situation if a person is acting aggressively, and return a few minutes later with a new, calmer approach to find the person with dementia cooperative, unaware that you were there before. Unfortunately, if a specific method of managing a person with dementia works one day, it may not work the next. Support for a person must always remain flexible and never follow rigid guidelines. If they do not wish to have a shower, offer a wash instead or try another time.

Screaming

A person with dementia has communication problems. At first, it is hard for the person to find the right word. As dementia progresses, the person speaks in short sentences or in single words. Often their speech cannot be understood. The person may scream to communicate. Screaming is common in people who are very confused and have poor communication skills. The person may scream a word or a name, or they may just make screaming or unintelligible sounds.

Possible causes include hearing and vision problems, pain or discomfort, fear and fatigue. Too much or not enough stimulation is another cause. The person may react to a carer or family member by screaming. Sometimes the following measures are helpful:

- providing a calm, quiet setting
- playing soft music
- having the person wear hearing aids and glasses
- having a family member or calm carer that knows the person well comfort and calm the person
- using touch to calm the person.

Abnormal sexual behaviours

Sexual behaviours are labelled abnormal because of how and when they occur. A person with dementia is not oriented to person, place or time. Sexual behaviour may involve the wrong person, the wrong place and/or the wrong time. They also cannot control the behaviour. A person with dementia may mistake someone else for a sexual partner. They may kiss and hug the other person. If the person's frontal lobe is affected, for example, in Alzheimer's disease or frontotemporal lobe dementia, inhibitions are decreased, so someone who feels too hot may simply take their clothes off so they can cool down.

Sometimes behaviours that look sexual are not. Touching, scratching and rubbing the genitals can signal infection, pain or discomfort in the urinary or reproductive systems. Poor hygiene is another cause. So is being wet or soiled from urine or faeces. Also, be vigilant in thoroughly cleaning and drying possible areas for fungal infections, such as the groin folds or folds under the stomach and breasts.

The person's sexual partner is encouraged to show affection, and their normal practices are encouraged. Examples include hand-holding, hugging, kissing and touching. If a person masturbates in public or removes their clothing, lead the person to their room and provide privacy and safety. Good hygiene prevents itching. Clean the person quickly and thoroughly after elimination. Do not let the person stay wet or soiled.

The registered nurse will assess the person for urinary or reproductive system problems and will contact the doctor as necessary.

Repetitive behaviour

Repetitive behaviour means to repeat something over and over again. A person with dementia may do the same motions repeatedly. For example, the person folds a napkin repeatedly, says the same words repeatedly or asks the same question. Such behaviours do not hurt the person. However, they can annoy carers and the family.

However, these acts sometimes indicate that there is a need; for example, the person is in pain or is thirsty. Music, picture books, especially photo albums with old photos, exercise and movies are distracting. Taking the person for a walk can help. Such measures also help when words or questions are repeated.

Sundowning

Sundowning is a frequently debated condition, with many researchers arguing that it does not exist while other people, particularly carers and healthcare staff, strongly assert that it certainly does exist. Sundowning describes an increase in the signs, symptoms and behaviours of dementia during the hours of darkness. It occurs in the late afternoon and evening hours. As daylight ends and darkness begins, the person's confusion and restlessness increase. So do anxiety, agitation and other symptoms. Behaviour is worse after the sun goes down and it may continue throughout the night. Sundowning may relate to being tired or hungry. Poor light and shadows may cause the person to see things that are not there. A person with dementia may be afraid of the dark. Carer fatigue may also contribute to an increase in dementia behaviours towards the end of the day if they also become tired or irritable. This would especially apply to those people being cared for at home by family members with minimal assistance. Exacerbations of the person's behaviours may also occur at other times and not just as the sun goes down.

Catastrophic reactions

A catastrophic reaction is an extreme response. The person reacts as if there is a disaster or tragedy and may scream, cry, become agitated or combative. These reactions are common and can result from too much sensory stimulation. Eating, music playing, having the television or radio on and being asked questions all at once could overwhelm the person.

STAGES OF DEMENTIA

Dementia has a number of stages that most of those affected go through. It has been identified that there are seven such stages regardless of the cause of the dementia. These are listed in Table 14.1.

Not everyone goes through these stages at the same time or stays in each stage for a predictable time. It varies between individuals and with the cause of the dementia.

Table 14.1
Seven stages of dementia

Stage No.	Diagnosis	Level of Cognitive Decline	Signs and Symptoms
Stage 1	No dementia	No cognitive decline	In this stage the person functions normally, has no memory loss and is mentally healthy. People with no dementia would be considered to be in Stage 1
Stage 2	No dementia	Very mild cognitive decline	This stage is used to describe normal forgetfulness associated with ageing. Symptoms are not evident to loved ones or the doctor
Stage 3	No dementia	Mild cognitive decline	This stage includes increased forgetfulness, slight difficulty concentrating, decreased work performance. People may be lost more often or have difficulty finding the right words
Stage 4	Early stage	Moderate cognitive decline	This stage includes difficulty concentrating, decreased memory of recent events and difficulties managing finances or travelling alone to new locations. People have trouble completing complex tasks efficiently or accurately, and may be in denial about their symptoms. They may also start withdrawing from family or friends
Stage 5	Mid-stage	Moderately severe cognitive decline	People in this stage have major memory deficiencies and need some assistance to complete their daily activities. Memory loss is more prominent and may include major relevant aspects of their current lives; for example, people may not remember their address or phone number and may not know the time or day or where they are
Stage 6	Mid-stage	Severe cognitive decline (middle dementia)	People in Stage 6 require extensive assistance to carry out daily activities. Many people can remember only some details of earlier life. They also have difficulty counting down from 10 and finishing tasks. Incontinence is a problem in this stage. Ability to speak declines. Personality changes, such as delusions, compulsions or anxiety and agitation, may occur.
Stage 7	Late-stage	Very severe cognitive decline (late dementia)	People in this stage have essentially no ability to speak or communicate. They require assistance with most activities (e.g. using the toilet, eating). They often lose psychomotor skills, e.g. the ability to walk.

Source: Adapted from Dementia Care Central (2020). Stages of Alzheimer's and dementia: durations and scales used to measure progression (GDS, FAST & CDR). Online 27 October 2021. Available: https://www.dementiacarecentral.com/aboutdementia/facts/stages

CARE OF THE PERSON WITH DEMENTIA

Person-centred care is a philosophy of care which is developed around the individual needs of a person and is ideal for people with dementia (Fazio et al 2018). The model ensures the person with dementia continues to be treated as an individual, recognising the person they are regardless of the stage of dementia. The premise that everyone needs to be recognised, respected and trusted is central to ensuring person-centred care is achieved. The person with dementia is central to the care planning and care receiving, and this continues even as they have decreased cognitive ability to plan. It is therefore imperative that the history of the person with dementia, important people and events throughout their life and preferences, are considered at all times. Most services now promote person-centred care as a philosophy. This includes advisory, home care, community and long-term services. As such, the person with dementia is central to care planning decisions and services planning. Routines that were familiar to a person with dementia prior to service provision are maintained as much as possible to recognise the person's preferences rather than those of the service provider. These should occur regardless of where the service is located.

Respite may help and often residential care is required during the late stages of the dementia progression. Sometimes hospital care is needed for other illnesses. The person and family need support and understanding. In fact, the inclusion of the family assists to ensure person-centred care is provided.

Respite day care

This is a planned program of activities usually run by health professionals such as diversional therapists. This is offered to those who live within the community alone or with family. Often they are linked to a residential aged care facility and offered within their settings. These programs provide socialisation and activities. They will also provide a meal and assistance with toileting if required. Not only are they beneficial for the older person, but they also provide caregivers with a break. It is reported that those who have dementia and attend day respite care have increased health, psychological and behavioural benefits (Ellen et al 2017).

People with dementia do not choose to be forgetful, incontinent, agitated or rude. Nor do they choose to have other behaviours, signs and symptoms of the disease. They cannot control what is happening to them (Box 14.5). The disease causes the behaviours. The disease is responsible, not the person.

BOX 14.5
Care of the person with Alzheimer's disease and other dementias

Environment

- Ensure the environment is not overstimulating, e.g. not too many bright lights, noises, etc
- Follow established routines
- Avoid changing rooms or roommates
- Place picture signs in rooms, bathrooms, dining rooms and other areas
- Keep personal items where the person can see them
- Do not invade the person's personal space
- Stay within the person's sight as much as possible
- Place memory aids (large clocks and calendars) where the person can see them
- Keep noise levels low
- Play music and show movies from the person's past
- Select tasks and activities specific to the person's cognitive abilities and interests.

Safety

- Remove harmful, sharp and breakable objects from the area. This includes knives, scissors, glass items, dishes, razors and tools
- Place safety plugs in electrical outlets
- Keep cords and electrical equipment out of reach
- Remove electrical appliances from the bathroom. Examples include hair dryers, curling irons, make-up mirrors and electric razors. Store personal care items (shampoo, deodorant, creams, etc) in a safe place
- Store household cleaners and medications in locked storage areas
- Store dangerous equipment and tools in a safe place
- Supervise the person who smokes
- Store cigarettes, cigars, pipes, matches and other smoking materials in a safe place
- Practise safety measures to prevent falls
- Practise safety measures to prevent fires
- Practise safety measures to prevent burns
- Practise safety measures to prevent poisoning
- Keep all doors to kitchens, utility rooms and housekeeping closets locked.

Basic needs

- Meet food and fluid needs. Provide finger foods. Cut food and pour liquids as needed
- Provide good skin care. Keep skin free of urine and faeces
- Promote urinary and bowel elimination
- Provide continence care as needed
- Promote exercise and activity during the day, as this helps reduce wandering and sundowning behaviours; the person may also sleep better
- Reduce intake of coffee, tea and cola drinks as they contain caffeine. Caffeine is a stimulant and can increase restlessness, confusion and agitation
- Provide a quiet, restful setting. Soft music is better than loud television programs
- Play soft music during care activities, such as bathing and during meals
- Promote personal hygiene. Do not force the person into a shower or bath tub. People with dementia are often afraid of bathing. Try bathing the person when they are calm. Use the person's preferred bathing method (bath, shower, bed bath). Provide privacy and keep the person warm. Do not rush the person
- Check the environment; for example, a person with **spatial perception** difficulties may interpret a tiled floor as having snakes/worms on it as they may see the lines between the tiles as moving
- Provide oral hygiene
- Choose clothing that is comfortable and simple to put on. Front-opening garments are easy to put on. Jumpers are harder to put on and the person may become frightened when their head is inside the jumper.
- Clothing that closes with Velcro is easy to put on and take off, particularly in the later stages if the person has contractures. Buttons, zippers, snaps and other closures can frustrate the person
- Offer simple clothing choices. Let the person choose between two shirts or blouses, two pants or slacks and so on
- Lay out clothing in the order it will be put on. Hand the person one clothing item at a time. Tell or show the person what to do. Do not rush them
- Have equipment ready for any procedure. This reduces the amount of time the person is involved in care measures
- Observe for signs and symptoms of health problems
- Prevent infection.

BOX 14.5
Care of the person with Alzheimer's disease and other dementias *continued*

Wandering

- Follow centre policy for locking doors and windows. In home settings, locks are often placed at the top or bottom of doors (Fig. 14.6). The person is not likely to look for a lock in such places
- Keep door alarms and electronic doors turned on. The alarm goes off when the door is opened
- Follow centre policy for fire exits. Everyone must be able to leave the building if a fire occurs
- Make sure the person wears a centre identification bracelet at all times if this is a facility policy
- Involve the person in activities – folding napkins, dusting a table, sorting socks, sweeping, sanding blocks of wood or watering plants
- Do not use restraints. Restraints require a doctor's order. They also tend to increase confusion and disorientation
- Do not argue with the person who wants to leave. The person frequently does not understand what you are saying. Distraction can be useful; for example, asking them to complete a task, e.g. sorting towels
- Go with the person who insists on going outside (Fig. 14.7). Make sure they are properly dressed. Guide the person inside after a few minutes
- Let the person wander in enclosed areas (Fig. 14.8). Many residential care services have enclosed areas where people can walk about. They provide a safe place for the person to wander. Make sure, however, they are not overexposed to sun for periods without sunscreen or appropriate fluids intake.

Hallucinations and delusions

- Make sure the person wears glasses or hearing aids as needed. Follow the care plan
- Do not argue with the person
- Reassure the person. Tell them that you will protect them from harm
- Distract the person with some item or activity. Taking the person for a walk may be helpful
- Use touch to calm and reassure the person (Fig. 14.9)
- Eliminate noises that the person could misinterpret. Television, radio, stereos, air conditioners, appliances and other things could affect the person
- Check lighting. Make sure there is no glare, shadows or reflections
- Cover or remove mirrors. The person could misinterpret their reflection.

Sleep

- Follow bedtime rituals
- Use night-lights so the person can see. They may help prevent accidents and disorientation
- Limit caffeine during the day
- Discourage naps during the day. However, during the later stages of dementia they will be sleeping more, especially during the day
- Encourage exercise during the day
- Reduce noises.

Sundowning

- Complete treatments and activities early in the day
- Provide a calm, quiet setting late in the day
- Play soft music
- Do not restrain the person
- Encourage exercise and activity early in the day
- Meet nutrition needs. Hunger can increase restlessness
- Promote elimination. The need to eliminate can increase restlessness
- Do not try to reason with the person. They may not understand what you are saying, although distraction may be helpful
- Ask the person what is bothering them. Communication may be impaired, but at times their answer or actions can indicate their problem.

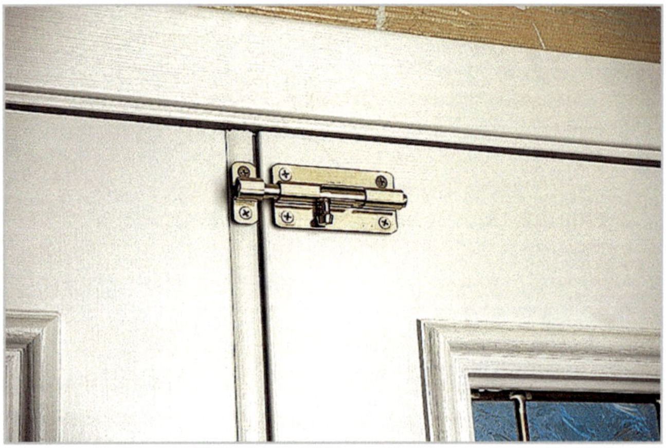

Fig. 14.6
A slide lock is at the top of the door.

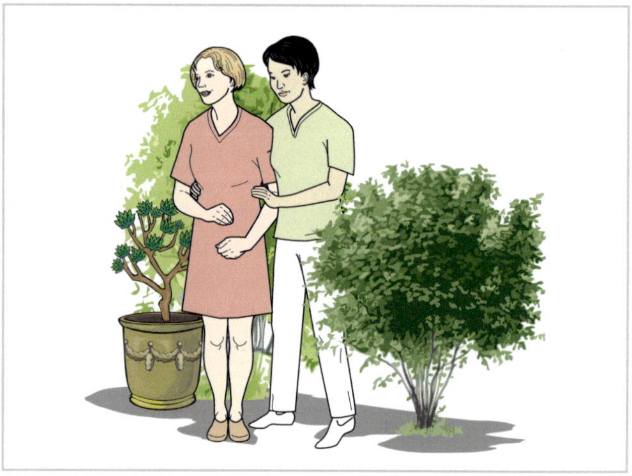

Fig. 14.7
Walk outside with the person who wanders. Then guide the person back inside after a few minutes.

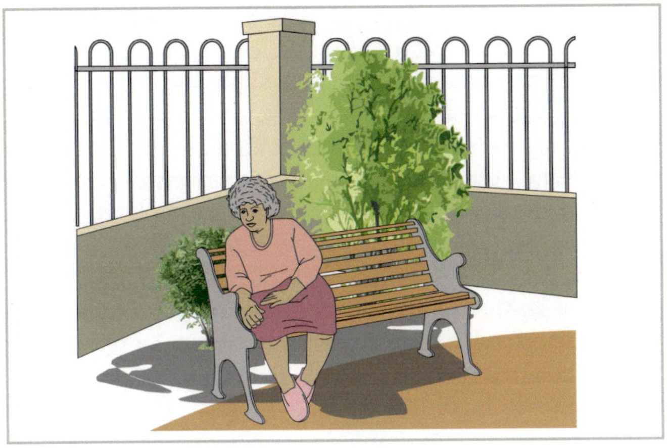

Fig. 14.8
An enclosed garden allows a person with Alzheimer's disease to wander in a safe setting.

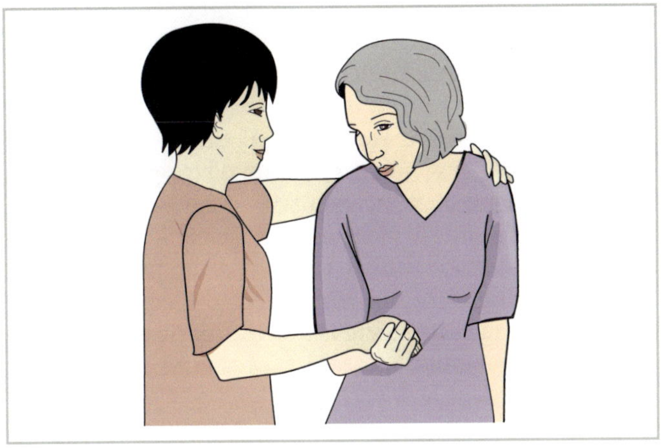

Fig. 14.9
Use touch to calm the person with Alzheimer's disease.

Currently, dementia has no cure and the symptoms worsen over many years. Dementia is a terminal disease. The rate of decline varies from person to person. Eventually, a person with dementia will come to depend on others for all care. Safety, hygiene, nutrition and fluids, elimination and activity needs must be met. So must comfort and sleep needs.

Comfort and safety are important. Good skin care and body alignment prevent skin breakdown and contractures. The carer must take special care to treat the person with dignity and respect. They have the same rights as those who are alert and active. Talk to them in a calm voice and always explain what you are going to do. Massage, soothing touch, music and aromatherapy are comforting and relaxing. Many facilities provide palliative/hospice care as death nears.

The person can have other health problems or injuries. However, they may not know they have pain, fever, constipation, incontinence or other signs and symptoms of illness. Often these issues will be apparent in varying behaviours. For example, often a urinary tract infection or constipation will be manifest with increased agitation or confusion. Carefully observe the person and report any change in the person's usual behaviour to the nurse.

Infection is a major risk. As the person cannot fully tend to self-care, infection can occur from poor hygiene. This includes skin care, oral hygiene and perineal care after bowel and bladder elimination. Inactivity and immobility can cause pneumonia and pressure ulcers.

Aside from physical needs, it is very important that the person feels useful, worthwhile and active. This promotes self-esteem. Diversional therapists and often carers work with one person, a small group or a large group of people with dementia. **Diversional therapies** and activities focus on the person's strengths and past successes. For example:

- a woman used to cook. She helps clean fruit or makes scones.
- a man was a good dancer. Activities are planned so he can dance.
- a woman likes to clean. She helps with dusting.

Supervised activities meet the person's needs and cognitive abilities. The person's interests are considered. Activities are based on what the person can do and what they enjoy. Some people like crafts, exercise, gardening and listening and moving to music. Others like sing-alongs, reminiscing and board games. Some like to string beads, fold towels or roll dough. Massage, range-of-motion exercises and touch are also important therapies. Most of these activities can be carried out by a carer, so be aware of your client's interests and you may be able to provide some meaningful activity that assists in maintaining a quality of life for the person with dementia.

Communication (verbal and non-verbal)

Regardless of what care is being provided, gentle, respectful communication is vital. A study by Ward and colleagues (2008), examining communication in an aged care facility, found:

- on average, each person with dementia spent no more than 2 per cent of the day communicating with a member of staff
- 78 per cent of interactions were concerned with specific care tasks and took place mainly in silence
- where there was verbal input, this was mostly routinised 'carespeak'
- encounters characterised by warmth were infrequent
- much of the behaviours of care staff seemed to avoid rather than encourage communication.

This is a common experience for the person with dementia living in an aged care facility. They are woken up by staff, frequently people they do not recognise. Staff are often focused on their tasks for the day and take no time to explain to the person who they are or what they want the person to do. You need to realise this when dealing with people with dementia or any other memory loss.

Verbal communication, particularly the choice of words when talking to a person with dementia, is important. It is possible to de-identify the person with dementia if the correct words are not used. As a result, language guidelines have been developed by Dementia Australia (2020b). The guidelines acknowledge that for people with dementia to be respected and recognised as an individual, language must be accurate, respectful, inclusive, empowering and non-stigmatising (Dementia Australia 2021). As a result, people with dementia are not referred to as demented, dementia sufferers or senile. These examples are among the many changes in verbal communication considerations for families and people with dementia.

In addition to the power of verbal communication, it is vital to remember that non-verbal communication can potentially be more powerful than verbal communication. As a result, it is important to have consistency in behaviour in order to communicate clearly. It is easy to provide a warm environment with a heart-felt smile. The list below offers more ideas about expressing verbal and non-verbal communication when caring for those who experience Alzheimer's disease.

- Approach the person in a calm, quiet manner.
- Approach the person from the front. Do not approach the person from the side or back, as this can startle them.
- Call the person by name.
- Identify other people by their names. Avoid pronouns (he, she, them and so on).
- Follow the rules of communication.
- Practise measures to promote communication.
- Use gestures or cues. Point to objects.
- Speak in a calm, gentle voice.
- Speak slowly. Use simple words and sentences. However, do not use childish or baby talk.
- Let the person speak. Do not interrupt or rush the person.
- Give the person time to respond.
- Do not criticise, correct or argue with the person.
- Present one idea, question or instruction at a time.
- Ask simple questions with simple answers. Do not ask complex questions.
- Do not present the person with many choices.
- Provide simple explanations of all procedures and activities.
- Give consistent responses.

Focus point: Remember that people with dementia retain their feelings and emotions, even though they may not understand what is being said – so it is important to always maintain their dignity and self-esteem. Your approach when assisting a person with dementia will greatly influence the effectiveness and quality of the interaction.

In addition to using standard good communication strategies that promote dignity and respect of the person with dementia, there are other possible strategies that can be used when communicating with a person with dementia. These include:

- *reminiscence:* the act of remembering and reflecting on previous life experiences, especially those with a personal significance. An example of **reminiscence** is going through a photo album that is full of old pictures, preferably in chronological order, highlighting the significant events and people in the life of the person with dementia. By sitting alongside the person with dementia and asking questions about the photos, they frequently remember one of the photos and will start talking about the event. Often, they re-live the experience in the photo as if it is in the present. Family members can also find this a useful way of communicating as it gives them an opportunity to talk about something they have in common and remember the person as the individual they are.
- *redirection:* the **redirection** of thoughts that are causing distress to something more pleasant and acceptable. An example is when someone wants to go home to mother or tend to their babies. By suggesting a cup of tea or a meal before they go and providing them with a drink and biscuit and an item they are connected to, for example, a book or picture, the 'distraction' is frequently effective. However, you must remember that body language, tone of voice and all non-verbals are important for it to work well. Other techniques that may assist are 'not being able to find' the hat (or favourite shoes) the person always wears when they go outside when they are insisting on going home, and then offering a distraction such as asking them to assist with completion of a task, e.g. putting out the placemats on the table.
- *validation:* this is similar to redirection, where painful or distressing emotions are redirected to less distressing thoughts; however, there is also **validation** or recognition of the emotions being experienced. Ask specific questions about how certain actions or situations make the person with dementia feel. After you receive an explanation of those feelings, validate them with phrases that show your support, such as, 'I'd be upset too, if that happened to me' or 'I understand why you feel that way'.
- *reality orientation:* orienting the person with dementia to where they are in time and their current stage in life has previously been recommended as useful, but it can in fact be detrimental if not done correctly. For example, it is distressing for a person who is looking for their spouse to be told by staff that they died several years ago. For them it is like being told for the first time. They have forgotten, so telling them now feels like it has just happened. This will cause significant distress and feelings of new loss and grief. You must ask yourself: 'What is the benefit to the person with dementia to be reoriented to the present?' If there is no benefit for them, then redirection and/or validation is usually the best for them.
- *using smell:* some of our strongest memories are triggered by odour. A smell can be associated with an event or moment in the past. Anything that has the power to channel reminiscences should be part of the daily life of the person with dementia. The smell of fresh bread or frying bacon can be a powerful trigger for the person and their families to reminisce.

Changed behaviours

Often the person with a dementia exhibits some changed behaviours. These may occur in isolation or in a combination. Changed behaviours can include:

- aggression
- agitation
- anxiety
- depression
- psychotic symptoms
- sleep disturbances
- wandering.

The management of and appropriate interventions to these behaviours will require an assessment process to identify triggers that may contribute to these behaviours. The more thoroughly the person is assessed for causes of the behaviour, the more likely it is that any interventions, psychosocial and/or pharmacological, will be appropriate. Managing these behaviours depends totally on the triggers.

Some management techniques may include:

- distraction
- diversion
- a peaceful environment
- music
- exercise
- avoidance of identified triggers
- appropriate levels of light
- reassurance with familiar objects
- family support
- noise and crowd reduction
- socialisation
- modification of the environment.

The family

The person with dementia may live at home or with children or other family members. Family members in the household give care or someone stays with the person. Healthcare is sought to provide assistance to the family to meet the person's needs. Home care and adult respite care are options. If you are caring for someone in the community, it is possible for the family to have some time out, or respite, via the home and community care options in both Australia and New Zealand, which support families. Respite care can be provided on a regular basis, even if only for a few hours per week. A designated carer will come to the family home and provide all necessary care to relieve the family of their responsibilities. In addition, family members can also access respite, usually in a residential facility, where the person with dementia has 'a holiday' for a week or two at a time, allowing a break for the carer from their carer duties.

As dementia progresses, long-term care may be required. It is usually needed when:

- family members cannot meet the person's needs
- the person no longer knows the carer
- family members have health problems
- money problems occur
- the person's behaviour presents a danger to the person or others.

Diagnostic tests, doctors' visits, medications and home care are costly. So is long-term care. The person's medical care can drain the family finances. As well as the person with dementia, the family also has specific needs. Caring for the person at home or in a residential care service is stressful. There are physical, emotional, social and financial stresses. Children are the 'sandwich' generation, as they are caught between their own children who need attention and an ill parent who needs care. Caring for two families is stressful. Often adult children also have jobs.

Family carers can suffer from anger, anxiety, depression and sleeplessness. In fact, **care-giver burden** is a recognised term used to describe the negative effects that many people experience as a direct result of constantly caring for someone at home. Some cannot concentrate or are irritable. They can develop health problems and need to take care of their own health. A healthy diet, exercise and plenty of rest are needed. Asking for help is important. The carer needs to be able to ask family and friends for help. Carer burnout is a significant problem for family members who care for a person with dementia in the community. This can result in significant depression and other health issues. Adequate respite care for them away from caring activities is essential (Hiyoshi-Taniguchi et al 2018).

Carers need much support and encouragement. Many join Alzheimer's disease support groups. Dementia Australia has a number of branches, providing a vast network of support groups around both Australia and New Zealand (see web links at the end of the chapter). It offers confidential counselling, workshops and information sessions. Support groups offer encouragement and advice. People in similar situations share their feelings, anger, frustration, guilt and other emotions. They also share coping and care-giving ideas. Online peer support groups are also an invaluable source of support, as caregivers can discuss with their peers similar issues and offer relevant advice.

The family often feels helpless. No matter what is done, the person only gets worse. Much time, money, energy and emotion are needed to care for the person. Anger and resentment may result, and feelings of guilt are very common, particularly in family members who were caring for them at home and can no longer continue to do so. The family knows that the person did not choose the disease or its signs, symptoms and behaviours, but sometimes behaviours are embarrassing. The family may be upset and angry that the loved one cannot show love or affection. Too often the effect that dementia has upon families, and specifically those caring for the person, is overlooked by the healthcare team.

Families are an important part of the health team. And can add considerable insight into understanding the person with dementia. They help plan the person's care whenever possible. Some take part in centre activities. For many people, family members provide comfort. They also need support and understanding from the health team. Too often the healthcare team overlook the expertise that family members have regarding care, preferences and interventions that do/do not work for the person with dementia.

The relationship between family members and healthcare professionals is very important and can benefit everyone. Communication strategies, such as reminiscence using a photo album of old pictures, for example, can be very helpful to the family member when they come to visit their loved one in an aged care facility.

The following poem was written by Anna Greening, a woman caring for her father with dementia. Within this poem she shares with us her observations of her father's decline as his dementia progresses.

ON THE WRONG FEET

Where did you go, Dad, where did you go?
When did your hair turn as white as fresh snow?
When did your spine cease to hold you upright?
When did your teeth start to come out at night?

Where did you go, Dad, when did it start?
It gradually crept in and pulled you apart
The talking in riddles, the anger, the fear
The volume up full blast yet still you can't hear.

Constantly losing things, ever distressed,
Putting your shirt on but under your vest,
Sitting in silence you stare into space,
Utter confusion so plain on your face.

Shuffling in slippers both on the wrong feet,
Wanting to know if it's soon time to eat?
Calling my name when I go out of sight,
Wandering around in the dead of the night.

No more enjoyment in watching TV,
No crossword, no reading. How bored you must be?
The days are so long, and you don't know the date,
You don't know the time, but you fear it's too late.

You've physically withered, your frailty is clear,
I'm crying inside, but I can't shed a tear.
Your tongue is so sharp it cuts deep as a knife
Harsh words from the man who gave me my life.

I know you don't mean it, you're terribly ill,
And you can't be cured by a prayer or a pill.
You'd always told me 'that life was unfair'
And I tell you what, Dad, you're bloody right there!

Where did you go, Dad, where did you go?
Wherever you are now there's one thing I know,
I'll be by your side through your sad misadventure
You won't be alone in your fight with dementia.

Anna Greening

Dementia-specific facilities

A number of facilities have dementia-specific units. Staff in these units are usually specially trained and the physical environments have been designed to meet the care needs of people with dementia. These units are secured. This means that entrances and exits are locked. People in these units have a safe setting to move about in and cannot wander away. Some people have aggressive behaviours that disrupt or threaten others, and they may need a secured unit. The units usually have a general environment conducive to people with dementia, often featuring walls painted in calming colours and equipment that may help distract clients should they become restless. This eliminates the need for any other form of restraint.

Approval for residential care through an NSAF (National Screening and Assessment Form) assessment is necessary for residential care in Australia, whether it be for low care, high care or dementia-specific care. In New Zealand, a gerontological review in conjunction with the Needs Assessment team will determine the level of care required, whether it is rest home level of care, hospital level of care or dementia. The person's rights are always protected.

At some point, the secured unit is no longer needed for safe care. For example, the person's condition progresses from moderate to severe stage. The person cannot sit or walk and is in bed. As wandering is no longer a concern, the person is usually transferred to another unit that specialises in 'high' care and is equipped with lifting hoists, etc.

The Aged Care Standards and Accreditation Agency has standards that are required to be met for residential and community care. Staff must have training in the care of people with dementia. Residential and community care centres must have programs that promote dignity, personal freedom and safety.

Dementia-friendly communities

In recognition of the increasing number of people with dementia and the importance of remaining within the general community for as long as possible, there has been an increased focus on ensuring communities in general are dementia-friendly. There are at least 13 countries (Lin & Lewis 2015) involved in developing dementia-friendly communities. According to Dementia Australia (2020a), 'A **dementia-friendly community** is a place where people living with dementia are supported to live a high quality of life with meaning, purpose and value'. There are a number of resources available for individuals, businesses, community groups and politicians to provide guidance on enhancing communities to a level that is dementia-friendly. Overall, dementia-friendly communities consider physical and social environments to promote inclusiveness and knowledge for health and community support service providers.

SELF-REFLECTION

Imagine the following scenario:

You are in a deep sleep when suddenly you are woken up by a person you don't know. They look as if they are in a great hurry and say something to you so quickly you don't understand it. They wave their hands around and then walk off, talking as they go. You lie in bed bewildered as you look around and have no idea where you are or how you got there. Suddenly the hurried looking person returns. She walks very briskly towards you, now looking cross, and quickly rips the blankets and sheet off the bed as she waves her arms around again. You stand up and start to follow, but you are afraid. You ask yourself: 'Where am I? Who is this? Where am I going?'

Now imagine experiencing this every day, over and over again. How would you feel?

FOCUS ON COMMUNITY CARE

Communication among health team members is needed. You may be required to give care to a client within the community who has early onset dementia. It is possible that your client may forget who you are between visits, even if you have been assisting with their care for a considerable period of time. It is important, therefore, to always introduce yourself when you arrive at the client's home. Always return your client's items to the same place each time, as they may become upset if they cannot find them after you have left.

There may be times when your client offers you a gift or small memento for giving care. Never take the item, as they may not remember having given it to you later, and be concerned as to where it has gone. If they insist and become upset at your refusal to accept the gift, advise your supervisor immediately. Your supervisor may suggest that you bring the item to the office and then have the family collect it, or perhaps leave the item in a safe place within the client's home.

Always observe your client carefully and report any signs of increasing dementia to your supervisor.

CASE STUDY

You have been assigned the care of Shane Worthington, an elderly man in his 80s with Alzheimer's disease. He is living at home and is cared for by his 83-year-old wife, who is experiencing significant stress related to his behaviours, especially when she tries to shower him. Last week she requested that his hygiene care be attended to by your community service due to his increasing resistance.

While you are preparing Shane for his morning shower, you notice that his wife is agitated and short-tempered with him. Therefore, so as not to increase the stress levels in the household, you decide to lead by example and demonstrate some of your communication techniques. During the shower you remain calm and give Shane a face washer of his own while you take your time to give Shane a nice back rub. He enjoys this and displays his happiness with a smile and seems to start relaxing. You provide lots of conversation with Shane, asking what football code and team he follows, and continue to chat as you wash his hair, covering his face with a washcloth to prevent too much water going over his face. Once the shower is finished you offer him a towel, which he continually rubs on his stomach while you dry the rest of him. Once dry, you hand him his clothes one at a time and provide him with assistance to put them on, gently prompting him as necessary; for example, helping him place his singlet over his head and providing the arm holes for him to see where to put his arms. You continue general conversation as you use the electric shaver to give him a shave and he combs his hair once all is done.

After the shower you assist Shane to sit in the living room with his wife, who has prepared a pot of tea for everyone. Shane's wife is surprised that he hasn't 'put on a turn', and that he seemed to actually enjoy his shower. At this point you find it appropriate to share some of your successful experiences when caring for people with dementia. Shane's wife is particularly interested in the fact that you did not voice step-by-step instructions throughout the shower, but rather 'just got on with it' while engaging him with conversation. Shane's wife is very pleased with this approach and acknowledges your calm nature. She looks forward to having you back soon. You leave feeling satisfied that you have developed a therapeutic rapport with the family and have paved the way for future guidance as needed.

QUALITY OF LIFE

Quality of life is important for all people with confusion and dementia. They may not know or be able to exercise their rights. However, the family know the person's rights and want those rights protected. They want respect and dignity for their loved one. As each person experiences dementia in their own individual way, you can help the person to make the best use of their particular skills and abilities as their condition changes. Be flexible in adapting activities, by encouragement, reassurance and common-sense measures.

People with dementia should be encouraged to communicate in whatever way seems most appropriate. To help preserve their sense of identity and improve their quality of life, activities that they enjoy should be encouraged. Also, seek ways to help the person you are caring for cope with memory problems, so that they can retain their confidence and independence for as long as possible.

The person has the right to privacy and confidentiality. Protect the person from exposure. Only those involved in the person's care are present for care and procedures. The person is allowed to have visitors in private. Space is provided for a private visit. Do not share information about the person's care and condition with others. Ensure that you only provide information to the next of kin or those who hold the enduring Power of Attorney. People with dementia can also have physical health problems and other mental illnesses, including depression. If neglected, these conditions can make the dementia worse and have a severely negative effect on the person's quality of life.

Personal choice is important. If possible, simple choices are encouraged. For example, a person chooses to wear a dress or slacks. Watching or not watching television may be a simple choice; however, caution must be taken with the types of programs available for watching by the person with dementia. The family makes choices if the person cannot. They choose bath times, menus, clothing, activities and other care. Even something as simple as making sure the right glasses and hearing aids are prescribed can make a striking difference.

The person has the right to keep and use personal items. Some items provide comfort. A pillow, blanket, rug or jumper may have meaning. The person may not know why or even recognise the item. Still, it is important. Personal items are kept safe. Protect the person's property from loss or damage.

People must be kept free from abuse, mistreatment and neglect. Caring for a person with confusion and dementia is often very frustrating and some behaviours are hard to deal with. Family and staff can become short-tempered and angry. Protect the person from abuse and report any signs of abuse to the nurse at once. Be patient and calm when caring for people with dementia. Talk with the nurse if you are becoming upset. Sometimes assignment changes are needed for a while.

All people have the right to be free from restraints. Restraints require a doctor's order and are used only if it is the best way to protect the person. They are not used for staff convenience. Restraints can make confused and demented behaviours worse. See Chapter 3 on legalities in the workplace for further information.

Activity and a safe setting promote quality of life. The person needs activities that are safe, calm and quiet. The recreational therapist and other health team members will find activities that are best for each person. These are part of the person's care plan.

ACCREDITATION

You are working in residential or home care and accreditors are at your service. Can you answer the following questions?

- What can you do as a carer to minimise the use of physical restraints?
- A person you are caring for is living with dementia and has moderate cognitive impairment. Give some strategies on how you would communicate with this person.
- How can an unmet need lead to aggressive behaviours, in those living with dementia?

REVIEW QUESTIONS

Circle T if the answer is true, or F if the answer is false:

1 T / F Confusion is a normal part of the ageing process.

2 T / F Everyone over the age of 80 years old gets dementia.

3 T / F Delirium is the start of dementia and can't be stopped.

4 T / F Dehydration can cause confusion that is easily fixed with fluids.

5 T / F Everyone with depression will eventually get dementia.

6 T / F People with Alzheimer's disease have the ability to plan behaviours to annoy their carer.

Circle the BEST answer:

7 Dementia is:

- a a condition of the brain that people wake up with one morning
- b a progressive decline of cognitive and social function due to changes in the brain
- c contagious to people who work in a dementia unit long-term
- d a result of long-term depression.

8 A person is confused after surgery. The confusion is likely to be:

- a permanent
- b temporary
- c intermittent
- d an indication of early dementia

9 Joe Dunn was diagnosed with Alzheimer's disease. Which of the following is true?

- a It occurs only in older people.
- b Diet and medications can stop the disease.
- c Alzheimer's disease and confusion are the same.
- d It is the most common form of dementia.

10 Which of the following is not common in people with Alzheimer's disease?

- a Memory loss, poor judgement and sleep problems
- b Loss of impulse control and poor communication
- c Wandering, delusions and hallucinations
- d Paralysis and pain

Answers to these questions are on p. 454.

References

Australian Bureau of Statistics (2017). Australian leading causes of death 2016. Online 7 October. Available: www.abs.gov.au/ausstats/abs@.nsf/Lookup/by%20Subject/3303.0~2016~Main%20Features~Australia%27s%20leading%20causes%20of%20death,%202016~3

Australian Institute of Health and Welfare (AIHW) 2021. Deaths in Australia 2019. Online 7 October 2021. Available: www.aihw.gov.au/reports/life-expectancy-death/deaths-in-australia/contents/leading-causes-of-death

Alzheimer's Association (2021). Parkinson's disease dementia. Online 8 October 2021. Available: www.alz.org/alzheimers-dementia/what-is-dementia/types-of-dementia/parkinson-s-disease-dementia

Alzheimers New Zealand (2021). Supporting someone. Online 7 October 2021. Available: alzheimers.org.nz/get-support/supporting-someone-with-dementia/

Brown L, Hansnata E, La H-A (2017). Economic cost of dementia in Australia 2016–2056. National Centre for Social and Economic Modelling (NATSEM), Canberra.

Dementia Australia (2021). Dementia statistics. Online 7 October. Available: www.dementia.org.au/statistics

Dementia Australia (2020a). Dementia-friendly communities. Online 7 October 2021 Available: www.dementia.org.au/resources/dementia-friendly-communities

Dementia Australia (2020b). Language guidelines. Online 7 October 2021 Available: www.dementia.org.au/resources/dementia-language-guidelines

Dementia Australia (2020c). Vascular dementia. Online 8 October 2021 Available: www.dementia.org.au/about-dementia/types-of-dementia/vascular-dementia

Dementia Australia (2018). Dementia prevalence data 2018–2058, NATSEM, University of Canberra. Online 7 October. Available: www.dementia.org.au/sites/default/files/documents/2018-2058_Dementia_prevalence_ST_1.pdf

Dementia Care Central (2020). Stages of Alzheimer's and dementia: durations and scales used to measure progression (GDS, FAST & CDR). Online 27 October 2021. Available: www.dementiacarecentral.com/aboutdementia/facts/stages

de Vugt ME & Verhey FR (2013). The impact of early dementia diagnosis and intervention on informal caregivers. Progress in Neurobiology 110:54–62.

Ellen M, Demaio P, Wilson M (2017). Adult day center programs and their associated outcomes on clients, caregivers, and the health system: a scoping review. The Gerontologist 57(6):e85–e94.

Fazio S, Pace D, Flinner J et al (2018). The fundamentals of person-centered care for individuals with dementia. The Gerontologist 58(suppl 1):S10–S19.

Hayo H (2015). Diagnosis and support for younger people with dementia. Nursing Standard 29(47):36–40.

Hiyoshi-Taniguchi K, Becker C, Kinoshita A (2018). What behavioural and psychological symptoms of dementia affect caregiver burnout? Clinical Gerontologist 41(3):249–254.

Lin S-Y, Lewis FM (2015). Dementia friendly, dementia capable, and dementia positive: concepts to prepare for the future. Gerontologist 55(2):237–244.

Scott TL, Kugelman M, Tulloch K (2019). How medical professional students view older people with dementia: Implications for education and practice. PLOS ONE. Online 26 October 2021. Available: https://doi.org/10.1371/journal.pone.0225329

The Australian Frontotemporal Dementia Association (2020). About FTD. Online 8 October 2021. Available: https://theaftd.org.au/about-afd/

The Lewy Body Society (2021). Symptoms. Online 7 October 2021. Available: www.lewybody.org/about-lbd/symptoms/

Ward R, Vass AA, Aggarwal N et al (2008). A different story: Exploring patterns of communication in residential dementia care, Ageing and Society 28(5):629–651.

World Health Organisation (WHO) (2021). Dementia key facts. Online 14 March 2021. Available: www.who.int/mediacentre/factsheets/fs362/en/

CHAPTER 15
Working with older clients with a disability

By Tara Kent

AFTER READING THIS CHAPTER, YOU SHOULD BE ABLE TO:

- define the key terms listed in this chapter
- identify issues affecting the older person with a disability
- identify the role of the Public Guardian
- identify lifestyle options
- have an understanding of the health issues for the elderly person with a disability
- know the importance of treating the person, not the disability
- speak in a manner that reflects respect and puts the person before the disability.

Key terms

acquired brain injury: Any type of brain damage that occurs after birth, which may occur due to infection, disease, head injury or lack of oxygen

autism spectrum disorder: Autism is a type of neurodiversity, which means the person experiences the world differently to an allistic person (person without autism). Autism can affect a person's speech, sensory processing and information processing. Autistic individuals prefer 'identity-first' language, which means you refer to them as an 'autistic person', not a 'person with autism'.

cognitive disability: A range of clinical diagnoses, including Down Syndrome, intellectual impairment, acquired or traumatic brain injury, some types of cerebral palsy and any other impairment that affects the cognitive capacity of the person.

National Disability Insurance Scheme (NDIS): The NDIS was set up to provide all Australians under 65 with a permanent disability reasonable support for themselves, their family and their carers.

polypharmacy: Using more than one medication to manage a health issue of an individual

Public Guardian: A statutory appointed substitute decision-maker for individuals with impaired capacity, subject to the provisions of the Guardianship and Administration Acts within the legislation of each individual state and territory

Queensland Civil and Administrative Tribunal (QCAT): An independent tribunal that actively resolves disputes in a way that is fair, just, accessible, quick and inexpensive. QCAT makes decisions on a range of matters for the first time (original decisions) and reviews decisions previously made by government agencies and statutory authorities

Supported independent living (SIL): This arrangement began with the NDIS; a situation where a small group of people live together and use their combined funds to ensure that there is sufficient access to support workers to meet their needs. This replaced the former SAU model.

When we care for the older person they will sometimes have a disability. This may have been present at birth – congenital – or have occurred across their lifespan – acquired. When caring for an older person with a disability it is important that we see that person as a whole person and not just as a 'disability'.

PRIMARY ISSUES AFFECTING INDIVIDUALS WITH A DISABILITY WHO ARE ELDERLY

Altered living situations and decreased functional ability and deterioration of mobility

As a person with a disability ages, at times their strategies for managing their disability may need to change. For example, the person who has been dependent on a wheelchair for mobility all their life may find they have increasing difficulty transferring to and from the wheelchair as they age. A loss of some muscle tone due to ageing may have left them with insufficient strength to manage these transfers unaided.

In some situations the ageing process, coupled with peripheral health and wellbeing issues, decreased carer capacity and varying daily interests, can lead to the need to make changes to the person's primary place of residence. In some situations this results in renovations being made to accommodate needs related to ageing, such as:

- reduced eyesight
- decreased mobility (Fig. 15.1)
- failing memory
- increased nutritional requirements
- altered, sometimes decreased functional ability
- confusion due to dementia or other cognitive impairment.

The complexity of this process is that any changes made to the residence need to also accommodate any other residents and must be within the financial limitations of the individual and their service provider. In some situations, the person may not own the property and the decision to renovate may fall to the service provider, other residents or family. One of the most common changes to arise as a person with a disability ages is to question the appropriateness of their current accommodation. Many supported independent living arrangements and large residential services are designed to consider the common interests of residents. For this reason, when people age, there is sometimes a subsequent effect upon the household and the support required. The elderly individual may no longer enjoy participating in the activities that all other residents have collectively enjoyed, yet without their participation the paid support may not be adequate to enable the activity to continue, and this could result in the other residents missing out. This type of issue contributes to the entire household being forced to live the lifestyle of the aged person, rather than just the person who is ageing. For this reason, the best option is to find a more suitable living situation that meets the changing needs of the ageing individual.

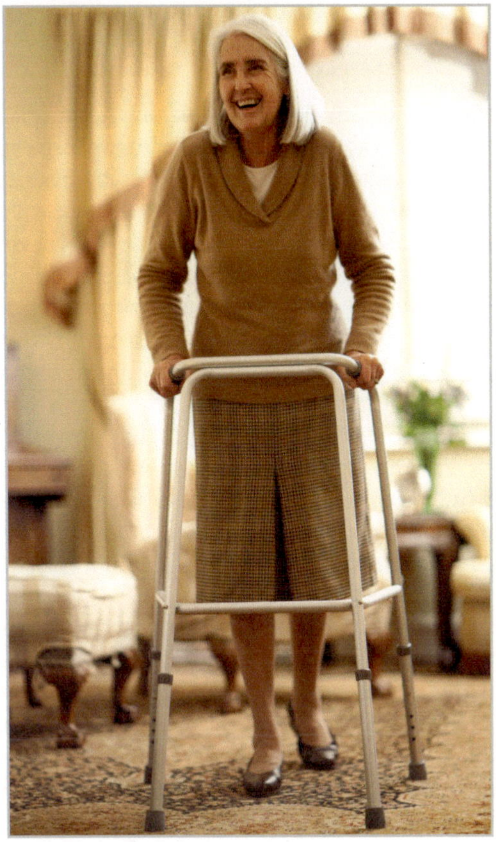

Fig. 15.1
Mobilising with a walking frame.

Options available to the person at this time are:

- to continue living in the current situation, with increased support (if available)
- to relocate to a larger residential facility with access to additional support from allied health professionals, increased staff and more frequent access by visiting medical practitioners
- to relocate to a nursing home that is aimed at supporting elderly individuals without an intellectual impairment, aside from those with cognitive impairments and cognitive disabilities that may occur to the aged person
- to move into a housing arrangement with family and/or a member of the individual's support network (if available).

These options require change to occur and can be traumatic to the individual. Increased funded support is not historically an accessible option to many, due to the limited funding available by the relevant government department and the complicated application process to access any increase to support. Within Australia, the **National Disability Insurance Scheme (NDIS)** is being rolled out across the country to support those with a disability and their families.

Different, sometimes increased, medical testing

As we age, our health decreases and our functional ability and mobility also show signs of deterioration. In anticipation of such health issues, medical practitioners recommend increased diagnostic testing to detect many age-related illnesses. For this reason, people with a disability who are ageing often have to endure increased tests and maintain frequent communication with their medical practitioner as they age. As discussed later in this chapter, there are various health issues that are more prevalent in people with a disability, alongside the health complications that affect all ageing people, including those with a disability. For this reason, vigilance is necessary when supporting individuals to receive appropriate healthcare to ensure a timely, proactive response to both the physiological issues relevant to their disability and the general issues associated with ageing.

One of the complexities associated with increased medical testing is the difficulty in supporting individuals to undergo the sometimes intrusive testing required to diagnose and treat various health issues. It is often necessary for a comprehensive health plan to be established and agreed to by all stakeholders, including the family or decision-maker for the individual, their doctor, their support service and any allied health practitioners involved. It is ideal for the social worker of the local hospital to be involved, as they are often able to negotiate multidisciplinary outcomes that are not apparent to those not directly involved in the hospital operation. In some situations, it has been necessary to liaise with the ambulance to enable a 'twilight' anaesthetic to be used for the trip from their residence to the hospital. This has been necessary in situations when the person requiring the medical treatment has a high likelihood of showing their fear through aggressive and potentially harmful behaviour.

- *Blood tests:* These require needles, which sometimes necessitate the use of force to encourage the person to remain still for testing. In some situations, the person needs to be chemically sedated to undergo certain medical testing, due to their fear and trepidation about the proposed procedure. In other situations, the nurses and/or support persons may need to physically support the person in such a way that they are unable to move while the needle is being inserted. Depending on how this is actioned, it may be determined to fall within the 'reasonable force' provisions of the Guardianship and Administration Acts or other relevant legislation from each state or territory. However, this is not the norm and many older people with a disability are as compliant as those who do not have a disability.
- *X-ray:* This often requires a person to lie down or stand perfectly still for a period of time to enable a radiographer to take a picture. Many people with a disability may be scared, feel threatened or are physically unable to stay still due to physiological complications of impairments such as cerebral palsy. Some people with an intellectual impairment, such as a **cognitive disability**, **acquired brain injury** or a neurodiversity such as **autism spectrum disorder (ASD)**, may demonstrate signs of being terrified of such procedures and blatantly refuse to undergo such treatment. For this reason, it may not be possible to perform such a test unless the person is sedated.
- *Ultrasound:* Similar to an X-ray, this type of test requires a person to lie down fairly still and have a wet gel placed on their body and pressure applied for the purposes of diagnosing internal complications. If the person undergoing this type of test is uncomfortable about the type of test being performed, or does not trust the radiographer performing the test, they are likely to not comply. Lack of compliance with such tests results in the inability to perform the test.
- *Colonoscopy and/or endoscopy:* These tests are highly intrusive and require sedation of some sort for most people, regardless of disability. However, people with intellectual impairments are most likely to require heightened sedation due to the potential trauma associated with their understanding of the presence of the tool used to perform the tests.
- *Medical check-up/general examination:* Depending on the relationship between the individual and the doctor, the success of having a thorough medical check-up can vary for each person. A check-up can involve blood pressure testing, requiring a tight cuff to be placed around the person's arm, a thermometer used to check temperature and physical manipulation to ascertain any internal injuries. In some situations, there might need to be significant preparation done to ensure the person receiving the examination is well informed about what might happen, what the doctor might ask and how certain things might feel.

In order to support people with disabilities to attend and participate in these examinations and/or diagnostic tests, it is important for support staff to:

- communicate effectively and consistently with the people they are supporting
- ensure that the medical practitioners have received all information they have requested and have the appropriate support to communicate with their patient
- use augmentative communication tools, such as pictures and social stories, to enable the person to understand what is expected of them and what might happen at the appointment
- have an 'exit strategy' in place to enable a quick and rapid termination of the appointment if necessary
- have the decision-maker informed prior to the appointment to enable a fast response to any decisions required, thus avoiding any further delays for the person
- ensure the medical practitioner is informed of the person's general capacity to manage complex medical testing and discuss possible contingency plans with the individual, their family or decision-maker, the medical practitioner and, if possible, the social worker of the hospital (if applicable).

DECISION-MAKING AND DECREASED CARER CAPACITY

Working with families and ageing carers

Factors such as whether the person with a disability has lived with their family or in a residential facility will contribute to varying degrees of dependence with their family members, friends and informal carers. Research indicates that 37 per cent more residents of group homes who have lived with family until middle age will have a family member take on a caring role in their life, compared to those who have lived the majority of their life in an institution.

Family relationships affect people with disabilities in a variety of ways, as the family may take on the roles of:

- providing emotional support
- providing physical support
- being someone to talk to
- taking the person to doctor and medical appointments
- helping to manage money
- providing social support and linking the person to the extended family and associated family functions.

A significant issue acknowledged in Queensland is the declining capacity of carers to provide support to their loved ones. A lifetime of advocacy, physical exertion and emotional support is leading to an increase in the exhaustion rates of carers. Some incorporated associations exist to support carers through the provisions of small emergency grants to enable respite, house-cleaning and other avenues of support that might provide the person and their family with some options regarding carer support.

A key issue for organisations and support workers is how to best support and facilitate the continued relationship between families and their loved one with a disability, without leading to an intrusion that places the service's needs above the family's natural authority to work towards solutions together. Service organisations have struggled to work out the parameters of this relationship (Fig. 15.2). Workbooks and questionnaires have been developed to encourage support staff to keep family members informed and develop frameworks of understanding regarding matters such as:

- how often the family member would like to be consulted and/or informed regarding matters affecting their loved one
- whether or not the family member wants to attend and/or organise all medical appointments, or if they would prefer to only be informed regarding outcomes?
- if there are any regular (e.g. weekly, fortnightly, monthly etc.) family gatherings that the person would like to attend, and, if so, what level of support is required to facilitate their participation?
- if there are any cultural, religious or spiritual requirements and/or norms that the service provider could support the person to maintain/practise?

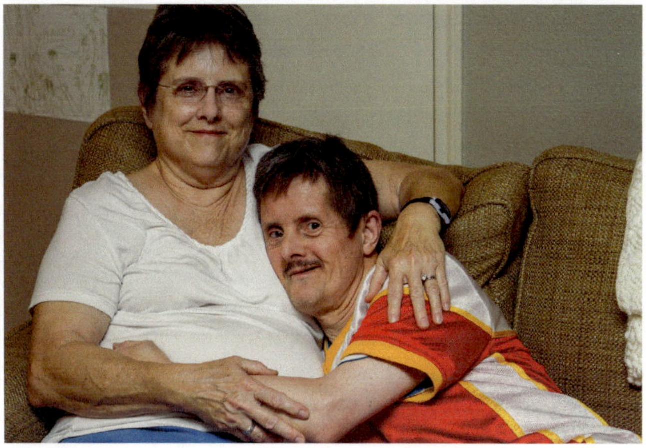

Fig. 15.2
Finding the best way to support older disabled adults is a key issue for organisations and support workers.

- whether or not the family member would like to be invited on a regular basis to the person's residence, or if they are happy to turn up at times suitable to them without invitation?
- when the family member visits the residential facility, would they like to be given private time with their loved one, or would they prefer support staff to remain with them and provide them with assistance when needed?
- the level of involvement (generally) the family wants and how this involvement is best maintained
- the best way to contact the family, to include and involve them: email, phone notifications or text messages?

Guardianship, and substitute decision-making

In some situations, individuals who don't have the capacity to make decisions require a substitute decision-maker. Ideally, this role is performed by a member of their family or informal support network, if there is someone who is willing and able to do so. In many situations there is either dispute within the family or no appropriate able or willing person to be responsible for decision-making. Each state or territory has an appropriate body that is able to manage these situations. For example, in Queensland it is the role of the **Queensland Civil and Administrative Tribunal (QCAT)** to make a determination regarding:

- whether a decision-maker is required
- if a decision-maker is required, for which matters the decision-maker is required
- who is the most appropriate person to make these decisions
- how long this person should be appointed as decision maker (Queensland Government 2021).

In situations where the appropriate state/territory body decides that there is no person in the individual's support network who is both willing and able to make decisions for them, this body may determine that the role of decision-maker will fall to a legally appointed decision-maker. All states and territories have statutory-appointed individuals with similar but slightly different roles. In Queensland this position is referred to as the **Public Guardian**. The Public Guardian is the decision-maker of last resort. Once appointed, the Public Guardian (or similar) is generally bound by the *Public Guardian Act* and/or the *Guardianship and Administration Act* of each state/territory to make decisions for the person.

It is considered best practice by the legally appointed guardian to always consult with family members, friends and any other informal support networks, medical practitioners and associated parties for an adult. However, they are not legally obliged to do so and their decisions can be made without such consultation if they have reasons to believe that this would be in the best interests of the adult for whom they have been made the appointed decision-maker.

LIFESTYLE OPTIONS

Residential aged care

Residential aged care is the name given to a large facility that houses numerous people who are ageing, with the purpose of meeting diverse health and lifestyle requirements, subsequently employing or contracting out the expertise of visiting medical practitioners, as well as allied health practitioners, including speech pathologists, physiotherapists, nurses and occupational therapists. The intention of such establishments is to provide a one-stop shop to people who are ageing to enable them to access diverse specialist services from their own home and have support staff and nurses readily available to them.

'Over 4500 people under 65 years of age live in residential care in Australia, and they experience poorer quality of life than people with similar disabilities in other settings' (Brown et al 2021). Aged care environments were never designed for young people; however, Australia has observed a significant shortage in suitable and appropriate accommodation options for young people with disability. As a result of this, numerous young people with disability have been housed in aged care environments out of necessity, due to a lack of other more appropriate options. Aged care residential facilities are staffed with skilled staff who are able to provide support to people with complex support needs and have therefore been considered a reasonable option in absence of few other available options. However, young people living in aged care environments have been the subject of considerable advocacy, as these environments are largely unsuitable to most young people and place a focus on health and care, rather than lifestyle and enjoyment. This has been recognised as an issue for many Australians and a variety of state and federal initiatives have highlighted this issue and strategised methods of responding to it in such a manner that aged care is not used for younger people with disability.

The NDIS has made a considerable impact in this space and provided a lot of alternative options to many participants who had no access to support before (Brown et al 2021). The NDIS promoted access to supported independent living (SIL) options, as well as specialist disability accommodation (SDA) options in response to the issues regarding service and appropriate housing shortages.

Further to this, the Younger People in Residential Aged Care Strategy 2020–2025 was put in place in response to the Royal Commission into Aged Care Quality and Safety and has set standards which are designed to reduce and limit the presence of younger people in aged care environments.

The benefits to living in residential aged care for a person with a disability who is elderly are:

- increased access to specialist health services
- ongoing monitoring and support from health professionals
- access to peers and planned social opportunities
- focus upon health implications of the elderly to enable better response times to likely issues
- an implemented routine
- access to friends and family for visitation (Fig. 15.3).

The potential difficulties and/or limitations are:

- regimented routine, which may be vastly different to the regimented routine the person has spent their last 50 years doing
- minimal focus on the specific necessities of disability-related health issues
- minimal understanding of the unique communication mechanisms of many people with disabilities
- residential aged care is based on a care model primarily, as compared to a lifestyle model, which is regarded as best practice in the disability sector
- the pace in residential aged care is often very different from the pace of a supported independent living arrangement aimed at people with a disability
- residential aged care services have significant similarities with hospital-type environments, which can be quite traumatic to people with a disability who are scared of or apprehensive about hospitals

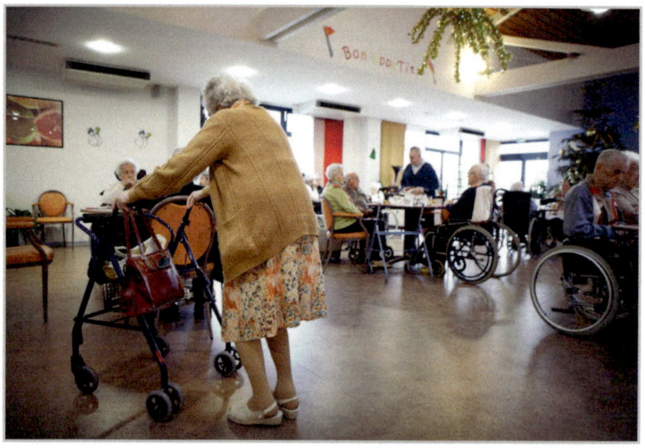

Fig. 15.3
A residential aged care facility can provide many benefits to older disabled residents.

- for those who are neurodiverse, such as those who are autistic or ADHD (attention deficit hyperactivity disorder), the change may be very difficult and they may find the aged care residential environment much noisier, with more people around them, making it very difficult to manage from a sensory perspective.

Supported independent living

Supported independent living (SIL) environments are living arrangements where between two and five people share a house in the community. The compatibility of residents is often linked to the funded support they each have access to and the subsequent merging of funded support for the purpose of enabling 24 hours per day, 7 days per week ('24/7') support from paid support workers.

SIL environments were created with the introduction of the NDIS. The NDIS provides the opportunity for each person to have an NDIS Plan which provides them with a certain amount of funds to use in certain categories of their lives. This can include:

- *Core Supports:* This funding is provided to pay for support workers, as well as consumable items such as incontinence aids, gloves and kylies (plastic-coated sheets to protect beds and chairs). Other items which can be billed from the Core Support category include transport, cleaning, gardening and home maintenance. There is also capacity for low cost assistive technology to be purchased from this category in some people's NDIS plans.
- *Capacity Building Supports:* This funding is for therapists or any initiatives which help the person build their skills and increase their capacity. Any allied health providers, such as speech and language pathologists and occupational therapists, are paid for under this category of funds. People who require specialised behaviour support will often have funding called 'Improved Relationships' funding within this category to meet those needs.
- *Capital Supports:* This category of funding allows the person to make capital purchases of items considered reasonable and necessary due to disability. Capital Supports has two sub categories of funding including:
  - assistive technology
  - home modifications.

  In most situations, quotes will be required for purchases to be made regarding capital supports. This is usually detailed on the person's NDIS plan (NDIS 2021).

Generally, NDIS funding will not continue once a person moves into an aged care environment; however there are many exceptions to this (general) rule. From December 2020, providers who are supporting residents using an NDIS package must also be registered as a provider with the NDIS (Australian Government, Aged Care Quality and Safety Commission 2021). This means that these providers are obliged to be registered with the Commonwealth NDIS framework, as well as the Commonwealth Aged Care framework. When providing a person with services under the NDIS framework, the provider is obliged to adhere to the NDIS rules and practice standards, as well as the Aged Care Standards.

Independent living options

Some individuals live with family or independently in the community. Depending on their access to funded support, they may be able to maintain a quality lifestyle by using a combination of family support and paid hours from staff through a funded disability service. Some people live in the family home for their entire life, only needing to move out when their primary carer and/or family member becomes unable to provide their care due to their own failing health.

Those who move to aged care from individual living situations have the greatest difficulties with change as their routine is so vastly different from what it was before. Communication between a family and an individual does not generally have to be 'effective' for it to be understood, therefore many family-understood communication methods are established but are unable to be understood by others.

HEALTH AND WELLBEING

Disability-related health issues for elderly people

People with disabilities are affected by a myriad of health issues. Some are similar to those encountered by people without disabilities, while others are specific to those living with an acquired or congenital impairment of some sort and are subsequently related to the way the impairment affects the individual.

However, research indicates that there are other common health issues that affect those with an impairment. Some of these occur due to the lack of attention provided to the health of people with a disability and some occur due to the lack of effective communication that can be understood by support staff and/or medical practitioners. Medical practitioners advise that it is important to be vigilant when supporting individuals with a disability to visit their doctor and ensure that a consistent relationship is developed between the individual and their doctor. Clear communication, appropriate information transfer and follow-up conversations, when necessary, will enhance the ability of a medical practitioner to diagnose, treat and manage health conditions appropriately.

Some of the following are health conditions that medical practitioners should pay attention to. As a support person of someone who has a disability, it's important that you acknowledge the presence of these as being common for people with a disability, regardless of their age:

- *Constipation:* This is prevalent in many people with an intellectual impairment, often due to use of medication such as anti-convulsants, benzodiazepines, H_2-receptor antagonists or proton pump inhibitors. Constipation can lead to further complexities for the person as it may contribute to immobility and food refusal.

- *Dental problems:* In tests performed on people with an intellectual disability, it was shown that 86 per cent of individuals were affected by dental problems. There have been numerous reports over the years of people who have been labelled as having 'challenging behaviour' due to frequent episodic aggression, who, upon testing, have been identified as suffering from significant pain due to dental health issues.
- *Mental illness:* People with an intellectual impairment have a higher likelihood of mental illness than the rest of the population, yet health services are significantly inadequate to respond to the increasing need for specialist psychiatric services.
- *Sensory, vision or hearing impairment:* Sensory impairments, including vision and hearing impairments, are highly prevalent in people with intellectual impairment. Studies indicate that sensory impairments often remain undiagnosed or are incorrectly diagnosed, and can affect the person's mobility, communication and social and functional ability.
- *Sensory processing issues, or having a heightened sensory profile:* Many individuals, especially those who are autistic or neurodivergent, might have a heightened sensory profile. This means that sensory input such as noise, touch, movement and vision may be craved or avoided in much more significant ways than their peers. This can make certain environments very difficult for some individuals as they struggle to manage the sensory input around them.
- *Gastro-oesophageal reflux disease (GORD) and* Helicobacter pylori*:* The prevalence of GORD is reported to affect a significantly higher percentage of people with an intellectual disability than that of the general population. It is recommended that frequent and ongoing testing is required to ensure that those who have GORD are responded to quickly and effectively to reduce the associated issues of peptic ulcer and gastric carcinoma.
- *Epilepsy:* There is a 20 per cent greater prevalence of epilepsy in people with an intellectual impairment; this subsequently requires the individual to be subject to anti-convulsant medication regimens and necessitates the use of complex planning when arranging community-based options to ensure safety is managed appropriately. Furthermore, medical practitioners, such as neurologists, are reliant upon the information presented at appointments, often by support staff accompanying the person. If adequate record keeping is not provided, then it is likely that the neurologist will have to rely upon opinions and assumptions of those present at the appointment.

Hospital experiences for people with an intellectual impairment have been reported as being quite negative due to inattention from hospital staff, over-sedation, patient fear and anxiety and poor discharge preparation. Literature indicates that many parents of people with disabilities have felt it necessary to remain in hospital with their loved ones for the entire duration of the hospital stay to make sure that they receive adequate care. Some of the primary issues experienced by people with a disability when staying in hospital include:

- ineffective communication capacity of staff to communicate with elderly patients with an intellectual impairment
- trepidation regarding diagnostic testing: even procedures as simple as blood tests have caused significant difficulties for all parties involved
- behavioural responses by patients with an intellectual impairment when experiencing pain which they cannot verbally articulate to medical professionals
- **polypharmacy** of patients already in place and complexities associated with adding further medication
- other patients in close proximity and the subsequent privacy issues
- overwhelming and different sensory input which the person is not used to and is not comfortable with
- unsuitable physical accommodation with individual needs not represented within the rooms that patients are staying in.

Some strategies that would help improve the hospital experience for individuals who are ageing and have an intellectual impairment include:

- education, information and support to the person prior to admission. Mechanisms such as social stories, picture cards and repetitive prompting can help the person to understand what they will be expected to do and what might happen to them during their visit
- the presence of people they are familiar with and minimal turnover of different hospital staff. This helps the person to feel more comfortable and enables their participation at a higher level
- bringing in objects from home that make them feel more comfortable. This can be particularly helpful to those experiencing anxiety about hospital stays
- the presence of communication partners, which enables staff to have a consistent dialogue with their patient and medical practitioners, and to receive information to enable decisions to be made regarding their wellbeing.

Testing for age-related health issues in people with a disability living in large residential services

The disability and ageing intervention study by Webber and colleagues (2012) tested people aged between the ages of 41 and 78 (average age of 55), and indicated that testing for general health issues, such as hearing, breast cancer (mammogram), cholesterol, blood glucose and blood pressure, was comparable to the rate for the general population of the same age who were living in large residential services. However, this same study indicated there was a significant disparity between the testing of faecal occult blood test (FOBT) and the Pap Smear test. Testing for FOBT was 19 per cent lower for people living in large residential services and 46 per cent lower for Pap Smear.

CRITICAL THINKING EXERCISE

Bridget and Megan are twin sisters, both living with cerebral palsy, along with a moderate vision impairment. Their mother, Mrs Franklin, has supported them in the family home for their whole lives. Bridget and Megan are now 58 years of age and their mother is 81. Mrs Franklin can no longer provide support to Bridget and Megan, and has had to acquire assistance from the carer respite centre to find a suitable house for them to live in. Bridget and Megan argue quite frequently but are very close as sisters and Mrs Franklin believes it is essential for them to have a residence together.

A medium-sized residential facility with seven other co-tenants is sourced and has two vacancies. The facility is quite close to Mrs Franklin and she is very happy that her twin daughters can continue living together. Mrs Franklin explains to the care manager that she needs a rest and will be visiting her daughters twice weekly, but that they can communicate well enough to assist the support staff to get to know them and help them meet their needs.

Mrs Franklin comes back four days later and finds that Megan has had a haircut, which is very short, and Bridget has a large bruise above her right eye. Mrs Franklin accesses the complaints department of the residential facility and demands to know what happened over the four days to lead to such concerning changes. The care manager and a representative from the complaints department meet with Mrs Franklin to discuss her concerns and provide some responses.

It is explained that shortly after Mrs Franklin helped her daughters move in, Megan made it quite clear she needed a haircut and, upon accessing a hairdresser, chose the short style. The support staff didn't feel it was appropriate for them to restrict her choice of hairstyle and Megan made it abundantly clear that this was the style she wanted. Bridget's bruise was due to her sitting up suddenly during an X-ray requested by her doctor and smacking her head on the overhead machinery in the hospital.

Mrs Franklin lodges a complaint that she was never consulted about Megan's haircut and she wasn't informed, nor consulted, about the doctor's appointment for Bridget or the required ultrasound; nor was she informed of the injury Bridget incurred.

With a group of colleagues, consider and discuss the following:

1. Did the support staff at the residential facility act appropriately?
2. What could the support staff have done differently to lead to a more positive outcome?
3. Was Mrs Franklin the one being unreasonable, or did the residential facility conduct themselves inappropriately and neglect to inform the key stakeholder appropriately?
4. What if the residential facility responds to Mrs Franklin's complaint by reminding her that she advised them she wanted to only visit twice weekly and inferred that any matters rested with the sisters, which was interpreted by the support to mean she didn't want to be contacted about every matter?

CARING ABOUT CULTURE

In the culture of many Indigenous Australians, there is no word for disability. The term has never been required, as people with disabilities are cared for by family members and friends. This is not looked upon as any kind of burden or weakness, just a family and community obligation.

It is important to be aware of this when supporting Indigenous Australians. Generally, the most important thing for them will be their family and community. Great measures must be taken to ensure that the person is surrounded by those close to them and immersed within their culture whenever possible. This will greatly assist them to be comfortable and feel familiar and at ease with their environment.

CASE STUDY 1

Ms Kitas is 62 years old and lives with her co-tenants, Mr Malczewski and Ms O'Halloran. This living arrangement has worked very well for the last 11 years and all three co-tenants seem to enjoy each other's company. However, over the last 3 years, Ms Kitas' eyesight has deteriorated significantly. As she moves around her home, she often bumps her arm or leg on furniture and has become incontinent on numerous occasions because of the trauma from her injury (at the time). Ms Kitas' support staff have been spending a lot of time supporting her and encourage her to gain help from them prior to moving around the house. However, although Ms Kitas' eyesight has become poor, her energy levels and enthusiasm remain constant and she is quite insistent that she doesn't need increased support. These complexities have been compounded by slight memory lapses that Ms Kitas has had. At times, she has left the oven on and once she left some eggs boiling, to the point that they were boiled dry and the smoke alarm went off.

Staff have begun moving the furniture around to reduce the likelihood of Ms Kitas bumping into it, but this has made it very hard for her housemates, Mr Malczewski and Ms O'Halloran, as they can no longer reach their chair to have their dinner and require increased assistance to pull the table out from near the wall when they want to eat. Support staff have also had to put some safeguards in place to support Ms Kitas in the kitchen as her kitchen skills were deteriorating to the point that they were becoming dangerous to her co-tenants.

Mr Malczewski's legal guardian (his brother) has become involved and requested that the furniture be put back into its regular position. Ms O'Halloran's mother supports Mr Malczewski's request and believes it is unfair to move the furniture, which is owned by the three residents, to a position preferred by only one consumer, but not by the other two.

The decision-makers of both Mr Malczewski and Ms O'Halloran have met and put forward a request for an 'urgent revision of the appropriateness of the shared co-tenancy' to occur as they no longer believe that Ms Kitas is an appropriate consumer due to her current age and subsequent deterioration of functional daily skills.

CASE STUDY 2

Ms Baker is 58 years old and enjoys antique dolls, travelling and trucks. Ms Baker has Down Syndrome and epilepsy and is known for eating inedible items (diagnosed as having 'pica'), and has endured frequent hospital stays due to the ingestion of items such as pen lids, small hats from her antique dolls and ribbons. Recently, Ms Baker has been demonstrating signs of extreme stomach pain, but despite four trips to the emergency room, she has refused to allow the doctor to touch her belly and attempt to ascertain the cause of her ongoing pain. After a very difficult night of screaming in pain, clutching her abdomen, her support staff phoned her doctor and begged him to help her somehow. Dr Naylor has agreed to help Ms Baker, but requested that she be sedated first as he's worried that he or others may be hurt as they try to perform diagnostic tests, such as an ultrasound and possibly an endoscopy.

Dr Naylor provides the contact details of Ms Hackett, the social worker, and Dr Blest, the anaesthetist, and requests that the support staff make contact with all practitioners who will be participating in the healthcare of Ms Baker at this time.

It is subsequently decided that it is necessary to place Ms Baker under a general anaesthetic (GA), due to the intrusive nature of the healthcare required. Dr Naylor then requests that Ms Hackett, the social worker, liaise with Ms Baker's guardian for the purpose of involving her dentist. It is believed that, if a GA is to be used, then it is best medical practice to perform all necessary tests and provide any potential healthcare that may be required in the foreseeable future to avoid having to put Ms Baker under a GA again in the near future.

Ms Baker is provided with twilight sedation by the ambulance officer at her home, then transported to the hospital. She is met at the hospital by Dr Blest who places her under a GA. After this, Dr Naylor performs a blood test; then she is transported for an X-ray and ultrasound. After this, Ms Baker's dentist performs some minor dental work and she then undergoes an endoscopy. During the endoscopy, a small blockage is found which appears to be a very small doll head, which she appears to have swallowed. Dr Blest is able to retrieve this and subsequently remove the reason for her pain.

When Ms Baker wakes up, she is greeted by her mother and her support staff, who inform her of the success of the procedure and help transport her home.

QUALITY OF LIFE

People with a disability who are ageing are subject to the perils of both disability-related health issues and age-related illness. In some situations, the ageing process will render the person's current accommodation inappropriate and further accommodation may need to be sought. Relationships with family members and carers, who may be ageing themselves, can become strained due to their decreasing capacity to meet the needs of their loved one with regard to funded support, appropriate accommodation, communication support and mobility assistance. In some situations, a decision-maker might be required, which will necessitate an application for a hearing to QCAT or similar organisations in other states and territories. At this hearing, it might be decided that a family member could continue or commence acting in the role of decision-maker, or it may be necessary to appoint the Public Guardian for matters, as listed on the Order.

Some of the most significant issues regarding individuals with disabilities who are ageing relate to the medical intervention required to respond in a timely manner to impending and current health issues, declining memory and decreased cognitive function and mobility. In some situations, increased medical testing can be a terrifying event for those with a disability and require intensive planning, support and management from all stakeholders. Access to suitable medical treatment is imperative and effective strategies for individuals to communicate with their medical practitioners must be put in place. In some situations, it may be necessary to acquire a communication partner to ensure that clear, consistent communication is available at all times.

REVIEW QUESTIONS

Circle T if the statement is true or F if the statement is false:

1 T / F One of the biggest challenges for an older person with a disability is the appropriateness of accommodation.

2 T / F Moving to new accommodation which has a different philosophy of care is not traumatic to the person.

3 T / F Testing the older person with a disability for age-related changes is not considered an essential activity.

4 T / F Sedation is sometimes used to assist in the performance of undertaking diagnostic testing.

5 T / F Every elderly person has access to government support.

6 T / F The Public Guardian is always the first choice as a decision-maker for the person who is unable to make their own decisions.

7 T / F Poor communication can impact on the health of the person.

Circle the BEST answer:

8 The benefits to living in residential aged care for a person with a disability who is elderly are:

a increased access to specialist health services
b access to peers and planned social opportunities
c access to friends and family for visitation
d all of the above

9 Supported independent living (SIL) are living arrangements with which of the following?

a 10–12 residents in a hospital-style environment
b family home environment
c a small group of residents who are living together to optimise the use of funding and access to support workers
d one consumer only living in independent accommodation

10 As the person with a disability ages:

a family relationships improve
b family relationships can become strained due to a decreased capacity to meet the person's needs
c younger family members automatically become the legal decision-maker for the person
d changes in family relationships are never compromised.

Answers to these questions are on p. 454.

Further reading

Department of Health, Victoria (1986). Guardianship and Administration Act 1986. Online 28 February 2021. Available: www.health.vic.gov.au/legislation/guardian-and-admin-act.htm

Nay R & Garratt S (2009). Older people: issues and innovations in care. 3rd edn. Elsevier, Sydney.

University of Hertfordshire (2002). Health guidelines for adults with an intellectual disability. Online 28 February 2021. Available: www.intellectualdisability.info/how-to-guides/articles/health-guidelines-for-adults-with-an-intellectual-disability

References

Australian Government, Aged Care Quality and Safety Commission (2021). Residential aged care providers delivering services to NDIS participants. Online 20 October 2021. Available: www.agedcarequality.gov.au/providers/residential-aged-care-providers-delivering-services-ndis-participants

Australian Government, Department of Social Services (2019a). Disability and Carers. Younger People in Residential Aged Care. Online 20 October 2021. Available: www.dss.gov.au/disability-and-carers/programmes-services/for-people-with-disability/younger-people-with-disability-in-residential-aged-care-initiative

Australian Government, Department of Social Services (2019b). Disability and Carers. Younger People in Residential Aged Care Strategy 2020–25. Online 20 October 2021. Available: www.dss.gov.au/disability-and-carers-programs-services-for-people-with-disability-younger-people-with-disability-in-residential-aged-care-initiative/younger-people-in-residential-aged-care-strategy-2020-25

Australian Institute of Health and Welfare (AIHW) (2012). Younger people with disability in residential aged care 2010–2011, Bulletin 103. Australian Government.

Brown M, Condi A, Davis E et al (2021). Young people in residential aged care: Is Australia on track to meet its targets? Australian Journal of Social Issues, Sept 21, doi.org/10.1002/ajs4.184

National Disability Insurance Scheme (NDIS) (2021). Support budgets in your plan. Online 20 October 2021. Available: www.ndis.gov.au/participants/using-your-plan/managing-your-plan/support-budgets-your-plan

Queensland Government, Queensland Civil and Administrative Tribunal (2021). About QCAT. Online 28 February 2021. Available: www.qcat.qld.gov.au/matter-types/decision-making-for-adults

Webber R, Bowers B, Bigby C (2012). Disability and ageing intervention study. Australian Catholic University, University of Wisconsin-Madison and La Trobe University.

CHAPTER 16
Working with older clients with a mental health issue

By Janet Kerswell Unnasch

AFTER READING THIS CHAPTER, YOU SHOULD BE ABLE TO:

- define the key terms listed in this chapter
- describe three types of anxiety disorders
- discuss how defence mechanisms relieve anxiety
- identify the common phobias
- recognise the behaviours seen with schizophrenia
- differentiate between bipolar disorder and depression
- describe three types of personality disorders
- discuss and evaluate the care required by people with mental health disorders
- know how to promote quality of life.

Key terms

affect: External representation of mood and feelings
anxiety: A vague, uneasy feeling in response to stress
bipolar disorder: Bipolar means two (*bi*) poles or ends (*polar*). In bipolar disorder, the person has extreme mood swings
cognitive: Knowledge or perception of something or a process
compulsion: The uncontrolled performance of an act
defence mechanism: An unconscious reaction that blocks unpleasant or threatening feelings
delirium: Acute disturbance of attention and cognition
delusion: A fixed false belief
delusion of grandeur: An exaggerated belief about one's own importance, wealth, power or talents
delusion of persecution: A false belief that one is being mistreated, abused or harassed
emotional illness: Mental illness, mental disorder, psychiatric disorder
hallucination: Seeing, hearing, tasting, smelling or feeling something that is not real
mental: Relating to the mind; something that exists in the mind or is done by the mind
mental disorder: Mental illness, emotional disorder, psychiatric disorder
mental health: In Western societies it means a person is able to cope with and adjust to everyday stresses in acceptable ways
mental illness: A disturbance in the ability to cope or adjust to stress; behaviour and functioning are impaired; mental disorder, emotional illness, psychiatric disorder
obsession: A thought or idea that is all-consuming
panic: An intense and sudden feeling of fear, anxiety, terror or dread
paranoia: A disorder (*para*) of the mind (*noia*); false beliefs (delusions) and suspicion about a person or a situation
phobia: Fear, panic or dread; an irrational fear
psychiatric disorder: Mental illness, mental disorder, emotional disorder
psychosis: A serious mental disorder; the person does not view or interpret reality correctly
schizophrenia: Split (*schizo*) mind (*phrenia*). A serious mental disorder; the person does not view or interpret reality as others do
stress: The response or change in the body caused by any emotional, physical, social or economic factor
stressor: Any factor that causes stress
the 3Ds: A term sometimes used to describe depression, delirium and dementia in the older population

Mental health can be viewed as a state of emotional and psychological wellbeing, but in reality this is seen on a continuum or as a journey, rather than as a finite destination. In accordance with *The Mental Health Act 2016*, mental illness is a condition that relates to the disruption or disturbance of one's mental function. This condition can impair a person's behaviour, mood, perception or memory. Effective mental health allows a person to experience a sense of satisfaction in their relationships with themselves, their environment and others.

A holistic approach to wellbeing considers the physical, social, psychological and spiritual dimensions of the individual. Each part affects the other. A physical problem has social, mental and spiritual effects. Likewise, mental health problems affect the person physically, socially and spiritually, and social problems can have physical, mental health and spiritual effects.

BASIC CONCEPTS

Mental relates to the mind, meaning something that exists in the mind or is influenced by the mind. Therefore, mental health involves the mind.

Mental health is an abstract concept that is subject to various cultural and societal interpretations. In Western society, mental health means the person copes with and adjusts to everyday stresses in ways accepted by society.

Mental health is not an absolute state. It has been described as a continuum between mental wellbeing and mental illness (Fig. 16.1). At one end of the continuum are healthy individuals and at the other end are individuals who have an acute mental illness. Our biological, psychological, social and spiritual resources, the number and severity of the stressors we encounter and our ability to cope determine where we sit on this continuum.

Between mental health and mental illness, there is a grey area. It is normal to have fluctuations in how we think, feel and behave. At times, it can be difficult to maintain positive mental health in the face of life's pressures and problems.

People encounter many **stressors** and hassles that test their ability to cope and function effectively in their everyday lives. Crises or sustained **stress** over a prolonged period can affect even the most balanced person. Events such as retirement, death of a spouse, illness, injury or change in residence can affect our emotional and psychological health. How we respond to these challenges depends on our biological, psychological and social resources.

It is essential that all those who care for a person with a mental health issue have some self-awareness of their own attitudes towards mental health. This self-awareness will contribute significantly to the caregiver's ability to provide effective care. This is knowing one's stand and views about mental health and being aware about it prior to looking after a person with a mental health condition.

Mental illness is a disturbance in the person's ability to cope or adjust to stress. Behaviour, function and relationships are impaired because of a significant alteration in an individual's **cognitive** abilities. The terms **mental disorder**, **emotional illness** and **psychiatric disorder** may also be used when referring to mental illness. The general term 'mental health problem' may be used to refer to the presence of any one or a number of mental health illnesses.

Stress may influence an individual's state of wellness. Stress may affect mental health and mental illness. Stress is a response or change in the body or mind caused by any emotional, physical, social or economic stressor.

Mental health disorders have many causes, including:

- being unable to cope or adjust (perhaps due to a lack of skills and knowledge) to stress
- chemical imbalances; for example, depression is often characterised by an increase in levels of noradrenaline and a decrease in serotonin
- genetics
- medication or substance abuse
- social and cultural factors.

Each state or territory has its own Mental Health Act and it is important that you understand the Act that is relevant to the state or territory you are working in, as there may be some minor differences. For example, in Queensland the Mental Health Act is as follows:

The *Mental Health Act 2016*

Despite the causes of mental illness, all care within Australia is governed by special laws and certain ethics. Due to growing societal awareness and concern about the treatment of those who experience mental illness, the Queensland *Mental Health Act 2000* has been reviewed and updated and is replaced by the *Mental Health Act 2016*. This Act now provides a modern-day template for the delivery of safe and ethical mental healthcare (Box 16.1). This is one example of a Mental Health Act in Australia and New Zealand. Links

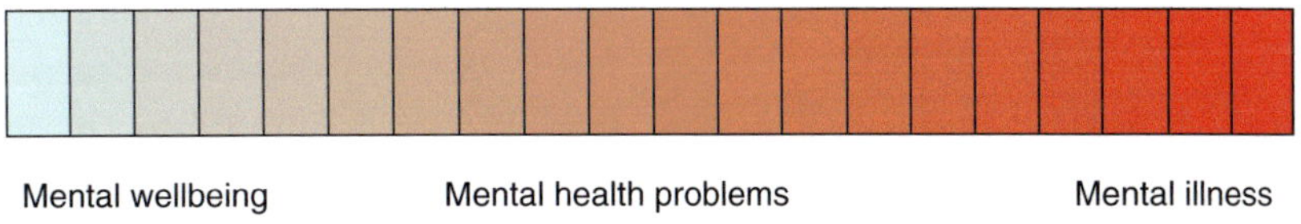

Fig. 16.1
The mental health continuum.

BOX 16.1
What is the purpose of the Mental Health Act?

The Queensland *Mental Health Act 2016* provides for the involuntary assessment and treatment, and the protection, of persons having a mental illness, while at the same time safeguarding their rights. The Act focuses on the aspects of mental illness that cannot be dealt with in other mainstream legislation. The Mental Health Act does not specifically provide for voluntary treatment of mental illness. Voluntary treatment for mental illness should be regarded in the same way as treatment for any other illness, with the protection of rights in other mainstream legislation. The Act also provides for the determination of a person's mental state when they have a mental illness and have been charged with a criminal offence, as well as their detention in a mental health service if necessary.

Why have objects and principles?

The principles are intended to underpin any decisions made, or actions carried out, under the Act. As a result, all users of the legislation should be familiar with the principles. They are consistent with national and international policy and principles, as well as other Queensland legislation (i.e. the *Guardianship and Administration Act 2000*, the *Public Guardian Act 2014* or the *Powers of Attorney Act 1998*).

What are the objects and principles?

- The Mental Health Act is based on objects and principles that respect basic human rights and ensure, to the greatest extent practicable, a person's participation in decisions made about them under the Act.
- The particular needs and circumstances of the person are to be taken into account, including the particular cultural, religious and language needs.
- Treatment given under the Act can only be provided if it is appropriate to promote and maintain the person's mental health and wellbeing.
- Chapter 1 of the *Mental Health Act 2016* deals with the purpose and application of the legislation. It contains a statement of objects and principles to guide the use of powers under the Act. Definitions for interpretation are also included in this chapter.
- A person's right to confidentiality must be recognised and taken into account, subject to specific provisions in this and other relevant legislation.
- Any power or function exercised under the Act must be exercised so that a person's liberty and rights are affected only if there is no less restrictive way to protect the person's health and safety or to protect others.
- If the person's liberty or rights are to be affected, the effect is to be the minimum necessary in the circumstances.

Source: *Mental Health Act 2016* © State of Queensland (Queensland Health).

to each state and territory and New Zealand legal portals are supplied at the end of this chapter.

Prior to reading further, take some time to reflect on your own values and attitudes towards mental health. Despite utmost vigilance, there are times when many healthcare workers can inadvertently transfer feelings of judgement. This in turn can sometimes perpetuate the notion of stigma within our community. The high level of stigma attached to mental illness has been brought to the attention of our society within recent times. Through dedicated educational and awareness programs, such as the National Mental Health Awareness Week, and other strategies such as R U OK? Day, there has been a slight shift in perspective regarding mental illness and thus some minimisation of stigma.

Pause to reflect on any occasions where you felt discriminated against or a sense of stigma that may have been attached to a condition or disorder you may have experienced. This is the kind of behaviour that all healthcare workers need to be aware of within their own practice and take steps to eliminate it.

CARING ABOUT CULTURE

Cultural and societal values influence how we view mental illnesses. A culture's religious and spiritual beliefs are strongly linked to the interpretation of mental illness. The explanation of *hallucinations* as symptoms of an illness or a spiritual experience will affect a community's reactions and the person's subsequent treatment.

In Western society, a person who hallucinates and behaves in a bizarre manner may alienate friends or family and finally come to the attention of the medical establishment. Their behaviour is viewed as a symptom of a mental illness that requires treatment.

In the non-Western world, however, the community may confer a supernatural explanation for a person who displays such behaviour. Some cultures may believe that mental health issues are a result of spirits or demons that have taken over the soul. Hallucinations and delusions might be viewed as visitations by spirits. Their accepted preference for treatment may be rituals or sacrifices to appease kindred spirits or gods who have been offended.

Puerto Rican schizophrenics are seen as having a supernatural capacity for communication with the spirit world. The community tolerates the symptoms of the disorder. Individuals with mental disorders are only treated if their behaviour is a danger to themselves or others. This lack of stigma and support from the community leads to a good outcome for the person.

The Chinese language does not contain any terms to describe psychological or psychosocial stressors. As Chinese culture does not differentiate between physical and mental health disorders, Chinese people may seek treatment for the physical manifestations of their stress. You should not express your personal views on a person's cultural beliefs.

As mental illness should always be considered in its cultural and social context, so too the reactions of clients and their families to the symptoms of mental illness are influenced by their cultural and religious beliefs. Culturally appropriate forms of care are necessary. This may include the use of an interpreter, culturally specific services for clients, involving the extended family or working alongside traditional healers. Sensitivity to the individual's cultural beliefs will ensure the best possible outcomes for your client.

ANXIETY DISORDERS

Anxiety is a vague, uneasy feeling in response to stress. The person may not know why or what has caused it. They may perceive that they are in danger or at risk of harm. The person acts to relieve the unpleasant feeling, perhaps seeking reassurance. Some anxiety is normal. When needs are not met, it is common for the person to experience anxiety.

Anxiety is linked to the fight or flight response, which is necessary to induce action in the face of a genuine physical or psychological threat. The physiological responses associated with anxiety are caused by the *autonomic nervous system*:

- *parasympathetic responses*, which conserve body responses
- *sympathetic responses*, which activate body processes
- the *limbic system*, which triggers the release of steroid hormones and neurotransmitters.

Anxiety produces symptoms such as heart palpitations, sweating and restlessness. Activity in the frontal lobe of the brain is suppressed, interfering with short-term memory, concentration and rational thought. This allows the person to react quickly to the threat. Mild anxiety can heighten physical and mental alertness; severe anxiety can produce unusual or irrational behaviour.

People with mental health disorders often experience anxiety, often at high levels. The effects that anxiety may have will depend on the degree of anxiety. Signs and symptoms include:

- a 'lump' in the throat
- 'butterflies' in the stomach
- pulse, respiration and blood pressure increases
- rapid speech and voice changes
- dry mouth
- sweating
- nausea
- diarrhoea
- urinary frequency and urgency
- poor attention span
- problems following directions
- difficulty sleeping
- loss of appetite.

Anxiety levels depend on the stressor or factor that causes stress. It can be emotional, physical, social or economic. Past experiences affect how a person reacts, as does the number of stressors. A stressor may produce only mild anxiety on one occasion, but at another time the same stressor may cause a greater degree of anxiety.

HINTS TO ASSIST A PERSON WITH ANXIETY

- The person with severe anxiety will need medical assistance. Medications will relieve the symptoms of anxiety but not the underlying cause
- A unique aspect of anxiety is that it is contagious. When interacting with an anxious person, the carer may also experience feelings of anxiety. It is not uncommon for the carer to feel irritated or frustrated because of their rising levels of anxiety
- Be patient and understanding
- Listen carefully
- Do not blame the person for their illness
- Relaxation promotes physical wellbeing, releases tension and reduces stress
- Massage and music can be soothing and aid relaxation
- Gentle exercise can also promote feelings of wellbeing and relieve tension
- Identify any environmental triggers that may precede the anxious feelings
- Coping mechanisms relieve anxiety. Some are healthy, whereas others may compromise wellbeing. Common coping mechanisms include:
  - eating and drinking
  - smoking
  - exercising
  - talking about the problem
  - playing music
  - going for a walk
  - taking a hot bath
  - wanting to be alone.

Defence mechanisms also relieve anxiety. Defence mechanisms are unconscious reactions. They block unpleasant or threatening feelings (Box 16.2). Everyone uses defence mechanisms as they protect the ego. Some use of defence mechanisms is normal, but at times they are poorly used in mental health disorders.

Panic disorder

Panic is the highest level of anxiety. Panic is an intense and sudden feeling of fear, anxiety, terror or dread. Onset is sudden, often with no obvious reason. The person usually cannot function adequately because the anxiety is so severe. Panic

BOX 16.2
Defence mechanisms

- *Compensation* – to make up for, replace or substitute. The person makes up for or substitutes strength for a weakness. Example: A boy is not good in sports. He learns to play music.
- *Conversion* – to change. An emotion is shown as or changed into a physical symptom. Example: A girl does not want to read out loud in school. She complains of a headache.
- *Denial* – refusing to accept or believe something that is true. The person refuses to face or accept unpleasant or threatening things. Example: A man has a heart attack. He continues to smoke after being told to quit.
- *Displacement* – to move or take the place of. An individual moves behaviours or emotions from one person, place or thing to a safe person, place or thing. Example: You are angry with your boss. You yell at a friend.
- *Identification* – to relate to or recognise. A person assumes the ideas, behaviours and traits of another person. Example: A little girl's neighbour is a high school cheerleader. The little girl practises cheerleading in her backyard.
- *Projection* – to blame another. An individual blames another person or object for one's own unacceptable behaviour, emotions, ideas or wishes. Example: A girl fails a test. She blames another girl for not helping her study.
- *Rationalisation* – 'rational' means sensible, reasonable or logical. An acceptable reason or excuse is given for one's behaviour or actions. The real reason is not given. Example: A man is often late for work. He did not get a raise. He says that this is because the boss does not like him.
- *Reaction formation* – a person acts in a way that is opposite to what he or she truly feels. Example: A man does not like his boss. He buys the boss an expensive gift for Christmas.
- *Regression* – 'regress' means to move back or retreat. The person retreats or moves back to an earlier time or condition. Example: A 4-year-old wants a baby bottle when a new baby comes into the family.
- *Repression* – 'repress' means to hold down or keep back. The person keeps unpleasant or painful thoughts or experiences from the conscious mind. They cannot be recalled or remembered. Example: A woman was sexually abused as a child. Now 33 years old, she has no memory of the event.

attacks can last for a few minutes or for hours and can occur frequently.

Phobic disorders

Phobia means fear, panic or dread. The person has an intense fear of an object or situation. These are the common fears experienced by people with a phobia:

- fear of being in an open, crowded or public place – agoraphobia
- fear of being in pain or seeing others in pain – algiophobia
- fear of water – hydrophobia
- fear of being in or being trapped in an enclosed or narrow space – stenophobia
- fear of talking because of the fear of stuttering – glossophobia
- fear of dirt or contamination – molysmophobia
- fear of night – noctiphobia
- fear of loud noises – ligyrophobia
- fear of fire – pyrophobia
- fear of strangers – xenophobia

Obsessive–compulsive disorder

An **obsession** is a recurrent thought, image or idea that is intrusive or inappropriate and may cause anxiety. A **compulsion** is an uncontrolled desire to perform a mental or physical act. The person experiences an overwhelming need or is compelled to carry out the activity. The person knows the act is wrong or unnecessary, but will experience much anxiety if they don't do it. Some eating disorders are obsessive–compulsive. The person is obsessed with thoughts of food. He or she may eat constantly or be ritualistic with eating; for example, they may only eat food items in groups of two. Constant handwashing is also common because of the fear of germs that may cause illness. Some obsessive–compulsive disorders involve violent acts.

Schizophrenia

Schizophrenia means split (*schizo*) mind (*phrenia*). It involves the following:

- **psychosis** – a serious mental disorder. The person does not view or interpret reality correctly
- **delusion** – a false belief. For example, a person believes he is God or a movie star
- **hallucination** – seeing, hearing or feeling something that is not real. A person may see animals, insects or people that are not real
- **paranoia** – a disorder (*para*) of the mind (*noia*). The person has false beliefs (delusions). He or she is suspicious about a person or situation. For example, a woman believes her food has been poisoned
- **delusion of grandeur** – an exaggerated belief about one's own importance, wealth, power or talents. For example, a man believes he is Superman or a woman believes she is the Queen of England
- **delusion of persecution** – the false belief that one is being mistreated, abused or harassed. For example, a person believes that someone is 'out to get' him or her.

The person with schizophrenia has a disorder of the mind (psychosis). Disturbances of thinking and behaviour can commonly occur. The person can have both delusions and hallucinations. They see, hear or feel things that are not real. The person has difficulty relating to others and may be paranoid or suspicious about a person or situation. Verbal and behavioural responses are inappropriate, and communication is disturbed. The person may ramble or repeat what another says. Sometimes their speech may not be understood. The person may withdraw, lacking interest or involvement with other people or society. He or she may sit for hours alone without moving, speaking or responding.

Hallucinations are false sensory experiences that can occur in any of the five senses. They seem very real, but exist only in the person's mind.

It is important to remember that:

- not all hallucinations are signs of a psychotic illness; they could be indicative of a delirium or an organic brain disease
- sensory impairment can also result in the person experiencing hallucinations
- in some cultures, visual and auditory hallucinations may be a normal part of religious experiences.

The person has no control over the hallucinations and to them they seem very real – so real that they can describe the situation in detail. Thus, if you keep telling the client that no one is there, you will only frustrate yourself because your client will insist that someone is there. The best management strategy in this instance is to acknowledge the client's feelings, provide empathy and assure them that, although you cannot see or hear what they are experiencing, you do indeed believe them. Being able to talk about the hallucinations may be reassuring for the person.

If your client is experiencing unpleasant hallucinations, let them know that you cannot see what they are seeing, but reassure them that they are safe with you. Some people find that noise and distraction help to decrease the hallucinations. Others respond to minimal environmental stimulation.

Delusions are fixed, false beliefs inconsistent with a person's educational and religious background. As with hallucinations, a delusion is not under the person's control and will not respond to logic. Delusions can be extremely upsetting to carers and are commonly linked to behavioural problems. A person with delusions may feel persecuted and fearful for his or her life, may believe that their spouse is unfaithful or that they are suffering from an imaginary disease. To the person, these ideas are very real, so they may respond with anger or fear. To the person with delusions, they are very real. Do not try to convince the client that their ideas are imaginary. This usually does not work and can annoy the client. Be aware of your own feelings towards the client. The client's loss of reality and associated behaviour can be distressing and frustrating for the carer.

SIMPLE BUT EFFECTIVE STRATEGIES TO HELP CLIENTS WITH SCHIZOPHRENIA

- Meet the client's physical needs for nutrition, hydration, rest and safety
- Establish a helping relationship by using effective communication strategies
- Maintain eye contact
- Call the client by name
- Be patient, use active listening skills and show acceptance
- If asked, indicate that you cannot see/hear the hallucination. Do not argue or agree with the client about the content of the hallucinations or delusional ideas
- Acknowledge the feelings attached to the delusion
- The person may be afraid or sad
- The person may need a referral for psychiatric evaluation and treatment
- Identify any environmental triggers that may precede the hallucinations. Increase lighting limit changes in the environment

AFFECTIVE DISORDERS

Affect relates to feelings and emotions. Affective disorders involve feelings, emotions and moods.

Bipolar disorder

Bipolar means two (*bi*) poles or ends (*polar*). The person with **bipolar disorder** has extreme mood swings. The person has emotional lows (depression) and highs (mania).

- When depressed, the person is beyond feeling sad. He or she feels guilty, lonely, worthless, empty and hopeless. Commonly the person experiencing this deep depression may have avolition; that is, lack of motivation. Avolition can present as the person not being able to get out of bed and being unable to attend to personal hygiene, nutrition and hydration. Avolition must not be confused with laziness as they appear similar. The personal carer may assist by prompting and encouraging the person to attend to their activities of daily living; however, it is often necessary for the personal carer to physically assist by helping to remove the consumer's clothing prior to a shower, setting up the bathroom with requirements and helping the person to wash. It is best practice to involve the consumer with personal choice, such as choosing clothes to wear. Frequently, though, the carer will be required to select clothing and assist the consumer to dress. Depression impairs the ability to communicate and respond to others. It is often difficult to know what to say to someone who is depressed.
- Acknowledge cultural needs. Be patient and show understanding. Listen carefully. Don't blame the person for their illness.

Sleep and appetite are disturbed and the person has problems concentrating. Self-esteem is low and they may have persistent, intrusive thoughts about suicide. If the consumer voices suicidal thoughts, it is appropriate to ask them further questions about this. Gain information, such as:

- has the consumer thought of a way to suicide?
- if so, ask them to tell you about it
- does the consumer have access to the means to carry out suicide, such as a gun, knife, rope, medications etc.?

This is imperative to ensuring the consumer's safety. If the consumer reports that they have a plan and the means to suicide, then they are at high risk of carrying it out. In this situation, the personal carer should remain with their patient if they feel safe to do so and immediately summon assistance from other members of the healthcare team. Depending on the situation, the personal carer may use the nurse call bell, a phone or even another patient to call for assistance.

In the manic phase, the person is excited and very busy. He or she has a lot of energy, speech is rapid and they cannot sleep. The person does not take time to eat or tend to self-care needs. Judgement is poor and the person is easily distracted. Delusions of grandeur are common. Mania may present as the consumer experiencing overwhelming euphoria, or at other times mania may present as the consumer experiencing overwhelming irritability.

Staff and client safety are the first priorities. The client may deliberately or accidentally harm themselves or others, because of psychotic symptoms or impaired judgement. Constant supervision may be required and medical assessment is indicated. The client may need further medication or hospitalisation.

Clients who are manic have an increased level of activity and usually ignore the need for rest, food and fluid. If left unassisted, the client may die from exhaustion and dehydration. Provide small, frequent meals, such as sandwiches, which can be 'eaten on the run'. Similarly, provide plastic water bottles and encourage the consumer to maintain their hydration level. Monitor food and fluid intake and sleep pattern.

Verbal or physical aggression can be a problem because of the client's irritability and poor impulse control. Do not attempt to hurry the client – quiet persuasion is the key to caring for a manic client.

The client's ability to deal with environmental stimuli is impaired. Group activities and excessive stimulation are best avoided during this time. As the client improves, their tolerance will increase. Implement strategies for hallucinations and delusions as previously discussed.

Major depression

Most people experience a fluctuation of mood in the course of day-to-day living. It is normal to feel sad, down in the dumps or blue in reaction to everyday hassles and stressors. Depressive feelings can vary in intensity and duration, from a brief reaction to an illness that affects all aspects of functioning. The term *depression* has been used collectively to describe a mood, a symptom or an illness.

Major depression is a serious illness where the person has either a depressed mood or a loss of interest or pleasure in nearly all activities, changes in appetite or weight, insomnia or hypersomnia, over- or under-activity, feelings of worthlessness or guilt, difficulty thinking, concentrating or making decisions, recurrent thoughts of death, suicidal ideation, plans or attempts and functional impairment.

Whether an individual is experiencing a depressed mood, depression as a symptom of another illness or a specific depressive disorder, the experience of depression is unique to that individual. The range of symptoms can be wide and varied. Some people emphasise physical complaints rather than feelings of sadness.

Suicidal thoughts may be present in those with moderate-to-severe depression, so safety is a priority. A severely depressed person may also be unable to maintain minimal personal hygiene due to apathy and loss of motivation. The appetite can be disturbed and constipation is a common problem. Sleeping patterns are commonly disturbed, including early morning waking, inability to fall asleep or stay asleep and, conversely, the desire to stay asleep for lengthy periods.

HINTS TO ASSIST A PERSON WITH DEPRESSION

- There is a direct link between depression and suicide. Take any comments about death or suicide seriously and seek immediate medical assessment
- A severely depressed person may be unable to maintain minimal personal hygiene due to apathy and loss of motivation. Appetite can be disturbed and constipation is a common problem. Insomnia occurs in 90 per cent of depressed people
- Depression impairs the person's ability to communicate and respond to others. It is often difficult to know what to say to someone who is depressed
- Be patient and understanding
- Listen carefully
- Don't blame the person for their illness
- Encourage decision-making about clothing, food and recreation
- Encourage activities that the person enjoys
- Acknowledge cultural needs

SAFETY ALERT

Unpredictable or challenging behaviour

Remember, anyone who is agitated, confused or feels threatened is capable of behaving in an aggressive or violent manner. You need to be able to leave the room quickly if necessary. It is safe practice to keep yourself between the exit door and the person exhibiting behaviours that may challenge your ability to respond effectively.

PERSONALITY DISORDERS

Personality disorders involve rigid and maladaptive behaviours. To *adapt* means to change or adjust. *Mal* means bad, wrong or ill. Maladaptive means to change or adjust in the wrong way. Because of their behaviours, those with personality disorders may not function well in society. Personality disorders include:

Cluster A personality disorders

Cluster A personality disorders are characterised by odd, eccentric thinking or behaviour. They include paranoid personality disorder, schizoid personality disorder and schizotypal personality disorder.

- *paranoid personality disorder* – the person is very suspicious. They do not trust others.
- *antisocial personality disorder* – people with this disorder have poor judgement. They lack responsibility and are hostile. They are not loyal to any person or group. Morals and ethics are lacking. They blame others for their actions and behaviours. They are not considerate of other people's rights and feel no guilt. They do not learn from experiences or punishment, and often find themselves in trouble with the police.
- *schizoid personality disorder* – the person has little desire for close relationships, including intimacy. The person prefers to be alone and shows little concern for feedback, including praise or criticism.
- *schizotypal personality disorder* – the person displays behaviours, such as believing that incidental objects or events have particular meaning for them. The person holds unusual beliefs and is seen as 'odd' by the community.

Cluster B personality disorders

Cluster B personality disorders are characterised by dramatic, overly emotional or unpredictable thinking or behaviour. They include antisocial personality disorder, borderline personality disorder, histrionic personality disorder and narcissistic personality disorder.

- *borderline personality disorder* – the person displays an intense fear of rejection and experiences extreme and unstable mood swings and forms relationships in a similar manner. The person can lack impulse control and exhibit self-destructive actions alongside suicidal behaviours.
- *histrionic personality disorder* – the person demands to be the centre of attention and usually has a dramatic element to their personality and appearance, including sexually explicit behaviour. This person can be easily influenced by others.
- *narcissistic personality disorder* – this person is preoccupied with self-importance and fantasies. The person strongly believes they are 'special' and should be treated accordingly, therefore displays a high level of arrogance and lacks empathy.

Cluster C personality disorders

Cluster C personality disorders are characterised by anxious, fearful thinking or behaviour. They include avoidant personality disorder, dependent personality disorder and obsessive-compulsive personality disorder.

- *avoidant personality disorder* – this person has a dire fear of rejection, therefore avoids close relationships, becomes easily embarrassed in social situations and is unlikely to take risks. This person usually holds onto an inferiority complex.
- *dependent personality disorder* – this person is reluctant to make decisions, needs reassurance and direction, lacks assertion and confidence, fears being alone and feels they need the security of always being in a relationship.
- *obsessive-compulsive personality disorder* – this person is compelled to comply with rules and a sense of organisation. They are often described as perfectionists and therefore are conscientious to their detriment. This person can also be a hoarder and is reluctant to spend money; they would rather work than socialise.
- *personality disorders not otherwise specified* – this person may exhibit characteristics of more than one disorder while not fulfilling all criteria in one or more areas.

THE 3Ds

This is a term that is often used to describe delirium, depression and dementia in the older person. Although these conditions have been discussed earlier, they are often linked together and described by the colloquial term '**the 3Ds**'. These conditions are often under-recognised within the older person, which impacts considerably on their quality of life, health and safety. When caring for the older person it is important that you have an understanding of the differences between each of the 3Ds and are able to report to your supervisor if you identify any. Table 16.1 clearly identifies the differences between each of these conditions.

TREATMENT

Treatment involves having the person explore their thoughts and feelings with the help of psychotherapy and group therapy. Occupational, art and family therapies are also useful. Medication can help with anxiety and depression. The care plan reflects the person's needs. It includes safety measures, particularly if suicide is a risk. Communication is an important tool in supporting a person's treatment. Be alert to the person's non-verbal communication and your own.

HINTS TO HELP A PERSON WITH A MENTAL HEALTH PROBLEM

- Use a warm, accepting, empathetic approach
- Accept the client as a worthwhile person through the use of non-judgemental communication and behaviour
- Encourage the client to share their thoughts and feelings
- Actively listen to the person's worries. This will communicate your interest and concern about their problems
- Give the person time to respond
- Be honest, dependable and constant in your interactions
- Maintain confidentiality and privacy

Table 16.1
The 3Ds

	Delirium	Depression	Dementia
Definition	Delirium is a medical emergency characterised by a sudden onset of confusion, disturbances in attention, disorganised thinking and/or decline in level of consciousness. Delirium cannot be accounted for by a pre-existing dementia; however, it can co-exist with dementia	Depression is a term used when a cluster of depressive symptoms is present on most days, for most of the time, for at least 2 weeks, and when the symptoms are of such intensity that they are out of the ordinary for that individual. Depression is a biologically-based illness that affects a person's thoughts, feelings, behaviour and even physical health	Dementia is a gradual and progressive decline in mental processing ability that affects short-term memory, communication, language, judgement, reasoning and abstract thinking. Dementia eventually affects long-term memory and the ability to perform familiar tasks. Sometimes there are changes in mood and behaviour
Onset	Sudden onset: hours to days	Recent unexplained changes in mood that persist for at least 2 weeks.	Gradual deterioration over months to years
Course	Often reversible with treatment Often fluctuates over 24-hour period and often worse at night	Usually reversible with treatment Often worse in the morning	Slow, chronic progression, and irreversible
Thinking	Fluctuations in alertness, cognition, perceptions, thinking	Reduced memory, concentration and thinking, low self-esteem	Cognitive decline with problems in memory
Psychotic Feature	Misperceptions and illusions	Delusions of poverty, guilt and often complaints of distressing physical symptoms. These are often accompanied by excessive fear and concerns.	Signs may include delusions of theft/persecution and/or hallucinations depending on type of dementia
Sleep	Disturbed but with no set pattern. Differs night to night	Disturbed Early morning awakening or insomnia	May be disturbed with an individual pattern occurring most nights
Mood	Fluctuations in emotions – outbursts, anger, crying, fearful	Depressed mood Diminished interest or pleasure Changes in appetite (over- or under-eating) Possible suicidal ideation/plan Hopelessness	Depressed mood especially in early dementia Prevalence of depression may increase in dementia; however, apathy is a more common symptom and may be confused with depression
Psychomotor activities	Hyperactive delirium: agitation, restlessness, hallucinations Hypoactive delirium: unarousable, very sleepy Mixed delirium: combination of hyperactive and hypoactive manifestations	Hyperactive: agitated depression Hypoactive: withdrawn, decreased motivation/ interest	Wandering/exit seeking or Agitated or Withdrawn (may be related to co-existing depression)

Source: Adapted from Dharia S, Verilla K, Breden EL (2011). The 3Ds of geriatric psychiatry: depression, delirium and dementia. The Consultant Pharmacist 26(8):566–578.

SPEAKING WITH A PERSON WHO HAS A MENTAL HEALTH PROBLEM

To promote effective communication, use active listening skills. Assume a neutral and encouraging approach. Acknowledge what the person expresses to you. The person may be hyper-aware of your response and will know if you do not believe them or if they are being patronised. Recognise your own limitations. If you are unsure of how to communicate with the person, or if you feel uncomfortable with the situation, seek assistance.

QUALITY OF LIFE

People with mental health problems have a right to quality of life. They have the same rights as any other member of society. Some people with mental health problems are very ill, and for a variety of reasons they cannot exercise their rights. In these cases, their legal representatives do so or they may be subject to provisions of the Mental Health Act.

Protect the person's right to privacy and confidentiality. The person may say or do something unusual. Share this when necessary, but ***only*** with those who are assisting in the person's care, such as members of the health team. No one else needs to know what the person said or did.

Protect their right to personal choice. The person may have problems making choices. Follow the care plan. Sometimes the number of choices may be limited. Making even a simple choice helps the person feel in control.

Protect the person from abuse, mistreatment and neglect. Some people cannot protect themselves and may not know that they are being mistreated. Report signs of abuse, mistreatment or neglect to the appropriate team member or authority.

Provide a safe setting. Some people who are mentally ill may be a danger to themselves or others. The care plan will include safety measures. If suicide or self-harm is a threat, remove all potentially harmful items from the person's setting as required. If you are unsure of what to do, seek assistance from others or be guided by the mental health regulations in your state.

The state of wellness does not necessarily mean the absence of a diagnosed disease. If managed effectively, people with a mental health problem can enjoy a positive, independent and satisfying life.

CRITICAL THINKING ACTIVITIES

Critical thinking 1

Mr Novak has experienced poor concentration, memory loss and confusion. Because of these symptoms he retired earlier than expected. Retirement was very difficult for Mr Novak, not only financially but also socially. His work colleagues were also his friends and now he was beginning to lose contact with them. Recently, he began to lose his temper at the slightest provocation and had accused his wife of having an affair. His appetite was poor and he had difficulty sleeping at night. After visiting his local GP he was diagnosed with depression and also a chest infection. He was commenced on a course of antidepressants and antibiotics.

1. Identify three symptoms that may indicate that Mr Novak is depressed.

Critical thinking 2

Mrs Samaras has a 50-year history of bipolar disorder and currently resides at home. When you visit, she presents as dishevelled and flamboyantly dressed, pacing around the room, waving her walking stick and laughing. Mrs Samaras reports feeling wonderful and appears elated. When asked about her mood, Mrs Samaras states that God has bestowed special powers on her, so she has just discovered the cure for cancer.

1. Identify three symptoms that may indicate Mrs Samaras is experiencing an acute episode of bipolar illness.

Critical thinking 3

Brian has regular visits to hospital for acute exacerbation of his chronic schizophrenic illness. His delusions centre on the belief that he can communicate with aliens. Although he feels he is an important person with a unique ability, he also becomes paranoid, complaining that the aliens are changing his thoughts and directing his behaviour. Compliance with treatment has been an issue as he denies that he is ill. Now that he is 69 years old, the negative symptoms of his illness have become more apparent. His physical hygiene has deteriorated, he is malnourished and has little energy or motivation. Most of his day is spent alone, smoking in the courtyard of the hostel where he resides.

1. Match the term to a description:

a	Belief that he can communicate with aliens	Schizophrenia
b	Complaining that the aliens are changing his thoughts	Denies he is ill
c	He feels he is an important person with a unique ability	Delusion
d	Does not take medication	Paranoid Delusion
e	A serious mental illness	Delusion

CASE STUDY

Last year, Katherine, 68, moved into a semi-independent living unit. She is divorced and had four sons. She has a close relationship with one, two live interstate and one died at age 36. Although Katherine has six grandchildren, only two live locally. She sees her sister only every 2 months. Katherine worked as a doctor's surgery receptionist before she retired. Although she knew many people through her work role, she says she now has few friends. Katherine has been expressing feelings of loneliness and uselessness since moving in. She is often heard to state that she 'can't be bothered with anything', feels tired and teary and avoids going out to shop and pay bills. Her son David says that Katherine had always been meticulous about her appearance, but lately has been less conscientious. He has also noticed that she appears to have lost weight. Her health problems include arthritis in her hip, which affects her mobility, psoriasis, which Katherine considers disfiguring, and macular degeneration, which has reached the point where she says she can no longer read or do crosswords – hobbies that she once enjoyed. Katherine seems to have difficulty concentrating when you speak with her. You have noticed that there are a number of empty wine bottles put out in her rubbish each week. You encourage Katherine to see her GP, outlining your concerns for her current state of wellbeing. Katherine is diagnosed with depression.

ACCREDITATION

You are working in residential or home care and accreditors are at your service. Can you answer the following questions?

- What are some ways in which you can support the mental health of your residents/consumers/clients in your role as a carer?
- One of your clients confides in you that they are thinking of taking their own life, as they are feeling very depressed. What would you do?

REVIEW QUESTIONS

Circle the BEST answer:

1 From the following descriptions, choose the best definition of mental health:
  a Mental health is a complete state of emotional and psychological wellbeing.
  b Mental health can only be achieved by adherence to the guidelines of the *Mental Health Act 2016*.
  c Mental health is a condition whereby a person's behaviour, mood, perception and memory are negatively impacted.
  d Mental health can be viewed as a state of emotional and psychological wellbeing on a continuum, whereby there are some normal fluctuations but the person leads a functioning life and is able to meet most needs.

2 From the following descriptions, choose the best definition of mental illness:
  a Mental illness is a complete state of emotional and psychological wellbeing.
  b Mental illness is experienced when there is diminished adherence to the guidelines of the *Mental Health Act 2016*.
  c Mental illness is a condition whereby a person's behaviour, mood, perception and memory are negatively impacted.
  d Mental illness is a disturbance in cognitive functioning.

3 Which of the following is a cause of mental illness?
  a Chemical imbalances in the brain
  b Lack of education
  c Lack of social network
  d Complicated family relationships

4 The primary role of the *Mental Health Act 2016* is:
  a to provide clinical guidelines for care
  b to safeguard the rights of mental health consumers
  c to provide evidence-based legislation within mental healthcare
  d to respect basic human rights

5 Which of the following statements is not consistent with the guidelines contained within the *Mental Health Act 2016:*
  a A person's right to confidentiality must be recognised.
  b Any power under the Act must be exercised so that the person's liberty and rights are affected only if there is no less restrictive way to protect the person's health and safety or to protect others.
  c Treatment given under the Act can only be provided if it is appropriate to promote and maintain the person's mental health and wellbeing.
  d If the person's liberty or rights are to be affected the use of restraint, chemical and physical can be implemented at the registered nurse's discretion.

6 Anxiety can be defined as:
  a a physical response to stress
  b hearing voices
  c an extreme panic attack
  d seeing visions of God

Circle T if the statement is true or F if the statement is false:

7 T/F Culture and social values do not affect how we see people with mental illness.

8 T/F Mild-to-moderate anxiety can heighten a person's capabilities.

9 T/F Anxiety is a general feeling of unease or apprehension.

10 T/F Physical illnesses can trigger depressive symptoms.

Answers to these questions are on p. 454.

Further reading

Queensland Government, *Mental Health Act 2016.* Online 28 February 2021. Available: www.legislation.qld.gov.au/view/pdf/asmade/act-2016-005

Australian and New Zealand legal links

The following links give access to the mental health Acts across Australia and New Zealand:

New Zealand
www.legislation.govt.nz/
Search Mental Health Act

Australian Capital Territory
www.legislation.act.gov.au/a/2015-38/

New South Wales
www.legislation.nsw.gov.au/view/whole/html/inforce/current/act-2007-008#frnt-lt

Northern Territory
https://legislation.nt.gov.au/en/Legislation/MENTAL-HEALTH-AND-RELATED-SERVICES-ACT-1998

Queensland
www.legislation.qld.gov.au/view/pdf/asmade/act-2016-005

South Australia
www.legislation.sa.gov.au/lz/c/a/mental%20health%20act%202009/current/2009.28.auth.pdf

Tasmania
www.legislation.tas.gov.au/view/html/inforce/current/act-2013-002

Victoria
https://content.legislation.vic.gov.au/sites/default/files/2020-02/14-26aa022%20authorised.pdf

Western Australia
www.legislation.wa.gov.au/legislation/prod/filestore.nsf/FileURL/mrdoc_41550.pdf/$FILE/Mental%20Health%20Act%202014%20-%20%5B01-g0-02%5D.pdf?OpenElement

References

Dharia S, Verilla K, Breden EL (2011). The 3Ds of geriatic psychiatry: depression, delirium and dementia, The Consultant Pharmacist 26(8):566–578.

Queensland Health (2017). A Guide to the *Mental Health Act 2016.* Queensland Government. Online 28 February 2021. Available: www.health.qld.gov.au/__data/assets/pdf_file/0031/444856/guide-to-mha.pdf

CHAPTER 17
Working with older clients requiring palliative care

By Janet Kerswell Unnasch

AFTER READING THIS CHAPTER, YOU SHOULD BE ABLE TO:

- define the key terms listed in this chapter
- understand reactions to grief, loss, death and dying
- be aware of attitudes to death and dying and how these attitudes are influenced by age, culture and religion
- know the stages of dying
- be aware of the legal issues in relation to the dying person
- know the signs of approaching death and the signs of death
- understand the aims of palliative care
- understand the care needs of the individual requiring palliative care
- assist with post-mortem care
- know how to promote quality of life.

Key terms

advance health directive: A document stating a person's wishes about healthcare when the person can no longer make their own decisions

Cheyne-Stokes respirations: Respirations that gradually increase in rate and depth and then become shallow and slow; breathing may stop for 10–20 seconds

euthanasia: When medical intervention takes place, at the patient's request, in order to end the patient's life

grief: An emotional response to loss and changes that have resulted because of that loss

loss: An actual or potential situation in which something or someone that is valued is no longer seen, felt, heard or experienced

palliative care: A philosophy of care for the person who has an incurable illness or injury

physician-assisted suicide: A doctor intentionally helping a person to terminate his or her life by providing drugs for self-administration, at that person's voluntary and competent request

post-mortem: After (*post*) death (*mortem*)

rigor mortis: The stiffness or rigidity (*rigor*) of skeletal muscles that occurs after death (*mortis*)

terminal illness: An illness or injury for which there is no reasonable expectation of recovery

Sometimes death is sudden and sometimes it is expected. The dying process can symbolise helplessness or a failure to cure. The dying person needs good palliative care, and the carer must carefully examine his or her own feelings about death and dying. Your opinions and thoughts will considerably affect the way you give care. As you will need to help meet the person's physical, psychological, social and spiritual needs, it is important that you have a thorough understanding of the dying process.

LOSS AND GRIEF

Loss, grief, death and dying are all part of the life cycle. Every person experiences these at different times during their own life. Each person's response to loss, grief, death and dying is individual. As a member of the healthcare team, personal carers will encounter clients and families experiencing these phenomena. Many people are uncomfortable with their feelings about loss, grief, death and dying. It is important that the personal carer has an understanding of these phenomena so that they understand their own feelings, but also, more importantly, so that they can assist the client and family who are experiencing loss, grief, death and bereavement.

There is nothing shameful or wrong in accepting that dealing with death and dying can have some impact on you personally. Speak with your supervisor and ask for some grief counselling to help you personally work through any issues.

Loss is an actual or potential situation in which something or someone that is valued is no longer seen, felt, heard or experienced. The loss may be temporary or permanent, complete or partial, physical or symbolic. It is important to understand that people will respond to loss in many different ways, but only the person experiencing the loss can determine the meaning of that loss.

Grief is the emotional response to the loss and the changes that have resulted because of that loss. Grief is a natural response to a loss. Responses can be complex and varied. When an individual is faced with a serious loss, the process of grieving may begin before the loss occurs. The process of grieving for the person who is dying may be a process of 'letting go'.

Reactions to loss and coping with grief are influenced by the type of loss experienced, the stage of growth and development of the person experiencing the loss and cultural, religious and spiritual beliefs. Mourning represents a period of time following the death of a loved one. Many cultures and religions have specific practices that are adhered to as part of the mourning process. Personal carers encounter clients and families who are experiencing loss and grief due to terminal illness, injury or death.

Responses to grief may include:

- emotional – anger, guilt, shame, relief, depression
- physical – nausea, lack of appetite, giddiness, headaches, shaking
- cognitive – preoccupation, lapse of memory, confusion.

TERMINAL ILLNESS

Many illnesses and diseases have no cure. Some injuries are so serious that the body cannot function and recovery is not expected. The disease or injury ends in death. An illness or injury for which there is no reasonable expectation of recovery is a **terminal illness**.

It is difficult to predict the duration of a terminal illness. A person may have years, months, weeks or days to live. The personal carer will encounter death at some time and it is important that you understand the dying process.

Attitudes to death and dying

Experiences, culture, religion and age influence people's attitudes to death and dying. Attitudes about death may change as a person grows older and as their health circumstances change. Some people view death and dying as a natural process that holds no fear. Some may experience anxiety and others may fear death. Common fears about death include:

- fear of pain or isolation while dying
- fear of non-existence
- fear of what happens after death
- fear of an unpleasant afterlife.

Care of the dying person can take place in traditional healthcare agencies, such as hospitals or aged care facilities, or in less traditional settings, such as hospices, palliative care units or the person's own home. The family is encouraged to be involved in the care of the dying person. However, many adults and children have not had experience with the process of dying and death. Therefore, it can be seen as a frightening process.

Age

Attitudes to death and dying may differ depending on the age of the person exposed to the death of another person. Adults may have more fears about death than children do. Adults fear pain and suffering, dying alone and the invasion of privacy. Loneliness and separation from loved ones are other fears. They worry about the care and support of those left behind. Adults often resent death because it affects their plans, hopes, dreams and ambitions.

Many people feel that discussing death and dying is morbid or in poor taste. However, it is important that the personal carer understands the attitudes that the person has to death and dying, in order to provide a caring and supportive environment for the client and their family.

Children's attitudes to death

Infants and toddlers have no concept of death. Between the ages of 3 and 5 years, children are curious and have ideas about death. They know when family members or pets die. They notice dead birds or bugs. They think death is temporary. Children often blame themselves when someone or something dies. To them, death is punishment for being bad. Answers to questions about death often cause fear and confusion. Children who are told 'he is sleeping' may become afraid to go to sleep.

Children between the ages of 5 and 7 years know death is final. They do not think they will die. Death happens to other people. It can be avoided. Children relate death to punishment and body mutilation and think that it may also involve monsters, ghosts and witches. These ideas come from fairy tales, cartoons, movies, video games and television.

Older people's attitudes to death

Older adults usually have fewer fears. They know death will occur. They have had more experiences with death and dying. Many have lost family members or friends. Some welcome death as freedom from pain, suffering and disability. Death may also mean a reunion with those who have died. Like younger adults, they often fear dying alone.

Carer's attitude to death

As a carer, you will have thoughts and feeling based on your own experiences and beliefs. At no time can you allow them to interfere with the care that you give. At all times you must follow the care plan and carry out the wishes and beliefs of your client. If you are unable to care for a dying or grieving client based on your own thoughts and feelings, you need to ask for supervision, guidance and support from a senior staff member or line manager.

Stages of grief

Although there are several theorists who discuss the grieving process and attitudes to dying, the foremost theorist of these subjects is Dr Elisabeth Kübler-Ross. She identified five stages of grief within her seminal text, *On Death and Dying* (1969):

1. *Denial* – the person refuses to believe they are dying. 'No, not me' is a common response. The dying person believes a mistake has been made. Information about the illness or injury is not heard. The dying person cannot deal with problems or decisions about the matter. This stage can last for a few hours, days or much longer. Some people are still in denial when they die.
2. *Anger* – the dying person thinks, 'Why me?' There is anger and rage. The dying person envies and resents those with life and health. Family, friends and the healthcare team are often targets of anger. The person blames others and finds fault with those who are loved and needed the most. It is hard to deal with the dying person during this stage. Anger is normal and healthy. Do not take the person's anger personally. Control any urge to attack back or to avoid the person.
3. *Bargaining* – anger has passed. The person now says, 'Yes, me, but ...'; often the person bargains with God for more time. Promises are made in exchange for more time. The person may want to see a child marry, see a grandchild, have one more Christmas or live for some other event. Usually, more promises are made as the dying person makes 'just one more' request. You may not see this stage. Bargaining is usually private and on a spiritual level.
4. *Depression* – the person thinks 'Yes, me' and is very sad. The person mourns things that were lost and future loss of life. The person may cry or say little. Sometimes the person talks about people and things that will be left behind.
5. *Acceptance* – the person is calm and at peace. They have said what needs to be said. Unfinished business is completed. The person accepts death. This stage may last for many months or years. Reaching acceptance does not mean that death is near.

A dying person does not always go through all five stages. A person may never get beyond a certain stage. Some move back and forth between stages. Some people stay in one stage until death (Kübler-Ross 1969). Some now dispute the work of Kübler-Ross, as dying and death cannot be easily staged in these five areas, but her work remains relevant today.

Culture and religion

The personal carer needs to understand and accept that there is a wide range of feelings and attitudes about death and dying based on personal, religious, cultural and spiritual needs and philosophies. These needs and philosophies include beliefs about the afterlife; for example, that in the afterlife one is free of suffering and hardship, or one is reunited with loved ones, or punished for one's sins or misdeeds, or that there is no afterlife and that death is just the end of life. There are religious beliefs about the body's form after death; for example, that the spirit or soul leaves the body and moves into the afterlife. Reincarnation is the belief that the spirit or soul is reborn in another human body or in another lifeform.

DEATH RITES

In discussing death with Indigenous Australians, many factors need to be considered: cultural beliefs, extended family and taboos about discussing death or a deceased person. The Indigenous person usually has a large extended family, which includes several mothers, fathers, brothers and sisters. Significant grief and loss responses can begin immediately the family is advised of an impending death. The concept of belonging to the land may be extremely important to the Indigenous person. They may wish to return to their own surroundings and be visited by their own kin.

After the Indigenous person has died, sorrow camps may be assembled. These camps differ between Indigenous groups. Grieving ceremonies are centred on the responsibility of the extended family to ensure that the spirit passes into the Dreamtime world. The person's room becomes 'taboo'. If it is in a hospital, the room becomes a place that can no longer be entered. If the person dies at home, the family moves. Indigenous communities may perform a smoking ceremony to ensure that the person's spirit moves on. The deceased person's name is no longer mentioned in some groups. This varies between groups, as spiritual beliefs differ from group to group.

It is important that the personal carer treats the Indigenous person and their family with respect, and acknowledges the significance of their culture.

The concept of kinship is very strong in Māori culture. When there is a death, Māori people mourn for three days. Death is very significant to the Māoris. When one person dies, the mourning affects everyone. After a death, visitors from far and wide will join the mourning ceremony. Special and treasured possessions may be laid in the grave with the person.

There are some very good resources available that examine different cultures and the rituals of dying and death. One such resource is *An outline of different cultural beliefs at the time of death* (see Further reading at the end of the chapter).

CARING ABOUT CULTURE

In Vietnam, quality of life is more important than length of life, because of beliefs about reincarnation. Less suffering in the next life is expected. Therefore, dying people are helped to recall past good deeds and to achieve a fitting mental state. Death at home is preferred over death in a hospital.

Upon death, the body is washed and wrapped in clean white sheets. In some areas, a coin or jewels (a wealthy family) and rice (a poor family) are put in the dead person's mouth. This is from the belief that they will help the soul go through encounters with gods and devils and that the soul will be born rich in the next life. Relatives sew small pillows to place under the body's neck, feet and wrists. The body is placed in a coffin for in-ground burial.

The Chinese have an aversion to death and to anything concerning death. Autopsy and disposal of the body are not prescribed by religion. Euthanasia is allowed. Donating body parts is encouraged. The eldest son makes all arrangements. The deceased is initially buried in a coffin. After seven years, the body is exhumed and cremated. The urn is reburied in the tomb. White clothing is worn for mourning.

Hindu people are often accepting of God's will. The person's desire to be clear-headed as death nears must be assessed in planning medical treatment. A time and place for prayer are essential for the family and the person. Prayer helps them deal with anxiety and conflict. The Hindu priest, or anyone present, may read from holy Sanskrit books. Some priests use strings (meaning a blessing) around the neck or wrist. After death, the priest pours water into the mouth of the deceased. Families may prefer that only Hindus touch the body and may wash the body themselves. Blood transfusions, organ transplants and autopsies are allowed. Cremation is preferred. Reincarnation is a Hindu belief.

PALLIATIVE CARE

Palliative care is a philosophy of care for the person who has an incurable illness or injury. The philosophy emphasises spiritual care, relief and management of symptoms, and the total care and support of the client and their family member during the terminal phases of illnesses. Palliative practices do not include **euthanasia** or **physician-assisted suicide**. The goal of palliative care is to achieve the best quality of life for the client and their family. The focus of care is the client and their family. Palliative care does not aim to hasten or postpone a person's death.

Aims of care

Caring is the essence of good palliative care. All the actions of the carer are focused on providing for the needs and comfort of the client and their family. The key aim of palliative care is the comfort of the client, including the control of symptoms, anticipating the physical changes and needs of the client and providing individualised care. The personal carer plays an important role in providing care and comfort for the terminally ill client. Wherever possible, it is important for the person receiving palliative care to be cared for in an environment of his or her own choice. In both Australia and New Zealand, there are national standards that outline the guidelines for the delivery of compassionate and appropriate end-of-life care. Take time to visit the websites and peruse the standards (see Further reading at the end of the chapter).

Delivery of palliative care

Palliative care can be delivered across a wide variety of healthcare environments. It is a complementary approach to traditional healthcare delivery for the terminally ill client. Different models of palliative care have evolved in response to the needs of the client and community. These models include dedicated palliative care units, community-based services, hospice-at-home services, inpatient care services and palliative care consultancy services. Within these services, the personal carer works as part of the larger multidisciplinary healthcare team to ensure a holistic, client-centred approach to care. Palliative care begins once a diagnosis of a terminal disease or injury has been made.

Palliative care team

The palliative care team is a multidisciplinary team that offers strategies and advice depending on the area of expertise and role in client care. The team may be made up of a general practitioner (GP), medical specialists, nurses, occupational therapist, dietitian, physiotherapist, speech therapist, counsellors, carers, family, friends and volunteers. As the carer, you will spend more time with the client than anyone else, so it is important that you recognise changes and report them to the appropriate person. You will also support and comfort the client and the family during this time. At no time should any member of the team impose their own personal opinions or beliefs onto the client's care plan.

PALLIATIVE CARE OF THE INDIVIDUAL

Palliative care of the terminally ill person is one of the most challenging skills faced by personal carers. It can be demanding and stressful, but it can also be very rewarding.

The healthcare team cannot control the inevitable death of the person, but the personal carer can do much to ensure that the final stages of life are as comfortable as possible for the dying person and their family.

The dying process may take place over a prolonged period. The body processes become slow and the person is weak. Changes occur in the level of consciousness. Promoting independence within the abilities of the client is encouraged. As the person becomes weaker, they may become dependent on others for basic needs and activities of daily living. The dying person may become angry or upset as they come to realise that they can no longer complete their own care needs and will now need to rely on others.

It is important to recognise that the person receiving palliative care has the same needs as other people; it is just that some needs take a greater priority than others. The overall aim of palliative care is to promote physical, psychological, emotional and spiritual support for the individual, while also preserving their self-esteem, dignity, individuality and cultural needs.

Physical comfort

It is imperative that a plan of care is developed and implemented that reflects specific and individual needs of the client. The dying process is often accompanied by discomfort and problems, including breathing difficulties and alterations in nutrition, hydration, elimination, mobility and sensory perception. At varying times during the process, the client may also experience acute or chronic pain. The care plan must be reviewed and altered in response to the client's changing needs in order to provide quality care.

Personal hygiene

Skin care, personal hygiene, back massages, good body alignment and oral hygiene promote comfort. Some people experience severe pain. The registered nurse or medical officer can give pain-relieving medications prior to attending to hygiene needs. Frequent position changes and supportive devices may also promote comfort. The personal carer may need help to turn the person slowly and gently. Semi-Fowler's position is usually best for breathing problems.

Oral hygiene promotes comfort. Routine mouth care is given whether the person can eat and drink or not. Frequent oral care is given as death nears and when taking oral fluids is difficult. Oral hygiene is needed if mucus collects in the mouth and the person cannot swallow.

Crusting and irritation of the nostrils can occur. Nasal secretions, an oxygen cannula or nasogastric tube are common causes. Regular nasal care is essential to the comfort of the client.

Circulation fails and body temperature rises as death nears, although the body may feel cold. The skin is cool, pale and mottled (blotchy). Perspiration increases. Skin care, bathing and preventing pressure ulcers are necessary. Linen and gowns are changed whenever needed. Although the skin feels cool, only light bed coverings are needed. Blankets may make the person feel too warm and cause restlessness.

Mobility and positioning

As the dying process progresses, the client will begin to have difficulty mobilising. They may require constant supervision and the use of mobility aids. Eventually, they will become unable to ambulate. It is important during this stage to maintain proper body alignment to prevent skin breakdown or contractures. The client should be positioned comfortably in bed or a chair with the support of pressure-relieving devices. Repositioning should take place at regular intervals at a time determined by the client's needs and comfort level. The client's wishes regarding repositioning must also be taken into consideration, such as at times preferring to remain as they are rather than being disturbed. Pain relief may be necessary prior to position changes.

Breathing difficulties

The client may experience shortness of breath, which increases significantly with minimal exertion. The personal carer should endeavour to minimise care activities that exacerbate breathing difficulties. The client may find it difficult to cough or expectorate to clear their airway. Aspiration of secretions is a potential problem, so the use of a semi-Fowler's or side-lying position can facilitate breathing. The personal carer must ensure that the airway is maintained. It may be necessary to perform oro-nasopharyngeal suctioning and apply oxygen therapy to promote ease of breathing. However, suctioning and oxygen therapy are usually attended to by the nurses – you must only do this if you have been given the delegated responsibility to do so. You must also be trained in these techniques prior to using them.

Nutrition and hydration

The client receiving palliative care may be unable to swallow safely and/or tolerate oral foods or fluids. The client may also require assistance with eating and drinking. They should be provided with food or beverages of their choice and within the limits of their tolerance for food or fluids. Regular mouth care is essential for such clients. Nausea and vomiting may be relieved by the use of anti-emetic medications.

If the client cannot swallow, nasogastric or percutaneous endoscopic gastrostomy feeding may be initiated dependent on the client's wishes. Subcutaneous fluid infusions are sometimes initiated. These options will have been previously discussed with the patient and their wishes should be documented in their advance health directive.

Medications

Pain is an individual experience, and it is often undertreated in the home, community and hospital settings. It is easy to underestimate or make false assumptions of an individual's pain. Pain is what the client feels and describes, not what you or others think. The client's perception of pain will depend on their mood, culture and what pain means to the individual client. It is important for the personal carer to observe their client for non-verbal signs of pain as some older clients will not complain of pain; however, they may admit to it if asked.

Medications to minimise pain and relieve symptoms associated with dying must be prescribed and administered. The nurses give these medications. These medications are usually opioids and include medications such as morphine and codeine. Medicated patches must only be removed by registered staff. If a patch is found to have come off, it is to be kept for registered staff for correct disposal. The registered staff member must be informed of this as soon as possible as the patient's pain management will be negatively affected.

When required, medications are also given to ease anxiety, depression or restlessness. Medications can be also used to help control some of the symptoms associated with the effects of terminal illness, such as constipation, nausea, terminal restlessness and anxiety.

Elimination

Common elimination problems experienced by clients include constipation, impacted faeces, urinary retention and urinary or faecal incontinence. Assessment by a continence adviser and the use of continence products may be recommended. Suppositories or enemas may be used to promote bowel evacuation. Appropriate incontinence aids, urinary catheters or stomal therapy appliances may also be used, depending on the underlying condition of the client. Perineal care is extremely important. Assisting the client with meeting their elimination needs, including perineal care, urinary catheter care or stomal therapy care, may be delegated to the personal carer. Clients often feel embarrassed during some procedures, so personal carers should endeavour to alleviate or minimise these feelings. Prompt and professional attention following episodes of incontinence will preserve your client's dignity.

Sensory perception

The client may experience diminishing sensory perception. Vision and touch may be affected. Vision blurs and gradually fails. Because of failing vision, it is important that the personal carer explains what is being done to the person whenever the carer is in the room. The room should be well lit, but avoid bright lights and glare.

Friends and family should be supported and encouraged to maintain gentle physical contact with the client.

Although the sense of touch may be diminished, the client can generally feel the pressure of touch.

The eyes may be half open. Secretions may collect in the corners of the eyes. Good eye care is essential. If the eyes stay open, the personal carer can be directed to apply a protective ointment or to apply moist eye pads to prevent further injury and discomfort. This treatment should be documented on the plan of care and reviewed by the registered nurse.

Hearing is not usually diminished. Many people hear until the moment of death. Even unconscious people may hear. It is important that the personal carer always assumes that the person can hear and speaks with a normal voice. Care strategies include providing reassurance and explanations about care, offering words of comfort and providing comfort measures, including playing favourite music. It is advisable to avoid topics that could upset the person.

Speech becomes difficult. It may be hard to understand the person. Sometimes the person cannot speak. Anticipate the person's needs. Do not ask questions that need long answers. Ask 'yes' or 'no' questions. These should be few in number. Despite the client's speech problems, the personal carer must continue to talk to the client.

Skin breakdown

Over time, the client may become emaciated and lose the adipose tissue that 'pads' bony prominences. The client may become unable to move, which increases the risk of pressure area development. Hygiene care and repositioning needs to be attended to regularly. Pressure-relieving devices and management of incontinence episodes are essential.

End-of-life care or advance care planning

As a person nears the end of their life, care changes will be necessary to support their needs. Clients' wishes need to be respected and care planned accordingly. Advance care planning is about making decisions now for future care and is carried out in consultation with the client and family. Advance care planning offers everyone – the client, their families and significant others – the opportunity to take control of decisions that affect their care. This includes determining the type and level of medical intervention that is to be undertaken.

Psychological, social and spiritual comfort

Clients receiving palliative care have psychological, social and spiritual needs. They may want family and friends to be present. They may want to talk about their fears, worries and anxieties. Some may want to be alone. Often people need to talk at night, when things are quiet and there are fewer distractions and more time to think.

Communication skills

The personal carer needs to use active listening and therapeutic touch skills.

- *Active listening* – the person needs to talk and share their worries and concerns. Let the person express feelings and emotions in their own way. Just being there and listening is helpful. Do not worry about saying the wrong thing or finding comforting words. Reassure the client that you hear and understand them; this can be simply accomplished by a nod of the head or quietly repeating what has been said. At times, the best communication strategy is silence. Being with the person is what is important.
- *Therapeutic touch* – this shows caring and concern when words cannot. Sometimes the person does not want to talk but wants you nearby. Physical presence is reassuring for the client. Therapeutic touch coupled with silence is

a powerful and meaningful means of communication. A gentle touch of the hand lets your client know they are not alone.

Spiritual needs

Personal carers must be sensitive to the spiritual needs of the client and promote actions that may help the client meet those needs. Clients receiving palliative care may want to see a religious or spiritual leader. They may wish to take part in religious or spiritual practices. The personal carer should respect the need for religious or spiritual comfort and ensure that the client has privacy during prayer or spiritual moments, and that religious or spiritual objects are nearby (e.g. medals, pictures, statues and religious writings).

The person's room

The person may wish to have palliative care delivered in their own home, or may wish to be in a hospital, aged care facility or hospice. It is important that the client's surroundings are pleasant and comfortable and reflect the person's needs and wishes. The room should be well lit and well ventilated. Unnecessary equipment is removed. Some equipment is upsetting to look at (e.g. suction machines, drainage containers). If possible, this equipment is kept out of the person's sight. Carers should also be mindful to ensure the surrounds are kept smelling fresh.

Mementoes, pictures, cards, flowers, religious items and other items are comforting. Arrange them within the person's view. The person and family arrange the room as they wish. This helps meet love, belonging and self-esteem needs.

The family

This is a hard time for the family. The personal carer's role is to assist the client and their family through the processes of grieving, loss, death and bereavement. It may be very hard to find comforting words. Show your feelings by being available, courteous and considerate. Use respectful touch to show your concern.

The family should be allowed to stay as long as they wish. Sometimes family members stay during the night. The health team helps make them as comfortable as possible.

You must respect the right to privacy. The person and family need time together. However, you cannot neglect care because the family is present. Most centres let family members help give care, or you can suggest that they take a break for a drink or a meal.

The family may be very tired, sad and tearful. Watching a loved one die is very painful. So is dealing with the eventual loss of that person. The family goes through stages, like the dying person. They need support, understanding, courtesy and respect. A spiritual leader may provide comfort. Communicate this request to the nurse at once.

Legal issues

Much attention is given to the right to die. Many people do not want machines or other measures keeping them alive. Consent is needed for any treatment. When able, the person makes care decisions. Some people make end-of-life wishes known. Each country and state has specific legal requirements (laws) that protect the terminally ill client and the care that they receive. The personal carer must be fully aware of and work within each of these legal boundaries.

The Powers of Attorney Acts (or similar) allow people to declare their health wishes in an advance health directive and enduring power of attorney. Under this form of legislation, the client or their legal representative can set out the wishes of the client with regard to their healthcare. The Powers of Attorney Acts include the provision of a statutory health attorney, who is appointed by the client to make decisions about healthcare needs in the event that the client is unable to tell others what they want.

An enduring power of attorney is a legal document that gives another person the power to make personal and/or financial decisions on behalf of the client in the event that the client loses the capacity to make decisions for themselves.

An **advance health directive** (also known as a living will) is a document in which the client gives instructions about their future healthcare. It comes into effect only when the client is unable to make their own decisions.

The client or their family representative must inform the healthcare agency or healthcare team that an advance health directive or enduring power of attorney has been made, to ensure that the client's wishes are respected.

SIGNS OF DEATH

As a person approaches death, physiological changes indicate that death is near. These signs may occur rapidly or slowly:

- Movement, muscle tone and sensation are lost. This usually begins in the feet and legs. It eventually spreads to other body parts. When mouth muscles relax, the jaw drops. The mouth may stay open. The facial expression is often peaceful.
- Peristalsis and other gastrointestinal functions slow. Abdominal distension, faecal incontinence, faecal impaction, nausea and vomiting are common.
- The person feels cool or cold, looks pale and perspires heavily.
- Circulation fails. The pulse is fast, weak and irregular. Blood pressure begins to fall.
- The respiratory system fails. **Cheyne-Stokes respirations**, which are slow or rapid and shallow respirations, are common. Mucus collects in the airway.
- Pain decreases as the person loses consciousness. However, some people are conscious until the moment of death.
- The signs of death include no pulse, respirations or blood pressure. The pupils are fixed and dilated. A doctor determines that death has occurred and pronounces the person dead. A registered nurse may complete a 'Life Extinct' form to allow funeral directors to undertake the ongoing care of the deceased person if a doctor is unavailable. This does not replace a death certificate.

DEATH AT HOME

The personal carer may encounter a death in the home setting. When the client is receiving palliative care, the death would be expected. The personal carer should contact their supervisor to discuss the actions to be taken. In some instances, the family GP or palliative care medical officer may be called to certify the death before the funeral director can take the body to the funeral home.

CARE OF THE BODY AFTER DEATH

Care of the body after (*post*) death (*mortem*) is called **post-mortem** care. The personal carer, as part of the healthcare team, may be required to perform post-mortem care. Post-mortem care begins when the doctor pronounces the person dead. Living in a diverse multicultural society, we must be sensitive to differing cultural or religious expectations following death. The individual preferences or rituals relating to cultural or religious observance should be explored with the person or the family well before death occurs. A detailed care plan should be completed in advance to avoid adding distress to the family at the time of death. Ensuring this documentation is available provides for best practice, care and respect for the deceased. In some centres, the body is prepared only for viewing. The funeral director completes post-mortem care. The death may occur in the home setting. Contact the healthcare team and advise them of the death. Follow the care plan, directions given by the healthcare team and the wishes of the family.

Post-mortem care is performed to maintain good appearance of the body. Within 2–4 hours after death, rigor mortis develops. **Rigor mortis** is stiffness or rigidity (*rigor*) of skeletal muscles that occurs after death (*mortis*). The body is positioned in normal alignment before rigor mortis sets in. Dentures should be placed in the mouth, if possible, to maintain the natural appearance of the face.

Post-mortem care may involve repositioning the body. For example, soiled areas are bathed and the body is placed in good alignment. Moving the body can cause remaining air in the lungs, stomach and intestines to be expelled. When air is expelled, sounds are produced. Do not be alarmed or frightened by these sounds. They are normal and to be expected.

The right to privacy and to be treated with dignity and respect apply after death. As the family may wish to see their loved one, the body should appear in a comfortable and natural position.

It is important that the personal carer is aware of the policies and procedures of the healthcare agency when performing post-mortem care.

ASSISTING WITH POST-MORTEM CARE

Quality of life

1 Remember to respect the client's privacy while doing any procedure.

Pre-procedure

2 Wash your hands.
3 Collect the following:
- post-mortem kit (shroud or body bag, gown, identification tags, gauze squares and safety pins); this will vary according to organisational/healthcare agency policy
- bed protectors
- washbasin
- bath towels and wash cloths
- tape
- dressings
- gloves
- cotton balls
- gown.

4 Provide for privacy.
5 Raise the bed for good body mechanics.
6 Make sure the bed is flat.

Procedure

7 Put on gloves.
8 Position the body supine (Fig. 17.1). Arms and legs are straight. A pillow is under the head and shoulders, and ensure pillowcase is clean and fresh.
9 Close the eyes. Gently pull the eyelids over the eyes. Apply moist cotton balls gently over the eyelids if the eyes will not stay closed.
10 Insert dentures if it is organisational/healthcare agency policy. If not, put them in a labelled denture container.
11 Close the mouth. If necessary, place a rolled towel under the chin to keep the mouth closed.
12 Follow organisational/healthcare agency policy about jewellery. Remove all jewellery, except for wedding rings, if this is policy. List the jewellery that you have removed. Place the jewellery and the list in a valuables envelope. When providing post-mortem care in the community or a home setting, jewellery can be directly passed on to the next of kin if present. Ensure this is clearly documented in the care record.
13 If a wedding ring remains, tape it in place.
14 Follow organisational/healthcare agency policy on drainage containers. Remove them if permitted. Ensure care is taken if removing infusion lines so as to avoid sustaining accidental needle stick injuries. All sharps are to be placed in a sharps container. Leave tubes and catheters in place if there will be an autopsy. Confirm with the registered nurse about removing tubes. Ensure sharps are removed and disposed of carefully. Follow organisational procedure for removal and disposal of infusions containing end-of-life medications.
15 Bathe soiled areas with plain water. Dry thoroughly.
16 Place a bed protector under the buttocks.
17 Remove soiled dressings. Replace them with a clean dressing.
18 Put a clean gown on the body. Position the body as in step 8.
19 Brush and comb the hair if necessary.
20 Cover the body to the shoulders with a sheet if the family will view the body.

21 Collect the person's belongings if appropriate. Put them in a bag labelled with the person's name.

22 Remove supplies, equipment and linen. Straighten the room. Provide soft lighting.

23 Remove the gloves and decontaminate your hands.

24 Let the family view the body. Provide for privacy. Return to the room after the family leaves.

25 Decontaminate your hands and put on gloves.

26 Fill out the identification tags. Attach one to an ankle or to the right big toe; alternatively some organisations prefer identification to be taped to the chest. Follow organisational policy.

27 Place the body in the body bag or cover it with a sheet. Alternatively, apply the shroud (Fig. 17.2).

- **a** Bring the top down over the head.
- **b** Fold the bottom up over the feet.
- **c** Fold the sides over the body.
- **d** Pin or tape the shroud in place.

28 Attach the second identification tag to the shroud, sheet or body bag.

29 Leave the denture cup with the body.

30 Pull the privacy curtain around the bed. Or close the door.

31 Remove the gloves and decontaminate your hands.

Post-procedure

32 Strip the unit after the body has been removed. Wear gloves for this step.

33 Remove the gloves and decontaminate your hands.

34 Document and report the following to the nurse:

- the time at which the body was taken by the funeral director
- what was done with jewellery and personal items
- what was done with dentures.

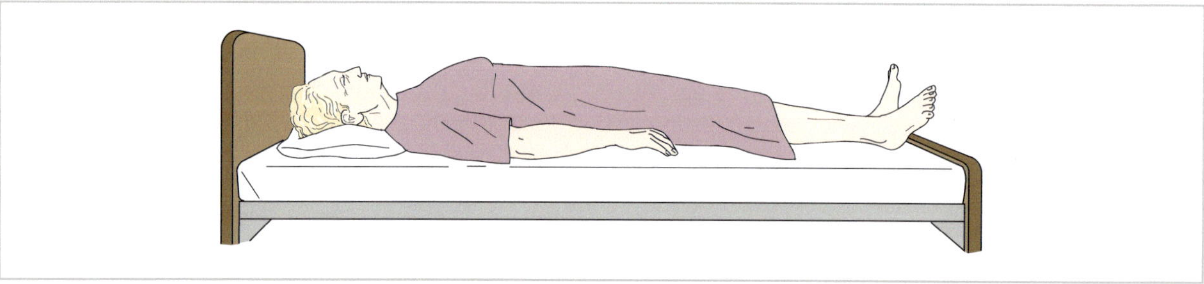

Fig. 17.1

The body is in the dorsal recumbent position. Arms are straight at the sides. A pillow is under the head and shoulders.

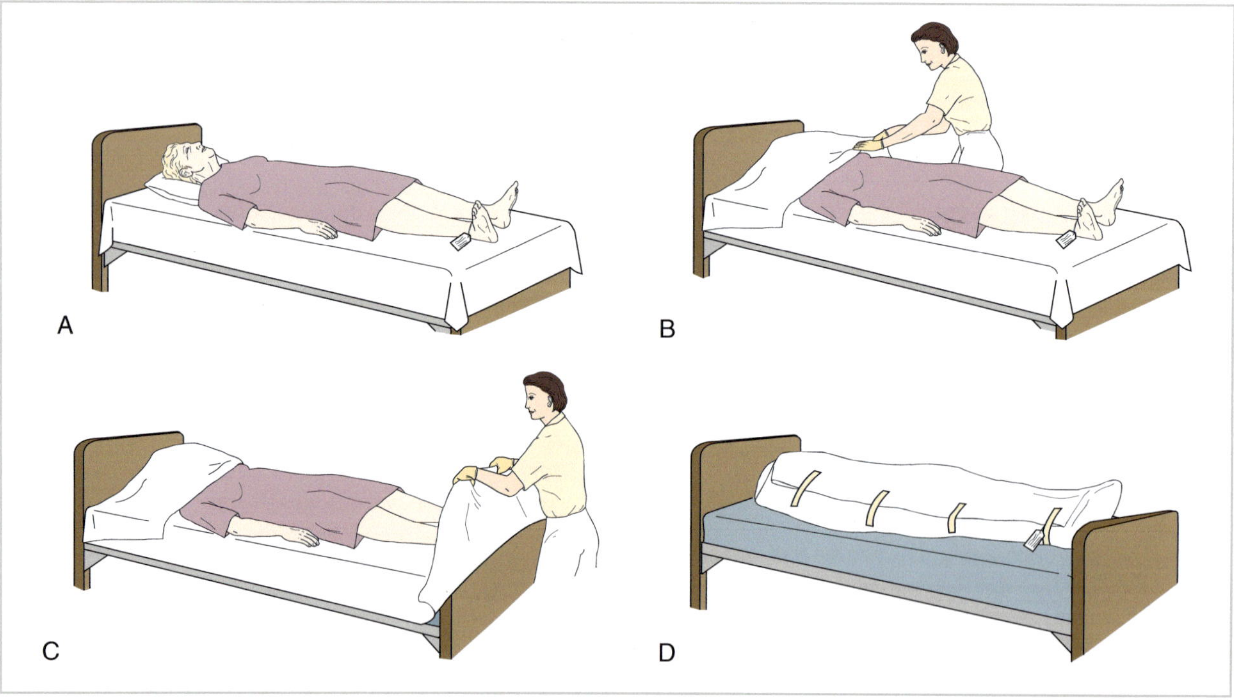

Fig. 17.2

Applying a shroud. **A.** Place the body on the shroud. **B.** Bring the top of the shroud down over the head. **C.** Fold the bottom up over the feet. **D.** Fold the sides over the body. Tape or pin the sides together. Attach the identification tag.

SAFETY ALERT

Post-mortem care

Standard Precautions are followed. You may have contact with infected blood, body fluids, secretions or excretions.

FOCUS ON COMMUNITY CARE

It is often a client's wish to have palliative care delivered within their own home rather than in a care facility. It is therefore important that you recognise you are working in the client's home and you must respect the client's property at all times. All home palliative care needs are planned with input from your client, their family and the care team. When delivering care within your client's home, always remember that your normal routine may be interrupted. Family members may wish to spend time with your client when you are there. You must be flexible to their needs at this time, and may have to compromise with your timetable. However, this must not be at your client's detriment. Always consider your client's wellbeing first.

While caring for your client, their family may ask you questions about the person's treatment, care and prognosis. Always refer them to either your supervisor or the medical team. There may be some issues or discussions that they wish to manage personally. Always answer truthfully about the care you personally give but do not discuss issues that you are unsure of. Refer to the registered nurse.

If family members wish to assist you to give care (and your client has agreed to this), let them help. It may assist these family members considerably with managing the situation.

There are a number of good internet sites on palliative care that you may also like to peruse to consolidate and extend your knowledge within this area. CareSearch, established by the Palliative Care Knowledge Network, is a good example of an Australian-based site. You will also find good data on the Department of Health website. Take time to search through these sites (see Further reading at the end of the chapter).

QUALITY OF LIFE

Quality of life is often described in very abstract terms. It is multidimensional and encompasses biological, psychological, environmental, social, economic, interpersonal and cultural dimensions. The personal carer needs to define quality of life in terms of those dimensions that are important to the dying person and their family. These factors will vary depending on the individual clients who are being cared for and impact on the care experienced by the client and their family.

CASE STUDY

Ravi Singh, a 53-year-old man, was diagnosed with an aggressive form of prostate cancer. He lived with his wife and had the support of his extended family (children, siblings and parents). His local doctor referred him to a specialist when he had a raised prostate-specific antigen (PSA) level. His specialist was attached to the local hospital. Surgery was performed and Ravi's prostate gland was removed.

Ravi then had radiotherapy and chemotherapy over a period of a couple of months. During this time he experienced incontinence of urine, erectile dysfunction, pain and depression. His specialist and local doctor managed his pain and other problems. Ravi's condition deteriorated and he was admitted to hospital for a palliative care team assessment. After the assessment, in consultation with Ravi, his wife and the palliative care team, it was decided that Ravi could return home. A full assessment was carried out of the home, and equipment necessary for Ravi to remain at home was provided. This included a hospital bed, walker, wheelchair, commode, bath chair and handrail in bathroom, toilet and entrance way. The palliative care team organised an education session for Ravi's wife and his family prior to his return home. Ravi was discharged to his home. The palliative care nurse was organised to visit Ravi, monitor his condition and provide him with pain relief. Ravi passed away 6 weeks after his discharge. He was at home with family and friends as he wished.

ACCREDITATION

You are working in residential or home care and accreditors are at your service. Can you answer the following questions?

- What is an advance care directive?
- How would you ensure that a consumer's end-of-life care requirements are followed?
- Who might be part of a multidisciplinary care team, when caring for a person at their end of life?

REVIEW QUESTIONS

Circle the BEST answer:

1 Which is true?

a The personal carer can do much to ensure that the final stages of life are as comfortable as possible for the dying person and their family.

b The personal carer is only able to offer comfort and support to their client, not their client's family.

c The personal carer only performs assistance with hygiene and nutritional needs for their client.

d The personal carer supports the client's family while the registered staff care for the client.

2 Which is true?

a Palliative care is commenced during the week before a person's death is anticipated.

b Palliative care is commenced when a person is diagnosed with a terminal illness.

c Palliative care is only offered if the patient's family request it.

d Palliative care is only offered to patients with private health insurance.

3 These statements relate to family involvement during the palliation of their loved one. Which is false?

a If the patient is agreeable, the family members may be allowed to take part in providing care.

b The family members should be allowed to visit with their loved one as long as they wish.

c The personal carer must recognise that the family need support, understanding, courtesy and respect.

d The family must ensure the family members leave at the closing of visiting hours.

4 It is important for the personal carer to assess their patient's level of pain and anxiety as:

a it may be possible for the registered nurse and doctor to administer extra or alternative types of medication to relieve pain and anxiety

b it means their time of death is imminent

c the family members need to be asked to leave so the patient can retain their dignity

d the personal carer can then perform tasks while the patient is already anxious and in pain

5 When attending post-mortem care all of the following are true EXCEPT:

a it is important to continue to treat your patient with dignity and respect

b it is important to place the body in good alignment

c dentures are to be placed in the mouth if possible

d eye glasses, if worn, should be put in place

6 An advance health care directive:

a is sometimes known as a living will

b contains the person's wishes regarding their future care

c should be acknowledged and complied with.

d All of the above

Circle T if the statement is true or F if the statement is false:

7 T/F A body should be placed in proper alignment after rigor mortis has commenced.

8 T/F The patient who is receiving palliative care must do so only in a hospital environment.

9 T/F The personal carer is an integral member of the palliative care team.

10 T/F A doctor must certify that the patient has died.

Answers to these questions are on p. 454.

Further reading

Australian Government, Department of Health (2017). Palliative care and planning for end-of-life care. Online 12 October 2021. Available: www.health.gov.au/palliativecare

CareSearch. Palliative Care Knowledge Network (2017). Online 12 October 2021. Available: www.caresearch.com.au/tabid/6129/Default.aspx

CareSearch. Palliative Care Knowledge Network (2017). Religious and cultural considerations. Online 12 October 2021. Available: www.caresearch.com.au/tabid/6329/Default.aspx

Centre for Cultural Diversity and Ageing (2017). An outline of different cultural beliefs at the time of death. Online 12 October 2021. Available: www.culturaldiversity.com.au/news/94-news-and-events/225-resource-an-outline-of-different-cultural-beliefs-at-the-time-of-death

Hospice New Zealand (2019). Standards for palliative care. Online 12 October 2021. Available: www.hospice.org.nz/resources/standards-for-palliative-care/

Kübler-Ross E (1969). On death and dying. Macmillan, New York.

Palliative Care Australia (2018). The National Palliative Care Standards, 5th edition. Online 12 October 2021. Available: www.palliativecare.org.au/Standards/Thenationalstandards.aspx

Palliative Care Australia 2017. Understanding grief. Online 12 October 2021. Available: palliativecare.org.au/wp-content/uploads/dlm_uploads/2015/05/PCA002_Understanding-Grief_W02.pdf

Parliament of Australia (2021). Euthanasia – The Australian law in an international context. Online 12 October 2021. Available: www.aph.gov.au/About_Parliament/Parliamentary_Departments/Parliamentary_Library/pubs/rp/RP9697/97rp4

CHAPTER 18
Assisting with medications

By Carla Unicomb and Penny Kraemer

AFTER READING THIS CHAPTER, YOU SHOULD BE ABLE TO:

- define the key terms listed in this chapter
- understand how to assist with and administer medications
- identify the effects of medications on older people
- discuss legal and other responsibilities of the personal care worker regarding medication administration
- describe the procedure for reporting medication errors
- identify adverse reactions
- identify reporting and recording requirements
- outline the procedure for assisting and administering medications
- understand how to handle medication contingencies

Key terms

adverse reaction: A reaction that occurs when a medication causes an unintended secondary effect

dose administration aid (DAA): An aid used to organise medicines according to the time and day when they should be taken

electronic medication management (EMM) system: A system that enables prescribing, supplying and administration of medications to be completed electronically

medication interaction: A reaction that can occur when one medication affects the actions of another

medication record: A legal record kept for each client detailing the medication requirements of each client

over-the-counter (OTC) medications: Medications available without a prescription (e.g. paracetamol, cough suppressants, vitamin supplements)

pill organiser: A device used to separate medication doses into days and times

polypharmacy: The use of five or more medications, including prescription, OTC and complementary medicines.

sachet packs: A pre-packed medication system packed by a packing machine, then checked by a pharmacist

self-administration: Managing and taking one's own medications

substance incompatibility: An undesirable reaction that may occur between two or more substances; for example, warfarin and aspirin. Both drugs have an anticoagulant action so can lead to increased risk of bleeding

therapeutic medications: Medications used to cure or maintain a condition, or medications that give relief (e.g. painkillers)

Issues related to assisting with medication administration are complex. They relate to both legalities and safety concerns. A registered nurse may delegate to you the responsibility of assisting people who cannot manage their own medication administration. Before you accept this responsibility, always ensure that you have the legal right to do so, that your organisational policy allows you to, that you have sufficient training and have been assessed as competent against your organisation's own medication procedures.

It is important that any care worker delegated the responsibility of assisting with medication administration should acknowledge the importance of this duty and act accordingly. Assisting with medications is something that a carer should never take lightly, as the consequences of any error may be lethal.

WHAT ARE MEDICATIONS?

We take medications every day without realising it. The caffeine in your coffee is a medication, so are the anthocyanins in a glass of red wine, and even the vitamin supplement you take can be classified as a medication. Medications can be used to cure or control a condition. They can also be used to give relief, as in the case of painkillers. These medications are called **therapeutic medications**. Some are prescribed by the doctor and others can be bought **over-the-counter (OTC)** from pharmacies or in supermarkets. Under legislation, the use and availability of all medications are identified under the *Scheduling of Medicines and Poisons Act* (see Box 18.3).

All medications have the capacity to both help and harm the client. Sometimes, very simple and common medications can cause potentially lethal **adverse reactions**, and high dosages of some vitamins can have harmful effects on the body. When more than five medications are taken by a client (**polypharmacy**), the risk of a **medication interaction** is significantly increased. For example, if a client is taking medication to prevent blood clotting, aspirin should not be taken as this can lead to bleeding. Even substances bought from health food shops can affect other medications taken by a client. It is also important to be aware of the effect even small amounts of alcohol can have on the actions of some medications.

THE EFFECTS OF MEDICATIONS ON OLDER PEOPLE

The ageing process alters the way in which medications are absorbed, broken down and excreted from our bodies. Therefore, medications are prescribed cautiously for the older client. Age-related changes in gastric acidity, gastric motility, kidney and liver function alter the way in which medications are absorbed, metabolised and excreted. A person's nutritional status and the presence of other chronic diseases also affect medications.

These changes can cause an overdose based on normal dosages or a reduced therapeutic effect. For example, age-related decline in kidney function can significantly reduce the excretion of medications, which can cause toxic effects.

If a client is experiencing diarrhoea, some medications that are administered can have a decreased therapeutic effect as the active ingredients do not stay in the client's system long enough to be absorbed, but are passed out quickly through the intestines. Therapeutic effectiveness can also be affected if a client has not been drinking enough fluids and becomes dehydrated. It is important to immediately report any changes in your client's physical state to the registered nurse, so that an appropriate assessment of their medication regimen can be undertaken. For example, **substance incompatibility** between warfarin and aspirin can lead to increased risk of bleeding as both drugs have an anticoagulant action.

MEDICATION ASSISTANCE

When a doctor prescribes a medication, specific instructions are given as to:

- when the medication is to be taken (a.m., noon, p.m.)
- how much of the medication is to be taken (dose, usually in milligrams)
- how the client is to take the medication (route)
- how much a day can be taken (as a dose in milligrams or as a number of tablets)
- whether it should be taken with food or on an empty stomach (some medications irritate the stomach lining)
- what other foods or medications must not be taken (e.g. alcohol).

These instructions can be found on the label of the bottle or packet or sometimes in writing on the dose administration aid (DAA) or sachet pack. Always follow these instructions. Never assist with medication administration if your instructions are contrary to what is written on the label, and never assist with medication administration if the label is defaced or unreadable. Are there any special considerations for the medications (Box 18.1)? Administration instructions should always be clear and consistent, and medications taken as prescribed.

If you assist someone with their medication, you must ensure that:

- it is the right medication (particularly if they are on multiple medications)
- the medication is given at the right time
- it is the right amount (dose)
- the medication is given via the right route (by mouth, injection, topically applied to the skin, inhalation, vaginally, rectally).

You must also ensure that you give the medication to the right client, particularly in a ward or institutional care situation where there are multiple clients. See the 'seven rights' of medication administration listed in Box 18.2 (overleaf).

BOX 18.1
Medication special considerations

- Unless a tablet is scored, it should never be broken to adjust dosage (breaking can cause incorrect dosage, intestinal irritation or drug destruction).
- Scored tablets may be split with a pill splitter.
- *Never* touch the medication with your fingers. *Always* wear gloves.
- In residential aged care facilities you cannot save split tablets as storage conditions are compromised. Generally, the pharmacy will pack in halves or quarters.
- Never substitute one medication for another unless told to do so by the registered nurse.
- Never give one client's medication to another.
- *Always* report errors to the registered nurse immediately.

BOX 18.2
The seven rights of medication administration

1. The right client.
2. The right drug.
3. The right time.
4. The right dose.
5. The right route.
6. The right reason.
7. The right documentation.

ALWAYS CHECK FOR ALLERGIES.

It is important to always check the expiry date on all medication packaging. Medications that have passed their expiry date can sometimes have a reduced, different or increased effect on the body. Never give any medication that has passed its expiry date.

SELF-ADMINISTRATION OF MEDICINES

Clients generally manage and take their own medications if they are able. This is called **self-administration**, where the client knows their own medications by name, colour and/or shape. The client knows what medications to take, the correct dosage and when and how to take them. In such cases, the client may question any changes to the usual medication routine. For example, they might comment that a pill is not broken in half if this is how it is usually administered, or notice that a pill looks different if it is sourced from a different manufacturer. Always report client comments or questions to the registered nurse.

Dose administration aids (DAAs), **sachet packs** and **pill organisers** are often used to make medication administration easier and more convenient. DAAs and sachet packs are common in aged care facilities and are now used in the community too. They have individual sections organised by day and time. The pharmacist prepares the DAA or sachet packs, which are sealed to indicate tamper-evidence (Fig. 18.1). Sometimes, family members will manually place medications in a plastic pill organiser. The client then takes the medications on the right day at the right time.

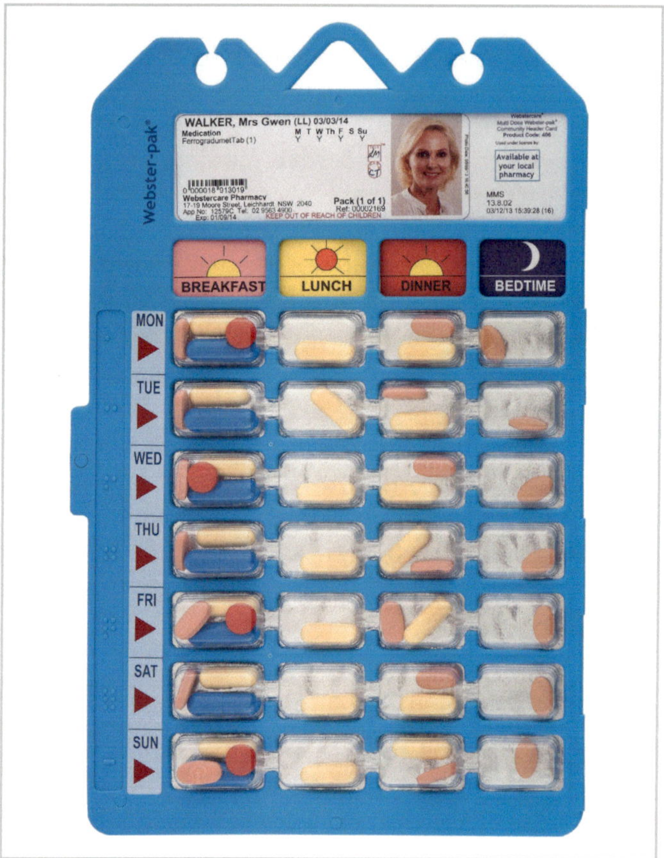

Fig. 18.1
Webster-pak® dose administration aid.

DAAs, sachet packs and pill organisers provide a visual reminder to take medication and show whether the medication has been taken. In some cases, extra assistance may be required with administration, as well as observing and recording that the medication has been taken.

Not all medications are oral tablets/capsules; for example, medications may also be administered by other routes, including inhaler devices, eye drops, medicated creams or transdermal patches.

Sachet packaging system

These are sachets that are pre-packed by a packing machine, then checked by a pharmacist.

The benefits of sachets are:

- the medication in each sachet is easy to identify and individually labelled and supplied in multi-dose sachets dispensed in a continuous roll

- medications are dispensed directly from the sachet
- you can crush medications directly in the sachet
- there is less handling so the risk of cross-contamination is reduced
- packed medications can be provided weekly
- sachets can be recycled and are environmentally friendly
- there are also medication charts provided as per facility requirements
- photo identification is placed on charts
- the medication sachet roll can be kept in a locked room and sachets to be used next can be placed in a tray or lockable trolley for the next medication round.

The sachets include up to five different tablets per dose time. Every sachet is clearly labelled with:

- the person's name
- the date and day of the week
- dose time
- names and physical descriptions (shape and colour) of the medicines
- the quantity of each tablet.

LEGISLATION AND DELEGATION

Commonwealth regulation

The Australian Government regulates the safety and efficacy of all medications. It does this under legislation, such as the *Therapeutic Goods Act 1989*, the *Poisons Standard* (under the *Legislative Instruments Act 2003*), the *Customs Act 1901* and the *National Health Act 1953*. New Zealand has its own set of national Acts and Regulations that control medications. If you travel and work between both countries, you will need to ensure that you know the relevant guidelines for each country.

State and local regulation

State, territory and local regulation control the advertising of medications in some areas, and the administration of medications by nurses. Each Australian state and territory has its own set of Acts and Regulations. If you move for work to another state or territory, it is important to understand what Acts and Regulations apply to your practice there. New Zealand does not have independent state guidelines, but has guidelines that can differ between each Health District.

Guiding Principles for Medication Management in Residential Aged Care Services

These guidelines from the Commonwealth Government (2021b) promote a Quality Use of Medicines (QUM) approach to the use of medicines and medication management in residential aged care services.

There are 17 guiding principles relating to medication management in residential aged care services. Guiding Principle 14 specifically relates to administration of medicines by residential aged care service staff (Department of Health 2021b). The registered nurse can delegate medicine administration tasks to appropriately trained and competent staff. The delegated staff should have formal training in medicine administration, be assessed by the residential aged care service and the registered nurse as competent to administer medicines, accept the delegation and be appropriately supervised. The residential aged care service should use ongoing quality improvement activities, such as staff education and training and ongoing competency assessment, developed in consultation with the Medication Advisory Committee, to support appropriate medicines' administration, monitoring and reporting practices.

Organisational policy

Each organisation has its own set of guidelines or policies for assisting with medications. Some organisations will allow carers to administer medications, while others will not. It is your responsibility to determine what you are expected to do, and what you are and are not permitted to do.

Delegation

Remember, it is your responsibility to find, read and understand your organisational policy. The policy tells you what you can and cannot do regarding assisting with medications. Never undertake assisting with medications if you have not been taught how to do so.

Your role in assisting with medications depends on your state's laws, organisational policy and your training and education. It may involve one or more of the following:

- reminding the client that it is time to take their medication
- reading the medication label to the client
- opening the containers for the client who cannot do so, or removing the medication from the DAAs or sachet packs for them
- checking the dosage against the medication label
- providing water, juice, milk or other fluids or foods as needed
- making sure the client takes the right medication, in the right amount, at the right time and in the right way
- reporting that the client took or did not take the medication according to organisational policy
- correctly storing medications.

If you are involved in administering medications, your role will involve following the seven rights of medication administration (see Box 18.2).

We also refer to the 'five rights' of delegation:

1. The right task – Can the task be delegated? Is the nurse allowed to delegate the task? Is the task in your job description?
2. The right circumstance – What are the person's physical, mental, emotional and spiritual needs at this time?
3. The right person – Do you have the training and experience to perform the task for this person?
4. The right directions and communication – Ensure that you have been given clear directions; the supervisor should tell you what observations to make, when to report back and allow questions and help you to set priorities.

BOX 18.3
Medicines and poisons schedules 2021

Schedule 1 – Not currently used
Schedule 2 – Pharmacy medicine – may be purchased without a prescription, but which may require advice from a pharmacist; only available in a pharmacy
Schedule 3 – Pharmacist-only medicine – requires professional advice or counselling by a pharmacist to ensure safe use
Schedule 4 – Prescription-only medicine or Prescription Animal remedy – require a prescription from a medical, dental or veterinary professional
Schedule 5 – Caution – substances with a low potential for causing harm, packaged appropriately with simple warnings and safety directions on the label
Schedule 6 – Poison – substances with a moderate potential for causing harm, packaged distinctively with strong warnings and safety directions on the label
Schedule 7 – Dangerous poison – substances with a high potential for causing harm at low exposure. Should only be available to specialised or authorised users. Availability, possession and storage may be restricted
Schedule 8 – Controlled drug – substances which require restriction of manufacture, supply, distribution and use to reduce abuse, misuse and physical or psychological dependence. Example: morphine.
Schedule 9 – Prohibited substance which may only be used for medical or scientific research or for analytical teaching or training purposes with approval from relevant authorities. Examples include heroin, cannabis
Unscheduled substances – Many of these preparations are sold in supermarkets. Examples include antacids, laxatives and paracetamol

Australian Government (2021). Federal Register of Legislation Poisons Standard October 2021. Online 13 October 2021. Available: www.legislation.gov.au/Details/F2021L01345

5 The right supervision – The supervisor/manager should guide, direct and evaluate the medication you are to give, they should demonstrate tasks as necessary and be available to answer questions.

There are also different schedules of medications, from medications that do not need a prescription (Schedule 2), to controlled drugs that can lead to dependence (Schedule 8), and thus have different requirements on how they are stored. Box 18.3 lists a common set of schedules.

SAFETY ALERT

Refusing a task

If a carer feels they are not competent to undertake the task, they have the right to refuse to do it. A carer can refuse the task of assisting or administering medications if:

- the task is beyond their limits of their role
- the task is not in their job description
- the carer is not prepared to perform the task
- the task could harm the person
- the person's condition has changed
- the carer doesn't know how to use the supplies or equipment
- the directions are unethical, illegal or against facility policy
- the directions are unclear or incomplete
- a supervisor is not available for supervision.

MEDICATIONS MANAGEMENT

Medication record

A **medication record** is kept for each client who needs help with medications. The record includes:

- the client's name
- any known allergies
- a list of medications, including the medication name, dose, directions and route of administration
- date and time to take the medication
- the doctor's name and signature
- the date and time at which help was given
- whether the medication was ingested or completed successfully
- any reaction the person had to the medication
- any further comments or observations you made
- whether the client refused the medication
- whether the medication was missing from its packaging or not able to be found, e.g. medicated cream
- the signature or initials of the person assisting.

This record will have an identifying picture of the client on the front. You must check this picture with the client you are assisting. If the picture is unclear or if you are unsure whether to proceed, report any issues with the registered nurse.

Electronic Medication Management (EMM) systems

Electronic medication management (EMM) systems support doctors, nurses and pharmacists to prescribe, order, check, reconcile, dispense and record the administration of medicines. EMM can assist in reducing the number of preventable adverse medication events and medication prescribing errors as the medication orders will be legible. An EMM system can improve the accuracy, visibility and legibility of medical information, so that the communication between professionals and consumers is clearer (ACSQHC 2019).

How does an EMM work?

- Authorised care staff will log in to the system at the start of a medication round and will only view the medication to be given within a particular time period.

- A digital photograph of each consumer ensures that the right medication is administered to the right person.
- Care staff can also select a reason for not administering the medication, such as consumer refused.
- All administered medications are stamped with a date, time and signature to create an electronic audit trail to confirm administration of each dose.
- Some EMM systems will issue an alert or warning to prompt staff to administer medications that are due or have been missed.
- EMM systems reduce medication errors such as omitted doses. They ensure stock levels of both prescribed and PRN medications are kept up to date. EMM systems also enhance stock auditing, disposing and re-ordering processes.

Reporting

You must report any medication errors and/or incidents to the registered nurse. You will also need to complete an incident report form. It is important to follow the organisational policy at all times.

Failure to report an error or incident could result in serious consequences for the client. Some medications need to be kept at certain levels in the bloodstream to maintain their effectiveness. If a medication is missed or vomited up, then the level in the bloodstream drops and the effectiveness of the medication is significantly decreased. Notify the registered nurse immediately if you notice any of these occurring. Do not wait until the end of your shift or when you next see the registered nurse. All incidents must be reported immediately as some medication errors can be corrected if assistance is given as soon as possible.

An error can include one or more of the following:

- the client takes another client's medication
- the client takes the wrong medication
- the client takes the wrong dose
- the client takes the medication at the wrong time
- the client takes the medication by the wrong route
- the client does not take the medication when ordered
- the medication is dropped on the floor
- the medication is vomited up after being taken
- you forget to assist with the client self-medication process
- the client takes the medication for the wrong reason.

Always indicate whether the client took the medication or refused it, or anything else that happened with the client or medication at this time.

Storing medications

Medications should always be kept in a secure place. This prevents someone else from taking them. In a residential facility they are kept in a locked container, cabinet or other area. In some places the medication is stored in a locked trolley or in a specific locked area. In residential aged care services, clients who self-administer are required to store their medications securely in their room in a locked drawer or cupboard. If the room is shared, each client's ability to safely store or keep medications must be assessed. In a home environment, medications should be stored in a safe place, particularly if children are visiting.

All medication must display the original pharmacy label and should be stored as directed on the label. For example, some medications are refrigerated; others are kept away from the light. The label also has an expiry date. Expired or discontinued medications are disposed of following organisational procedures. If you are working within somebody's home, you will need to have such medications returned to the local pharmacy. Under no circumstances are medications to be removed from their original container. They are not to be taken from one bottle and placed in another.

Routes of administration

Medications are taken in various ways (Box 18.4). The doctor determines which way they are to be taken. Many medications are taken by mouth. Others are taken via inhalation, through the skin, injection or as suppositories into the vagina or rectum. Medicines can also be applied directly (topically) where the result is required; for example, eye drops, ear drops, creams and lotions. As a carer, you should never assist in the administration of a medication by any route for which you have not received specific training. This includes the giving of rectal suppositories and application of patches.

TYPES OF MEDICATIONS

Medication comes in different forms. Often the form determines how it is to be administered. Sometimes a doctor will order a different form of medication to better suit the client's needs (Box 18.5). For example, a client with problems swallowing will not be prescribed a tablet but a liquid medication instead. If medication is to be given

BOX 18.4
Routes for medication administration

- *Aural:* Drops or creams placed in the ear canal
- *Cutaneous:* Applied to the surface of the skin
- *Eye:* Drops or creams placed directly into the eye, usually just under the eyelid
- *Inhalation:* Breathed directly into the lungs
- *Injection:* Injected into the body by breaching the skin's surface with a sharp needle (e.g. intramuscular – injected into the depth of the muscle; subcutaneous – injected just under the skin; intravenous – injected into the blood vessels)
- *Nasal:* Drops, creams or sprays placed inside the nostrils of the nose
- *Oral:* Given by mouth and swallowed
- *Rectal:* Inserted through the anus into the rectum
- *Sublingual:* Placed in the mouth under the tongue for absorption
- *Vaginal:* Inserted within the vagina

BOX 18.5
Clients with special needs

Dementia

Care workers who have completed a Certificate IV level qualification with the unit Administer and Monitor Medication administer medications to people with dementia. Special consideration should be applied as people with dementia are at times unable to ask for assistance or observe any errors in medications. If you are assisting a client with dementia to take their medications, always observe the safety rules.

Swallowing difficulties

If you notice that a client is experiencing swallowing difficulties and oral medication needs to be administered, you must report this immediately to the registered nurse. This will also need to be assessed and documented. It may also be necessary to check under the tongue and sides of the mouth to be certain that the client has swallowed the oral medication. Never leave medications at the bedside.

Older adults

Older adults often have dry mucous membranes in their mouth, so it may be necessary to offer fluids before administering tablets or capsules to prevent them from sticking to the sides of the client's mouth. Offer sufficient fluids after the medication has been taken. Clients who wear dentures may not be able to feel medication in their mouth, so inspecting the mouth to ensure all medication has been swallowed may be necessary.

through the rectum, a suppository is ordered rather than a tablet. Ensure that the client not only has the right medication, but also has the medication in the right form. Box 18.6 describes some common forms of medications that can be prescribed.

In general, if the person becomes upset, combative or refuses to take their medication, report this to the registered nurse immediately. You are not permitted by law to force any person to take medications if they choose not to do so.

BOX 18.6
Common forms of medications

- *Caplet:* Solid dosage form for oral use; similar to a tablet but compressed into a capsule shape and coated for ease of swallowing.
- *Cream:* A soft, water-soluble preparation that may contain medication and is applied to the skin. It is thicker than a lotion, spreads easily, is moisturising and requires a preservative to extend the shelf life.
- *Drops:* A liquid preparation used to administer medication in small quantities to the eyes, ears or mouth
- *Lotion:* A low-viscosity topical preparation that may contain medication and is intended for application to the skin. Lotions are more readily applied to regions of hairy skin such as the scalp.
- *Ointment:* A thick semi-solid, oil-based preparation that may contain medication and is applied to the skin. Ointments feel greasy and are 'occlusive', meaning they stay on the surface of the skin, trap moisture and are not well absorbed
- *Capsule:* Solid dosage form for oral use; medication in powder, liquid or oil form and encased by a gelatin shell.
- *Elixir:* Clear fluid containing water and/or alcohol for oral use, usually has sweetener added. This medication should not be diluted.
- *Emulsion:* Liquid or semi-solid medication where an insoluble liquid is dispersed within a carrier liquid and may separate out on standing. Emulsifiers may sometimes be added to prevent separation. Always shake this medication well before administering.
- *Enteric-coated tablet:* Tablets for oral use coated with materials that do not dissolve in the stomach; coating dissolves in the intestine where medication is absorbed. This medication should not be crushed.
- *Inhaled medication:* There are many different types of inhaler devices that allow for medication to be delivered directly to the lungs.
- *Lozenge:* Solid medicated tablets intended to be slowly dissolved in the mouth, sometimes under the tongue. Liquids should not be taken for at least 18 minutes after administration to prevent dilution from area.
- *Transdermal patch:* Medication contained within a semi-permeable membrane patch, which allows the medication to be absorbed through the skin slowly over a long period.
- *Tablet:* Powdered dosage form compressed into a solid round disc or cylinder.
- *Syrup:* Liquid medication dissolved in a concentrated sugar solution; may contain flavouring to make medication more palatable. This medication may be diluted.
- *Suspension:* Finely powdered solid medication particles dispersed in a liquid medium for both oral and topical use. When a suspension is left standing, the particles settle to the bottom of the container. Always shake this medication well before administering.
- *Suppository:* Solid dosage form mixed with gelatine and shaped in the form of a pellet for insertion into a body cavity (rectum/vagina); melts when it reaches body temperature, releasing medication for absorption.
- *Wafer:* A very thin, compressed biscuit-like medication; dissolves quickly in the mouth.

Medication groups – Medications listed under generic names not brand names

From 1 February 2021 prescribing in Australia was required to be by active ingredient and not brand name (PBS 2021). This has been done to assist consumers, so that they know what medications they are taking, with the aim of reducing confusion and better informing consumers.

- Central and peripheral nervous system:
  - Anti-anxiety (diazepam)
  - Sedative/hypnotic (temazepam)
  - Antiepileptic drugs (sodium valproate)
  - Antipsychotics (risperidone)
  - Antidepressants (sertraline)
  - Stimulants (methylphenidate)
  - Migraines (sumatriptan)
- Musculoskeletal system
  - Anti-inflammatory drugs (meloxicam)
  - Non-opioid analgesics (paracetamol)
  - Opioid (buprenorphine)
- Neurodegenerative disorders (donepezil), muscle relaxants (baclofen)
- Endocrine system – thyroid (thyroxine), insulin, oral hypoglycaemic drugs (metformin)
- Cardiovascular system and blood – anticoagulants (warfarin, apixaban), antiplatelets (aspirin), cardiac glycosides (digoxin), antiarrhythmic drugs (amiodarone), anti-anginal agents (glyceryl trinitrate), antihypertensives (ramipril), lipid lowering drugs (atorvastatin)
- Respiratory system – asthma management agents (salbutamol, ipratropium, fluticasone/salmeterol)
- Gastrointestinal system – antacids (magnesium hydroxide), proton pump inhibitors (pantoprazole), antiemetics (metoclopramide), laxatives (docusate + senna, macrogol), antidiarrhoeal agents (loperamide)
- Renal/urinary system – diuretics (furosemide (frusemide)), anticholinergics (oxybutynin)
- Reproductive systems – contraceptives (levonorgestrel + ethinyloestradiol), female hormones (tibolone)
- Immune system – immunosuppressant medications (azathioprine)

Dose administration aids

- Dosette box – a common way of packaging pills to organise people's medication; the days of the week and times to take the pills are printed on the box.
- Dose administration aids (DAAs), 'such as the Webster-Pak system', are filled by a pharmacist and are the most commonly used in the community services and health industry.

Table 18.1 provides a list of equipment needed for medication administration.

Table 18.1
Equipment required for medication administration

Equipment	Use
Medication chart	To identify the person Check for allergies Record medication given and the date and time given
Keys	To open a cupboard or trolley where the medication is stored
Apron	To wear during procedures to protect clothing
Disposable gloves	To wear when you apply topical treatments
Medicine cups	To dispense medication from original container just prior to the person taking it
Spoon in the correct measurement	To mix medication with small amounts of stewed fruit To hand to the person to take medication
Tumblers, glasses, paper cups	To give water to the person to swallow oral medication
Water jug	To keep water to serve the person
Pill crusher/mortar and pestle	To crush medication for a person who finds it hard to swallow
Measuring cups	To measure liquid medication
Tablet divider or pill cutter	To cut scored tablets in half for a person who finds it hard to swallow larger tablets
Paper towels and tissues	To dry any equipment To wipe any spills
Nebuliser	To add air to medication (mostly used for bronchodilators or mucolytic medication, e.g. Ventolin)
Containers for used equipment	To store all used equipment prior to washing, for example, teaspoons
Containers for used paper goods and disposable items	To dispose of used equipment and paper goods
Trolley	The trolley will be taken from room to room

SAFETY ALERT

Medications

All medications that are designated to heal also have the capacity to cause substantial harm to the individual.

SAFETY ALERT

Altering medications

Sometimes patients are unable to swallow their medications whole. They may chew their tablets or they may require you to crush the tablets or open the capsules to assist swallowing. Not all tablets and capsules are made in a way that safely allows them to be altered and doing so may increase the risk of adverse effects and compromise patient safety. Always follow the instructions on the medication chart and on the dose administration aid. Notify the registered nurse if the patient is unable to swallow their medications whole or you observe them chewing their medications. There are different types of crushing devices, but if using a mortar and pestle it must be cleaned in between each use to make sure there are no remnants of previously crushed medications.

Table 18.2
Metric conversion chart

Weight	1000 micrograms (mcg)	equals	1 milligram (mg)
	1000 milligrams		1 gram (g)
	1000 grams		1 kilogram (kg)
Volume	1000 millilitres (mL)	equals	1 litre (L)

Example

Mr Jones is ordered 500 mg of Epilim Syrup. Strength supplied is 200 mg per 5 mL.

$$\frac{500}{200} \times \frac{5}{1}$$
$$= 12.5 \text{ mL}$$

MEDICATION ADMINISTRATION

There are times when drug dosages need to be calculated prior to administration (Table 18.2).

Formula for drug calculation

$$\text{Volume required} = \frac{\text{Strength required}}{\text{Strength in stock}} \times \frac{\text{Volume of stock}}{1}$$

SAFETY ALERT

Medication assistance

Remember, you *do not* administer medications. The personal care worker assists a client to self-medicate only. This task will be delegated to you by a registered nurse. *Never* undertake this task if you have not received training to do so, and never undertake this task if you are unsure of what you are doing.

ASSISTING A CLIENT WITH THEIR ORAL MEDICATION

Oral medications include those that come as tablets or capsules. It is important to respect the client's privacy while carrying out a procedure. It is also essential to address the client by name and ensure that they know your name. If you are unfamiliar with the client, ask another staff member to identify the client for you.

The process of assisting a client with their oral medications can be organised into three main steps:

Step 1: Preparation

The client or a registered nurse may request your assistance with client self-medication. It is important that you complete the following steps:

1. Check the delegation guidelines (state and organisational) to ensure that you are allowed to assist with medications.
2. Wash your hands thoroughly.
3. Identify the correct client and call them by name.
4. Ensure there is adequate lighting and minimal noise.
5. Be attentive and discourage interruptions.

Step 2: Procedure for packed oral medications

6. Collect all equipment needed, such as: medication trolley and keys, medicine cups, the client's medication chart, DAA/sachet pack, water or liquid for swallowing, container for dirty equipment, paper towel or tissues, tablet divider and/or tablet crusher, handwash (see Table 18.1).
7. Correctly locate the client's orders for packed oral medications by logging onto the e-tablet or referring to current medication record.
8. Remove the client's DAA or sachet pack from the medication cupboard or trolley and relock the cupboard/trolley.
9. Read the instructions on the label of the bottle, the medication chart or the blister/sachet pack. Some facilities require carers to check the DAA/sachet pack instructions against those on the medication record before every episode of medication administration.

10 Check the seven rights of medication administration to ensure that the right medication will be taken as prescribed (Box 18.2).
11 Only administer those medicines that you have prepared personally or received from the pharmacy.
12 Check the expiration date of the medication. Do not use discoloured medication or those with damaged labels. Always check with the registered nurse for clarification.
13 Wash hands or use hand sanitiser.
14 Place tablets or capsules into the cap of the container and then empty the cap into a clean medication cup. Never touch the medication with your hands at any stage.
15 Check that the number of tablets in the medication cup matches the number of tablets on the medication sheet or e-tablet.
16 Pour a quantity of water into a glass and place it within reach of the client.
17 Offer the medication to the client.
18 Observe as the client takes the medication and assist the client with a drink.
19 If you are assisting with liquid medications, hold the medicine cup at eye level or place it on a flat surface at eye level to pour the medication. The lower curve of the liquid (meniscus) should be at the calibration line indicating the correct dosage.
20 Pour liquids from the bottle on the opposite side from the label (in case of spillage) and wipe the bottle after pouring the liquid.
21 If any liquid medication is poured in excess, do not return any excess to the original container. Discard it.
22 Remove the medicine cup and dispose of the cup as per organisational policy.

Step 3: Aftercare

When you have completed assisting the client with self-medication, you will need to complete the following steps:

23 Replace the DAA/sachet pack in a safe place.
24 Ensure that you have not left any medicines unattended.
25 Lock medication trolley and return it to locked, secure area.
26 Wash your hands thoroughly.
27 Observe the client for any unusual reaction to the medications.
28 Report any unusual occurrence to the supervisor.
29 Document the medication taken in the medication record. You must always sign the record after administration and never before. This document is a legal record and can be used in a court of law if required as evidence. Your signature must be signed in ink and be clearly recognisable.

Assisting with non-packed and non-oral medications

Not all medications are tablets/capsules.

Other forms of medications

- Ear drops
- Eye drops
- Nose drops and nasal sprays
- Inhaled medications
- Transdermal patches
- Medicated creams
- Vaginal creams and pessaries
- Suppositories
- Injection, such as insulin.

It is important to be competent in the administration of these other forms of medications; for example, ensuring a client takes their inhaled medication properly. Failure to administer these medications correctly can compromise their efficacy as well as increase the risk of side effects.

OBSERVING FOR CHANGES IN A CLIENT'S CONDITION

As a care worker it is important to observe changes in the client's condition. You need to assess your client prior to administering medication and if you notice any changes report them to the supervisor or registered nurse prior to giving the medication.

It is also important to observe the client for changes after you have administered medications. Some changes that you would need to report verbally to a registered nurse/supervisor and in writing are:

- Are they sweating?
- Do they look confused or drowsy?
- Are they scratching themselves?
- Do they have a different skin colour?
- Are they slurring their speech more than usual?
- Are they walking well?
- Has their behaviour changed? Do they seem more depressed?

Listen to the person. The older person may tell you that they feel different or feel concerned that their medication is making them feel worse. Encourage them to talk to you. Get them to describe exactly how they feel. Ask questions that follow up what the person is saying to gain clarification and to gain more information that may be required. It is your job to record this clearly so the doctor can follow it up.

There are many reasons why an older person's condition may have changed:

- Their existing health condition may have worsened.
- The doctor may have changed their medication.
- The person may have mixed up their medications.
- The person may have forgotten or chosen not to take their medications (if they self-medicate).
- The person may have developed another condition, such as the flu.
- The person may be unable to sleep, which makes it harder for them to think clearly.

SIDE EFFECTS OF MEDICATIONS

We have discussed observing a client for changes in their condition. We must also observe for medication side effects.

A side effect is an unwanted symptom caused by the medication. Side effects can be mild, such as feeling nauseous, to severe, such as anaphylaxis. Some examples of side effects of medications are:

- dizziness
- falls
- swallowing difficulties
- weight loss
- incontinence
- constipation.

Note: medications can cause a whole range of things that affect an older person's quality of life and increase morbidity and mortality.

PROCEDURES FOR REPORTING A CLIENT'S RESPONSE TO ADMINISTERED MEDICATION

If you are working in a community setting you should immediately contact the person in charge if a person has had a reaction to an administered medication. Clearly explain the situation. Do not proceed with giving any medication until you receive further directions from them. You must write the changed situation in the older person's care or progress notes. Remember to record the date, time, details of the changed condition and who you have reported it to.

If you are working in a client's home, telephone your supervisor straight away. If you are working in a residential aged care service you must report to your supervisor or registered nurse and document as set out above in the client's progress notes or on the client's electronic reporting system.

Disposal of unused or expired medications

Unused drugs or expired medication must be returned to the pharmacy for safe disposal. Some environmental health units will have specific guidelines in relation to this; for example, there may be a requirement for Schedule 8 drugs to be dealt with in a different manner. Check with your supervisor if your organisation has any specific guidelines for the disposal of Schedule 8 drugs. Always check with the pharmacist if you are not sure.

Providing accurate information about medications

- *Side effects* – known effects of a medication. For example, if you are taking a cold and flu preparation the package might state that a side effect of this medication is drowsiness.
- *Adverse reactions* – an unexpected response to the medication; for example, dizziness. Sometimes two clients might take the same medication; one client has an adverse response while the other does not.
- *Allergic reactions* – a reaction a person has to a medication due to sensitivity to the substance. It may be mild, such as a rash, or life threatening, such as anaphylactic shock (Box 18.7).
- *Anaphylactic shock* – a severe whole-body allergic reaction. The reaction is sudden, severe and involves the whole body.

BOX 18.7
Symptoms of drug allergy

- Hives (a less common type of rash)
- Itching of the skin or eyes (common)
- Skin rash (common)
- Swelling of the lips, tongue or face
- Wheezing

SAFETY ALERT

Cytotoxic medication handling precautions

A cytotoxic drug is one that interferes with cell division in rapidly growing tissues, such as cancer. Cytotoxic drugs should be dispensed in a purple pack; use universal precautions and avoid touching the tablet/capsule. When administering wear purple gloves. Empty containers, gloves and medicine cups should be disposed of in the purple contaminated waste bin.

If there is ever any doubt, never give the medication. Speak to the registered nurse immediately.

HANDLING CONTINGENCIES

There must be protocols/plans in place to handle contingencies. A contingency is a future event or circumstance that may occur but cannot be predicted. Even though a contingency is unlikely to occur, it still must be prepared for. A contingency plan is designed to take account of a possible future event or circumstance.

Things that might occur are:

- the client refuses to take the medication
- incomplete ingestion of medication
- medications are out of date or contaminated
- there is a missing or an extra tablet in a DAA pack
- medication falls on the floor
- medication is past its expiry date
- the photo of the client is out of date or not identifiable
- the staff member's signature is missing and you are not sure if the medication has been given
- the doctor has not signed the chart.

CASE STUDY 1

You have been delegated the task of assisting Mrs Bellini with her medications. Mrs Bellini is 87 years old and taking medications for a heart problem and diabetes. You have previously checked and know that the legislation within your state allows you to assist with medication. At your orientation, you were given documentation that discussed the organisational policies on assisting with medications. Your facility allows carers to do so.

After washing your hands, you take Mrs Bellini's medication chart and her DAA/sachet packs to her. After checking her identity against the picture on the pack and greeting her by name, you begin to check the medications required. You check the time they are to be given, and you check the number of tablets. You check that she is to have tablets and not a liquid; and you check that you are helping her with the right medication. All your checks are positive and you proceed to help her with her medications.

Without touching the medication, you push her tablets out from the DAA/sachet pack into a small container and hand them to her. She has a small glass of water next to her, which she uses to wash down the tablets. After she has taken the medication, you sign on the medication chart that she has taken her medications and return the DAA/sachet pack to the locked cupboard.

By following all the appropriate steps for safe medication administration, you have ensured the safety of Mrs Bellini and avoided unnecessary and potentially fatal adverse reactions.

CASE STUDY 2

You are assisting with care for Mrs Burns in an aged care facility. The registered nurse has instructed you to assist with the medication administration for this client. Your shift commenced at 0700 and it is documented on Mrs Burns' medication record that she is due for oral medication at 0800. The oral medication you will be assisting with administering is paracetamol. It is Monday and the DAA for Mrs Burns has two (2) paracetamol tablets assigned for Monday at 0800. The medication record also states two (2) paracetamol to be taken at 0800. Your first medication check is in process. You will need to remember your five rights. Do you have the right person? (Mrs Burns), right medication? (paracetamol), right route? (oral), right dose? (two (2) tablets) and right time (0800)? The organisational policy and procedures allow carers to assist in medication administration and you have had the education and training needed to assist the client with medication administration. You also know that it is extremely important to check the expiry date on all medications that will be administered.

QUALITY OF LIFE

Clients often rely on medications to maintain quality of life, such as relief from pain or to treat a disease process. Medications can also provide relief for a number of symptoms, such as pain or swelling. The client must, therefore, have the right medication at the right time, in the right dose and via the right route. When a client needs assistance to take medications, a carer may be delegated this responsibility. To do this task safely the carer needs to be appropriately trained and assessed. They also need to know what to report and when to report to the registered nurse.

Given that all medications have the potential to harm, the carer must be continuously vigilant and observe for any reaction that may be caused by the medication regimen.

As a carer, it is extremely important that you do not work outside your scope of practice. Always know what your state and local regulations and organisational guidelines are regarding carers and medication assistance. Never assist with medication if you have not had training to do so or have any doubts about what you are doing.

FOCUS ON COMMUNITY CARE

When assisting your client with their medications at home, you must always follow the same safety guidelines as outlined in this chapter. It is important to check the storage requirements of all medications to ensure that they are appropriately stored. Some clients may place them on window sills or in cupboards, or in the refrigerator or bathroom sink. While some medications may be stored in these places, it is not suitable for others.

After assisting with medications, always return the medication to an appropriate place. Never leave them on benches or tables, where visitors, especially children, may have access to them. Never assist with medication administration if the medication is not labelled for that particular client. Never speak in public of the medications your client is taking. This places your client at considerable risk of theft and undermines the client's right to privacy.

ACCREDITATION

You are working in residential or home care and accreditors are at your service. Can you answer the following questions?

- How you do ensure that the correct consumer receives the correct medications?
- What do you do if you find a medication error when assisting a consumer to take their medications?

REVIEW QUESTIONS

Circle T if the statement is true or F if the statement is false:

1 T / F Carers are permitted to assist with medications in all facilities.

2 T / F Carers administer medications.

3 T / F It is okay to substitute one medication for another.

4 T / F Medication adverse reactions can be lethal.

5 T / F All medications need to be crushed to enable easier swallowing, especially in older people.

6 T / F Allergic reactions to medications can be fatal.

7 T / F Assisting with oral medication administration does not require the carer to observe the client taking the medication.

Circle the BEST answer:

8 The seven rights of medication assistance are:
 a The right medication, right route, right dose, right time, right person
 b The right classification of medication, the right route, the right dose, right time, right person
 c The right disease, for the right medication, at the right time, right route, right person
 d The right client, right medication, right route, right time, right dose, right documentation, right reason

9 When a client has run out of a medication, you should:
 a ask another consumer for one of theirs
 b get the client to ask another consumer for one of theirs
 c miss the dose and tell the nurse within 24 hours
 d tell the nurse or your supervisor immediately

10 When someone refuses an essential medication, you should:
 a get someone to help you give it
 b open the person's mouth and put the medication at the back of their throat
 c give the medication in a different form (e.g. injection)
 d tell the nurse or supervisor immediately

Answers to these questions are on p. 454.

References

Australian Commission on Safety and Quality in Health Care (ACSQHC) (2019). Electronic Medication Management Systems – a guide to safe implementation. Online 12 October 2021. Available: www.safetyandquality.gov.au/sites/default/files/2019-08/sq19-030_emms_functional_requirements_acc_01n_5_aug_2019.pdf

Australian Government, Department of Health (2021). Guiding principles for medication management in residential aged care facilities. Australian Government. Online 7 March 2021. www.health.gov.au/internet/main/publishing.nsf/Content/nmp-pdf-resguide-cnt.htm

Australian Government, Department of Health (2006). Guiding Principle 12 – Risk management in the administration and use of medicines in the community. Online 12 October 2021. Available: www1.health.gov.au/internet/publications/publishing.nsf/Content/nmp-guide-medmgt-jul06-contents~nmp-guide-medmgt-jul06-guidepr12

The Pharmaceutical Benefits Scheme (PBS) (2021). Active ingredient prescribing. Online 13 October 2021. Available: www.pbs.gov.au/info/general/active-ingredient-prescribing

APPENDIX A
Web links

AUSTRALIA

- Australian Council on Healthcare Standards
  www.achs.org.au
- The Australian Resuscitation Council
  www.resus.org.au/
- The Department of Health
  www.health.gov.au
- Health Direct
  www.healthdirect.gov.au/
- Home Care Packages
  www.myagedcare.gov.au/help-home/home-care-packages
- Indigenous information
  www.indigenous.gov.au/
- Institute for Health and Ageing
  acuresearchbank.acu.edu.au/research-institute/802xw/institute-for-health-and-ageing
- My Aged Care Australia
  www.myagedcare.gov.au
- National Ageing Research Institute
  www.nari.net.au/
- National Disability services
  www.nds.org.au/
- Rural and Remote Health
  www.aihw.gov.au/reports/australias-health/rural-and-remote-health
- Seniors information (My Aged Care)
  www.myagedcare.gov.au
- Wounds Australia
  www.awma.com.au

NEW ZEALAND

- Enable New Zealand
  www.enable.co.nz/
- HealthEd
  www.healthed.govt.nz
- Health Information
  www.healthnavigator.org.nz/
- Māori Health
  www.health.govt.nz/our-work/populations/maori-health
- Ministry of Social Development
  www.msd.govt.nz/
- NZ Ministry of Health
  www.moh.govt.nz/moh.nsf
- NZ Positive Ageing Strategy
  www.msd.govt.nz/about-msd-and-our-work/publications-resources/planning-strategy/positive-ageing/
- Office for Disability Issues
  www.odi.govt.nz
- Office for Senior Citizens
  www.osc.govt.nz

INTERNATIONAL SITES

- Australian and New Zealand Society for Geriatric Medicine
  www.anzsgm.org/
- International Federation on Ageing
  www.ifa-fiv.org/
- US National Institute on Aging
  www.nia.nih.gov/
- World Health Organisation
  www.who.int/en/

APPENDIX B
Answers to review questions

CHAPTER 1
1 T
2 F
3 T
4 T
5 F
6 T
7 T
8 T
9 T
10 T

CHAPTER 2
1 F
2 T
3 T
4 F
5 T
6 T
7 T
8 T
9 D
10 C

CHAPTER 3
1 F
2 F
3 T
4 T
5 T
6 F
7 F
8 C
9 A
10 A

CHAPTER 4
1 F
2 T
3 F
4 T
5 F
6 T
7 A
8 D
9 A
10 B

CHAPTER 5
1 D
2 D
3 D
4 D
5 B
6 D
7 A
8 C
9 B
10 D

CHAPTER 6
1 T
2 T
3 F
4 T
5 T
6 T
7 T
8 T
9 T
10 F

CHAPTER 7
1 T
2 T
3 T
4 T
5 T
6 F
7 T
8 F
9 T
10 T

CHAPTER 8
1 F
2 T
3 F
4 F
5 F
6 T
7 B
8 D
9 C
10 A

CHAPTER 9
1 D
2 A
3 C
4 D
5 C
6 B
7 D
8 T
9 F
10 F

CHAPTER 10
1 C
2 A
3 C
4 D
5 B
6 B
7 C
8 D
9 C
10 A

CHAPTER 11
1 C
2 B
3 D
4 C
5 A
6 B
7 B
8 C
9 T
10 T
11 F

CHAPTER 12
1 D
2 C
3 A
4 B
5 C
6 D
7 C
8 F
9 F
10 T

CHAPTER 13
1 C
2 D
3 D
4 D
5 D
6 D
7 B
8 A
9 B
10 D

CHAPTER 14
1 F
2 F
3 F
4 T
5 F
6 F
7 B
8 B
9 D
10 D

CHAPTER 15
1 T
2 F
3 F
4 T
5 F
6 F
7 T
8 D
9 C
10 B

CHAPTER 16
1 D
2 C
3 A
4 B
5 D
6 A
7 F
8 T
9 T
10 T

CHAPTER 17
1 A
2 B
3 D
4 A
5 D
6 D
7 F
8 F
9 T
10 T

CHAPTER 18
1 F
2 F
3 F
4 T
5 F
6 T
7 F
8 D
9 D
10 D

GLOSSARY

abbreviation: A shortened form of a word or phrase
abducted: To draw away from the midline of the body
Aboriginal Australians: The original inhabitants of the Australian continent and nearby islands, excluding the Torres Strait Islands; the First Nations people of Australia
abrasion: A partial-thickness wound caused by the scraping away or rubbing of the skin
abuse: Actions which lead to the mistreatment or harm of another person
accountable: Being responsible for one's actions and the actions of others who perform delegated tasks; answering questions about and explaining one's actions and the actions of others
accreditation: A series of standards and processes that aged care services must meet and go through in order to ensure continued admission of clients to that service. It ensures standards of care for older people
acetone: Ketone body that appears in the urine from the rapid breakdown of fat for energy
acquired brain injury: Any type of brain damage that occurs after birth, which may occur due to infection, disease, head injury or lack of oxygen
acute illness: A sudden illness from which the person is expected to recover
acute pain: Pain that is felt suddenly from injury, disease, trauma or surgery; it lasts for less than 6 months
additional precautions: Infection control precautions that are applied in the care of a client who is known to have a communicable disease or to be in an infectious state
admission sheet: A sheet that is completed when a person is first admitted to a service and contains important information about the person
advance health directive: A clear statement of a person's directions and wishes on medical treatment when they are no longer able to make these decisions themselves
adverse reaction: A reaction that occurs when a medication causes an unintended secondary effect
advocacy: Providing support and/or representation on behalf of another person to ensure that their rights are upheld
affect: External representation of mood and feelings
afternoon care: Care given after lunch or after the evening meal
Aged Care Assessment teams (ACATs): Teams of medical, nursing and allied health professionals who assess the physical, psychological, medical, restorative, cultural and social needs of frail older people and help them and their carers to access appropriate levels of support
aged care funding instrument: A system of classification that is based primarily on the resident's dependency (need for care), rather than on care planning or care provided by an aged care home; it determines the amount of federal funding that a residential care service receives
aged care service: A service that provides healthcare services to residents who require regular or continuous care; with registered nursing, care, allied health and diversional therapy staff
alopecia: Hair loss
Alzheimer's disease: A disease that is the most common form of dementia and causes progressive damage to brain cells resulting in impaired memory, thinking and potential changes to behaviour
ambulation: The act of walking
anal incontinence: Faecal incontinence
anorexia: Loss of appetite
anticoagulant: A medication that prevents or slows (*anti*) blood clotting time (*coagulate*)
anxiety: A vague, uneasy feeling in response to stress
aphasia: The inability (*a*) to speak (*phasia*)
arterial ulcer: An open wound on the lower legs and feet caused by poor arterial blood flow
arteries: Blood vessels that carry blood away from the heart
arthritis: Joint (*arthr*) inflammation (*itis*)
aspiration: Breathing fluid or an object into the lungs
assault: Intentionally attempting or threatening to touch a person's body without the person's consent
assessment: Collecting information about the client
assisted living: Living in a home environment with some assistance from informal (family and friends) and/or formal (paid) support, depending on the person's needs. Most commonly used in an aged care context where the older person requires support to live safely in their own home or accommodation
atelectasis: A complete or partial collapse of a lung or lobe of a lung
atrophy: A decrease in size or a wasting away of tissue
autism spectrum disorder: Autism is a type of neurodiversity, which means the person experiences the world differently to an allistic person (person without autism). Autism can affect a person's speech, sensory processing and information processing. Autistic individuals prefer 'identity-first' language, which means you refer to them as an 'autistic person', not a 'person with autism'
autonomy: The ability of a person to make decisions for themselves

base of support: The area on which an object rests
battery: Touching a person's body without their consent
behavioural psychological symptoms of dementia (BPSD): Used to describe a broad range of psychological reactions, psychiatric symptoms and behaviours occurring in people with any form of dementia
beneficence: Any action that is taken to prevent harm, done for the benefit of or to improve the situation of another
biculturalism: The existence of two distinct cultural groups within the one nation
bioethics: The rights and duties of clients and healthcare professionals, including how health research is conducted
bipolar disorder: Bipolar means two (*bi*) poles or ends (*polar*). In bipolar disorder the person has extreme mood swings

blood glucose level: Glucose that the bloodstream carries to all the cells in the body to supply energy
blood pressure: The amount of force exerted against the walls of an artery by the blood
body alignment: The way in which the head, trunk, arms and legs are aligned with each other
body language: Messages sent through facial expressions, gestures, posture and body movements; non-verbal communication
body mechanics: Using the body in an efficient and careful way
body temperature: The amount of heat in the body, which is a balance between the amount of heat produced and the amount lost by the body
body work: Any therapeutic technique that involves working with the human body in a form involving manipulative therapy, such as massage
BPSD (behavioural psychological symptoms of dementia): Used to describe a broad range of psychological reactions, psychiatric symptoms and behaviours occurring in people with any form of dementia
bradycardia: A slow (*brady*) heart rate (*cardia*); the rate is less than 60 beats per minute
Braille: A tactile writing and reading system that uses raised dots; used by blind and vision-impaired people
bruise: A contusion
Buddhism: A religion and philosophy founded in India by Siddhartha Gautama, called the Buddha
bullying: A form of harassment that consists of repeated, health-harming mistreatment of a person by one or more perpetrators
burn: Injury to the skin or mucous membranes caused by heat, cold, electricity, chemicals, gases, friction or radiation

CALD: Culturally and linguistically diverse
capillaries: Tiny blood vessels; food, oxygen and other substances pass from the capillaries to the cells
care plan/comprehensive care plan: A written guide about the care a consumer should receive
care/case manager: Someone who provides individually planned and coordinated, flexible packages of care to provide for the complex care needs of older people
care-giver burden: Negative physical or psychosocial effects experienced by a person as a direct result of looking after someone in need of care; often seen in family members caring for their loved one at home when no or limited support services are used
Carer Counselling Program: works to improve the health, wellbeing, resilience and financial security of carers and to ensure that caring is a shared responsibility of family
carrier: A human or animal reservoir for microorganisms not showing signs or symptoms of infection
catheter: A tube used to drain or inject fluid through a body opening
catheterisation: Inserting a catheter
cell: The basic unit of body structure
central nervous system (CNS): Part of the nervous system which controls, directs and coordinates body functions; consists of the brain and spinal cord
chair position: A position that ensures good body alignment for a client sitting in a chair
Cheyne-Stokes respirations: Respirations that gradually increase in rate and depth and then become shallow and slow; breathing may stop for 10–20 seconds
chromosomes: Thread-like structures within the cell that carry genes and transmit hereditary information
chronic illness: An illness, slow or gradual in onset, for which there is no known cure; the illness can be controlled and complications prevented
chronic pain: Pain lasting longer than 6 months; it may be constant or occur on and off
chronic wound: A wound that does is slow to heal
circadian rhythm: Daily rhythm based on a 24-hour cycle; the day–night cycle or body rhythm
circulatory ulcer: An open wound on the lower legs and feet caused by decreased blood flow through arteries or veins; vascular ulcer
clean-contaminated wound: An infection following surgical entry of the urinary, reproductive, respiratory or gastrointestinal systems, which are not sterile
clean wound: A wound that is not infected; microbes have not entered the wound
closed fracture (simple fracture): The bone is broken but the skin is intact
closed wound: A wound in which tissues are injured but the skin is not broken
code of practice: Practical guidance for people who have work health and safety duties about how to achieve the standards required under the *Work Health and Safety Act 2011*, and effective ways to identify and manage risks
cognition: The process of thinking, learning and remembering. This includes the ability to plan, manipulate information, start and end activities and recognise errors
cognitive: Knowledge or perception of something or a process
cognitive disability: A range of clinical diagnoses, including Down Syndrome, intellectual impairment, acquired or traumatic brain injury, some types of cerebral palsy and any other impairment that affects the cognitive capacity of the person
colloquial language: Informal language that should not be used in formal situations
colostomy: A surgically created opening (*stomy*) between the colon (*colo*) and the abdominal wall
coma: The state of being unaware of one's surroundings and unable to react or respond to people, places or things
comatose: Being unable to respond to verbal stimuli
comfort: A state of wellbeing; the person has no physical or emotional pain and is calm and at peace
Commonwealth Home Support Programme (CHSP): Entry-level support at home for older people who need some help with daily tasks so they can live independently
communicable disease: A disease that can be spread from person to person; caused by pathogens
communication: The exchange of information; a message sent is received and interpreted by the intended person
communication barriers: Barriers that prevent us from sending and receiving messages effectively, such as using unfamiliar language, acknowledging cultural differences and failing to listen
complementary therapies: Practices and products that are not generally considered to be part of conventional medicine

compulsion: The uncontrolled performance of an act
confidentiality: Entrusting others with personal and private information
conflict: A clash between opposing interests and ideas
constipation: Defecation blocked by a hard, dry stool
Consumer Directed Care (CDC) model: A way of delivering care that gives individuals choice and flexibility
contaminated wound: A wound that has been contaminated by infection
contamination: The process of becoming unclean and contaminated with microorganisms
contracture: The lack of joint mobility caused by abnormal shortening of a muscle
contusion: A closed wound caused by a blow to the body; bruise
country/nation: Interchangeable terms used to identify the land of ancestral origin
criminal law: Laws concerned with offences against the public and society in general
cultural awareness: A basic understanding of the differences between cultures
cultural competence: The ability to interact effectively with people of different cultures and backgrounds
cultural safety: Safe care provided to those of all cultures as defined by the recipients of that care
cultural sensitivity: An understanding of your own cultural values and perceptions and how these have shaped your opinions of other cultures
culture: The behaviours, beliefs and characteristics of particular social and ethnic groups, including language, values, beliefs, habits, likes and dislikes
customs: Traditions passed on from one generation to the next

dandruff: An excessive amount of dry, white flakes from the scalp
database: A collection of data or information that is stored electronically in a structured format
deconditioning: The process of becoming weak from illness or lack of exercise, with muscle wastage
defamation: Injuring the name and reputation of a person by making false statements to a third person
defecation: The process of excreting faeces from the rectum through the anus; a bowel movement
defence mechanism: An unconscious reaction that blocks unpleasant or threatening feelings
dehiscence: The separation of wound layers
dehydration: A decrease in the amount of water in body tissues
delegating: Authorising another person to perform a task
delirium: A temporary state of acute mental confusion
delusion: A fixed false belief
delusion of grandeur: An exaggerated belief about one's own importance, wealth, power or talents
delusion of persecution: A false belief that one is being mistreated, abused or harassed
dementia: A set of chronic signs and symptoms in which memory and the ability to think and reason are lost
dementia-friendly community: A community that assists people with dementia to remain included through consideration of physical and social factors and education of health providers
dementia with Lewy bodies (DLB): a type of dementia characterised by Lewy bodies, microscopic protein deposits that develop within the nerve cells involved in thinking, memory and motor control
diarrhoea: The frequent passage of liquid stools
diastole: The period of heart muscle relaxation
diastolic pressure: The pressure in the arteries when the heart is at rest
digestion: The process of physically and chemically breaking down food so that it can be absorbed for use by the cells
dirty wound: An infected wound
disability: A lost, absent or impaired physical or mental function
disaster: A sudden catastrophic event in which many people are injured and killed, and property is destroyed
discomfort: A feeling of aching, hurting or soreness; pain
disinfectant: A liquid chemical that destroys microorganisms and viruses, as opposed to an antiseptic which prevents the growth and spread of microorganisms
distraction: Something that changes a person's centre of attention
diversional therapy: Participation in leisure-type activities that promote a feeling of wellbeing or positive experience based on the person's interests
do not resuscitate: A written directive, usually within an advance health directive, to provide palliative care for a person rather than resuscitating them
documentation: The process of creating written records of processes, care and observation; also known as written recording
dorsal recumbent position: The back-lying or supine position
duty of care: A legal term based on the principle of reasonableness; founded in the law of negligence; the responsibility of carers to protect the health and safety of others in the workplace where reasonable and practical
dysphagia: Difficulty (*dys*) swallowing (*phagia*)
dyspnoea: When difficult, laboured or painful breathing occurs with activity
dysuria: Painful or difficult (*dys*) urination (*uria*)

earth: Lead that carries leaking electricity to the earth and away from an electrical item
effective communication: When a message sent is received and interpreted by the intended person
elder abuse: Physical, psychological, financial, sexual or verbal abuse or neglect within a relationship with an older person
Elders: Highly regarded keepers of knowledge, including lore, language, customs, beliefs and creation stories, among Torres Strait Islander and Aboriginal communities
electric shock: When electric current passes through the body
electronic medication management (EMM) system: A system that enables prescribing, supplying and administration of medications to be completed electronically
embolus: A blood clot that travels through the vascular system until it lodges in a distant vessel

emotional illness: Mental illness, mental disorder, psychiatric disorder
empowerment: The process by which an individual gains control over the decisions that shape their life and treatment
enema: The introduction of fluid into the rectum and lower colon
Enable New Zealand: An organisation that supports disabled people to access health and disability services, equipment and information, enabling them to live the lives they want to lead
enrolled nurse (EN): An individual who has studied nursing and is registered with a national authority to practise as an EN; also called a registered nurse (Division 2) in some states of Australia; also called a nursing assistant in New Zealand
enteral nutrition: Giving nutrients through the gastrointestinal tract (enteral)
enuresis: Urinary incontinence in bed at night
esteem: The worth, value or opinion one has of another person
ethics: Knowledge of what is right and wrong conduct
ethnicity: A sense of peoplehood or nationhood in which a person or group's ethnic background is reflected in their identity, history, language, nationality and religion
euthanasia: When medical intervention takes place, at the person's request, in order to end the patient's life
evaluation: A review of whether the goals in the planning step of the nursing process have been met
evening care: Care given in the evening at bedtime
evisceration: The separation of a wound along with the protrusion of abdominal organs
expressive aphasia: Difficulty expressing or sending out thoughts; thinking is clear
expressive–receptive aphasia: To have both expressive and receptive aphasia – difficulty expressing thoughts and receiving information
external rotation: When the legs and hips turn outwards

faecal impaction: The prolonged retention and build-up of faeces in the rectum
footdrop: The foot falls down at the ankle (permanent plantar flexion)
Fowler's position: A semi-sitting position; the head of the bed can be raised between 45 and 90 degrees
fracture: A broken bone. Tissues around the fracture (muscles, blood vessels, nerves and tendons) are injured
friction: The rubbing of one surface against another
full-thickness wound: The dermis, epidermis and subcutaneous tissue are penetrated; muscle and bone may be involved

gangrene: A condition in which there is death of tissue, caused by infection, injuries and circulatory disorders
gastrostomy: A surgically created opening (*stomy*) in the stomach (*gastro*)
gavage: Tube feeding
glucosuria: Sugar (*glucose*) in the urine (*uria*); also called glycosuria
goal: A desired aim by a person who requires nursing care
graduated jug/measuring container: A container used to measure fluids
grief: An emotional response to loss and changes that have resulted because of that loss
guided imagery: Creating and focusing on an image

haematuria: Blood (*haem*) in the urine (*uria*)
haemoglobin: The substance in red blood cells that carries oxygen and gives blood its colour
hallucination: Seeing, hearing, tasting, smelling or feeling something that is not real
hapū: Sub-tribe
harassment: To trouble, torment, offend or worry a person by one's behaviour or comments, including workplace bullying
hazardous substance: Any chemical that presents a physical hazard or a health hazard in the workplace
health literacy: For individuals, health literacy is the ability to obtain and understand basic health information and services required to make informed and appropriate health decisions. For those who work in health fields, health literacy is about their ability to convey health information and to support those they work with to build their skills and knowledge
healthcare assistant: Staff member who provides basic task-oriented care under a nurse's supervision. May also be called a personal care worker or assistant in nursing
hemiplegia: Paralysis on one side of the body
hirsutism: Excessive body hair in women and children
holism: A concept that considers the whole person; that each person has physical, social, psychological, emotional and spiritual parts that are woven together and cannot be separated
home care packages (HCP): Coordinated care that enables older people to continue living at home, who might otherwise require residential aged care services
homeopathy: Based on the principle of 'like cures like', remedies are chosen that would cause symptoms in large doses, but in small doses trigger the body to use its own process of healing
hormone: A chemical substance secreted by the glands into the bloodstream
hospice: A healthcare agency or program for people who are dying
hygiene: A set of practices performed for the promotion and preservation of health
hyperglycaemia: High (*hyper*) sugar (*glyc*) in the blood (*aemia*)
hypertension: Persistent blood pressure measurements above (*hyper*) the normal systolic (140 mmHg) or diastolic (110 mmHg) pressures
hypoglycaemia: Low (*hypo*) sugar (*glyc*) in the blood (*aemia*)
hypotension: When the systolic blood pressure is below (hypo) 110 mmHg and the diastolic pressure is below 60 mmHg

immunity: Protection against a certain disease, either through the human body's own mechanism or through vaccination
implementation: Performing or carrying out nursing interventions in the care plan
incision: An open wound with clean, straight edges; usually intentionally produced with a sharp instrument

Indigenous Australians: The original inhabitants of the Australian continent and nearby islands, and these people's descendants; Indigenous Australians are distinguished as either Aboriginal Australians or Torres Strait Islanders. First Nations people
infected wound: A wound containing large amounts of bacteria and showing signs of infection; a dirty wound
infection: A disease state resulting from the invasion and growth of microorganisms in the human body
informed consent: A client is able to refuse or accept treatment based upon the information provided by a healthcare professional, which may be either verbal or written
insomnia: A chronic condition in which the person cannot sleep or stay asleep for the entire night
Islam: A monotheistic religion that originated with the teachings of the prophet Muhammad, having the same roots as Christianity and Judaism; its revelatory scripture is the Koran (Qur'an); its followers are called Muslims
iwi: Tribe

jejunostomy: An opening (*stomy*) into the middle part of the small intestine (*jejunum*)
job description: A list of the responsibilities and functions the centre expects a worker to perform
justice: The administration of fairness and equity

kapa haka: Māori performing arts
karakia: Incantation or prayer
karanga: Ceremonial call
kaumātua: Male elders (*koroua*) and female elders (*kuia*)
kaupapa Māori: Provision within a Māori worldview, e.g. kaupapa Māori health services
ketone bodies: Acetone
kilojoule: A measure of the amount of energy produced when the body burns food
kōhanga reo: Māori language preschools
korowai: Traditional cloak
kura kaupapa Māori: Māori language schools at the primary and secondary levels of provision

laceration: An open wound with torn tissues and jagged edges
laryngeal mirror: An instrument used to examine the mouth, teeth and throat
lateral or side-lying position: Lying on one side or the other
law: A rule of conduct made by a government through legislation and enacted by the court system
lexical gap: The absence of a word form in a particular language
libel: Making false statements in print or writing, or through pictures or drawings
lifestyle facilitator: Someone employed to facilitate a person's lifestyle; involves creating opportunities and taking a pragmatic, values-based approach to community development; also called a support worker
log rolling: A method of turning a person as a unit, in alignment, with one motion
loss: An actual or potential situation in which something or someone that is valued is no longer seen, felt, heard or experienced

manual handling: Any activity in which force is exerted to lower, carry, push, pull or otherwise manipulate a person or an object
marae: Customary Māori community centres
mechanical lifter or hoist: A piece of equipment that is used to raise the client from their bed, chair, bath or the floor
medical diagnosis: The identification of a disease or condition by a doctor
medical record: A written account of a client's illness and response to the treatment and care given by the health team; chart
Medicare: The Australian federal health insurance program for Australian citizens, New Zealand citizens and permanent visa holders
medication interaction: A reaction that can occur when one medication affects the actions of another
medication record: A legal record kept for each client detailing the medication requirements of each client
mental: Relating to the mind; something that exists in the mind or is done by the mind
mental disorder: Mental illness, emotional disorder, psychiatric disorder
mental health: In Western societies it means a person is able to cope with and adjust to everyday stresses in acceptable ways
mental illness: A disturbance in the ability to cope or adjust to stress; behaviour and functioning are impaired; mental disorder, emotional illness, psychiatric disorder
metabolism: The burning of food for heat and energy by the cells
microorganism: A small (*micro*) living plant or animal (*organism*) seen only with a microscope; a microbe
micturition: The process of emptying urine from the bladder; urination or voiding
mirimiri: Massage
mob: Colloquial term used by many Aboriginal peoples to define their country, or family of origin
modified left lateral recumbent position: A left side-lying position in which the upper leg is sharply flexed so that it is not on the lower leg and the lower arm is behind the person
monkey bar: Triangular-shaped attachment that hangs over the client's bed, used by the client to shift their weight in the bed or to steady themselves as they get into or out of bed
morning care: Care given before or after breakfast
multiculturalism: The acceptance of multiple ethnic cultures into one nation
multidisciplinary healthcare team: The many healthcare workers whose skills and knowledge focus on the person's total care
Multi-Purpose Services (MPS) Program: Provides integrated health and aged care services to regional and remote communities in areas that can't support both a separate aged care home and a hospital
muscle atrophy: Loss of muscle strength from inactivity
My Aged Care: An Australian Commonwealth government website and contact centre facilitating access to all government-subsidised aged care services

nasal speculum: An instrument used to examine the inside of the nose

nasogastric (NG) tube: A tube inserted through the nose (*naso*) into the stomach (*gastro*)
National Aboriginal and Torres Strait Islander Aged Care Strategy: The National Aboriginal and Torres Strait Islander Health Plan 2013–2023 is an evidence-based policy framework designed to guide policies and programs to improve Aboriginal and Torres Strait Islander health over the decade from 2013 to 2023
National Disability Insurance Scheme (NDIS): Commonwealth Government scheme providing a range of supports for people under 65 with a permanent disability to help them live an ordinary life; may include personal care and support, access to the community, therapy services and essential equipment. This may be at home or in residential aged care
National Relay Service (NRS): The person placing the call accesses the NRS from any TTY or standard phone by calling 711. The caller is connected to a communications assistant, who relays communication between the caller and the recipient
National Respite for Carers Program: Program that aims to give the carer a break; achieved by taking the carer or care recipient out of the carer environment
naturopathy: A system of healing that aims to provide holistic or whole body healthcare by drawing on treatment methods from several traditional systems of medicine
need: Something necessary or desirable for maintaining life and mental wellbeing
negligence: A situation when a person's acts or omissions result in a person not receiving a reasonable level of care, which causes harm to a person and/or their property
neutral detergent: A cleaning fluid that is used to maintain high standards of cleanliness for reusable items
nocturia: Frequent urination (*uria*) at night (*noct*)
non-maleficence: The act of intentionally avoiding harm or injury
non-pathogen: A microbe that does not usually cause an infection. Non-pathogens can and do become pathogens
non-REM (NREM) sleep: The phase of sleep when there is no rapid eye movement (REM) sleep
non-verbal communication: Communication that does not involve words
normal flora: Microorganisms that live and grow in a certain area and cause no harm if left undisturbed
nosocomial infection: An infection acquired after admission to an aged care service, hospital or healthcare service
nursing diagnosis: A statement describing a health problem that can be treated by nursing measures
nursing intervention: An action or measure taken by the nursing team to help the consumer reach a goal
nursing process: The method used by registered nurses to plan and deliver nursing care; its five steps are: assessment, nursing diagnosis, planning, implementation and evaluation
nursing/caring team: The individuals involved in providing nursing care: registered nurses, enrolled nurses and personal carers
nutrient: A substance that is ingested, digested, absorbed and used by the body
nutrition: The many processes involved in the ingestion, digestion, absorption and use of foods and fluids by the body
objective data: Information that can be seen, heard, felt or smelt by another person; signs; also known as factual data
observation: Using the senses of sight, hearing, touch and smell to collect information about a consumer
obsession: A thought or idea that is all-consuming
oedema: Swelling caused by fluid collecting in tissues
oliguria: Scant amount (*olig*) of urine (*uria*); usually less than 500 mL in 24 hours
open fracture (compound fracture): The broken bone has come through the skin
open wound: The skin or mucous membrane is broken
ophthalmoscope: A lighted instrument used to examine the internal structures of the eye
optimal level of functioning: A person's highest potential for mental and physical performance
oral hygiene: Mouth care
organ: A group of tissues with the same function
organelles: Tiny structures in the cell that perform specialised functions
orthostatic hypotension: A drop in (*hypo*) blood pressure when the person stands (*ortho* and *static*); postural hypotension
otoscope: A lighted instrument used to examine the external ear and the eardrum (tympanic membrane)
over-the-counter medications: Medications available without a prescription (e.g. paracetamol, cough suppressants, vitamin supplements)

pain: A feeling of aching, hurting or being sore
palliative care: A philosophy of care for the person who has an incurable illness or injury
panic: An intense and sudden feeling of fear, anxiety, terror or dread
papakāinga: Village-style housing on Māori land, such as on marae
paranoia: A disorder (*para*) of the mind (*noia*); false beliefs (delusions) and suspicion about a person or a situation
paraphrasing: Restating a message in your own words
paraplegia: Paralysis from the waist down; cervical injuries cause loss of function to the arms, chest and below the chest
partial-thickness wound: A wound in which the dermis and epidermis of the skin are broken
pathogen: A microbe that is harmful and can cause an infection or a disease
pediculosis: Lice infestation
penetrating wound: An open wound in which the skin and underlying tissues are pierced
percussion hammer: An instrument used to tap body parts to test reflexes; reflex hammer
percutaneous endoscopic gastrostomy (PEG) tube: A tube inserted into the stomach (*gastro*) through a stab or puncture wound (*stomy*) made through (*per*) the skin (*cutaneous*); a lighted instrument (*scope*) allows the doctor to see inside a body cavity or organ (*endo*)
perineal care: Cleaning the genital and anal areas
peripheral nervous system: Part of the nervous system which controls, directs and coordinates body functions; involves nerves throughout the body

peristalsis: Involuntary muscle contractions in the digestive system that move food through the alimentary canal
personal care worker: A person who provides basic personal care under a nurse's supervision; also called personal care assistant, personal carer or personal care attendant
personal protective equipment (PPE): Gloves, protective eye wear and a plastic apron to protect from body fluids or hazardous chemicals
person-centred care: An approach recognising that caring for a person with dementia needs to be approached holistically, recognising the person with dementia, their values, beliefs and preferences, rather than a biomedical approach emphasising the effects of dementia
phantom pain: Pain felt in a body part that is no longer there
phlebitis: Inflammation (*itis*) of a vein (*phleb*)
phobia: Fear, panic or dread; an irrational fear
physician-assisted suicide: A doctor intentionally helping a person to terminate his or her life by providing drugs for self-administration, at that person's voluntary and competent request
phytotherapy: Herbal medicine
pill organiser: A device used to separate medication doses into days and times
plantar flexion: Bending the foot
plaque: A thin film that sticks to the teeth; it contains saliva, microbes and other substances
poisoning: Occurs when a substance that is harmful to the body is swallowed, inhaled, injected or absorbed
polypharmacy: The administration of more than one medication at the same time; also using more than one medication to manage an individual's health issue
polyuria: Abnormally large amounts (*poly*) of urine (*uria*)
post-mortem: After (*post*) death (*mortem*)
postural hypotension: Orthostatic hypotension
posture: Body alignment
pouri-pouri: Traditional form of Indigenous black magic; involves supernatural concepts of spirits, mostly bad spirits; although it was forced into secrecy by the church, pouri-pouri is still practised today
prefix: A word element placed at the beginning of a word that alters its meaning
presbyopia: Age-related far-sightedness
pressure injury: Any injury caused by unrelieved pressure; may also be called a decubitus ulcer, bedsore or pressure sore
pressure ulcer: A wound that occurs because of poor skin care and immobility
privacy: The state in which a person or a person's actions are not observed or supervised by other people
private hospital: A service owned by a for-profit, not-for-profit or a charitable organisation
private insurance: Insurance bought by individuals and families
progress notes: A written description of the care given and the client's response and progress
prone position: Lying on the abdomen with the head turned to one side
proprioceptive devices: Pieces of equipment designed to balance the abdominal and back muscles
psychiatric disorder: Mental illness, mental disorder, emotional disorder
psychosis: A serious mental disorder; the person does not view or interpret reality correctly
Public Guardian: A statutory appointed substitute decision-maker for individuals with impaired capacity, subject to the provisions of the Guardianship and Administration Acts within the legislation of each individual state and territory
public hospital: A service owned, operated or funded by the state/territory/country
pulse: The beat of the heart felt at an artery as a wave of blood passes through the artery
pulse rate: The number of heartbeats or pulses felt in 1 minute
puncture wound: An open wound made by a sharp object; entry of the skin and underlying tissues may be intentional or unintentional
purulent drainage: Thick green, yellow or brown drainage

Queensland Civil and Administrative Tribunal (QCAT): An independent tribunal which actively resolves disputes in a way that is fair, just, accessible, quick and inexpensive. QCAT makes decisions on a range of matters for the first time (original decisions) and reviews decisions previously made by government agencies and statutory authorities

race: Group of persons belonging to the same genetic group
radiating pain: Pain felt at the site of tissue damage and in nearby areas
range of motion (ROM): The movement of a joint to the extent possible without causing pain
raranga: Weaving
receptive aphasia: Difficulty receiving information; the person has trouble understanding what is said or read
recording: Writing an account of care and observations
redirection: The redirection of thoughts that are causing distress to something more pleasant and acceptable
Regional Assessment Service (RAS): A service for older people who have lower care needs, but still require a little help around the home
registered nurse (RN): An individual who has studied nursing for a minimum of three years and is registered with a national licensing authority to practise as an RN
regurgitation: The backward flow of food from the stomach into the mouth
relaxation: To be free from mental or physical stress
religion: Spiritual beliefs, needs and practices
REM sleep: The phase of sleep when there is rapid eye movement (REM)
reminiscence: The act of remembering and reflecting on previous life experiences, especially those with a personal significance
reporting: Giving an oral account of care and observations
reservoir: The environment in which microorganisms live and grow (e.g. a host)
residential aged care service: A service that provides 24-hour aged care services
respiration: The act of breathing air into (inhalation) and out of (exhalation) the lungs

respiratory rate: The number of respirations undertaken in 1 minute
rest: A state of calmness, ease and relaxation, free from anxiety and stress
restraint: The use of any force or control that intentionally removes a person's right to freedom
retirement village: A complex made up of self-care accommodation; it may or may not include hostel-type accommodation and an aged care service
rheumatoid arthritis (RA): An inflammatory disease that causes joint pain, swelling and stiffness
rigor mortis: The stiffness or rigidity (*rigor*) of skeletal muscles that occurs after death (*mortis*)
rongoā: Māori traditional healing system that includes the use of plant-based remedies
root: A word element containing the basic meaning of the word
Royal Flying Doctor Service: A non-profit organisation that provides emergency and primary health care services for those living in rural, remote and regional areas of Australia

sachet packs: A pre-packed medication system packed by a packing machine, then checked by a pharmacist
safe patient handling: Formerly known as the 'no lift policy', where manual lifting in all but exceptional cases is replaced by the use of lifting machines, people-moving aids and self-mobilisation
safety: To achieve an acceptable level of risk by identifying and controlling recognised hazards
sanguineous drainage: Bloody (*sanguis*) drainage
schizophrenia: Split (*schizo*) mind (*phrenia*). A serious mental disorder; the person does not view or interpret reality as others do
seclusion: The state of being isolated from other people; may be voluntary or involuntary
self-actualisation: Reaching one's full potential
self-administration: Managing and taking one's own medication
self-esteem: Thinking well of oneself, seeing oneself as useful and being well thought of by others
semi-Fowler's position (semi-upright): The head of the bed is raised 45 degrees and the knee portion is raised 15 degrees; or the head of the bed is raised 30 degrees and the knee portion is not raised
serosanguineous drainage: Thin, watery drainage (*sero*) that is blood-tinged (*sanguineous*)
serous drainage: Clear, watery fluid (*serum*)
service delivery plan: A plan used by services to detail the use of funding assigned to support a person. It can include information about all facets of the person's life and the type of support required for them to continue their lifestyle
serviced apartment: An apartment in a safe setting, where supervision is provided with support but not 24-hour nursing care for residents assessed as requiring a low level of care
sexual harassment: Unwanted sexual behaviours by another
shearing: When skin sticks to a surface and the muscles slide in the direction the body is moving in
short-term restorative care: Supports people to be independent again after a setback, such as an illness or a fall, allowing them to stay in their own home
side-lying position: Lying on one side or the other; also known as the lateral position
signs: What you observe when caring for a client; an indication or characteristic based on physical observation, examination or treatment of a client; objective data
skin tear: A break or rip in the skin; the epidermis separates from the underlying tissue
slander: Making false statements verbally
sleep: A state of unconsciousness, reduced voluntary muscle activity and lowered metabolism
slide sheet: A sheet used to slide and reposition the client without unnecessary pulling or dragging of the client in their bed, chair or other surface
spatial perception: The ability to evaluate how things are arranged in space and recognise their relations in the environment, for example, the space between a cup and table when putting the cup down on it
sphygmomanometer: A cuff and measuring device used to measure blood pressure
standard of care: The skills, care and judgement required of health team members under similar conditions
standard precautions: Precautions that prevent the spread of infection within a healthcare setting
standing lifter: A lifter used for clients who can bear their weight and stand up
stasis ulcer: An open wound on the lower legs and feet caused by poor blood return through the veins; venous ulcer
stethoscope: An instrument used to listen to the sounds produced by the heart, lungs and other body organs
stress: The response or change in the body caused by any emotional, physical, social or economic factor
stressor: Any factor that causes stress
stroke: A cardiovascular disease affecting the blood vessels that supply blood to the brain
subjective data: What is reported by a consumer and cannot be observed by using the senses; symptoms; also considered as a person's opinion
substance incompatibility: An undesirable reaction that may occur between two or more substances; for example, warfarin and aspirin. Both drugs have an anticoagulant action so can lead to increased risk of bleeding
suffix: A word element placed at the end of a root to change the meaning of the word
suffocation: When breathing stops from lack of oxygen
sundowning: Signs, symptoms and behaviours of a person with dementia that increase as the sun goes down
supine position: The back-lying or dorsal recumbent position
supported accommodation unit (SAU): A purpose-built unit or house where a group of people with funding packages combine their funded support to facilitate a living situation that allows them 24-hour care
Support Needs Assessment Unit: Successful health needs assessments require a practical understanding of what is involved, the time and resources necessary to undertake assessments, and sufficient integration of the results into planning and commissioning of local services
Support Services for Remote and Indigenous Aged Care: Services that provide specialised care services that

respect culture as well as meeting care needs. These include employing Aboriginal or Torres Strait Island people to provide care; including the local community in aged care planning and providing care; having buildings for cultural ceremonies and family visits
symptoms: A physical or mental feature that may indicate a person has a disease or a condition; a consumer's description of what they are experiencing
syncope: A brief loss of consciousness; fainting
system: Organs that work together to perform special functions
systole: The period of heart muscle contraction
systolic pressure: The amount of force needed to pump blood out of the heart into the arterial circulation

tachycardia: A rapid (*tachy*) heart rate (*cardia*); the heart rate is over 100 beats per minute
tartar: Hardened plaque
task: A function, procedure, activity or work that does not require the knowledge or judgement of a registered nurse
terminal illness: An illness or injury for which there is no reasonable expectation of recovery
terra nullius: A Latin expression deriving from Roman law meaning 'land belonging to no one' (or 'no man's land'), which is used in international law to describe territory that has never been subject to the sovereignty of any state, or over which any prior sovereign has expressly or implicitly relinquished sovereignty; sovereignty over territory that is terra nullius may be acquired through occupation
tetraplegia: (formerly quadriplegia) Paralysis of both arms and legs
the 3Ds: A term sometimes used to describe depression, delirium and dementia in the older population
therapeutic medications: Medications used to cure or maintain a condition, or medications that give relief (e.g. painkillers)
thrombus: A blood clot
tinnitus: Ringing in the ears
tino rangatiratanga/rangatiratanga: Self-determination
tissue: A group of cells with similar functions
tohunga: Māori specialists in a range of areas who are traditional leaders
Torres Strait Islanders: The original inhabitants of the Torres Strait Islands
transition care: Time-limited, goal-oriented and therapy-focused services available to eligible older people after a hospital stay
trapeze: Triangular-shaped attachment that hangs over the client's bed, used by the client to shift their weight in the bed or to steady themselves as they get into or out of bed; also known as a monkey bar
trauma: An accident or violent act that injures the skin, mucous membranes, bones and internal organs
triggers: Clues for the client assessment
tuning fork: An instrument vibrated to test hearing

unintentional wound: A wound resulting from trauma
urinary frequency: Voiding at frequent intervals
urinary incontinence: The inability to control the loss of urine from the bladder; loss of bladder control
urinary urgency: The need to void immediately
urination: The process of emptying urine from the bladder; micturition or voiding

vaccine: A preparation that contains dead or weakened microorganisms given to produce immunity against an infectious disease
vaginal speculum: An instrument used to open the vagina so it and the cervix can be examined
validation: Similar to redirection where painful or distressing emotions are redirected to less distressing thoughts; however, there is also validation or recognition of the emotions being experienced
vascular ulcer: An ulcer due to vascular insufficiency
vein: A blood vessel that carries blood back to the heart
venous ulcer: A stasis ulcer
verbal communication: Communication that can involve the spoken and written word
vertigo: dizziness
vicarious liability: A form of secondary liability in which the employer is liable for the negligent acts or omissions made by their employees
vital signs: The basic signs of life, which include: temperature, pulse, respirations, oxygen saturation and blood pressure
voiding: Urination or micturition

waiata: Song
waka ama: Outrigger canoeing
walking belt: A belt used to transfer a person who is unsteady or disabled
whaikōrero: Formal speech-making
whakapapa: Genealogy or lines of descent from ancestors
whānau: Extended family
word element: A part of a word
workplace-related violence: Any act or threat of physical violence, harassment, intimidation or other threatening behaviour that occurs at work and can affect and involve employees, clients and visitors
wound: A break in the skin or mucous membrane
written communication: Communication that can be read

INDEX

A

C

D

E

F

G

H

J

K

L

N

O

Q

R

S

T

U

V

Made in the USA
Las Vegas, NV
03 November 2026

57423144R00305